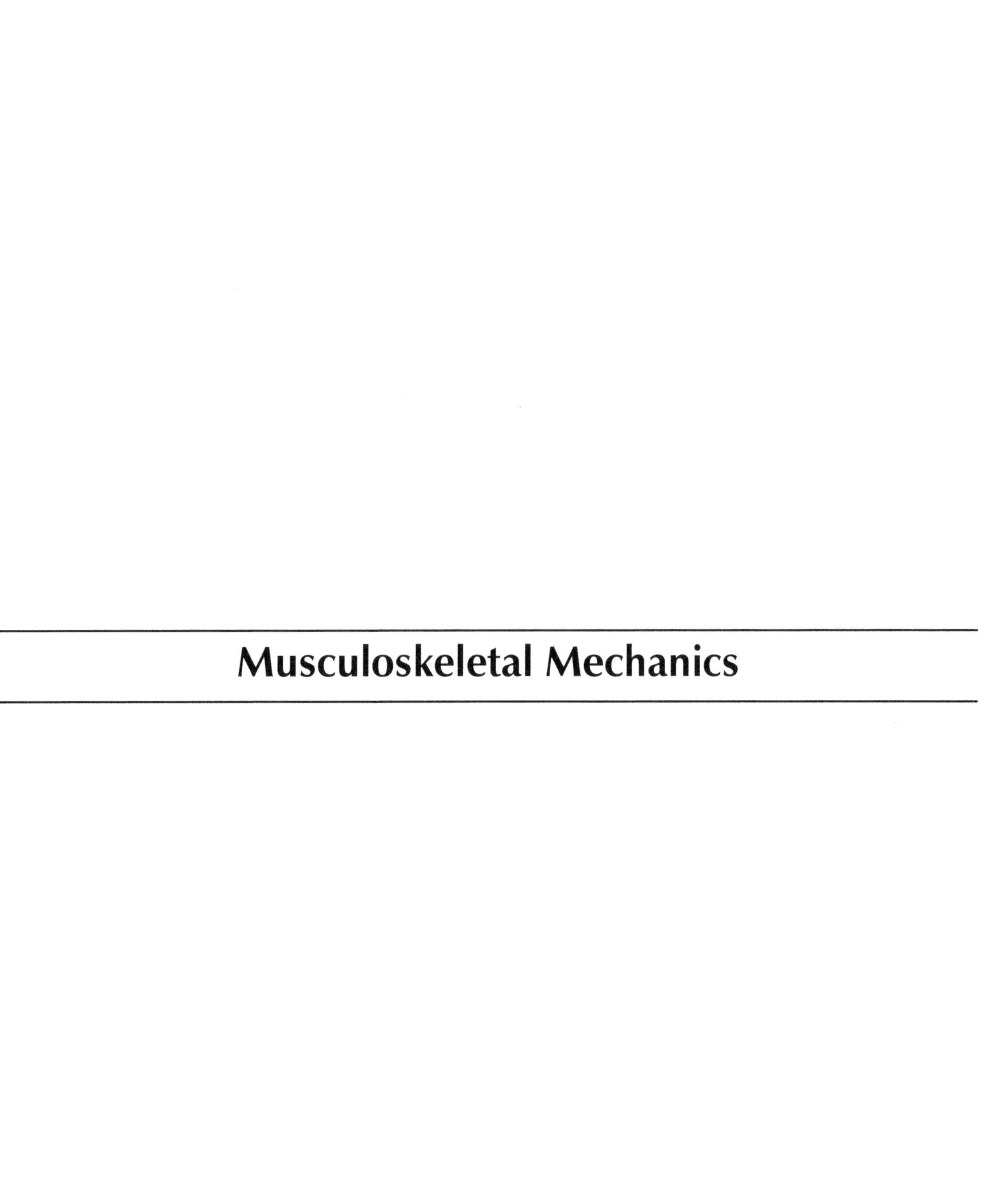

Musculoskeletal Mechanics

Musculoskeletal Mechanics

Editor: Newman Wagner

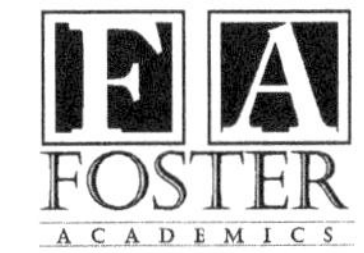

www.fosteracademics.com

www.fosteracademics.com

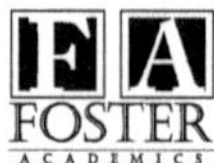

Cataloging-in-Publication Data

Musculoskeletal mechanics / edited by Newman Wagner.
p. cm.
Includes bibliographical references and index.
ISBN 978-1-63242-491-4
1. Musculoskeletal system--Mechanical properties. 2. Human mechanics. 3. Biomechanics. I. Wagner, Newman.
QP303 .M87 2017
612.76--dc23

Foster Academics,
118-35 Queens Blvd., Suite 400,
Forest Hills, NY 11375, USA

ISBN 978-1-63242-491-4 (Hardback)

Printed and bound in the United States of America.

Contents

Preface

The human musculoskeletal system provides the ability to effectively use the muscular and skeletal systems as well as give the body stability and motor skills. This book on musculoskeletal mechanics discusses the mechanisms of the musculoskeletal system as well as the malformations and diseases that affect those parts. Physiotherapy, pain medication, orthopedic surgery, etc. are common treatments in this field. Back-pain, carpel tunnel syndrome, tendinitis and sprains are common musculoskeletal disorders. Contents in this book seek to provide knowledge about the diagnosis and treatment of these disorders. Coherent flow of topics, student-friendly language and extensive use of examples make this book an invaluable source of knowledge. It aims to serve as a resource guide for students and experts alike and contribute to the growth of the discipline.

This book is the end result of constructive efforts and intensive research done by experts in this field. The aim of this book is to enlighten the readers with recent information in this area of research. The information provided in this profound book would serve as a valuable reference to students and researchers in this field.

At the end, I would like to thank all the authors for devoting their precious time and providing their valuable contributions to this book. I would also like to express my gratitude to my fellow colleagues who encouraged me throughout the process.

Editor

1

Uncoordinated Transcription and Compromised Muscle Function in the *Lmna*-Null Mouse Model of Emery-Dreifuss Muscular Dystrophy

Viola F. Gnocchi[1], Juergen Scharner[1], Zhe Huang[1], Ken Brady[2], Jaclyn S. Lee[1], Robert B. White[1], Jennifer E. Morgan[3], Yin-Biao Sun[1], Juliet A. Ellis[1,9], Peter S. Zammit[1*,9]

1 The Randall Division of Cell and Molecular Biophysics, King's College London, New Hunt's House, Guy's Campus, London, United Kingdom, **2** Centre for Ultrastructural Imaging, King's College London, New Hunt's House, Guy's Campus, London, United Kingdom, **3** The Dubowitz Neuromuscular Centre, Institute of Child Health, University College, London, United Kingdom

Abstract

LMNA encodes both lamin A and C: major components of the nuclear lamina. Mutations in *LMNA* underlie a range of tissue-specific degenerative diseases, including those that affect skeletal muscle, such as autosomal-Emery-Dreifuss muscular dystrophy (A-EDMD) and limb girdle muscular dystrophy 1B. Here, we examine the morphology and transcriptional activity of myonuclei, the structure of the myotendinous junction and the muscle contraction dynamics in the *lmna*-null mouse model of A-EDMD. We found that there were fewer myonuclei in *lmna*-null mice, of which ~50% had morphological abnormalities. Assaying transcriptional activity by examining acetylated histone H3 and PABPN1 levels indicated that there was a lack of coordinated transcription between myonuclei lacking lamin A/C. Myonuclei with abnormal morphology and transcriptional activity were distributed along the length of the myofibre, but accumulated at the myotendinous junction. Indeed, in addition to the presence of abnormal myonuclei, the structure of the myotendinous junction was perturbed, with disorganised sarcomeres and reduced interdigitation with the tendon, together with lipid and collagen deposition. Functionally, muscle contraction became severely affected within weeks of birth, with specific force generation dropping as low as ~65% and ~27% of control values in the extensor digitorum longus and soleus muscles respectively. These observations illustrate the importance of lamin A/C for correct myonuclear function, which likely acts synergistically with myotendinous junction disorganisation in the development of A-EDMD, and the consequential reduction in force generation and muscle wasting.

Editor: Sean Lee, The National Institute of Diabetes and Digestive and Kidney Diseases, United States of America

Funding: VFG was supported by The Medical Research Council project grant G0700307 (http://www.mrc.ac.uk/) awarded to PSZ, JEM and JAE. JS received funding from the Biomedical School, King's College London and the EC Network of Excellence MYORES (contract 511978). RBW and JSL were supported by The Wellcome Trust project grant 085137/Z/08/Z (http://www.wellcome.ac.uk/), JEM is financed by a Wellcome Trust University Award (084241/Z/07/Z), Y-BS has a British Heart Foundation Senior Research Fellowship (FS/09/001/26329) and ZH is funded by Medical Research Council grant G0601065, awarded to Professor Malcolm Irving. The laboratory of PSZ is also supported by OPTISTEM Grant Agreement number: 223098, from the European Commission 7th Framework Programme and The Muscular Dystrophy Campaign. The funders had no role in study design, data collection and analysis, decision to publish, or preparation of the manuscript.

Competing Interests: The authors have declared that no competing interests exist.

* E-mail: peter.zammit@kcl.ac.uk

9 These authors contributed equally to this work.

Introduction

Muscular dystrophies are a clinically heterogeneous group of diseases characterised by progressive muscle weakness and wasting of variable distribution and intensity [1]. They are subdivided into groups with respect to the age of onset, and in accordance with the primary muscle groups affected [1]. In many instances, a severe cardiomyopathy is also present, sometimes in the absence of the myopathy. The genes responsible for muscular dystrophies encode proteins that form a disparate group, both in function and location within the cell. For example, dystrophin is associated with the cytoskeleton and its absence causes Duchenne muscular dystrophy (DMD) [2], while emerin is located in the nuclear membrane and its deficiency underlies X-linked Emery-Dreifuss muscular dystrophy (X-EDMD) [3]. Also located in the nuclear envelope are lamin A and lamin C, mutations in which are responsible for autosomal-Emery-Dreifuss muscular dystrophy (A-EDMD) [4] and limb girdle muscular dystrophy (LGMD) 1B [5], in addition to several other degenerative diseases [6].

The A-type (lamin A/C) and B-type (lamin B1 and B2) lamins are type V intermediate filament proteins, which are major components of the nuclear lamina: proteinaceous network underling the inner nuclear membrane. Along with associated nuclear envelope proteins such as emerin, nesprin isoforms and SUN 1 and 2 (Sad1 and UNC84 domain-containing 1 and 2), lamins contribute to maintaining the structural integrity of the cell by cross-linking the nuclear envelope to the cytoskeletal network via the link of nucleoskeleton and cytoskeleton complex (LINC) [7]. All A-type lamins are encoded by *LMNA* by alternative splicing, and mutations in this gene give rise to 16 tissue-specific degenerative diseases collectively known as laminopathies [6]. Two non-mutually exclusive hypotheses have been proposed to explain this repertoire. The first underlines the importance of lamin A/C as structural proteins in maintaining nuclear architecture, since their absence results in sensitivity to mechanical stress [8]. The second focuses on the role of the nuclear lamina as a transcription platform, since nuclear lamins interact with a variety of transcription factors such as c-Fos [9,10] and disruption to such interactions lead to anomalous down-stream gene expression [10].

The majority of laminopathies arise from dominant missense or frameshift mutations (e.g. [4,11]), whereas mouse models to date, need to be homozygous for a *lmna* mutation to display a phenotype [12]. A patient reported to have a complete lack of *LMNA* function had a severe phenotype and died at birth [13], so the *lmna*-null also provides a useful model for A-EDMD [14]. *Lmna*$^{-/-}$ mice are viable, but exhibit growth retardation from 2–3 weeks of age, and stop growing after ~4 weeks. At 4–6 weeks of age, the mice develop a rapidly progressive dilated cardiomyopathy (DCM), with death usually around 8 weeks [15]. By 3–4 weeks, an abnormal posture and gait develops, with many skeletal muscles exhibiting dystrophic features, including the presence of centrally located myonuclei, variability in myofibre diameter, signs of atrophy and hyaline or flocculent cytoplasm. Muscle involvement is not uniform however, with muscles of the head, tongue and diaphragm largely unaffected in mutant mice [14]. As observed in A-EDMD patients, myonuclei in *lmna*-null mice exhibit both structural and antigen distribution abnormalities (e.g. LAP2, lamin B, emerin). *Lmna* heterozygous mice do not show any overt signs of growth retardation or dystrophic muscle, but develop atrio-ventricular defects as early as 10 weeks of age [16].

Myonuclei are often analysed using muscle sections from patients and mouse models. However, this technique does not allow accurate enumeration of myonuclei per myofibre, analysis of their distribution along a myofibre, or determination of the proportion with abnormal morphology or function. To address these limitations, we examined complete isolated myofibres from mutant mice, allowing the ready scrutiny of all myonuclei and satellite cells (the resident stem cells of adult muscle [17]). We found fewer myonuclei present in myofibres from *lmna*-null mice, many of which had morphological abnormalities, with variability in size, shape and chromatin distribution. Assaying both epigenetic modifications and the transcriptional machinery, revealed distinct differences in the transcriptional activity between myonuclei within a myofibre. Myonuclei with abnormal morphology and decreased transcriptional activity were distributed along the length of the myofibre, but were particularly evident at the myotendinous junction. Indeed, the structure of the myotendinous junction was generally disturbed, with less inter-digitations between myofibre and tendon, disorganised sarcomeres and collagen/lipid deposition. Investigation of muscle contraction dynamics showed that function in *lmna*$^{-/-}$ muscles was dramatically impaired at 4–5 weeks of age, as shown by the reduction in muscle specific force. Thus there are clear structural myofibre abnormalities and deregulation of gene expression between individual myonuclei distributed throughout a myofibre, which likely contribute to the marked decline in muscle contractile ability observed.

Materials and Methods

Ethics statement

Mice were bred, and experimental procedures carried out, in accordance with British law under the provisions of the Animals (Scientific Procedures) Act 1986, under project license PPL0672, as approved by the King's College London Ethical Review Process committee.

Mouse models

A heterozygous breeding colony of mice with a null allele of *lmna* [14] was established to obtain *lmna*$^{-/-}$, *lmna*$^{-/+}$ and *lmna*$^{+/+}$ (wild-type), from mice supplied by Carlos Lopez-Otin (University of Oviedo, Spain). Mice were genotyped by PCR on genomic DNA obtained from the tail using the Manual ArchivePure DNA Purification Kit (5Prime, Gaithersburg, MD, USA) with the following primers:

Forward: 5′ CGATGAAGAGGGAAAGTTCG 3′

Mutant-specific reverse: 5′ GCCGAATATCATGGTGGAAA 3′

Wild-type-specific reverse: 5′ CCATGGACTGGTCCTGAA-GT 3′

Cycling parameters were 95°C/30 s, 60°C/30 s, 72°C/60 s for 35 cycles. PCR produced a 750 bp amplicon from the mutated allele and a 520 bp amplicon from wild-type.

Myofibre isolation

Mice aged 4–6 weeks were killed by cervical dislocation and the extensor digitorum longus (EDL) and/or soleus muscles removed from the hind limb. Muscles were incubated in 0.2% collagenase Type I/DMEM with 400 mM L-Glutamine (Sigma, Dorset, UK) and 1% (v/v) penicillin/streptomycin solution (Sigma, Dorset, UK) for 1.5 hour at 37°C. Collagenase was then inactivated and individual myofibres liberated by trituration, as described in detail elsewhere [18,19]. Selected myofibres were free of capillaries or residual connective tissue. 15 or more isolated myofibres from at least 3 mice per genotype were analyzed for each experiment.

In order to determine the total number of myonuclei, myofibres were immunostained for Pax7 (to identify satellite cells, [20]) and 4,6-diamidino-2-phenylindole (DAPI) to visualize all nuclei (both myonuclei and satellite cells). EDL myofibres were isolated from 5 wild-type, 5 *lmna*$^{-/+}$ and 7 *lmna*$^{-/-}$ age-matched mice and multiple myofibres analyzed per type.

Antibodies and immunostaining

Myofibres were fixed in 4% paraformaldehyde/PBS for 10 minutes, permeabilised with 0.5% (v/v) Triton X-100 in PBS and then blocked using 10% (v/v) goat serum and 10% (v/v) swine serum (DakoCytomation, Ely, UK) in PBS.

Primary antibodies used were monoclonal mouse anti-Pax7 (Developmental Studies Hybridoma Bank, Iowa, USA), polyclonal rabbit anti-acetylated (K9 and K14) -Histone H3 (Millipore, Watford, UK) and monoclonal rabbit anti-PABPN1 (clone EP3000Y, Epitomics, CA, USA). Primary antibodies were visualized with species-specific highly adsorbed Alexafluor-conjugated secondary antibodies (Cell Signalling, MA, USA) before mounting on slides with VECTASHIELD Mounting Medium containing 1.5 mg/ml of DAPI (Vector Laboratories, Peterborough, UK).

Images were acquired using a LSM 5 *EXCITER* confocal microscope equipped with a water immersion LD C-Apochromat 40x/1.1 W Corr objective with acquisition software ZEN 2007 LSM (Zeiss), or a Zeiss Axiophot 200 M microscope with a Charge-Coupled Device (Zeiss AxioCam HRm). Images were adjusted globally for brightness and contrast and assembled into figures using Adobe Photoshop CS.

Transmission electron microscopy

Six EDL and soleus muscles from age-matched (35±1 days) wild-type (n = 3) and *lmna*-null (n = 3) mice were fixed in 2.5% phosphate buffered glutaraldehyde (pH 7.3, 0.1 M) for 4 hours at 4°C. The samples were then washed and post-fixed in 1% OsO_4 in

0.1 M Milloning's phosphate buffer pH 7.3 for 1.5 hour at 4°C. Dehydration in ascending grades of ethanol and resin impregnation at room temperature occurred prior to embedding in epoxy resin TAAB Premix Medium Resin Kit (TAAB Laboratories Equipment Limited, Berks, UK). Ultra-thin sections (~80 nm thick) were stained with a saturated solution of uranyl acetate and 0.17% lead citrate in 0.1 N sodium hydroxide. At least 3 sections per muscle per mouse were analyzed and viewed at 75 Kv in a Hitachi H7600 Transmission Electron Microscope.

Image analysis

Image J software (http://rsb.info.nih.gov/ij) was used to measure the length, width, area and perimeter of myonuclei on confocal images from multiple EDL myofibres. Images of myonuclei from soleus muscles acquired by TEM were also analyzed with Image J software to measure length and width of nuclei, together with the amount of highly condensed nuclear chromatin. TEM images from 22 myonuclei from 3 wild-type, and 32 myonuclei from 3 *lmna*-null mice (6 muscles per genotype) were analyzed.

Muscle mechanical force evaluation

Three EDL and three soleus muscles were dissected from wild-type, $lmna^{-/+}$ and $lmna^{-/-}$mice aged 4 and 5 weeks (3 mice per genotype per age) and their contractile properties were measured in an experimental chamber filled with an oxygenated Krebs-Henseleit solution at 25°C. The chamber was perfused continuously with 95% O_2/5% CO_2. One end of the muscle was attached to the force transducer (300B, Aurora Scientific Inc., Ontario, Canada) and the other end to a fixed steel hook. The muscles were stimulated by an electric field generated between two platinum electrodes placed longitudinally on either side of the muscle. Square wave pulses 0.2 ms in duration were generated by a stimulator to produce a maximum isometric twitch force. Muscles were adjusted to the optimum length for the development of maximum isometric tetanic contraction. After the experiment, the muscle was blotted dry and weighed, and the mean cross-sectional area was calculated assuming a muscle density of 1.06 mg mm^{-3} [21]. The muscle specific force at optimum length was expressed as the maximum isometric tetanic force per unit cross-sectional area of muscle.

All statistics are given as mean ± SEM. Unpaired *t*-test was used, where $p<0.05$ (two-tailed) was considered statistically significant.

Results

Myofibres from *lmna*-null mice have fewer myonuclei and satellite cells

We used the EDL and soleus muscles from the crural hind limb, since lower leg muscles are among those more severely affected in human EDMD patients [22]. In addition, the EDL is mainly composed of fast type IIx and IIb fibre types, while soleus comprises slow type I and fast type IIa fibres [23,24], allowing assessment of the major extrafusal muscle fibre types in mouse.

To first determine if *lmna*-null mice had as many myonuclei and satellite cells as controls, myofibres were isolated from the EDL muscle of $lmna^{-/-}$, $lmna^{-/+}$ and $lmna^{+/+}$ (wild-type) mice and immunostained for Pax7 to identify satellite cells, then counterstained with DAPI to distinguish myonuclei [25]. EDL myofibres from $lmna^{-/-}$ mice contained significantly fewer myonuclei (201.1±3.8 versus 289.5±7.7 in wild-type) and satellite cells (3.3±0.2 versus 4.6±0.3 in wild-type) than either $lmna^{-/+}$ or wild-type; which had similar numbers (Table 1). Interestingly, the ratio of satellite cell number to total nuclei number per myofibre, remained constant at ~1.6±0.1 for each genotype (Table 1).

Myonuclear morphology is abnormal in *lmna*-null mice

To next examine the morphology and chromatin distribution in myonuclei, myofibres were isolated from both the EDL and soleus muscles of $lmna^{-/-}$, $lmna^{-/+}$ and $lmna^{+/+}$ (wild-type) mice, together with those from *mdx* mice (a model of DMD [26,27]). In both $lmna^{-/+}$ and wild-type mice, 98% of myonuclei were of a regular oval shape, similar in size and evenly distributed along the entire length of the myofibre (Figure 1a and 1d). The long and short axes of myonuclei in wild-type EDL myofibres were 13.1±0.2 μm and 6.8±0.1 μm respectively, and the length/width ratio was 2±0.1. Their contour ratio (4π area/perimeter^2 - a measure of how close to round a structure is) was 0.8±0.01. By contrast, myonuclei in $lmna^{-/-}$ mice varied greatly in size, were irregularly shaped, and often were unusually elongated along the long axis of the myofibre (Figure 1b and 1e). The long and short axes of myonuclei of *lmna*-null EDL myofibres were 16.1±1.2 μm and 4.6±0.3 μm, respectively, and their length/width ratio was 4.5±0.7 ($p<0.01$ compared to wild-type) with a contour ratio of 0.6±0.02. All *lmna*-null myofibres analyzed had regions containing abnormal myonuclei and DAPI-stained fragments, but there was no evidence of myofibre branching or organized chains of centrally located myonuclei, indicative of muscle regeneration (Figure 1b and 1e). While myofibres from the soleus of *lmna*-null mice clearly contained many myonuclei with an abnormal morphology (Figure 1e), it was often difficult to delimit individual myonuclei to get a representative sample for detailed measurements, as performed for EDL myofibres. There was also a higher variability in EDL and soleus myofibre length and diameter between $lmna^{-/-}$ mice compared to those from either $lmna^{-/+}$ or wild-type (data not shown).

Condensed chromatin amount and distribution are altered in myonuclei lacking lamin A/C

DAPI binds to double-stranded DNA and is routinely used to examine condensed chromatin (heterochromatin) distribution

Table 1. Total nuclei and satellite cells in EDL myofibres from *lmna*-null mice.

	Total nuclei per EDL myofibre	Satellite cells per EDL myofibre	Satellite cell/total nuclei ratio
Wild-type (n = 67)	289.5±7.7	4.6±0.3	1.6±0.1
$lmna^{-/+}$ (n = 68)	268.9±5.4	4.4±0.6	1.6±0.1
$lmna^{-/-}$ (n = 97)	201.1±3.8*	3.3±0.2*	1.6±0.1

20 myofibres from 3 mice per genotype were analyzed. Total number of myofibres analyzed is indicated in parenthesis. Values are mean ± SEM. An asterisk denotes $p<0.01$ compared to wild-type using Student's t-test.

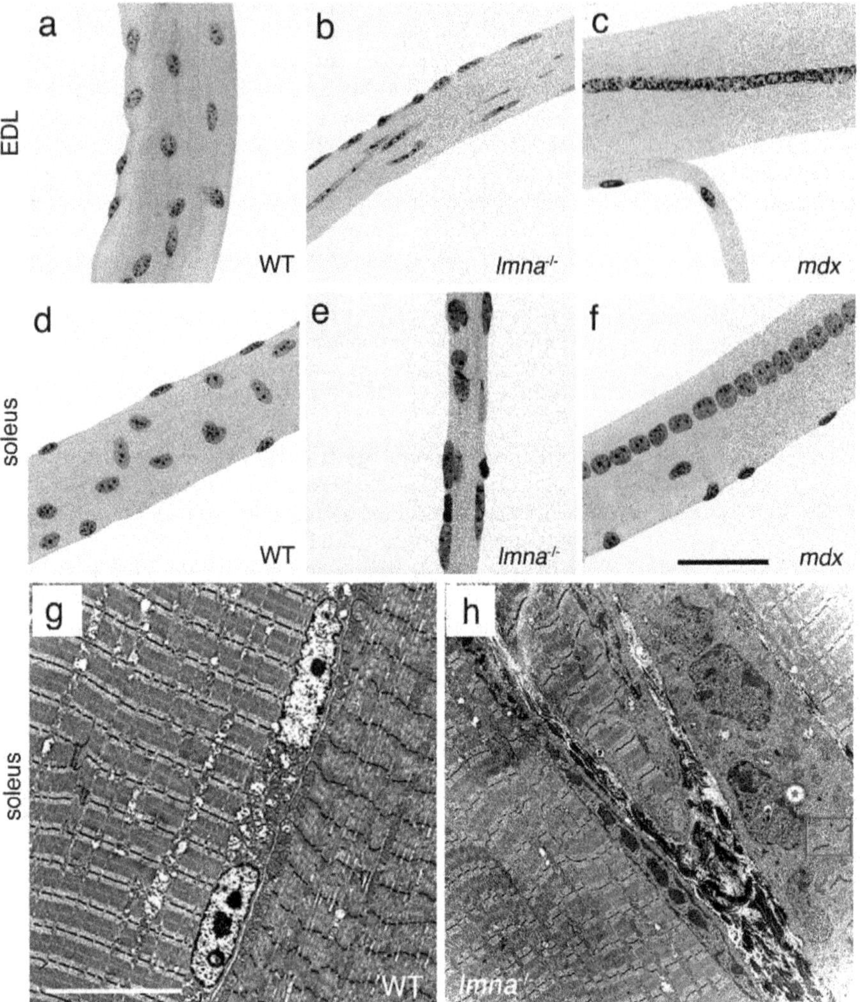

Figure 1. Myonuclear morphology is abnormal in *lmna*-null mice. DAPI staining of representative EDL and soleus myofibres from wild-type (WT) $lmna^{+/+}$mice show that myonuclei are evenly distributed and have similar shape, size and heterochromatin content (**a and d**). By contrast, myonuclei in $lmna^{-/-}$ myofibres are unevenly distributed, with variable size and shape, and heterogeneous chromatin content and distribution (**b and e**). Myofibres isolated from the *mdx* mouse model of DMD contain myonuclei of a more regular size, shape and heterochromatin organization (**c and f**). Unlike in $lmna^{-/-}$ myofibres, myonuclei in *mdx* mice are often located in a chain in the centre of the myofibre, indicative of a recent regenerative event (**c and f**). Representative TEM images of longitudinal sections of soleus muscle from wild-type $lmna^{+/+}$ (**g**) and $lmna^{-/-}$ (**h**) mice. WT myonuclei (thin red arrows) are regularly shaped, and have an even layer of highly condensed chromatin around the nuclear rim, in addition to centrally located condensations (**g**). Myonuclei (thin red arrows) from *lmna* null mice are irregularly shaped and have disorganized chromatin throughout with occasional vacuoles (**h** - red *). A thick red arrow indicates an abnormally elongated myonucleus. Note connective tissue between myofibres and the disruption of the sarcomeric arrangements near the abnormal myonuclei (red open square). Scale bar for (**a–f**) is 50 μm and 10 μm for (**g and h**).

[28]. In wild-type EDL and soleus myofibres, the DAPI staining was similar in all myonuclei, with strongly stained chromatin regions regularly distributed throughout the myonucleus (Figure 1a and 1d). By contrast, *lmna*-null mice exhibit differential DAPI staining between myonuclei, with variable amounts of irregularly distributed, and highly condensed, chromatin (Figure 1b and 1e).

To increase resolution, we used Transmission Electron Microscopy (TEM) on ultra-thin sections of soleus muscle from wild-type $lmna^{+/+}$ and *lmna*-null mice (Figure 1g and 1h). The ratio of nuclear length to width showed that myonuclei from soleus were significantly more elongated (7.1±0.8 compared to 2.7±0.2 - Table 2). Myonuclei from wild-type mice possessed a condensed chromatin layer directly inside the nuclear membrane. In addition, there were one or more round central clumps of condensed chromatin, indicative of nucleoli, together with occasional smaller accumulations (Figure 1g). In ~85% of *lmna*-null myonuclei analyzed by TEM, such highly organized chromatin distribution was lost (Figure 1h). Furthermore, it was no longer completely juxtaposed to the inner nuclear membrane. Such a distribution of heterochromatin can be a sign of DNA fragmentation and a key feature of the early stages of apoptosis [29]. Measuring the area of the myonucleus occupied by electron dense chromatin, revealed that it was significantly higher in $lmna^{-/-}$ mice (63.4±2.2% versus 49.4±2.1% in wild-type - Table 2). Moreover, ~24% of the analyzed myonuclei contained vacuoles (labelled with an asterisk in Figure 1h). Interestingly, myofibres often displayed disorganized sarcomeres in close proximity to the most affected myonuclei (Figure 1h - residual sarcomeres in an highly disorganized area are shown in the red box).

Table 2. Morphological and chromatin content alterations in soleus myonuclei of *lmna*-null mice.

	Length (μm)	Width (μm)	Length/Width ratio	Percentage of nuclear volume occupied by condensed chromatin
Wild-type myonuclei (n = 22)	8.4±0.5	3.4±0.3	2.7±0.2	49.4±2.1%
***lmna*-null myonuclei** (n = 32)	12.5±1.1	2.2±0.2	7.1±0.8*	63.4±2.2%*

7 myonuclei from 3 mice per genotype were analyzed by TEM. Total number of myonuclei analyzed is indicated in parenthesis. Values are mean ± SEM. An asterisk denotes $p<0.01$ compared to WT using Student's *t*-test.

Abnormal myonuclei are not a hallmark of all dystrophic muscle

To determine whether our observations on the myonuclei of *lmna*-null myofibres were a general feature of dystrophic muscle, or specific to the dystrophic phenotype associated with a lack of lamin A/C, we also isolated myofibres from the *mdx* mouse model of DMD [26,27]. Myofibres from EDL and soleus of *mdx* mice had highly variable lengths and diameters (data not shown), more so than $lmna^{-/-}$ myofibres, and were occasionally split and branched (Figure 1c and 1f). However, myonuclei had a regular shape and size, and were evenly distributed, although there were many areas containing chains of centrally located myonuclei (Figure 1c and 1f), indicative of muscle regeneration. Moreover, DAPI staining of *mdx* myonuclei revealed an overtly normal chromatin distribution.

Abnormal myonuclei accumulate at the myotendinous junction. The myotendinous junction is a specialised structure where the muscle connects to the tendon, and is the principal site of longitudinal force transmission across the muscle cell membrane [30,31]. Myonuclei at the myotendinous junction of wild-type $lmna^{+/+}$ myofibres were indistinguishable from those located elsewhere along the fibre (Figure 2a and d). By contrast, many myonuclei at the myotendinous junction of $lmna^{-/-}$ mice were clearly structurally abnormal, with aberrant chromatin accumulations (Figure 2b and e). Measuring the 10 myonuclei closest to the myotendinous junction (from at least 5 myotendinous junctions from 5 mice per genotype) we found that the average length and width of wild-type myonuclei were 11.1±0.2 μm and 6.1±0.1 μm, respectively; whereas the average length and width of the 10 *lmna*-null myonuclei closest to the myotendinous junction were 16.5±0.9 μm and 4.7±0.2 μm. Thus, the length/width ratio for *lmna*-null myotendinous junction myonuclei was 4.0±0.3, significantly different ($p<0.01$) from the wild-type ratio of 1.9±0.1. The average contour ratio was 0.6±0.02 for *lmna*-null myonuclei at the myotendinous junction versus 0.8±0.01 for wild-type ($p<0.01$). Importantly, ~85% of myofibres from *lmna*-null mice had myotendinous junctions at which myonuclei were clustered (Figure 2b and e). Again, we examined whether this was a common feature of muscular dystrophy. Myotendinous junctions of *mdx* myofibres did not accumulate myonuclei, and when present, chains of centrally located myonuclei often remained in register until the extremity of the myotendinous junction (Figure 2c and f).

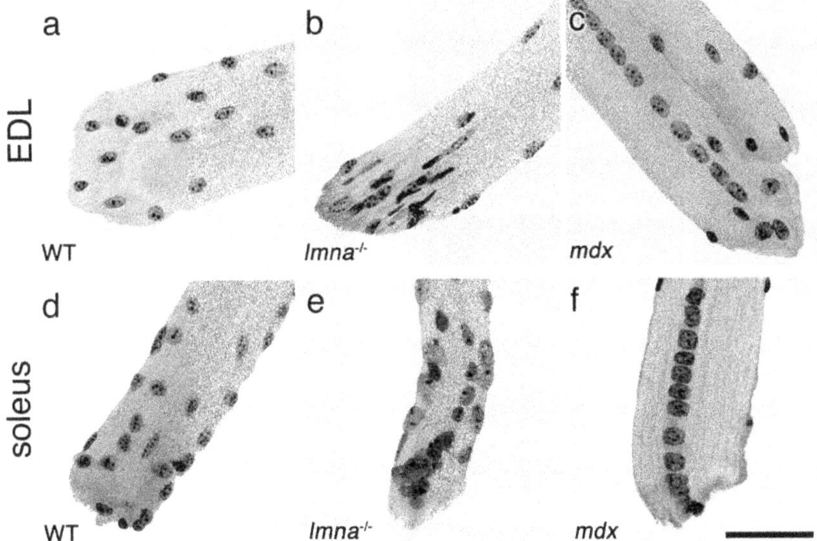

Figure 2. Myonuclei cluster at the myotendinous junctions of $lmna^{-/-}$ myofibres. DAPI staining at the myotendinous junction from wild-type (WT) $lmna^{+/+}$ EDL and soleus myofibres show that myonuclei are evenly distributed, with similar shape, size and chromatin organization (**a and d**). Myonuclei tend to cluster at the myotendinous junction from $lmna^{-/-}$ mice, and are unevenly distributed with varying sizes, shapes and condensed chromatin content (**b and e**). Myonuclei of the myotendinous junction from *mdx* mice have an overtly normal morphology, although often in centrally located chains that continue to the end of the myofibre (**c and f**). Scale bar 50 μm.

Heterogeneous transcriptional activity of myonuclei in *lmna*-null mice

Abnormal chromatin distribution in the *lmna*-null mice may indicate compromised transcription. Histones can be epigenetically modified by site-specific combinations of phosphorylation, acetylation and methylation, which correlate with specific biological readouts, such as transcriptional activation or repression, chromatin remodelling or stabilization [32]. In particular, acetylation of histones H3 and H4 positively correlates with active gene transcription [33,34].

As an assessment of transcriptional activity of myonuclei, we immunostained for acetylated histone H3 (K9 and K14). Largely homogeneous immunostaining of acetyl-H3 was observed in myonuclei from freshly isolated EDL myofibres of wild-type $lmna^{+/+}$ mice, indicating coordinated transcriptional activity (Figure 3a-c). By contrast, myonuclei in *lmna*-null myofibres had heterogeneous levels of histone H3 acetylation, with some myonuclei virtually unstained, while others exhibited normal, or even apparently increased, levels of immunostaining. These varying levels of histone H3 acetylation indicate that transcriptional activity differs between individual, often adjacent, myonuclei (Figure 3d–f). Approximately 50% of myonuclei were clearly misshapen in EDL *lmna*-null myofibres, compared to ~2% for those of wild-type. While severely misshapen myonuclei were most

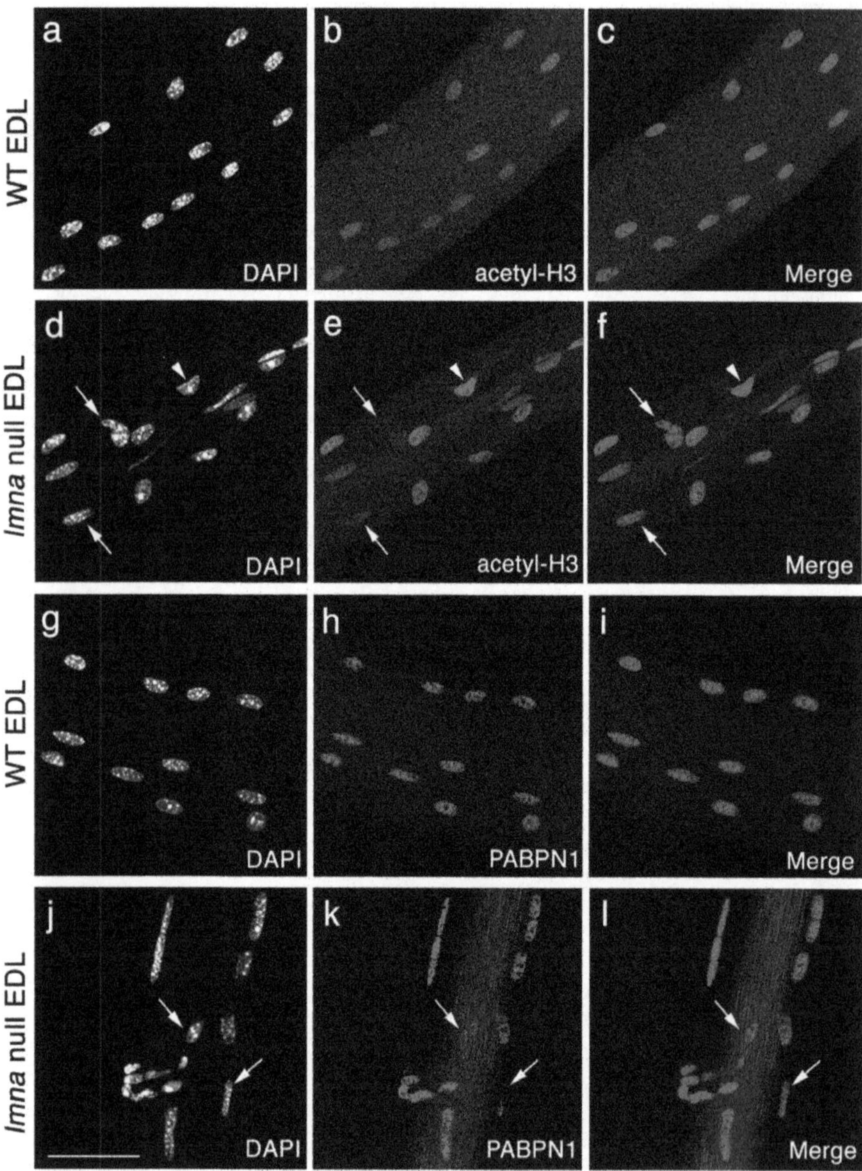

Figure 3. Variable transcriptional activity and mRNA processing between myonuclei of *lmna*-null mice. Representative images of wild-type (WT) $lmna^{+/+}$ EDL myofibres, immunostained for acetyl-histone H3 (red) and counter-stained with DAPI (white), with merged images (**a–c**). Myonuclei in WT myofibres have near uniform acetyl-histone H3 immunostaining, suggesting similar transcriptional activity. By contrast, immunostaining of $lmna^{-/-}$ EDL myofibres showed that myonuclei clearly have varying acetyl-histone H3 levels, indicating heterogeneous transcriptional activity, with some immunostaining at near background levels (**d–f** - arrows) while others appear hyperacetylated (**d–f** - arrowhead). WT myonuclei also show virtually homogeneous PABPN1 immunostaining (**g–i**), while in many myonuclei of $lmna^{-/-}$ EDL, PABPN1 is either reduced, or absent (**j–l** - arrows). Scale bar 50 μm.

likely to exhibit background levels of acetyl-histone H3 immunostaining (~26% of the 50% misshapen, so ~13% of total nuclei were hypoacetylated), there were also a significant number of overtly morphologically normal myonuclei that were hypoacetylated (~7%, i.e. ~3.5% of total). Western Blot analysis of EDL myofibres showed that global acetyl-histone H3 levels were significantly increased (~2.5 fold) in *lmna*-null myofibres compared to wild-type (data not shown).

Next, we assessed the state of the transcriptional machinery: poly(A) binding protein nuclear 1 (PABPN1) is an abundant nuclear protein that is part of the polyadenylation complex and integral for completion of messenger RNA maturation [35]. Myonuclear PABPN1 immunostaining was virtually homogeneous in wild-type $lmna^{+/+}$ myofibres (Figure 3g–i), whereas it varied greatly between individual, often adjacent, myonuclei in *lmna*-null myofibres (Figure 3j–l). Together with the epigenetic changes indicated by variable histone acetylation, the distribution of PABPN1 further indicates that gene expression is deregulated in the absence of lamin A/C. The wide variation in transcriptional activity both between individual myonuclei and myofibres is consistent with the transcriptional deregulation observed in patient muscle [10]. Unfortunately, we were unable to co-immunostain

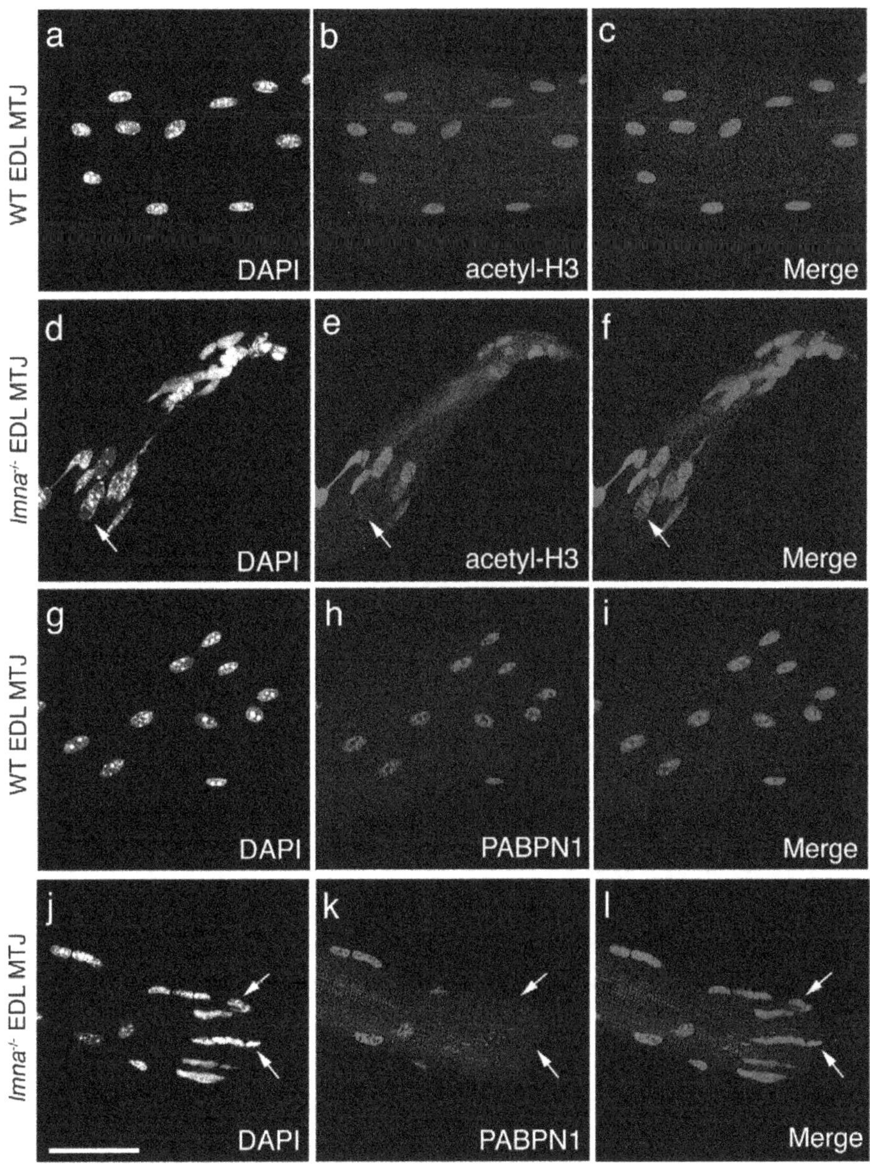

Figure 4. Transcriptional activity and mRNA processing are often impaired in myonuclei at the myotendinous junctions of *lmna*-null mice. Representative images of wild-type (WT) $lmna^{+/+}$ EDL myofibres immunostained for acetyl-histone H3 (red) and counter-stained with DAPI (white), with merged images (**a–c**). Myonuclei at the myotendinous junction (MTJ) in WT myofibres have near homogeneous acetyl-histone H3 immunostaining, as observed along the myofibre, indicating similar levels of transcriptional activity. By contrast, immunostaining of $lmna^{-/-}$ EDL myofibres revealed that myonuclei at the myotendinous junctions clearly had varying acetyl-histone H3 levels, indicating heterogeneous transcriptional activity, ranging from virtually inactive (background levels - arrow in **d–f**), to hyperacetylated, myonuclei (**d–f**). WT myonuclei also exhibit regular and homogeneous PABPN1 immunostaining at the myotendinous junction (**g–i**). In myonuclei at the myotendinous junctions of $lmna^{-/-}$ EDL however, varying PABPN1 levels are observed, with many being virtually unstained (**j–l** - arrows), indicating an impairment of mRNA processing and maturation. Scale bar 50 µm.

for acetyl-histone H3 and PABPN1 because both antibodies were raised in rabbit, and were of the same isotype.

Consistent with myonuclei distributed along the myofibre, myonuclei at the myotendinous junctions in wild-type *lmna*$^{+/+}$ mice had near homogeneous immunostaining for acetyl-H3 (Figure 4a–c) and PABPN1 (Figure 4g–i). However, myonuclei at the myotendinous junctions of *lmna*-null mice exhibited heterogeneous immunostaining, with a majority being hypoacetylated (Figure 4d–f) or having a marked reduction in PABPN1 protein levels (Figure 4j–l).

The structure of the myotendinous junction is severely perturbed in *lmna*-null mice

Examining the ultrastructure of both EDL and soleus muscles using TEM, we found that the myotendinous junctions from wild-type *lmna*$^{+/+}$ mice had myonuclei with normal morphology, a regular sarcomeric organization, and marked interdigitations between the myofibre and tendon (Figure 5a–c and 5g–i). In *lmna*$^{-/-}$ mice however, ~90% of myotendinous junctions in EDL (Figure 5d–f) and all examined in soleus (Figure 5j–l) exhibited structural abnormalities including: myofibril loss in the proximity of

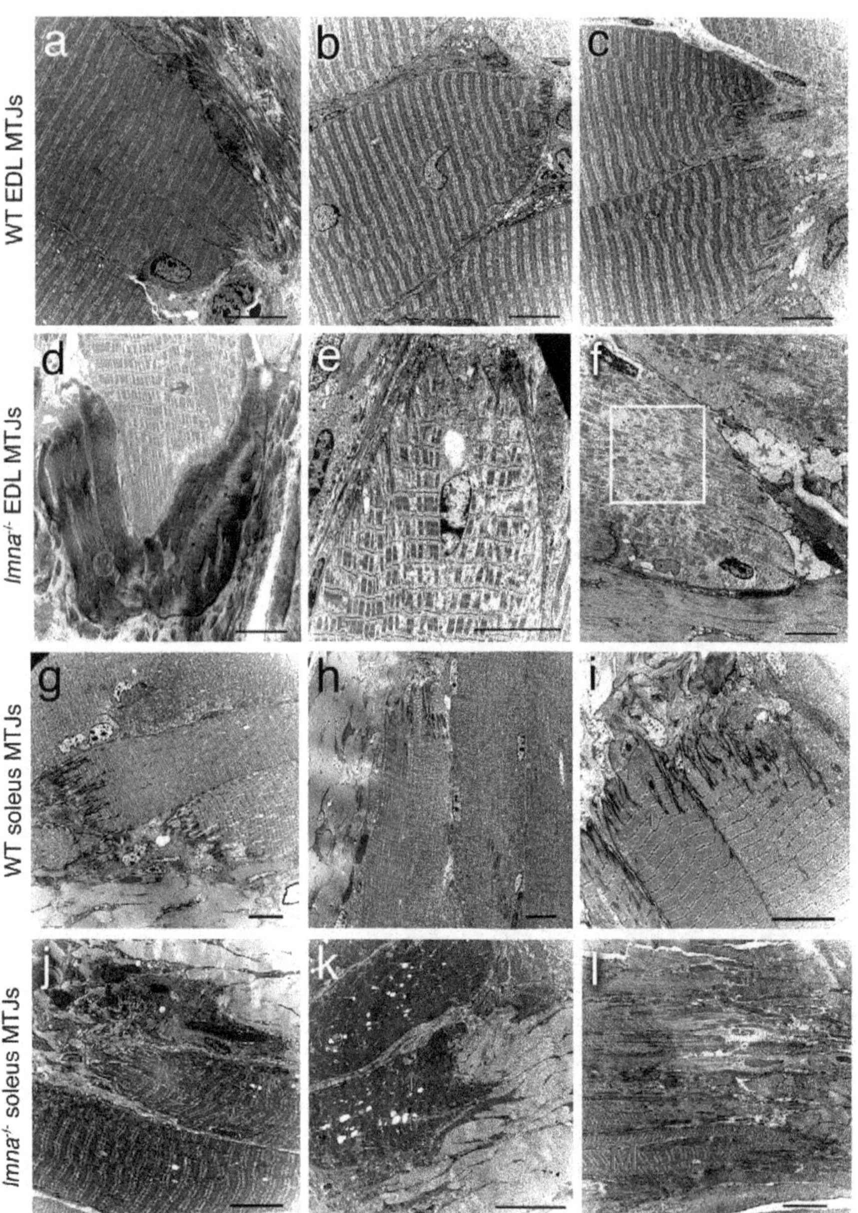

Figure 5. Myotendinous junction structure is abnormal in *lmna*$^{-/-}$ mice. Representative TEM images of longitudinal sections of myotendinous junction (MTJ) from EDL (**a–c**) and soleus (**g–i**) myofibres of wild-type (WT) *lmna*$^{+/+}$ mice. Myonuclei (red arrows) and sarcomere organisation appear normal. Note the extensive inter-digitations between the myofibre and tendon. TEM images of longitudinal sections of myotendinous junctions from EDL (**d–f**) and soleus (**j–l**) myofibres from *lmna*$^{-/-}$ mice. Myonuclei with abnormal shape, size and chromatin organization are evident (red arrows). There is a lack of inter-digitations, abnormal connective tissue (C in panel **d**) and fat accumulations (asterix in panel **f**) and sarcomeric disorganisation (boxed area in panel **f**). Myotendinous junctions in soleus muscle are particularly badly affected (**j–l**). The tissue architecture in (**l**) is so disrupted that the muscle region (M) and the connective tissue region (C) are barely distinguishable. Scale bar in each image equals 10 µm.

the plasmalemma (~92% EDL and ~95% soleus - Table 3); increased fibrotic and adipose deposition (~83% EDL and ~92% soleus - Table 3); reduced and irregular interdigitation (~75% EDL and ~82% soleus - Table 3) and presence of vacuoles (~42% EDL and ~63% soleus - Table 3). Disorganised sarcomeres were regularly observed at the myotendinous junction, which was more pronounced in the proximity of abnormal myonuclei. Myotendinous junctions in soleus were more disrupted than those of the EDL (Table 3), often showing a complete loss of the organized transition between muscle and tendon (as illustrated in Figure 5l).

Lmna-null mice have delayed growth and decline in weight after a month of age

Lmna-null mice show post-natal growth retardation with weight ~50% of their wild-type littermates at 28 days of age [14]. Similarly, we found that wild-type and *lmna*$^{-/+}$ mice were indistinguishable 24 days after birth, whereas *lmna*$^{-/-}$ mice were approximately half their size (6.3±1.2 g). Both wild-type and *lmna*$^{-/+}$ mice increased their body mass by ≥0.5 g per day, whereas *lmna*-null body mass increased by only ~0.2 g per day, and reached a maximum by day 29 to 32, after which it declined by ~0.3 g per day. By day 37 *lmna*$^{-/-}$ mice were less than one third the size of wild-type and heterozygous littermates (6.3±0.9 versus 20.6±0.7 and 20.2±0.9 g respectively). Generally, between day 34 and 37 *lmna*-null mice stopped moving and were sacrificed.

Lmna-null muscles generate less force

To examine if the structural and transcriptional changes we identified correlate with compromised muscle function, we measured force generation in EDL and soleus muscles at 4 and 5 weeks of age. Muscle contractile properties were tested in terms of muscle specific force, which was measured at 25°C and calculated by dividing maximum isometric tetanic force by mean muscle cross-sectional area. Three EDL and three soleus muscles removed from wild-type *lmna*$^{+/+}$, *lmna*$^{-/+}$ and *lmna*$^{-/-}$ mice (n = 3 per age group) aged 4 weeks (mice still growing and active) and compared to those from 5 weeks old mice (mice no longer growing, often barely active). EDL and soleus muscle mass was reduced in *lmna*-null mice, in accordance with the reduced total body mass. Moreover, the muscle mass actually declined between 4 and 5 weeks, with EDL and soleus of *lmna*-nulls ~80% of wild-type and heterozygous at 4 weeks, and ~35% by 5 weeks.

Soleus muscles from 4 week old *lmna*$^{-/-}$ mice showed a significant reduction in force generation, with muscle specific force only ~70% of controls (Figure 6a). The muscle specific force in both EDL and soleus from 5 week old *lmna*$^{-/-}$ mice was significantly reduced. Mean P_0 of soleus muscles was only ~27% of age-matched controls, while it was ~65% for the EDL (Figure 6a). There was no reduction in the force generation ability of muscles from *lmna*$^{-/+}$ mice at either age.

Importantly, the reduction in muscle specific force of *lmna*-null muscle was not accompanied by changes in force generation profile, with the soleus muscle still showing the force generation profile typical of a slow muscle and the EDL, that of a fast muscle (Figure 6b).

Discussion

EDMD and LGMD1B are characterised by muscle weakness and wasting, with abnormal myonuclear morphology. However it is unclear how many myonuclei are actually affected, with estimates ranging from 10%–90% for those having morphological and/or chromatin irregularities [36–38]. These observations have been largely made using muscle sections however, which makes it is extremely difficult, if not completely impractical, to examine all myonuclei in a given myofibre: the basic functional unit of skeletal muscle. Furthermore, three dimensional myonuclear morphology and distribution are also not easily analysed. These limitations however, can be overcome by isolating entire myofibres where possible.

Myofibres from the *lmna*-null mouse model of A-EDMD varied in size, but were generally smaller than controls, containing ~30% fewer myonuclei. Importantly, each myofibre contained myonuclei with abnormal morphology and chromatin distribution, which equated to ~50% of the entire population in the EDL. These pathological hallmarks were even more widespread in the soleus, where altered chromatin distribution and increased compacted and clumped chromatin were evident using TEM. Interestingly, chains of centrally located myonuclei were not seen in adult *lmna*-null mice, while this hallmark of muscle regeneration is apparent in many myofibres of *mdx* mice [26].

Our findings are consistent with reports of the morphology and chromatin distribution in myonuclei from other skeletal muscles, cardiomyocytes and embryonic fibroblasts in *lmna*-null mice [15,39] and in patients, where an overall decrease of condensed heterochromatin, focal loss of chromatin and increased clumping away from the myonuclear rim have been described [36–38,40]. Similarly, ~10% of myonuclei in the H222P mouse model of EDMD (containing a pathogenic point mutation at residue 222 in the *lmna* gene that causes familial A-EDMD and dilated cardiomyopathy in man) exhibit structural abnormalities and heterochromatin redistribution when examined using muscle sections [41]. Since similar changes occur in cardiomyocytes of *syne1* null mouse (lacking nesprin 1) [42], this indicates that disruption of different components of the LINC complex cause a common phenotype.

It is well established that lamin A/C have a crucial role in chromatin organization [43,44] and gene transcription [45]. To understand how such morphological changes affect myonuclear function, we examined the transcriptional state of myonuclei by assessing both epigenetic modifications indicative of an active

Table 3. Quantification of myotendinous junction abnormalities in *lmna*-null mice.

	Myofibril loss	Increased fibrosis	Decreased interdigitation	Vacuoles
Wild-type EDL myotendinous junction	2/33 (6.1%)	1/33 (3.0%)	2/33 (6.1%)	2/33 (6.1%)
***lmna*-null EDL myotendinous junction**	22/24 (91.7%)	20/24 (83.3%)	18/24 (75.0%)	10/24 (41.7%)
Wild-type soleus myotendinous junction	2/35 (5.7%)	0/35 (0%)	1/35 (2.9%)	2/35 (5.7%)
***lmna*-null soleus myotendinous junction**	38/38 (100%)	35/38 (92.1%)	31/38 (81.6%)	24/38 (63.1)

TEM images of 33 wild-type EDL myotendinous junctions, 24 *lmna*-null EDL myotendinous junctions, 35 wild-type soleus myotendinous junctions and 38 *lmna*-null soleus myotendinous junctions were acquired from a minimum of 7 myotendinous junctions from 3 mice per genotype.

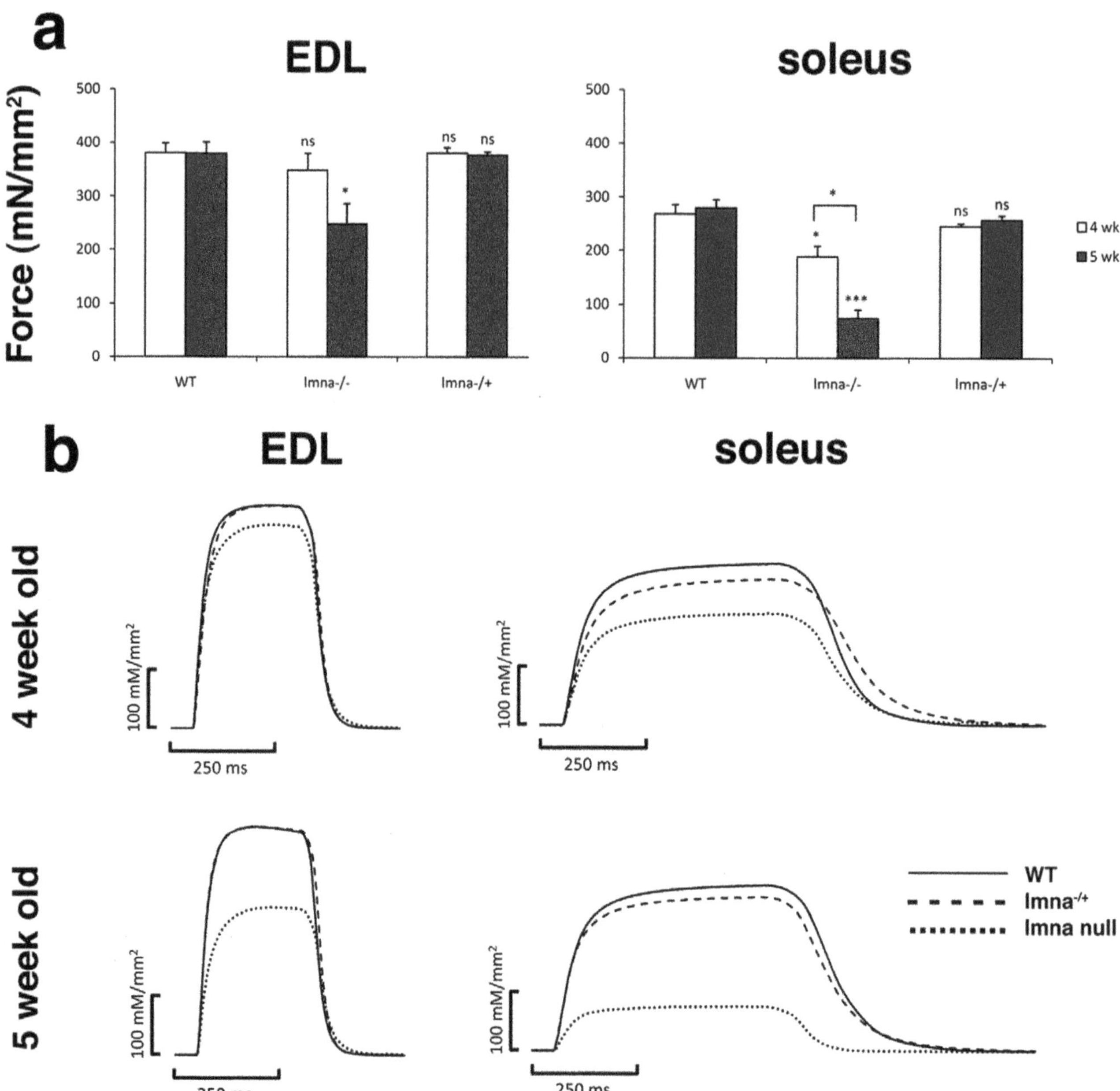

Figure 6. Force generation is impaired in EDL and soleus muscles lacking lamin A/C. Muscle specific force produced by EDL (left panel) and soleus (right panel) from wild-type (WT) *lmna*$^{+/+}$, *lmna*$^{-/-}$ and *lmna*$^{-/+}$ mice at 4 (white bars) and 5 (grey bars) weeks of age (**a**). Generation of isometric tetanic force at optimim length by EDL and soleus from WT (—), *lmna*$^{-/+}$ (---) and *lmna*$^{-/-}$ (····) mice at 4 and 5 weeks of age (**b**). 3 muscles from 3 mice per genotype per age were analyzed. Values are mean ± SEM from three muscles. An asterisk denotes significance level using Student's *t*-test. *** $p<0.001$; * $p<0.05$; ^{ns} $p>0.05$. Each value is compared with that of age-matched WT. The muscle specific force was also significantly different for soleus muscles from *lmna*$^{-/-}$ mice between 4 and 5 weeks of age.

transcriptional state (histone H3 acetylation - [33,34]) and PABPN1, a component of the transcriptional machinery. PABPN1 is an abundant nuclear protein that binds the poly(A) tail of pre-mRNA and is part of the polyadenylation complex through interactions with poly(A) polymerase and cleavage and adenylation specificity factor. PABPN1 stimulates the polymerization of the tail by poly(A) polymerase, thus controlling the length of the poly(A) tail [35].

Absence of lamin A/C caused heterogeneous levels of both acetylated histone H3 and PABPN1 between myonuclei, indicating that transcriptional activity varied and revealing a lack of coordinated transcriptional control. Importantly, altered acetyl-histone H3 patterns were not always linked to aberrant morphology, with many apparently 'normal' myonuclei being completely hypoacetylated, and so presumably transcriptionally inactive. Assessing global acetyl-histone H3 levels by Western blot, we found a significant increase (~2.5 fold) in *lmna*-null myofibres compared to wild-type. Histone H3 hyperacetylated fibres have also been observed in the tibialis anterior muscles *of lmna*-null mice [46]. Therefore, the marked reduction/absence of acetyl-histone H3 from a significant number of *lmna*-null myonuclei was more than counterbalanced by the relative hyperacetylation in other myonuclei. Global epigenetic defects have been reported in myoblasts from A-EDMD patients carrying either the R377H or R545C mutations [47,48], and also occur following over-expression of the A-EDMD-causing lamin A mutation R453W in C2 myoblasts [49]. Epigenetic modifications are also found in fibroblasts from patients with the premature aging disorder Hutchinson-Gilford progeria syndrome [50], indicating that it may be a feature common to laminopathies in general.

Lamin A/C not only binds chromatin and chromatin-associated proteins [51,52], but can also associate with specific transcription factors. For example, lamin A/C-mediated c-Fos sequestration at the nuclear envelope and their interactions with ERK1/2, regulate AP1 (Activating Protein 1) activity [9,53]. Thus regulation of transcription mediated by A-type lamins can operate through at least two inter-dependent mechanisms: firstly, through direct binding of chromatin and chromatin-associated proteins, the nuclear lamina can regulate chromatin positioning, promote silencing at the periphery and induce global epigenetic changes; secondly, by interaction with specific transcription factors and signal transduction components, it can mediate the fine tuning of tissue specific transcriptional programs and signalling pathways. Indeed, general disturbances of the transcriptome in A-EDMD and X-EDMD patient muscle have been reported using microarrays [10], with a number of signal transduction pathways being affected including Rb1/MyoD, MAPK/ERK, PI3K/Akt and TGFβ/Smad [10,54–57].

A striking finding was that myonuclei of *lmna*-null mice not only clustered at the myotendinous junction, as previously reported [58], but were consistently abnormal, with irregular shape, chromatin distribution and importantly, reduced transcriptional activity. Thus, this myonuclear clustering may be a response to the compromised transcriptional activity of many myonuclei, and the necessity to reduce the average myonuclear domain. There were also more widespread structural defects at the myotendinous junction, including increased fibrotic and adipose tissue, loss of myofibrils and sarcomeric organization, the presence of vacuoles in the cytoplasm and a lack of interdigitation between the muscle fibre and tendon. EDMD is unique amongst muscular dystrophies in that contractures develop early, notably in the Achilles tendons and elbow, prior to any clinically significant muscle weakness. Since myotendinous junctions are the main point of force transmission between fibre and tendon, and the primary site of lesion in many muscle tears [30,59,60], we speculate that defects at the myotendinous junction could be in part responsible for the functional failure contributing to joint contractures. In particular, the lack of interdigitations and cytoplasmic splitting could significantly reduce the area over which the transmitted force is distributed [59,60], and accumulation of connective tissue on the tendon side could cause stiffness and, ultimately, contractures. Myofibres from *mdx* mice have blunt myotendinous junctions, lacking the digit-like processes typical of wild-type myofibres [61], but we did not observe myonuclear clustering at the myotendinous junction in *mdx*. Thus, while these two mouse models share some pathophysiological changes at the myotendinous junction, myonuclei clustering is a specific feature of lamin A/C-deficient muscles. Interestingly, myonuclear positioning at the neuromuscular junction is also affected in *lmna*-null mice, and myonuclei also showed hyperacetylation of histone H3 lysine 9, a hallmark of muscle denervation [46].

The myotendinous junction is the essential force-transmitting component of the musculoskeletal system, and so their perturbed structure could affect force generation in muscles. While muscle specific force was reduced in both the EDL and soleus by 5 weeks of age, the soleus was more precociously and severely affected than EDL. This may correlate with the more widespread and greater disturbances in myonuclei and structure of the myotendinous junction in *lmna*-null soleus muscle. A drop in twitch and tetanic force generation in soleus and diaphragm muscle from *lmna*-null was previously reported [62]. However, soleus and diaphragm both consist of slow and fast muscle fibre types, and so we compared soleus with the EDL, which is almost exclusively composed of fast muscle fibre types [23]. It is important to note that the reduction in force generation was not accompanied by a change in the overall fibre type distribution, with the soleus still generating a typical tetanic force curve of a slow muscle and the EDL, that of a fast muscle. Although other factors probably contribute, such as the variable transcriptional status, the perturbed myotendinous junction structure is likely to be a significant factor.

In conclusion, analyzing myofibres from the *lmna*-null mouse model of A-EDMD revealed that compromised myonuclear structure and transcriptional deregulation were widespread. Abnormal myonuclei accumulate at the myotendinous junction, the structure of which is clearly perturbed. Combined, these changes presumably result in the rapid decline in force generation. Therefore, myonuclear and myotendinous junction dysfunction may act synergistically to produce the dystrophic phenotype in A-EDMD.

Author Contributions

Conceived and designed the experiments: PSZ JAE VFG. Performed the experiments: CGF JS ZH KB JSL RBW YBS. Analyzed the data: PSZ JAE YBS VFG. Wrote the paper: PSZ VFG JAE YBS.

References

1. Sewry CA (2010) Muscular dystrophies: an update on pathology and diagnosis. Acta Neuropathol 120: 343–358.
2. Hoffman EP, Brown RH, Jr., Kunkel LM (1987) Dystrophin: the protein product of the Duchenne muscular dystrophy locus. Cell 51: 919–928.
3. Bione S, Maestrini E, Rivella S, Mancini M, Regis S, et al. (1994) Identification of a novel X-linked gene responsible for Emery-Dreifuss muscular dystrophy. Nat Genet 8: 323–327.
4. Bonne G, Di Barletta MR, Varnous S, Becane HM, Hammouda EH, et al. (1999) Mutations in the gene encoding lamin A/C cause autosomal dominant Emery-Dreifuss muscular dystrophy. Nat Genet 21: 285–288.
5. Muchir A, Bonne G, van der Kooi AJ, van Meegen M, Baas F, et al. (2000) Identification of mutations in the gene encoding lamins A/C in autosomal dominant limb girdle muscular dystrophy with atrioventricular conduction disturbances (LGMD1B). Hum Mol Genet 9: 1453–1459.
6. Scharner J, Gnocchi VF, Ellis JA, Zammit PS (2010) Genotype-phenotype correlations in laminopathies: how does fate translate? Biochem Soc Trans 38: 257–262.
7. Crisp M, Liu Q, Roux K, Rattner JB, Shanahan C, et al. (2006) Coupling of the nucleus and cytoplasm: role of the LINC complex. J Cell Biol 172: 41–53.
8. Lammerding J, Schulze PC, Takahashi T, Kozlov S, Sullivan T, et al. (2004) Lamin A/C deficiency causes defective nuclear mechanics and mechanotransduction. J Clin Invest 113: 370–378.
9. Gonzalez JM, Navarro-Puche A, Casar B, Crespo P, Andres V (2008) Fast regulation of AP-1 activity through interaction of lamin A/C, ERK1/2, and c-Fos at the nuclear envelope. J Cell Biol 183: 653–666.
10. Bakay M, Wang Z, Melcon G, Schiltz L, Xuan J, et al. (2006) Nuclear envelope dystrophies show a transcriptional fingerprint suggesting disruption of Rb-MyoD pathways in muscle regeneration. Brain 129: 996–1013.
11. Scharner J, Brown CA, Bower M, Iannaccone ST, Khatri IA, et al. (2010) Novel LMNA mutations in patients with Emery-Dreifuss muscular dystrophy and functional characterization of four LMNA mutations. Hum Mutat. DOI 10.1002/humu.21361.
12. Cohen TV, Stewart CL (2008) Fraying at the edge mouse models of diseases resulting from defects at the nuclear periphery. Curr Top Dev Biol 84: 351–384.

13. van Engelen BG, Muchir A, Hutchison CJ, van der Kooi AJ, Bonne G, et al. (2005) The lethal phenotype of a homozygous nonsense mutation in the lamin A/C gene. Neurology 64: 374–376.
14. Sullivan T, Escalante-Alcalde D, Bhatt H, Anver M, Bhat N, et al. (1999) Loss of A-type lamin expression compromises nuclear envelope integrity leading to muscular dystrophy. J Cell Biol 147: 913–920.
15. Nikolova V, Leimena C, McMahon AC, Tan JC, Chandar S, et al. (2004) Defects in nuclear structure and function promote dilated cardiomyopathy in lamin A/C-deficient mice. J Clin Invest 113: 357–369.
16. Wolf CM, Wang L, Alcalai R, Pizard A, Burgon PG, et al. (2008) Lamin A/C haploinsufficiency causes dilated cardiomyopathy and apoptosis-triggered cardiac conduction system disease. J Mol Cell Cardiol 44: 293–303.
17. Morgan JE, Zammit PS (2010) Direct effects of the pathogenic mutation on satellite cell function in muscular dystrophy. Exp Cell Res 316: 3100–3108.
18. Rosenblatt JD, Lunt AI, Parry DJ, Partridge TA (1995) Culturing satellite cells from living single muscle fiber explants. In Vitro Cell Dev Biol Anim 31: 773–779.
19. Collins CA, Zammit PS (2009) Isolation and grafting of single muscle fibres. Methods Mol Biol 482: 319–330.
20. Zammit PS (2008) All muscle satellite cells are equal, but are some more equal than others? J Cell Sci 121: 2975–2982.
21. Mendez J, Keys A (1960) Density and composition of mammalian muscle. Metabolism 9: 184–188.
22. Emery AE (2000) Emery-Dreifuss muscular dystrophy - a 40 year retrospective. Neuromuscul Disord 10: 228–232.
23. Rosenblatt JD, Parry DJ (1992) Gamma irradiation prevents compensatory hypertrophy of overloaded mouse extensor digitorum longus muscle. J Appl Physiol 73: 2538–2543.
24. Girgenrath S, Song K, Whittemore LA (2005) Loss of myostatin expression alters fiber-type distribution and expression of myosin heavy chain isoforms in slow- and fast-type skeletal muscle. Muscle Nerve 31: 34–40.
25. Gnocchi VF, White RB, Ono Y, Ellis JA, Zammit PS (2009) Further characterisation of the molecular signature of quiescent and activated mouse muscle satellite cells. PLoS One 4: e5205.
26. Bulfield G, Siller WG, Wight PA, Moore KJ (1984) X chromosome-linked muscular dystrophy (mdx) in the mouse. Proc Natl Acad Sci U S A 81: 1189–1192.
27. Watchko JF, O'Day TL, Hoffman EP (2002) Functional characteristics of dystrophic skeletal muscle: insights from animal models. J Appl Physiol 93: 407–417.
28. Kapuscinski J (1995) DAPI: a DNA-specific fluorescent probe. Biotech Histochem 70: 220–233.
29. Sandri M, Carraro U (1999) Apoptosis of skeletal muscles during development and disease. Int J Biochem Cell Biol 31: 1373–1390.
30. Tidball JG (1991) Force transmission across muscle cell membranes. J Biomech 24(Suppl 1): 43–52.
31. Monti RJ, Roy RR, Hodgson JA, Edgerton VR (1999) Transmission of forces within mammalian skeletal muscles. J Biomech 32: 371–380.
32. Munshi A, Shafi G, Aliya N, Jyothy A (2009) Histone modifications dictate specific biological readouts. J Genet Genomics 36: 75–88.
33. Allfrey VG, Mirsky AE (1964) Structural Modifications of Histones and their Possible Role in the Regulation of RNA Synthesis. Science 144: 559.
34. Hebbes TR, Thorne AW, Crane-Robinson C (1988) A direct link between core histone acetylation and transcriptionally active chromatin. Embo J 7: 1395–1402.
35. Kuhn U, Wahle E (2004) Structure and function of poly(A) binding proteins. Biochim Biophys Acta 1678: 67–84.
36. Sabatelli P, Lattanzi G, Ognibene A, Columbaro M, Capanni C, et al. (2001) Nuclear alterations in autosomal-dominant Emery-Dreifuss muscular dystrophy. Muscle Nerve 24: 826–829.
37. Sewry CA, Brown SC, Mercuri E, Bonne G, Feng L, et al. (2001) Skeletal muscle pathology in autosomal dominant Emery-Dreifuss muscular dystrophy with lamin A/C mutations. Neuropathol Appl Neurobiol 27: 281–290.
38. Park YE, Hayashi YK, Goto K, Komaki H, Hayashi Y, et al. (2009) Nuclear changes in skeletal muscle extend to satellite cells in autosomal dominant Emery-Dreifuss muscular dystrophy/limb-girdle muscular dystrophy 1B. Neuromuscul Disord 19: 29–36.
39. Galiova G, Bartova E, Raska I, Krejci J, Kozubek S (2008) Chromatin changes induced by lamin A/C deficiency and the histone deacetylase inhibitor trichostatin A. Eur J Cell Biol 87: 291–303.
40. Fidzianska A, Hausmanowa-Petrusewicz I (2003) Architectural abnormalities in muscle nuclei. Ultrastructural differences between X-linked and autosomal dominant forms of EDMD. J Neurol Sci 210: 47–51.
41. Arimura T, Helbling-Leclerc A, Massart C, Varnous S, Niel F, et al. (2005) Mouse model carrying H222P-Lmna mutation develops muscular dystrophy and dilated cardiomyopathy similar to human striated muscle laminopathies. Hum Mol Genet 14: 155–169.
42. Puckelwartz MJ, Kessler E, Zhang Y, Hodzic D, Randles KN, et al. (2009) Disruption of nesprin-1 produces an Emery Dreifuss muscular dystrophy-like phenotype in mice. Hum Mol Genet 18: 607–620.
43. Vaughan A, Alvarez-Reyes M, Bridger JM, Broers JL, Ramaekers FC, et al. (2001) Both emerin and lamin C depend on lamin A for localization at the nuclear envelope. J Cell Sci 114: 2577–2590.
44. Schirmer EC (2008) The epigenetics of nuclear envelope organization and disease. Mutat Res 647: 112–121.
45. Andres V, Gonzalez JM (2009) Role of A-type lamins in signaling, transcription, and chromatin organization. J Cell Biol 187: 945–957.
46. Mejat A, Decostre V, Li J, Renou L, Kesari A, Hantai D, et al. (2009) Lamin A/C-mediated neuromuscular junction defects in Emery-Dreifuss muscular dystrophy. J Cell Biol 184: 31–44.
47. Reichart B, Klafke R, Dreger C, Kruger E, Motsch I, et al. (2004) Expression and localization of nuclear proteins in autosomal-dominant Emery-Dreifuss muscular dystrophy with LMNA R377H mutation. BMC Cell Biol 5: 12.
48. Kandert S, Wehnert M, Muller CR, Buendia B, Dabauvalle MC (2009) Impaired nuclear functions lead to increased senescence and inefficient differentiation in human myoblasts with a dominant p.R545C mutation in the LMNA gene. Eur J Cell Biol 88: 593–608.
49. Hakelien AM, Delbarre E, Gaustad KG, Buendia B, Collas P (2008) Expression of the myodystrophic R453W mutation of lamin A in C2C12 myoblasts causes promoter-specific and global epigenetic defects. Exp Cell Res 314: 1869–1880.
50. Shumaker DK, Dechat T, Kohlmaier A, Adam SA, Bozovsky MR et al (2006) Mutant nuclear lamin A leads to progressive alterations of epigenetic control in premature aging. Proc Natl Acad Sci U S A 103: 8703–8708.
51. Glass CA, Glass JR, Taniura H, Hasel KW, Blevitt JM, et al. (1993) The alpha-helical rod domain of human lamins A and C contains a chromatin binding site. Embo J 12: 4413–4424.
52. Taniura H, Glass C, Gerace L (1995) A chromatin binding site in the tail domain of nuclear lamins that interacts with core histones. J Cell Biol 131: 33–44.
53. Ivorra C, Kubicek M, Gonzalez JM, Sanz-Gonzalez SM, Alvarez-Barrientos A, et al. (2006) A mechanism of AP-1 suppression through interaction of c-Fos with lamin A/C. Genes Dev 20: 307–320.
54. Worman HJ (2006) Inner nuclear membrane and regulation of Smad-mediated signaling. Biochim Biophys Acta 1761: 626–631.
55. Muchir A, Pavlidis P, Decostre V, Herron AJ, Arimura T, et al. (2007) Activation of MAPK pathways links LMNA mutations to cardiomyopathy in Emery-Dreifuss muscular dystrophy. J Clin Invest 117: 1282–1293.
56. Muchir A, Pavlidis P, Bonne G, Hayashi YK, Worman HJ (2007) Activation of MAPK in hearts of EMD null mice: similarities between mouse models of X-linked and autosomal dominant Emery Dreifuss muscular dystrophy. Hum Mol Genet 16: 1884–1895.
57. Marmiroli S, Bertacchini J, Beretti F, Cenni V, Guida M, et al. (2009) A-type lamins and signaling: the PI 3-kinase/Akt pathway moves forward. J Cell Physiol 220: 553–561.
58. Mittelbronn M, Sullivan T, Stewart CL, Bornemann A (2008) Myonuclear degeneration in LMNA null mice. Brain Pathol 18: 338–343.
59. Tidball JG, Quan DM (1992) Reduction in myotendinous junction surface area of rats subjected to 4-day spaceflight. J Appl Physiol 73: 59–64.
60. Tidball JG, Quan DM (1992) Modifications in myotendinous junction structure following denervation. Acta Neuropathol 84: 135–140.
61. Ridge JC, Tidball JG, Ahl K, Law DJ, Rickoll WL (1994) Modifications in myotendinous junction surface morphology in dystrophin-deficient mouse muscle. Exp Mol Pathol 61: 58–68.
62. Grattan MJ, Kondo C, Thurston J, Alakija P, Burke BJ, et al. (2005) Skeletal and cardiac muscle defects in a murine model of Emery-Dreifuss muscular dystrophy. Novartis Found Symp 264: 118–133;discussion 133–119,227–130.

2

Treatment of Mouse Limb Ischemia with an Integrative Hypoxia-Responsive Vector Expressing the Vascular Endothelial Growth Factor Gene

Eduardo Gallatti Yasumura, Roberta Sessa Stilhano, Vívian Yochiko Samoto, Priscila Keiko Matsumoto, Leonardo Pinto de Carvalho, Valderez Bastos Valero Lapchik, Sang Won Han*

Research Center for Gene Therapy, Department of Biophysics, Universidade Federal de São Paulo, São Paulo, São Paulo, Brazil

Abstract

Constitutive vascular endothelial growth factor (VEGF) gene expression systems have been extensively used to treat peripheral arterial diseases, but most of the results have not been satisfactory. In this study, we designed a plasmid vector with a hypoxia-responsive element sequence incorporated into it with the phiC31 integrative system (pVHAVI) to allow long-term VEGF gene expression and to be activated under hypoxia. Repeated activations of VEGF gene expression under hypoxia were confirmed in HEK293 and C2C12 cells transfected with pVHAVI. In limb ischemic mice, the local administration of pVHAVI promoted gastrocnemius mass and force recovery and ameliorated limb necrosis much better than the group treated with hypoxia-insensitive vector, even this last group had produced more VEGF in muscle. Histological analyses carried out after four weeks of gene therapy showed increased capillary density and matured vessels, and reduced number of necrotic cells and fibrosis in pVHAVI treated group. By our study, we demonstrate that the presence of high concentration of VEGF in ischemic tissue is not beneficial or is less beneficial than maintaining a lower but sufficient and long-term concentration of VEGF locally.

Editor: Holger K. Eltzschig, University of Colorado Denver, United States of America

Funding: This work was supported by Fundação de Amparo à Pesquisa do Estado de São Paulo (FAPESP) 2006/59630-0 and 2011/00859-6. EGY was a recipient of FAPESP scholarship 08/52381-0. The funders had no role in study design, data collection and analysis, decision to publish, or preparation of the manuscript.

Competing Interests: The authors have declared that no competing interests exist.

* E-mail: sang.han@unifesp.br

Introduction

Peripheral arterial disease (PAD) is characterized by arterial narrowing that reduces oxygen supply to the extremities resulting in severe pain, non-healing ulcers and possible loss of the affected limb. The incidence of PAD is high at about 1000 affected per million individuals, and this incidence increases in individuals over 70 years of age and in diabetics [1]. According to the Transatlantic Inter-Society Consensus, approximately 25% of patients with advanced PAD will suffer amputation because conventional medical and revascularization treatments are not feasible. The prognosis for these patients is bad; after one year, about 25% of them will die, and 20% will still have PAD [1]. Therefore, it is necessary to continue the search for new therapies.

The main cause of PAD is atherosclerosis, which leads to narrowing and malfunctioning of arteries, *i.e.*, ischemia. Consequently, current therapies promote new vessel formation by administering growth factors, which can be provided in protein or gene form or even as cells that produce these factors naturally or after genetic modification [2–4]. Among several growth factors used for angiogenic therapy, vascular endothelial growth factor (VEGF) has been the most extensively studied because it is a potent mitogenic factor that also has anti-apoptotic and vessel dilation activities [5,6]. This factor acts primarily on endothelial cells through the VEGFR1 and VEGFR2 receptors, but it also promotes chemotaxis of smooth muscle cells, monocytes and bone marrow progenitor cells [6–8]. In animal studies, VEGF has been shown to improve perfusion and to increase capillary density in ischemic limbs [9–15]. Many of these studies have advanced to clinical trials, but most of the results have not been satisfactory.

To date, all clinical trials on limb ischemia treatment have used plasmid or adenoviral vectors designed to express transiently and locally [2–4], and muscle has been the favorite target tissue. Transgene expression is transient because the genes are not integrated into the host genome. In clinical trials, these vectors are injected directly into the muscle at high enough doses to express high levels of angiogenic factors due to the characteristics of these vectors. As the angiogenic factor concentration required in loco to induce a therapeutically beneficial amount of angiogenesis is variable depending on the degree of ischemia, angiogenic gene therapy in some tissues can induce hemangioma due to the exaggerated production of growth factors [16,17], and in other tissues, it cannot ameliorate ischemia due to insufficient production of the angiogenic factor. Thus, the ideal vector system should have a mechanism to allow for the long-term production of angiogenic factors according to the local degree of ischemia.

To obtain a vector that is responsive to ischemia and is capable of long-term VEGF expression, we designed an integrative plasmid vector based on the ΦC31 integrase system that contains an HRE (hypoxia-responsive element) sequence. The HRE consensus sequence, isolated from the 3′ end of the erythropoietin (Epo) gene, is present in many genes involved in erythropoiesis, angiogenesis and glycolysis [18] that are activated during hypoxia. Cells and tissues exposed to hypoxia trigger an adaptive response driven by hypoxia induced factor 1 (HIF-1), which binds to the HRE sequence located in the enhancer regions of these genes. It has been demonstrated that vectors constructed with an HRE sequence provide enhanced transgene expression under hypoxic conditions through HIF-1 binding to the HRE [18,19]. In addition, to allow for integration of the vector, the attB sequence from phage ΦC31 was included. The integrase from ΦC31 recognizes plasmids with the attB sequence and inserts them into genomic regions containing pseudo-attP sequences [20], which are present in mammalian genomes. Because the integration process is unidirectional, once the plasmid is inserted into the genome, it is maintained stably [21]. In our study, we found that limb ischemic mice treated with our integrative vector that is responsive to variations in oxygen concentration had a better therapeutic response than mice treated with other delivery vectors.

Materials and Methods

Vector construction

The commercially available pVAX vector (Invitrogen, Carlsbad, EUA) was cut with HincII enzyme, and a cassette containing 9 copies of the HRE sequence (CCGGGTAGCTGGCG-TACGTGCTGCAG) from the AAV-H9-lacZ vector (kindly provided by Dr Hua Su, The Cardiovascular Research Institute, University of California, USA [22], which was obtained by digesting with EcoRI and BglII and treating with Klenow polymerase, was ligated to make pVAX-HRE. This vector was digested with NruI and was ligated with the attB sequence from the pTA-attB vector (kindly provided by Dr Michele P. Calos, Genetics department of Stanford University, USA [20]), which was previously digested with BamHI and EcoRV and treated with Klenow polymerase, to make pVAX-HRE-attB. Finally, to insert the human VEGF165 sequence into pVAX-HRE-attB, both it and the uP-VEGF vector [23], which expresses human VEGF165, were digested with HindIII and ApaI and ligated together to make pVAX-HRE-attB-VEGF. The integrase expression vector uP-INT was constructed by inserting the ΦC31 integrase gene into the uP vector. The p-INT vector has a construction similar to uP-INT, but it does not have a CMV promoter; therefore, it does not express integrase (Fig. 1).

Cell culture under normoxia and hypoxia

The human embryonic kidney cell line HEK293T [24] was maintained in DMEM supplemented with 10% fetal bovine serum (DMEM+). For transfection, in a 6-well plate 1×10^5 HEK 293 cells were seeded. Twenty-four hours later, 2.5 μg of the donor plasmid containing $hVEGF_{165}$ and 2.5 μg of pVAX or p-INT or uP-INT plasmids were mixed for transfection by the calcium-phosphate co-precipitation method. After 24 h, the medium was replaced with a fresh one, and at the indicated time, the supernatant was collected to determine VEGF levels by ELISA.

To establish hypoxic condition in vitro, the cells were cultured with DMEM+ containing 100 μM cobalt chloride [25]. To test the toxicity of the cobalt, HEK293 cells were cultured with 0, 200 or 400 μM cobalt chloride, and cell viability was assessed using the Trypan blue method.

The mouse myoblast cell line (C2C12) was also maintained in DMEM+, but for transfection the Amaxa NHDF Nucleofector kit and Nucleofector Amaxa (Lonza, Basel, Switzerland) were used following the provided protocol.

Ischemic hind limb model and muscular transfection

All procedures involving animals were approved by the Research Ethics Committee of the Federal University of São Paulo, Brazil (Approval number: CEP 0729/08). Initially, 10–12 week-old Balb/c male mice were anesthetized with an intraperitoneal injection of ketamine (40 mg/kg) and xylazine (20 mg/kg). Hind limb ischemia was induced surgically as previously described [26,27]. Briefly, the femoral artery was excised from its origin at the external iliac artery branch to its bifurcation into the saphenous and popliteal arteries without damaging the femoralis vein or nerves. Branches including the circumflex artery were also obstructed completely to avoid retrograde flow. Gene therapy was performed by injecting 50 μg of each vector in 100 μl of phosphate-buffered saline (PBS) into the middle of the quadriceps muscle soon after ischemic surgery. After plasmid injection, 3 electric pulses of 80 V/cm and 20 ms in duration were applied using needle electrodes (Electroporator T820; BTX Genetronics, San Diego, USA). After gene therapy, the animals were kept under analgesia with daily peritoneal injections of 5 mg/kg carprofen. In our study, the following groups were included with 7–10 animals per group: normal, ischemic and ischemic treated with vector.

Visual assessment of necrosis

Limb ischemia was visually evaluated 30 days after treatment. The following four grades were used to measure the degree of limb necrosis: grade 0, absence of necrosis; grade 1, necrosis limited to the toes; grade 2, necrosis extending to the dorsum pedis; grade 3, necrosis extending to the crus [26].

Muscle force determination

Isometric gastrocnemius muscle contraction was performed 30 days after treatment based on a previous study [28]. The animals

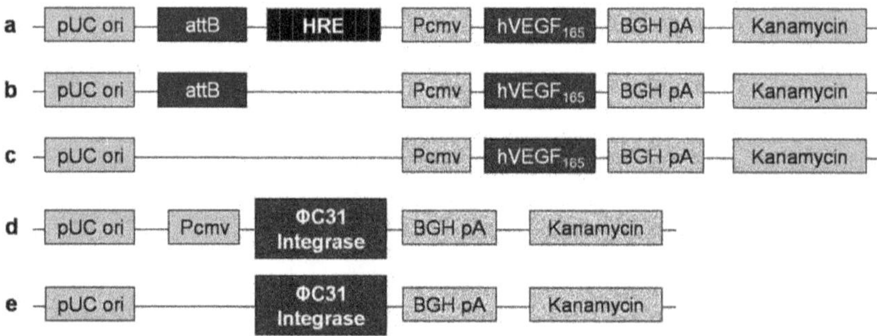

Figure 1. Schematic vector diagrams. (A) pVAX-HRE-attB-hVEGF165; (B) pVAX-attB-hVEGF165; (C) pVAX-hVEGF165; (D) uP-INT; (E) p-INT. pUC ori: replication origin. Pcmv: human cytomegalovirus promoter. BGHpA: polyadenylation signal of the bovine growth hormone. Kanamycin: kanamycin resistance gene.

were anesthetized and maintained at 37°C on a temperature-controlled plate. The leg and knee were fixed on the plate with the gastrocnemius muscle exposed. The Achilles tendon was cut and attached to a wire connected to a force transducer (MLT 1030/D - ADInstruments, Bella Vista NSW, Australia). The lateral gastrocnemius and soleus muscles were removed; the vascular and nerve systems were kept intact. Medial gastrocnemius muscles were left free from the surrounding tissue to minimize effects from the contraction of other muscles. The sciatic nerve was isolated and placed in contact with a bipolar silver electrode for electro-stimulation. One stimulus of 5 volts at a frequency of 60 Hz was applied for 10 ms with a 1 minute interval between stimulations. The isometric contractions were measured as the highest force stretching the wire. All collected data were recorded and analyzed using the PowerLab 8/30 system and LabChart Pro software (ADInstruments, Bella Vista NSW, Australia). After force determination, the animals were subjected to euthanasia, and their medial gastrocnemius muscles were then removed for mass measurement and histological analysis.

Determination of $hVEGF_{165}$ by ELISA

Supernatant from cultured cells was collected periodically to determine the concentration of $hVEGF_{165}$ using a DuoSet ELISA kit (R&D Systems Inc., Minneapolis, USA) following the manufacturer's instructions. To determine $hVEGF_{165}$ levels in muscle, the quadriceps muscle was removed after muscle force measurement. The middle part of the gastrocnemius muscle was mechanically homogenized using lysis buffer (25 mM Tris-HCl, pH 7.4, 50 mM NaCl, 0.5% Na-deoxycholate, 2% NP-40, 0.2% sodium dodecyl sulfate, 1 mM phenylmethylsulphonyl fluoride). The homogenized tissue was centrifuged at 4500× g for 10 min at 4°C, and the supernatant was recovered. Total protein and $hVEGF_{165}$ concentrations were determined using the Bio-Rad Protein Assay (BioRad, California, USA) and a DuoSet ELISA Kit, respectively.

Gene expression analysis by quantitative reverse transcription polymerase chain reaction (qRT-PCR)

Total RNA from C2C12 or HEK293 cells was extracted with Trizol reagent (Invitrogen, Carlsbad, CA, USA) and treated with DNAse I (Invitrogen). cDNA was synthetized using High Capacity cDNA Reverse Transcription kit (Invitrogen) and qRT-PCR was conducted using QuantiFast SYBR Green RT-PCR Kit (Qiagen, Hilden, Germany) in the Rotor Gene-Q (Qiagen). The following primers were used to quantify mouse HIF1- α (m HIF1- α), human HIF1- α (h HIF1- α) and human VEGF (hVEGF): mHIF1-α_F (gca gca gga att gga acat t), mHIF1-α_R (gcat gct aaa tcg gag ggta), hHIF1-α_F (caa gaa cct act gct aat gc), hHIF1-α_R (tta tgt atg tgg gta gga gat g), hVEGF_F (ttc tgc tgt ctt ggg tgc att gg), hVEGF_R (gaa gat gtc cac cag ggt ctc g). Relative gene expression was calculated by $2^{-\Delta CT}$. The changes in mRNA expression were expressed as fold-changes relative to control, which was the RNA from C2C12 or HEK293 cells without cobalt and transfection. As normalizer of qRT-PCR, the ribosomal gene hRPS29 was used with primers hRPS29_F (gag cca ccc gcg aaa at) and hRPS29_R (ccg tgc cgg ttt gaa cag) for HEK 293 and the murine β-actin gene with primers mβ-actin_F (gct cct cct gac cgc aag) and mβ-actin_R (cat ctg ctg gaa ggt gga ca) for C2C12. Each reaction was carried out in duplicate and all experiments were carried more than three times. Values were expressed in the mean ± standard error of the mean. One way ANOVA with Bonferronis's multiple comparison was used to statistical analysis.

Vector integration analysis by PCR

Genomic DNA was extracted from quadriceps muscles or from transfected HEK293 cells using the QIAMP DNA Mini Kit (QIAGEN Inc., Valencia, USA). To check for vector integration into the host genome, a PCR reaction was carried out using a pair of primers, CMV reverse 5′-TCATTATTGACGTCAA TGGGC-3′ and attB sense 5′-CTCCACCTCACCCATCT-3′, at a final concentration of 0.5 μM. The PCR reaction was performed by programming a thermocycler to 94°C for 1 min and 35 cycles of 94°C/1 min, 52°C/1.5 min and 72°C/1 min. After the final cycle, the reaction continued for 7 min at 72°C, and the tubes were then maintained at 4°C. As an internal control for the PCR, the glyceraldehyde-3-phosphate dehydrogenase (GAPDH) housekeeping gene was used with GAPDH sense (5′-ACCA-CAGTCCATGCCATCAC-3′) and GAPDH antisense (5′-TCCACCACCCTGTTGCTGTA-3′) primers. The PCR products were analyzed by 1% agarose gel electrophoresis with ethidium bromide staining.

Histological analysis

Muscle samples were fixed in 10% formaldehyde, dehydrated and embedded in paraffin. Four micrometer sections were obtained and stained with hematoxylin-eosin (HE) and picrosirius. The extent of necrosis, muscle regeneration and fibrosis were analyzed from 20 fields and quantified using Image Pro Plus software (Media Cybernetics, Inc., Bethesda, USA). Other sections were collected in poly L-lysine coated slides and submitted for immunohistochemistry with biotinylated Griffonia (bandeiraea) simplicifolia lectin I (1:100) (Vector Laboratories, Peterborough, UK) or anti-alpha smooth muscle actin antibody (1:50) (Vector Laboratories, Peterborough, UK) followed by incubation with streptavidin conjugated peroxidase (Sigma-Aldrich, Saint Louis, USA) and detection with diaminobenzidine chromogen. Vessel and capillary densities were quantified from 20 random fields per slide. The results were expressed as the average number per square millimeter.

Statistical analysis

The results were expressed as mean ± standard error of the mean. Analysis of variance (ANOVA) was performed using a Bonferroni correction for multiple comparisons or a Mann-Whitney test for a comparison of two groups. Visual assessment of necrosis was analyzed by the one way ANOVA with Tukey's multiple comparison tests. Only $P<0.05$ was considered significant.

Results

In vitro evaluation of VEGF gene expression

To assess the functionality of the constructed vectors (Fig. 1), HEK293T cells were transfected with these vectors, and VEGF gene expression was monitored for more than 90 days (Fig. 2). The calcium co-precipitation method was used to transfect HEK293T cells because this method achieves more than 90% transfection efficiency in this cell line (data not shown). To induce hypoxia, $CoCl_2$ was added to the medium at a final concentration of 100 μM, which is a concentration commonly used to mimic hypoxia [24]. HEK293T cells incubated with 100 μM $CoCl_2$ for nine days retained about 90% cell viability (data not shown).

Under normoxia conditions, all groups showed a peak of VEGF gene expression at 48 hours post-transfection, which is a well-known transient gene expression pattern, but by the 14th day, VEGF expression in all groups had returned to basal levels (Fig. 2). Cells transfected with the integrative vectors pVAVI and pVHAVI

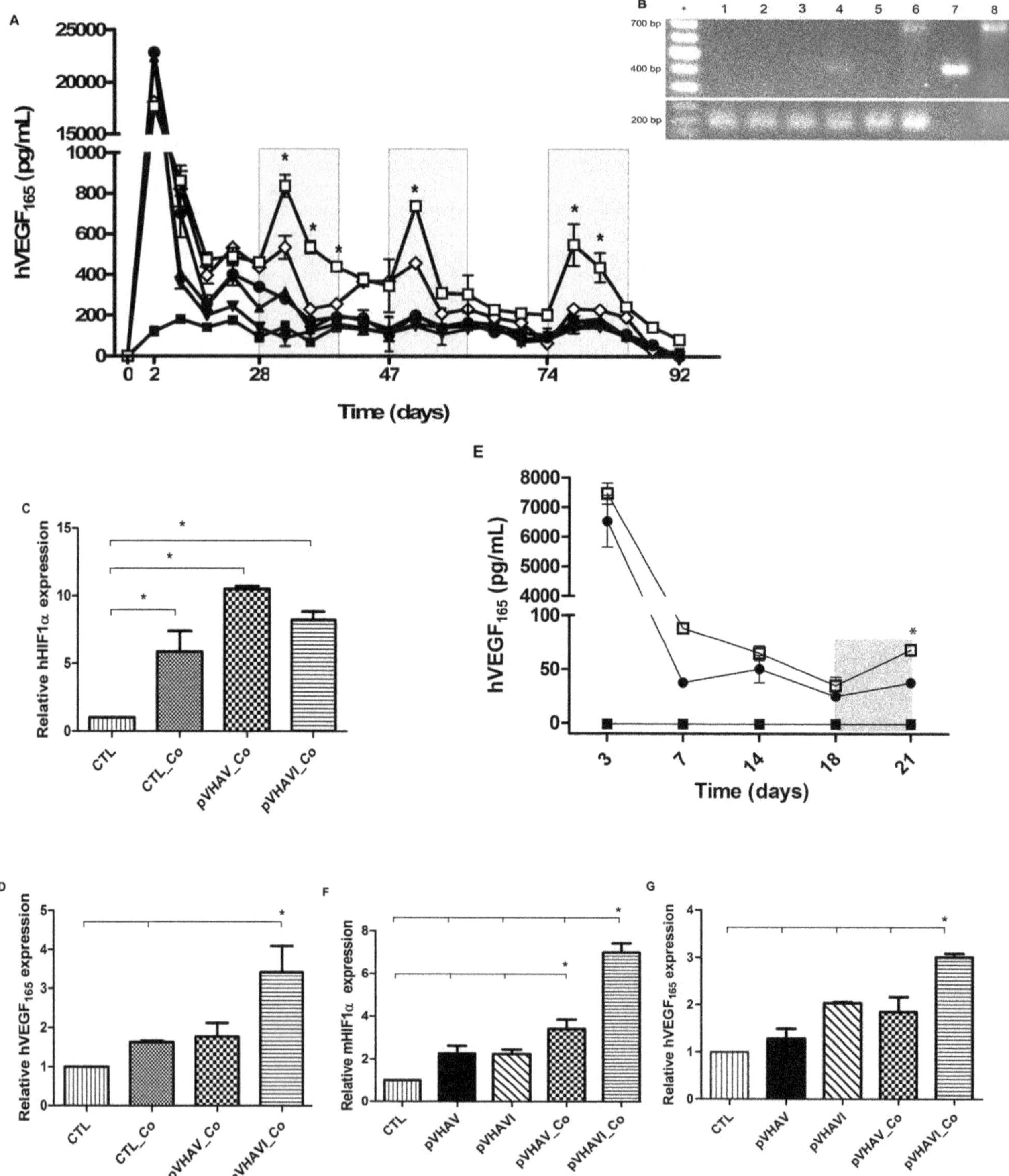

Figure 2. Assessment of VEGF expression vectors. (A) $hVEGF_{165}$ production under hypoxia and normoxia in HEK293 cells. On days 28, 47 and 74, $CoCl_2$ was added to a final concentration of 100 μM, and the medium was replaced every 3 days with fresh medium containing $CoCl_2$ for 9 days (gray bars). -■- no transfection; -▲- pVV; -▼- pVAV; -◇- pVAVI; -●- pVHAV; -□- pVHAVI. * $p<0.001$, pVHAVI in comparison to all groups. (B) Genomic DNA PCR after 4 weeks of transfection. 1: no transfection; 2: pVV; 3: pVAV; 4: pVAVI; 5: pVHAV; 6: pVHAVI; 7: pVAX-attB-$hVEGF_{165}$ (432 bp); 8: pVAX-HRE-attB-$hVEGF_{165}$ (725 bp). The 200 bp band is from GAPDH. * 100 bp ladder. pVV: pVAX-$hVEGF_{165}$ + pVAX; pVAV: pVAX-attB-$hVEGF_{165}$ + p-INT; pVAVI: pVAX-attB-$hVEGF_{165}$ + uP-INT; pVHAV: pVAX-HRE-attB-$hVEGF_{165}$ + p-INT pVHAVI: pVAX-HRE-attB-$hVEGF_{165}$ + uP-INT (C) HIF1α and (D) $hVEGF_{165}$ expression in HEK293 cells. On day 15 the HEK293 cells from the experiment (A) were collected for analysis by qRT-PCR. CTL: control; Co: $CoCl_2$; * $p<0.05$. (E) $hVEGF_{165}$ production under hypoxia and normoxia in C2C12 cells. On day 18 $CoCl_2$ was added to a final concentration of 100 μM and 3 days later the medium was collected for VEGF quantification by ELISA. -■- no transfection; -●- pVHAV; -□- pVHAVI. * $p<0.05$. (F) HIF1α and (G) $hVEGF_{165}$ expression in C2C12 cells. On day 15 the C2C12 cells from the experiment (C) were collected for analysis by qRT-PCR. CTL: control; Co: $CoCl_2$; * $p<0.05$ of pVHAVI_Co group versus all other groups.

still maintained about 500 pg/ml VEGF expression, whereas those transfected with non-integrative vectors expressed about half of this value. On the 28th day, $CoCl_2$ was added to the culture medium and maintained for 9 days. Three days after $CoCl_2$ addition, VEGF production was found to be enhanced only in the pVHAVI transfected cells; it reached about 900 pg/ml but returned to basal levels later. The pVAVI group did not show any increase in VEGF levels during the first 3 days, and these levels diminished even more in subsequent days. Upon removing $CoCl_2$, VEGF gene expression levels returned to their initial status.

Activation of VEGF gene expression by $CoCl_2$ was repeated on the 47th and 74th days and resulted in a very similar pattern of gene expression. After the third stimulation, the experiment was stopped because most of the cells became unviable. Long-term cell culturing with $CoCl_2$ seems to affect cell viability. These results clearly demonstrate that the vectors functioned correctly, particularly the pVHAVI system, which is the only system that is expected to be hypoxia-responsive.

To verify genomic integration of the pVHAVI and pVAVI vectors, genomic DNA was extracted 30 days after transfection, and a known region of the vectors was amplified by PCR. Fig. 2B shows the amplification of 735 bp and 432 bp products, which correspond to the pVAX-HRE-attB-hVEGF$_{165}$ and pVAX-attB-hVEGF$_{165}$ vectors, respectively. DNA from the other vectors was not amplified by PCR.

To demonstrate the activation of HIF1α by $CoCl_2$, the expression of HIF1α and hVEGF genes was evaluated by qRT-PCR at the 15th day. Irrespective of the presence or not of vectors, the presence of $CoCl_2$ in the medium elevated HIF1α gene expression 7 to 11 folds in relation to cells without $CoCl_2$ (Fig. 2C); however, only those cells transfected with pVHAVI had elevated VEGF gene expression in the presence of $CoCl_2$ (Fig. 2D), indicating the correct functioning of the pVHAVI system.

To strengthen these findings, we tested pVHAVI system in the murine myoblast cell line C2C12, which is the main cell type present in skeletal muscles. To transfect this cell line we chose nucleofection method, because we had very low level of transfection with calcium phosphate co-precipitation method (not shown). Even using nucleofection the VEGF gene expression levels were lower than HEK293 cells, but the profile of gene expression over 21 days was very similar (Fig. 2E). At the 3rd day after transfection, VEGF gene expression reached about 7,000 pg/ml by both pVHAVI and pVHAV systems, but in a week it dropped to basal level and, at 14th day, there was no significant difference of gene expression between these two systems.

$CoCl_2$ was added to cell culture media at the 18th day, but only those cells transfected with pVHAVI had increased hVEGF gene expression, meanwhile the cells transfected with pVHAV or non-transfected ones did not have any significant alterations. Activation of HIF1α by $CoCl_2$ was also seen in C2C12 cells (Fig. 2F), which was about 7 and 4 folds higher than control group by pVHAVI and pVHAV systems, respectively, but only pVHAVI transfected cells had increased hVEGF gene expression (Fig. 2G).

Visual, functional and molecular analyses of muscles after gene therapy

Visual assessment is an easy method to carry out and provides consistent and relevant information. To make this type of assessment quantitative, the degree of necrosis was scored as described in the "Materials and Methods" section. All animals in the ischemic group without gene therapy presented grade 1 or 2 necrosis. Two animals from the pVV group presented no necrosis, demonstrating the therapeutic effect of the treatment, but the rest of group still showed some degree of necrosis. The pVAVI-treated animals had a better outcome than the pVV group because about half of them had no necrosis. However, the best result was obtained with pVHAVI treatment, which resulted in no visual necrosis in any animals in the group (Fig. 3).

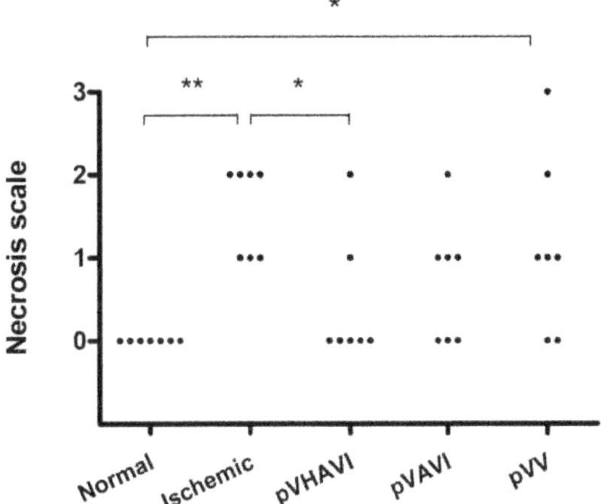

Figure 3. Visual assessment of ischemic limbs after gene therapy. Four weeks after gene therapy, limbs were evaluated according to the following necrosis scale: grade 0: absence of necrosis; grade I: necrosis limited to the toes; grade II: necrosis extending to the dorsum pedis, grade III: necrosis extending to the crus. * $P<0.05$; ** $P<0.005$.

To assess muscle functioning, the gastrocnemius muscle force was determined after 4 weeks of gene therapy. Ischemic limbs showed a drastically reduced force from 1.04 N to 0.12 N, but pVHAVI-treated animals exhibited a force of about 0.46 N, which is equivalent to a 400% improvement. pVV- and pVAVI-treated animals reached an intermediate score of 0.3 N (Fig. 4A). The weight of the gastrocnemius muscle varied among the groups in a pattern similar to that of the muscle force variation. In the pVHAVI-treated animals, this weight was about 50% that of the non-ischemic animals, whereas in the other groups, it was only about 36% (Fig. 4B). It is important to note that the untreated ischemic animals had a similar muscle weight compared to those treated with pVV or pVAVI, but in terms of muscle force, the untreated ischemic group had a much lower value. Muscle force depends on the number and volume of correctly functioning muscle fibers, whereas muscle mass encompasses the mass of all tissues including non-contractile fibrotic tissues, the amount of which varies with disease evolution. Therefore, a minor variation between muscle mass and force after 4 weeks of ischemia is expected.

The pVAVI and pVHAVI vectors are integrative systems, and consequently, gene delivery using these vectors is expected to result in long-term gene expression. To validate the correct functioning of these vectors, VEGF gene expression was evaluated in both serum and muscle tissue. In serum, VEGF was not detected at any time in any group. Muscle extracts obtained after 30 days from the pVHAVI and pVAVI groups had about 3.3 and 4.2 pg/mg of VEGF, respectively, and the ischemic and pVV-treated groups had less than 1.5 pg/mg (Fig. 5A). As 1.5 pg/mg is at the limit of VEGF detection by ELISA, we considered this to be a null value.

To check for vector integration in host cells, PCR was performed using genomic DNA obtained from muscles as a

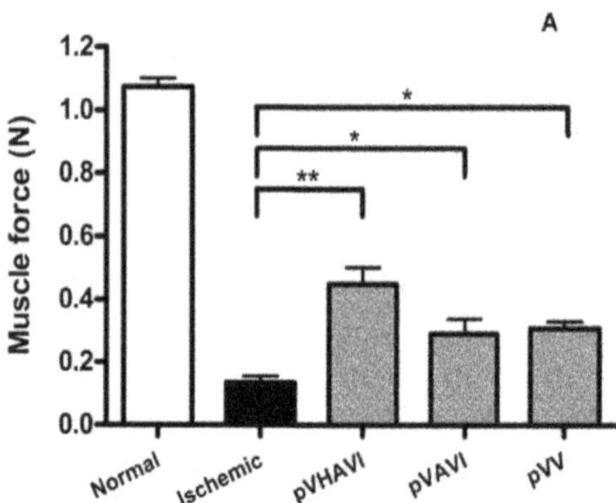

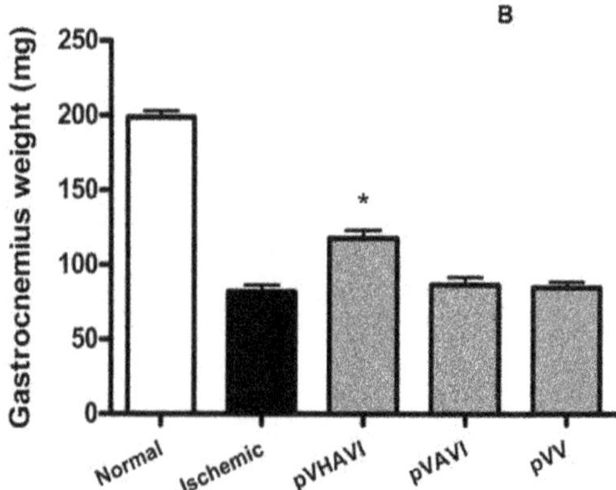

Figure 4. Determination of the mass and force of the gastrocnemius muscle. Muscle force (A) and mass (B) were measured 4 weeks after gene therapy. For each group, seven mice were used. The sham-operated and non-ischemic groups showed no difference in their results and are denoted here as normal. (A) * $P<0.05$; ** $P<0.005$. (B) * $P<0.05$, pVHAVI in comparison to each group.

template. DNA bands of 735 bp and 432 bp were detected in the pVHAVI and pVAVI groups, respectively, and these correspond to the pVAX-HRE-attB-hVEGF$_{165}$ and pVAX-attB-hVEGF$_{165}$ vectors, respectively (Fig. 5B). Other groups showed no amplification, indicating that no vector integration had occurred after 30 days.

Histological analyses

Gastrocnemius muscles were stained with HE, and the numbers of necrotic, normal and regenerative cells were quantified (Fig. 6A and 6B). The ischemic group showed about 15 cells/mm^2 of necrotic cells, and this was reduced to 5 cells/mm^2 in the pVHAVI-treated group. Moreover, the normal cell count increased from 5 cells/mm^2 in the untreated ischemic group to almost 20 cells/mm^2 in the pVHAVI-treated group. The groups treated with the other vectors showed intermediate values. In terms of regenerative cell count, the pVHAVI group (12 cells/mm^2) had a smaller count than the pVAVI group (18 cells/mm^2) but a much higher count than the ischemic group (4 cells/mm^2).

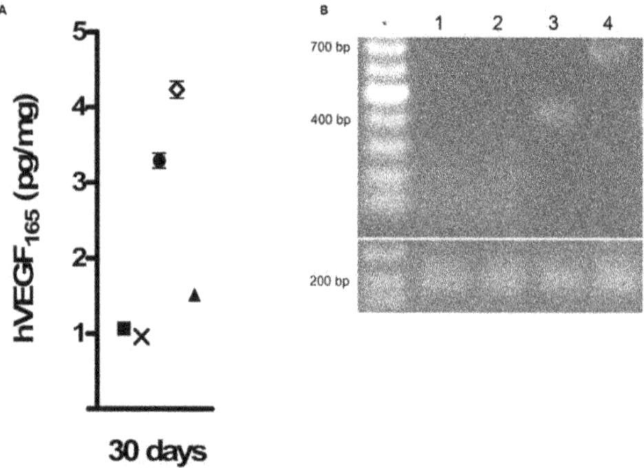

Figure 5. Assessment of VEGF expression vectors after gene therapy. (A) Concentration of hVEGF$_{165}$ in the quadriceps muscle: -x- Ischemic; -■- Normal; -▲- pVV; -●- pVHAVI; - ◇ - pVAVI. (B) Genomic DNA PCR after four weeks of gene therapy. 1: normal; 2: pVV; 3: pVAVI (432 bp); 4: pVHAVI (725 bp). The 200 bp band is from GAPDH. * 100 bp ladder.

A similar order of fibrotic area was seen after staining with Picrossirus (Fig. 6C): ischemic>pVV>pVAVI>pVHAVI>normal. These findings corroborate the previously obtained results demonstrating that the therapeutic effect of pVHAVI is better than that of either the non-integrative pVV system or the integrative and constitutive pVAVI system.

To evaluate angiogenic activity promoted by VEGF, vessels were stained with lectin Griffonia, which recognizes endothelial vessels and macrophages. This staining system was chosen over staining with an anti-CD31 antibody to allow both vessels and infiltrated macrophages to be visualized in the same section. Macrophages and endothelial cells can be differentiated easily by optical microscopy using high magnification. In addition, the anti-alpha-actin antibody was used to localize mature and larger vessels. The number of vessels stained with the two systems was similar (Fig. 6D and 6E). The pVHAVI-treated group had the highest number of vessels followed by the pVAVI and the pVV groups. Even though the difference between the pVHAVI and pVAVI groups was not statistically significant, the pVHAVI treatment tended to be superior.

Discussion

Since the first clinical trial of gene therapy for the treatment of ischemic limbs (which used a plasmid vector expressing the VEGF gene) by Jeffrey Isner in 1996 [29], more than 150 gene therapy trials have been initiated, and about half of them are still opened (http://www.wiley.co.uk/genetherapy/clinical/). The VEGF gene has been widely used in preclinical and clinical assays to treat ischemic diseases because it is a pleiotropic factor involved in many cellular activities, most of which are closely related to angiogenesis. In most of the animal studies, vectors expressing VEGF have been injected directly into the ischemic tissue, and this was found to improve blood flux and transiently augment vessel density [2]. However, we and other groups have demonstrated that long periods of high expression of this gene in ischemic tissue can lead to deleterious effects, such as a decrease in capillary density, the loss of muscle mass and force and the augmentation of limb necrosis [27,30,31]. It is likely that the high concentration of VEGF provided by the ischemic tissues together with the transfected cells promotes fast endothelial cell proliferation and vessel formation, which are not followed by adequate vessel maturation. These premature vessels in muscles can be easily disassembled by muscular movements, potentially leading to

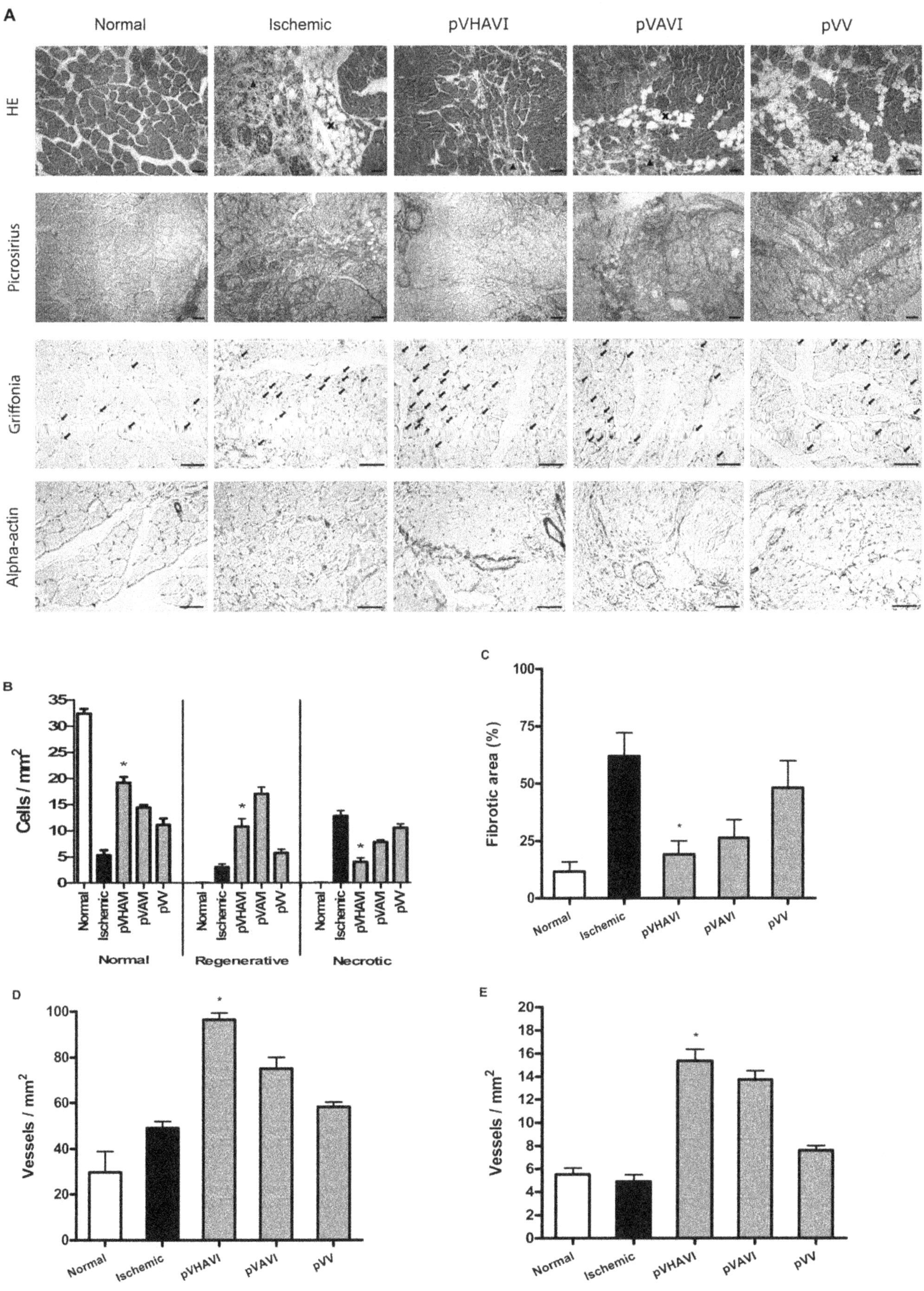
A
Normal
Ischemic
pVHAVI
pVAVI
pVV
HE
Picrosirius
Griffonia
Alpha-actin
B
Cells / mm²
Normal
Regenerative
Necrotic
Normal
Ischemic
pVHAVI
pVAVI
pVV
C
Fibrotic area (%)
D
Vessels / mm²
E
Vessels / mm²

Figure 6. Morphometric analysis of limb muscles. The gastrocnemius muscle was collected from mice after four weeks of gene therapy. Tissue samples were stained with HE (A) and used to quantify necrotic, regenerative and normal areas (B). The sham-operated and non-ischemic groups showed no difference in their results and are denoted here as normal. Fibrotic area, capillary density and mature vessel density were determined after staining with Picrosirius (C), Griffonia (D) and alpha-actin antibody (E), respectively. Bar = 50 μm. * $p<0.05$. ▲, Infiltrated mononuclear cells; X, adipocytes; →, capillary; In the figure B, pVHAVI was different statistically in comparison to all groups.

edema and cell death. Using VEGF together with either the stem cell mobilizing factor G-CSF (granulocyte colony stimulating factor) or the arteriogenic and vasculogenic factor GM-CSF (granulocyte macrophage-colony stimulating factor) to treat mouse ischemic limbs has resulted in much better outcomes than treatment with VEGF alone [26,27]. Our interpretation of these results is that, to make a stable and functional vessel, it is necessary to recruit more growth factors and cells in an adequate time frame and at adequate concentrations, as happens physiologically.

In angiogenic gene therapy assays, plasmid and adenoviral vectors are primarily used because they provide efficient gene transfer to muscles in vivo and express transgenes transiently. Most (if not all) of these vectors are designed to express transgenes highly and continuously using strong constitutive promoters, with the expectation that the secreted angiogenic factors will be spread around the whole ischemic area. However, most angiogenic factors like VEGF contain a heparin-binding domain in their structure [32–34], which causes these factors to be retained around the production area. Consequently, an area with cells transfected with VEGF produces this factor continuously irrespective of the local production due to ischemia, making the local concentration higher than necessary after a certain period of time. Such a condition usually leads to the formation of unstable, immature and hypofunctional vessels [16,35]. The best way of expressing VEGF for therapy is ideally by using vectors that respond to the requirements of the local tissue, *i.e.*, vectors that are regulated by the local degree of ischemia, as normal cells are.

Physiological VEGF gene expression is modulated by the local oxygen concentration. In ischemic tissue, the oxygen supply is limited, and oxygen distribution occurs mostly by passive diffusion from arteries to tissues [36]. This is one of the reasons that limbs distant from the obstructed artery are more affected than proximal limbs. Therefore, it is expected that the degree of ischemia, or the degree of oxygenation, will be variable in different parts of ischemic tissue. In this manner, VEGF production should correlate with either the degree of ischemia or the oxygen concentration. In humans, to overcome the ischemic condition, the ischemic tissues naturally express angiogenic factors based on the local oxygen concentration, such as VEGF, which is monitored by HIF-1 [37]. HIF-1α translocates to the nucleus during hypoxia, where it associates with HIF-1β to make a dimer, which in turn activates genes containing HRE (hypoxia responsive element) sequences. Genes involved in survival under hypoxic conditions, such as those that regulate angiogenesis, vessel dilation, erythropoiesis and glycolysis, are regulated by the binding of HIF to the HRE [19,37].

To make a VEGF-expressing vector responsive to hypoxia, we used nine repeats of the HRE sequence, which is responsive to HIF. A vector with nine repeats was used because it functioned better than vectors with fewer repeats [38]. In addition, with the goal of making an integrative vector capable of providing long-term VEGF expression, the phiC31 integrase system was used. This system allows integration of the vector in one direction, *i.e.*, once the vector is integrated into the host genome it cannot be removed enzymatically [20,21]. Using this system, our expectation was that one treatment of an ischemic limb with the vector (pVHAVI) would be sufficient for a long period, and VEGF gene expression would be regulated by the vector itself.

To demonstrate that the pVHAVI system was functioning correctly, these vectors were tested *in vitro* using HEK293T cells and myoblast cell line C2C12 and *in vivo* using a mouse ischemic limb model. In our *in vitro* study, HEK293T cells were transfected with several vectors (Fig. 1), and VEGF gene expression was followed for more than 90 days. The pVHAVI system was the only one that responded to hypoxia, which was induced by $CoCl_2$ to stabilize HIF1α from degradation. It is important to note that hypoxia was induced at three different times and the cells modified with pVHAVI responded precisely to the hypoxic signal each time. A very similar result was also seen in C2C12 cell line. These results demonstrate clearly that VEGF expression can be activated at any moment by hypoxia, as we predicted.

Correct functioning of the pVHAVI system, as indicated by the induction of VEGF gene expression by hypoxia, was observed for a month. In this study, we opted to use the limb ischemia model rather than administration of $CoCl_2$ because the first model is much more similar to human ischemic disease, and it is a well-established animal model [26,27,39]. Additionally, we have not found a method for using $CoCl_2$ to induce ischemia in vivo or any other method that can induce limb ischemia repeatedly without significantly affecting the animal's physiology. As a result, we could not induce hypoxia repeatedly in animals to evaluate the functioning of the pVHAVI system over a long period as we could for the in vitro model. Consequently, we chose to evaluate the system indirectly after gene therapy by examining therapeutic parameters such as alterations in muscle mass, force and histology and by visually assessing muscle necrosis. For in vivo gene transference, electroporation was used because in our previous studies, we demonstrated that this method is reproducible and results in high levels of transfection [26,27].

The first important step in our in vivo study was to demonstrate that the pVHAVI and pVAVI systems were integrated into muscle cells by phiC31 integrase after one month, and this was proven by PCR (Fig. 5B). It is also very important to note that both systems produced VEGF at a similar level (Fig. 5A), but the physiological response was quite different between them, as follows: 1) most of the animals treated with pVHAVI showed no necrosis, whereas half of those treated with pVAVI had some degree of necrosis (Fig. 3); 2) muscle weight and force were higher in animals treated with the pVHAVI system (Fig. 4A and 4B) and 3) the degree of angiogenesis and fibrosis was better with the pVHAVI system than the pVAVI system (Fig. 6).

Even though the VEGF concentration in muscles was similar in both systems, it is important to note that this concentration was determined from the whole muscle only once, at the 4th week, due to limitations of the method. Therefore, whether any variation in VEGF gene expression occurred in different parts of the muscle after transfection with either vector system during the 4 weeks is unknown. However, it is reasonable to assume that the pVHAVI system, which mainly expresses VEGF during hypoxia, acted differently than the pVAVI system, which expresses VEGF constitutively. We have no direct evidence to support this assumption, but the in vitro data and the improvement of animals treated with the pVHAVI system allow us to make this interpretation.

In this study, the viral CMV promoter was used to construct pVHAVI, which promoted hVEGF expression for three months in vitro and one month in vivo, at least. However, it is a well-known phenomenon that viral promoters, used to express mammalian genes, are frequently silenced during long-term studies. The use of muscle specific promoters like MCK (muscle creatine kinase) in construction of pVHAVI can bring better benefit to PAD patients in long-term treatment.

In conclusion, we demonstrated that a plasmid vector with an HRE sequence incorporated into it provides hypoxia-inducible VEGF expression. This vector, produced with the phiC31 integrative system, allowed for long-term VEGF gene expression, which was only activated under hypoxic conditions. For the treatment of mouse limb ischemia, the hypoxia-sensitive vector pVHAVI ameliorated the symptoms much better than the hypoxia-insensitive vector pVAVI. This last result corroborates the idea that the presence of high concentrations of VEGF in ischemic tissue is not beneficial or is less beneficial than maintaining a lower but sufficient and long-term concentration of VEGF locally.

Author Contributions

Conceived and designed the experiments: SWH. Performed the experiments: EGY RSS VYS PKM LPC VBVL. Analyzed the data: EGY RSS VYS PKM LPC VBVL SWH. Contributed reagents/materials/analysis tools: VBVL SWH. Wrote the paper: EGY SWH.

References

1. Norgren L, Hiatt WR, Dormandy JA, Nehler MR, Harris KA, et al. (2007) Inter-Society Consensus for the Management of Peripheral Arterial Disease (TASC II). Eur J Vasc Endovasc Surg 33 Suppl 1: S1–75.
2. Hammond HK, McKirnan MD (2001) Angiogenic gene therapy for heart disease: a review of animal studies and clinical trials. Cardiovasc Res 49: 561–567.
3. Gupta R, Tongers J, Losordo DW (2009) Human studies of angiogenic gene therapy. Circ Res 105: 724–736.
4. Rissanen TT, Yla-Herttuala S (2007) Current status of cardiovascular gene therapy. Mol Ther 15: 1233–1247.
5. Carmeliet P, Collen D (2000) Molecular basis of angiogenesis. Role of VEGF and VE-cadherin. Ann N Y Acad Sci 902: 249–262; discussion 262–244.
6. Ferrara N, Gerber HP, LeCouter J (2003) The biology of VEGF and its receptors. Nat Med 9: 669–676.
7. Grosskreutz CL, Anand-Apte B, Duplaa C, Quinn TP, Terman BI, et al. (1999) Vascular endothelial growth factor-induced migration of vascular smooth muscle cells in vitro. Microvasc Res 58: 128–136.
8. Barleon B, Sozzani S, Zhou D, Weich HA, Mantovani A, et al. (1996) Migration of human monocytes in response to vascular endothelial growth factor (VEGF) is mediated via the VEGF receptor flt-1. Blood 87: 3336–3343.
9. Bauters C, Asahara T, Zheng LP, Takeshita S, Bunting S, et al. (1995) Site-specific therapeutic angiogenesis after systemic administration of vascular endothelial growth factor. J Vasc Surg 21: 324–315.
10. Becit N, Ceviz M, Kocak H, Yekeler I, Unlu Y, et al. (2001) The effect of vascular endothelial growth factor on angiogenesis: an experimental study. Eur J Vasc Endovasc Surg 22: 310–316.
11. Takeshita S, Rossow ST, Kearney M, Zheng LP, Bauters C, et al. (1995) Time course of increased cellular proliferation in collateral arteries after administration of vascular endothelial growth factor in a rabbit model of lower limb vascular insufficiency. Am J Pathol 147: 1649–1660.
12. Takeshita S, Weir L, Chen D, Zheng LP, Riessen R, et al. (1996) Therapeutic angiogenesis following arterial gene transfer of vascular endothelial growth factor in a rabbit model of hindlimb ischemia. Biochem Biophys Res Commun 227: 628–635.
13. Takeshita S, Zheng LP, Brogi E, Kearney M, Pu LQ, et al. (1994) Therapeutic angiogenesis. A single intraarterial bolus of vascular endothelial growth factor augments revascularization in a rabbit ischemic hind limb model. J Clin Invest 93: 662–670.
14. Tsurumi Y, Takeshita S, Chen D, Kearney M, Rossow ST, et al. (1996) Direct intramuscular gene transfer of naked DNA encoding vascular endothelial growth factor augments collateral development and tissue perfusion. Circulation 94: 3281–3290.
15. van Weel V, Deckers MM, Grimbergen JM, van Leuven KJ, Lardenoye JH, et al. (2004) Vascular endothelial growth factor overexpression in ischemic skeletal muscle enhances myoglobin expression in vivo. Circ Res95: 58–66.
16. Schwarz ER, Speakman MT, Patterson M, Hale SS, Isner JM, et al. (2000) Evaluation of the effects of intramyocardial injection of DNA expressing vascular endothelial growth factor (VEGF) in a myocardial infarction model in the rat–angiogenesis and angioma formation. J Am Coll Cardiol 35: 1323–1330.
17. Lee RJ, Springer ML, Blanco-Bose WE, Shaw R, Ursell PC, et al. (2000) VEGF gene delivery to myocardium: deleterious effects of unregulated expression. Circulation 102: 898–901.
18. Semenza GL (1999) Perspectives on oxygen sensing. Cell 98: 281–284.
19. Semenza GL (2004) Hydroxylation of HIF-1: oxygen sensing at the molecular level. Physiology (Bethesda) 19: 176–182.
20. Calos MP (2006) The phiC31 integrase system for gene therapy. Curr Gene Ther 6: 633–645.
21. Chalberg TW, Portlock JL, Olivares EC, Thyagarajan B, Kirby PJ, et al. (2006) Integration specificity of phage phiC31 integrase in the human genome. J Mol Biol 357: 28–48.
22. Su H, Arakawa-Hoyt J, Kan YW (2002) Adeno-associated viral vector-mediated hypoxia response element-regulated gene expression in mouse ischemic heart model. Proc Natl Acad Sci U S A America 99: 9480–9485.
23. Sacramento CB, Moraes JZ, Denapolis PM, Han SW (2010) Gene expression promoted by the SV40 DNA targeting sequence and the hypoxia-responsive element under normoxia and hypoxia. Braz J Med Biol Res 43: 722–727.
24. DuBridge RB, Tang P, Hsia HC, Leong PM, Miller JH, et al. (1987) Analysis of mutation in human cells by using an Epstein-Barr virus shuttle system. Mol Cell Biol 7: 379–387.
25. Yuan Y, Hilliard G, Ferguson T, Millhorn DE (2003) Cobalt inhibits the interaction between hypoxia-inducible factor-alpha and von Hippel-Lindau protein by direct binding to hypoxia-inducible factor-alpha. J Biol Chem 278: 15911–15916.
26. Sacramento CB, Cantagalli VD, Grings M, Carvalho LP, Baptista-Silva JC, et al. (2009) Granulocyte-macrophage colony-stimulating factor gene based therapy for acute limb ischemia in a mouse model. J Gene Med 11: 345–353.
27. Sacramento CB, da Silva FH, Nardi NB, Yasumura EG, Baptista-Silva JC, et al. (2010) Synergistic effect of vascular endothelial growth factor and granulocyte colony-stimulating factor double gene therapy in mouse limb ischemia. J Gene Med 12: 310–319.
28. Hourde C, Vignaud A, Beurdy I, Martelly I, Keller A, et al. (2006) Sustained peripheral arterial insufficiency durably impairs normal and regenerating skeletal muscle function. J Physiol Sci 56: 361–367.
29. Isner JM, Pieczek A, Schainfeld R, Blair R, Haley L, et al. (1996) Clinical evidence of angiogenesis after arterial gene transfer of phVEGF165 in patient with ischaemic limb. Lancet 348: 370–374.
30. Masaki I, Yonemitsu Y, Yamashita A, Sata S, Tanii M, et al. (2002) Angiogenic gene therapy for experimental critical limb ischemia: acceleration of limb loss by overexpression of vascular endothelial growth factor 165 but not of fibroblast growth factor-2. Circ Res 90: 966–973.
31. Ozawa CR, Banfi A, Glazer NL, Thurston G, Springer ML, et al. (2004) Microenvironmental VEGF concentration, not total dose, determines a threshold between normal and aberrant angiogenesis. J Clin Invest 113: 516–527.
32. Nugent MA, Edelman ER (1992) Kinetics of basic fibroblast growth factor binding to its receptor and heparan sulfate proteoglycan: a mechanism for cooperactivity. Biochemistry 31: 8876–8883.
33. Maciag T, Mehlman T, Friesel R, Schreiber AB (1984) Heparin binds endothelial cell growth factor, the principal endothelial cell mitogen in bovine brain. Science 225: 932–935.
34. McCaffrey TA, Falcone DJ, Du B (1992) Transforming growth factor-beta 1 is a heparin-binding protein: identification of putative heparin-binding regions and isolation of heparins with varying affinity for TGF-beta 1. J Cell Physiol 152: 430–440.
35. von Degenfeld G, Banfi A, Springer ML, Wagner RA, Jacobi J, et al. (2006) Microenvironmental VEGF distribution is critical for stable and functional vessel growth in ischemia. FASEB J 20: 2657–2659.
36. Wittenberg BA, Wittenberg JB (1989) Transport of oxygen in muscle. Annu Rev Physiol 51: 857–878.
37. Wang GL, Semenza GL (1993) General involvement of hypoxia-inducible factor 1 in transcriptional response to hypoxia. Proc Natl Acad Sci U S A 90: 4304–4308.
38. Ruan H, Su H, Hu L, Lamborn KR, Kan YW, et al. (2001) A hypoxia-regulated adeno-associated virus vector for cancer-specific gene therapy. Neoplasia 3: 255–263.
39. Goto T, Fukuyama N, Aki A, Kanabuchi K, Kimura K, et al. (2006) Search for appropriate experimental methods to create stable hind-limb ischemia in mouse. Tokai J Exp Clin Med 31: 128–132.

3

A Sub-Cellular Viscoelastic Model for Cell Population Mechanics

Yousef Jamali*, Mohammad Azimi, Mohammad R. K. Mofrad

Molecular Cell Biomechanics Laboratory, Department of Bioengineering, University of California, Berkeley, California, United States of America

Abstract

Understanding the biomechanical properties and the effect of biomechanical force on epithelial cells is key to understanding how epithelial cells form uniquely shaped structures in two or three-dimensional space. Nevertheless, with the limitations and challenges posed by biological experiments at this scale, it becomes advantageous to use mathematical and *'in silico'* (computational) models as an alternate solution. This paper introduces a single-cell-based model representing the cross section of a typical tissue. Each cell in this model is an individual unit containing several sub-cellular elements, such as the elastic plasma membrane, enclosed viscoelastic elements that play the role of cytoskeleton, and the viscoelastic elements of the cell nucleus. The cell membrane is divided into segments where each segment (or point) incorporates the cell's interaction and communication with other cells and its environment. The model is capable of simulating how cells cooperate and contribute to the overall structure and function of a particular tissue; it mimics many aspects of cellular behavior such as cell growth, division, apoptosis and polarization. The model allows for investigation of the biomechanical properties of cells, cell-cell interactions, effect of environment on cellular clusters, and how individual cells work together and contribute to the structure and function of a particular tissue. To evaluate the current approach in modeling different topologies of growing tissues in distinct biochemical conditions of the surrounding media, we model several key cellular phenomena, namely monolayer cell culture, effects of adhesion intensity, growth of epithelial cell through interaction with extra-cellular matrix (ECM), effects of a gap in the ECM, tensegrity and tissue morphogenesis and formation of hollow epithelial acini. The proposed computational model enables one to isolate the effects of biomechanical properties of individual cells and the communication between cells and their microenvironment while simultaneously allowing for the formation of clusters or sheets of cells that act together as one complex tissue.

Editor: Nick Monk, University of Nottingham, United Kingdom

Funding: Financial support by National Science Foundation is gratefully acknowledged. Dr. Jamali was supported by a generous fellowship support from the Institute for Research in Fundamental Sciences. The funders had no role in study design, data collection and analysis, decision to publish, or preparation of the manuscript.

Competing Interests: The authors have declared that no competing interests exist.

* E-mail: mofrad@berkeley.edu

Introduction

One of the important phenomena in cell engineering and developmental biology is the shape of tissue and the cell's organization. Depending on the cell type and environmental conditions, cells can create unique shapes such as flat sheets, self-enclosed monolayers, cysts, or elongated tubes. The more important question is how these cells interact and how their local interaction causes a global geometrical distinctive shape for tissues like the heart or kidney [1–6]. The geometrical interactions and coordinated adhesion among neighboring cells and between the cells and local environment are critical for structure and function of epithelial tissue [7–13]. Any perturbation of these orchestrated interactions can cause abnormality in behavior and function of tissue and often lead to initiation of tumor growth and invasion [14–15]. Another interesting subject is embryogenesis, when a stem cell with consecutive rapid divisions and differentiation can create different tissues, wherein the interactions between cells and environmental biochemical and biomechanical signals have critical, yet nearly unknown roles [16–17]. However, in the last two decades, improved experimental techniques and developments in new laboratory instruments have allowed for more detailed understanding of cell-cell communication and the cell's response to biochemical and biomechanical environmental signals. Nevertheless, biological experiments are expensive and depend on many parameters that are mostly difficult to control and test in isolation. As a complementary method, mathematical modeling and '*in silico*' (computational) experiments are a good candidate to help explore the behavior of the individual tissue cells along with investigating their response to environmental cues. Due to easy isolation in *in-silico*, computational models, incorporating the related fundamental physical and biological parameters can explain how specific biochemical or biomechanical parameters may affect the tissue cells and their arrangement. Such a model can help reduce the number of experiments required to obtain meaningful observations by eliminating unlikely hypothesis while providing a better explanation of observations.

For example, to investigate how individual cells cooperate and contribute to the overall structure and function of a particular tissue, a proper computational model must be capable of allowing cells to be defined as individually deformable shapes, time- and space-dependent individually regulated cell turnover, and cell-cell and cell-ECM interaction. Many models have been developed to mimic cell behavior, such as response to external mechanical and biochemical signals, cell-cell interaction, cell motility, and cell morphology. For example, some models have attempted to mimic cell collection behavior such as cancer invasion through the use of continuum and/or discrete approaches [18–19] (Figure 1; Method 1), where each cell is represented by a finite element and follows a cellular automata (CA) method [14,20–24]. Several models are based on the extended Cellular Automata method (Figure 1; Method 2), e.g. the lattice-gas based cellular automata (LGCA), and the cellular potts model (CPM) [25] (Figure 1; Method 3). In other approaches, cells are modeled as colloidal objects capable of interacting with their environment [26–29]. In such models, cells are capable of migrating, growing, dividing, and changing their orientation. For example, in a model proposed by Galle, Loeffler et al. (2005), the cells move according to the Langevin dynamics framework and can interact based on a combination of attractive and repulsive forces (Figure 1; Method 4). The aim of these models is to replicate the multi-cellular growth phenomena. By focusing on monolayer culture, Galle et al. [29] have investigated the effect of key factors on rate and quality of culture growth. They also analyzed the underlying processes involved in multi-cellular spheroids, intestinal crypts, and other aspects of developmental biology. These models are robust in mimicking various aspects of cell population, but fail to examine the effects of cell deformation and morphology on pattern formation and growth processes. To investigate the effects of cell morphology on a multi-cellular structure, Newman and colleagues [30–31] developed a phenomenological model involving a number of identical sub-cellular elements, whose dynamics and interactions are defined by intracellular potentials, which are stronger and bind elements belonging to the same cell as well as intercellular potentials, which are weaker and bind elements of neighboring cells (Figure 1; Method 5). This model can simulate cell growth and division, and when modeling the growth of a multi-cellular cluster from a single cell, this algorithm simulates cellular shapes and multi-cellular structures in 3D. Some models are based on the viscoelasticity of cells [32–37], where each cell includes certain elastic and viscous elements. Such models lend themselves to easy incorporation of the cell-cell adhesion and repulsion, and various forces acting on individual cells in the cluster. For example, a 3D deformable cell model with cell adhesion and signaling was developed by Palsson and colleagues [32–33], where each cell is taken as an ellipsoid, with its axis composed of a combination of springs and viscous elements (Figure 1; Method 6). This model was used to investigate the role of cell signaling, cell adhesion, chemotaxis, and coordinated differentiation in the morphology of a developed organism. Another biomechanical approach developed by Rejniak and colleagues [35–37] represents cells as deformable viscoelastic objects that can be arranged into tissues of various topologies. Rejniak's model employs an immersed boundary method with distributed sources (Figure 1; Method 7). This approach joins elastic cell dynamics with a continuous representation of a viscous incompressible cytoplasm. The model covers many aspects of cellular behavior such as cell growth, division, apoptosis and polarization. With this model it is possible to investigate the biomechanical properties of cells and cell-cell interaction, the effects of the microenvironment on a cellular cluster, and how

	Method	Morphology of Cell	Intracellular Elements	Adhesion	Growth	Division	Movement	Polarization	Nucleus	Cell-Environment Interaction	Biomechanical Behavior	Computational Efficiency	Scale	Ref
1	Continuum and/or Discrete	N	N	N	N	S	N	N	N	S	N	L	mm	[18-19]
2	Cellular Automata (CA)	N	N	N	N	N	S	N	N	S	N	L	mm	[14,20-24]
3	Cellular Potts (CPM)	A	N	A	A	N	S	N	N	S	N	H	µm-mm	[25]
4	Cell Based Langevin Dynamics	N	N	A	A	A	A	N	N	S	N	M	mm	[26-29]
5	Sub-cellular Elements with Phenomenological Potentials	A	A	A	A	A	N	N	N	A	A	H	µm-mm	[30-31]
6	Cells with Viscoelastic Axis	S	S	A	N	N	A	A	N	A	A	M	µm-mm	[32-37]
7	Immersed Boundary Method with Distributed Sources	S	A	A	A	A	A	A	A	A	N	H	µm-mm	[35-37]
8	Sub-Cellular with Multiple Viscoelastic Elements	S	A	A	A	A	A	A	A	A	A	M	µm-mm	Present model

Figure 1. A comparison of existing models for cell morphology based on model realism and computational cost. A = Advanced, S = Simple, N = None; L = Low, M = Moderate, H = High.

individual cells work together and contribute to the structure and function of a particular tissue. Some applications of this model include the following: the folding of a trophoblast bilayer [38], tumor growth [35] and self-arrangement into a hollow acinus [36]. More recently, Coskuna et al. [34] developed a mathematical model for ameboid cell movement in which a viscoelastic (spring–dashpot) system was used to represent the cytoskeleton. This model was used to solve an inverse problem of amoeboid cell motility and to find the variation of spring and dash-pots parameters in time. The research shows that the model and the solution to the inverse problem for simulated data sets are highly accurate. In general, cell mechanics has been modeled based on non-living structures using different approaches [39] ranging from the soft glassy material model [40–41], to the cortical shell–liquid core model [42–43], and tensegrity architecture [44–51]. Few of the theoretical models that have been proposed for analyzing the mechanical properties of adherent living cells are capable of simultaneously incorporating (i) the discrete nature of the cytoskeleton, (ii) cell–cell and/or cell–extracellular matrix (ECM) interactions, and (iii) the cellular pre-stress [48]. To address this shortcoming, a new biomechanical model for the cell is proposed here that is able to incorporate all these properties of the cell simultaneously. In this model, inspired by the tensegrity concept, each cell is capable of changing its morphology, and performing various cellular processes such as growth, division, death, and polarization. The modeled cells are able to interact with each other and with their environment. Each cell in this model is an individual unit containing several subcellular elements, such as the elastic plasma membrane, encompassed by viscoelastic elements that perform the function of the cytoskeleton, and the viscoelastic elements of the cell nucleus (Figure 1; Method 8). Additionally, the cell membrane is divided into segments where each segment (or point) incorporates the cell's interaction and communication with its environment, such as adherens junctions. The qualities of the various models discussed above are summarized in Figure 1. The remainder of this paper is organized as follows. In Methods, the mathematics of the model have been discussed. In Result and Discussion, the model has been used to mimic several relevant biological examples to show validity and the capabilities of the model. In Conclusions, the model and its capabilities are summarized and future steps for improving the model have been suggested.

Methods

The details of our computational model are outlined here while Table 1 summarizes the parameters of this paper and Table 2 provides quantitative values that were used in this model that are valid for a typical cell. In this model, cells are represented as objects with initial circular structures. The cell and nuclear membranes are initially discretized, arbitrarily, into N_0 nodes (points), where a mass is associated with each point representing altogether the total mass of the nucleus and cytoskeleton. Each point on the cell and nuclear membranes is then $1/N_0$ of the mass of the cytoskeleton and nucleus, respectively (Figure 2). Hereafter, unless explicitly mentioned, the subscripts of parameters refer to the cell number and point number. Superscript m indicates that the point is on the cell membrane, and superscript n represents a point on the nuclear membrane. If neither m nor n is specified, the given point can be assumed to lie on either the cell membrane or nucleus. For example, the $k'th$ membrane point of the $i'th$ cell is represented by $P^m_{i,k}$, the corresponding point in the nucleus is represented by $P^n_{i,k}$, and $P_{i,k}$ represent the general point k of $i'th$ cell.

Force balances at each point have been considered as follows. The total force $F^{tot}_{i,k}$, acting on $P^m_{i,k}$ is calculated according to

$$F^{tot}_{i,k} = F^{inner}_{i,k} + F^{cell\_cell}_{i,k} + F^{cell\_ECM}_{i,k} + F^{ext}_{i,k} + F^{mitosis}_{i,k} \quad (1)$$

Here $F^{inner}_{i,k}$ is the total force that acts on $P_{i,k}$ due to the inner structure of the cell (Figure 3 and Figure 4), i.e. the cytoskeleton, membrane, and the cytoplasm, $F^{cell\_cell}_{i,k}$ is the total force resulting from the interaction with other cells (cell-cell interaction), $F^{cell\_ECM}_{i,k}$ is the force due to an interaction with a substrate(cell-ECM interaction), $F^{ext}_{i,k}$ represents the external forces, (as described below) and $F^{mitosis}_{i,k}$ is the sum of the forces acting on $P_{i,k}$, when the cell undergoes the cell division process (Figure 5). This force is due to the shortening of the spindle fibers; a contractile ring is formed by contractile forces acting on opposite sides of the cell boundary. In the following subsections, these forces will be discussed and described further in the context of various cellular events.

a. Inner cell structure

To model the inner cell structure, a viscoelastic Voigt model, represented by a purely viscous element (a damper) and purely elastic element (a spring) connected in parallel, is used (see Figure 2). The force of a Voigt subunit connected to points $P_{i,k}$ and $P_{j,l}$ is given as:

$$f^v_{i,k}(P_{j,l},\mu,k_s,l) = k_s \frac{|R_{i,k}(t) - R_{j,l}(t)| - l}{|R_{i,k}(t) - R_{j,l}(t)|}(R_{i,k}(t) - R_{j,l}(t)) + \mu\big(V_{i,k}(t) - V_{j,l}(t)\big) \quad (2)$$

Here $R_{i,k}(t)$ and $V_{i,k}(t)$ are the position and velocity corresponding to $P_{i,k}$ respectively, l is the rest length of the spring, k_s is the spring constant, and μ represents viscosity. It should be noted that μ, k_s and l vary with time and position and depend on i^{th}, j^{th} cells and k^{th}, l^{th} points, i.e. the two points that are connected by this element (see Figure 2). The inner force $F^{inner}_{i,k}$ (see Figure 3 and Figure 4) can be represented by the equation:

$$F^{inner}_{i,k} = F^{csk}_{i,k} + F^{mem}_{i,k} + F^{p}_{i,k},$$

where $F^{csk}_{i,k}$ is the force from the cytoskeleton, $F^p_{i,k}$ is the force due to liquid in the inner cell, i.e. cytoplasm, and $F^{mem}_{i,k}$ is the force from the membrane acting on $P_{i,k}$.

Cytoskeleton. The mechanical properties of the cytoskeleton, like elasticity and viscosity, are critical to the validity of the model. Voigt subunits are effective for modeling a viscoelastic system; the spring constants of the model are linear approximations to the elasticity of the inner cell. Additionally, all springs are subjected to a damping force resulting from the viscosity of the cytoplasm, where linear dash-pots are used to approximate the viscosity of the cytoskeleton. In the present model, the cytoskeleton is divided into N uniformly radial distributed parts, each of which is represented by a Voigt subunit radiating from the nucleus (Figure 3, blue subunits). Each subunit connects two points of the cell and nuclear membrane, which are aligned in a radial direction from the center of the nucleus. The nucleoskeleton is represented as a viscoelastic model involving an actomyosin system (Figure 3, red subunits). The model also contains N Voigt subunits in the nucleus (Figure 3, red subunits), each of which connects two nuclear membrane points n and n' in which $n' - n$ equal to $[N/3]$

Table 1. List of variables and their definitions used in this paper.

Subscripts		**Parameters**	
i,j	$i'th$ and $j'th$ cells	N_0	number of nodes (points) on the perimeter of the cell and nucleus (i.e. their membranes)
k,l	$k'th$ and $l'th$ points	P	point
a	anterior region of cell	F	force
p	posterior region of cell	$f^{v}_{i,k}$	force of a Voigt subunit acting on $P_{i,k}$
		μ	viscosity of a Voigt subunit
		k_s	spring constant of a Voigt subunit
		$R_{i,k}$	position of $P_{i,k}$
Superscripts		$V_{i,k}$	velocity of $P_{i,k}$
m	cell membrane	Pr_{os}	inner pressure
n	cell nucleus	Pr_0	environmental pressure
tot	total of all related parameters	V_s	stop volume region
$inner$	inner cell	V_g	growth volume region
$cell\_cell$	cell-cell interactions	V_c	current volume of the cell
$cell\_ECM$	cell-ECM interactions	V_r	rest volume of the cell
ext	external parameters	α_s	stop volume region coefficient
$mitosis$	mitosis process	α_g	growth volume region coefficient
csk	cytoskeleton	f^{n}_{div}	dividing force that acts on nucleus points
$ncsk$	nucleus cytoskeleton	f^{m}_{con}	dividing force that acts on membrane points
mem	membrane	d_{sep}	distance separating two daughter cells
p	pressure	D	drag coefficient of each point
adh	adhesion	d^{adh}_0	maximum separation between two points for initiating adhesion
rep	elastic cell-cell or cell-ECM repulsion	d^{adh}_{hys}	minimum separation between two points for disrupting adhesion
		d^{rep}_0	maximum separation between two points for elastic interaction
		$d^{j}_{i,k}$	distance between $P_{i,k}$ and the membrane surface of $j'th$ cell or ECM
		k_f	form factor
		Ω	total occupied area of cells
		n_{cell}	number of cells
		ρ	cell edge density
		L_b	sum of the lengths of all internal cell boundaries plus half of the perimeter of the patch

(Figure 3). This allows the nucleus to show more resistance to changes in its shape and volume due to exterior pressures when compared to simply connecting opposing points on the cell membrane. Only elements from the cytoskeleton act on each point in the cell membrane, therefore, it can be said (see Figure 3):

$$F^{m,csk}_{i,k} = f^{v}_{i,k}(P^{n}_{i,k}, \mu^{csk}, k^{csk}_{\mu}, l^{csk}) \tag{3}$$

For nuclear membrane points (see Figure 3):

$$\begin{aligned} F^{n,csk}_{i,k} = {} & f^{v}_{i,k}(P^{m}_{i,k}, \mu^{csk}, k^{csk}_{\mu}, l^{csk}) + f^{v}_{i,k}(P^{n}_{i,k+[N/3]}, \mu^{ncsk}, k^{ncsk}_{\mu}, l^{ncsk}) \\ & + f^{v}_{i,k}(P^{n}_{i,k-[N/3]}, \mu^{ncsk}, k^{ncsk}_{\mu}, l^{ncsk}) \end{aligned} \tag{4}$$

Where $ncsk$ refers to the nuclear cytoskeleton.

As a note, the inclusion of additional cellular elements into a biomechanical model should be justified. In our model, an additional yet key biomechanical element that is considered is the structure of the nucleus' cytoskeleton (actin filaments [52] and nuclear lamina) which is connected to the cytoplasm cytoskeleton via connected proteins (LINC) [53]. Our model attempts to incorporate key aspects of the cell that play an important role in cell biomechanics while maintaining simplicity. Additionally, not all cells are flat nor are their nuclei positioned in the center of the cell. The fact that the nucleus is not positioned in the center of the cell plays an important role in the shape of the cell (e.g. satellite shape of fibroblasts). Furthermore, under some mechanical conditions, the nucleus plays an important role in the final shape of the cell. Moreover, the mechanical behaviors of the nuclear region (e.g. kinetochore microtubule shortening) play a key role in mitosis. Inclusion of the nucleus in the model helps substantially in modeling the dynamics of mitosis based on what happens in the real cell during this process. In cellular mechanotransduction, the nucleus itself may play an important role in the response of the cell to force [54] and the forces acting on the nucleus are believed to be important in eliciting events such as gene expressionas shown by Wang *et al* [55]. Subsequently, through inclusion of the nucleus in our model, we can investigate the effect and intensity of forces that act on the nucleus from the external environment through the cytoskeleton. The inclusion of the nucleus is ultimately necessary in multi-scale modeling of the cell. From a modeling point of view, if we were to ignore the nucleus, we would need to connect all of

Table 2. The parameters for a typical cell, most of the parameters adopted from [34].

P	Definition of Parameters	Units	Value
K^{cyt}	Radial spring constants	kg/s^2	4.0×10^{-18}
B^{cyt}	Damping constants for radial springs	kg/s	1.5×10^{-15}
K^{ncyt}	Nucleus spring constants	kg/s^2	3.0×10^{-16}
B^{ncyt}	Damping constants for nucleus springs	kg/s	0
$K_{i,k}^{m,adh}$	Adhesion spring constants	kg/s^2	4.0×10^{-17}
$B_{i,k}^{m,adh}$	Damping constants for adhesion spring	kg/s	0
$K_{i,k}^{m,mem}$	Cell membrane spring constants	kg/s^2	6.5×10^{-17}
$B_{i,k}^{m,mem}$	Damping constants for cell membrane springs	kg/s^2	2.0×10^{-15}
$D_{i,k}^{m,mem}$	Drag coefficients at the cell membrane	kg/s	13.5×10^{-16}
$K_{i,k}^{n,mem}$	nucleus membrane spring constants	kg/s^2	3.0×10^{-16}
$B_{i,k}^{n,mem}$	Damping constants for the springs	kg/s	1.0×10^{-14}
$D_{i,k}^{n,mem}$	Drag coefficients at the nucleus membrane	kg/s	2.5×10^{-15}
N_0	Number of initial points		30
$l_{i,k}^{ad}$	Adhesion spring rest lengths	μm	0
R_{cell}	Cell radius	μm	5.0
R^n	Nucleus radius	μm	1.0
M_{cell}	Cell mass	Kg	1.0×10^{-12}
M_{nuc}	Nucleus mass	Kg	1.0×10^{-13}
α_s	Percent of rest volume where growth ends under this volume		85
α_g	Percent of rest volume that growth continues above this volume		95
dt	Time step	s	10
T	Temperature	$^\circ k$	300

the end points of the cytoskeleton elements to each other at a single central point. In this situation this point will play a critical role in simulations and can cause some singularities and abnormal behavior during simulation and impose many limitations on the model. Conversely, with the current structure, the force is distributed around the nucleus and the whole system is more stable (A possible alternative is to connect each point on the membrane to the point on the opposing side of the membrane; in this case each force on one point is directly transmitted to the other side of the cell and causes artificial behavior).

Membrane. To represent the viscoelasticty of the membrane, or, more correctly, the viscoelasticty of the cortical cytoskeleton, two consecutive membrane points are connected with a Voigt subunit (Figure 4, a and b, green subunits); hence the model includes N Voigt subunits on the cell membrane and N subunits on the nuclear membrane.

$$F_{i,k}^{mem}=f_{i,k}^{v}(P_{i,k+1},\mu^{mem},k_{\mu}^{mem},l^{mem})+f_{i,k}^{v}(P_{i,k-1},\mu^{mem},k_{\mu}^{mem},l^{mem}) \quad (5)$$

Cytoplasm. The cytoplasm is a viscous incompressible fluid, naturally hindering the cell's shape and volume changes. On the other hand, osmotic pressures caused by the relatively higher concentrations of proteins and other molecules inside the cell compared to its external environment [56] act on the membrane. This internal pressure is involved in the determination of cell shape and morphology and affects the driving force of cell movement [57–60]. In addition, the curved shape of microtubules in the cell (despite their large effective persistence length compare to the length of the cell [39,61]) implies that they must push the cell membrane outward [39]. To represent these, a normal stress (pressure) field acting on each point of the cell membrane is defined, whose direction is outward and perpendicular to the cell membrane (Figure 4c):

$$F_{i,j}^{m,p}=(\mathrm{Pr}_{os}-\mathrm{Pr}_{0})\frac{dR}{2}$$
$$dR=|R_{i,j}(t)-R_{i,j+1}(t)|+|R_{i,j}(t)-R_{i,j-1}(t)| \quad (6)$$

where Pr_{os} and Pr_0 are the inner pressure and environmental pressure, respectively. However, we make the approximation that pressure in the cell is constant and independent of volume in equilibrium conditions. This approximation is not very speculative as various membrane channels allow for the flow of intracellular fluid into or out of the cell at equilibrium, not allowing for the buildup of hydrostatic pressure due to intracellular fluid accumulation.

b. Cellular processes

Growth. To implement cell growth in the proposed model, the number of membrane points, i.e. the number of viscoelastic compartments, is allowed to increase as follows. First an integer random number in the range $(1,N)$ is generated, say j, providing the location of the point j on the perimeter, then a point between $j'th$ and $(j+1)'th$ points in the cell membrane is added and the

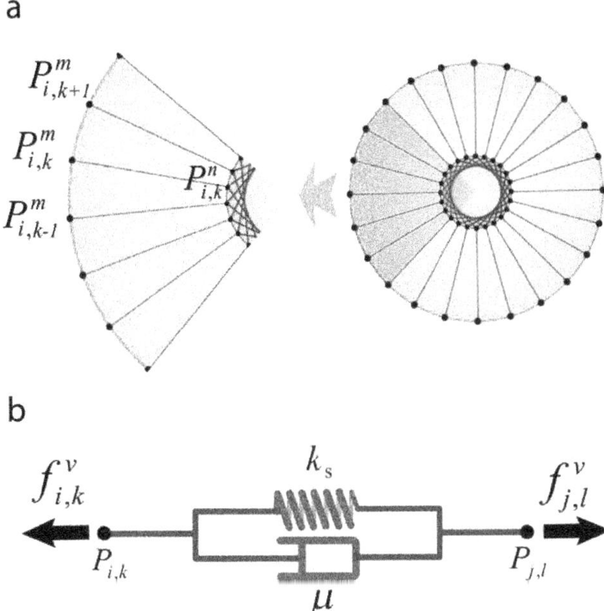

Figure 2. Cell structural model. a) The perimeter of the cell and nucleus (i.e. their corresponding membranes) are initially discretized into N_0 nodes (points). The superscript m indicates that the point is on the cell membrane and superscript n represents a point on the nuclear membrane. If neither m nor n are specified, the given point can be assumed to lie on either the cell membrane or nucleus. For example, the $k'th$ membrane's point of $i'th$ cell represented by $P^m_{i,k}$. Each line that connects two points (red, green and blue lines) refers to a Voigt subunit. The total force that acts on each point is F^{tot} and is calculated by Eq(1) b) Voigt subunit. A linear Kelvin-Voigt solid element, represented by a purely viscous element (a damper) and purely elastic element (a spring) connected in parallel. The force that is exerted on $P_{i,k}$ from this subunit is $f^v_{i,k}$ (Eq.(2)). k_s is the spring constant and μ represents viscosity.

same is done for the nuclear membrane. As a result, four subunits are added to the system, one Voigt subunit for each the cell membrane, nuclear membrane, inner nucleus, and cytoplasm). The parameters of these new subunits are calculated from the average of the first neighboring homogeneous subunit parameters. With the additional 'growth' point, the circumferential length of the membrane increases in proportion to $\frac{N+1}{N}$. Hence, the rest volume (in 2D), i. e. the volume of cell when it grows freely without any inner or outer constraint, must increase proportional to $\left(\frac{N+1}{N}\right)^2$, therefore the rest length of radial springs is increased proportionally to $\frac{N+1}{N}$. Two regions of volume, stop volume region, V_s, and growth volume, V_g are defined as:

$$\begin{aligned} V_c \in V_s \quad &if \quad V_c < \alpha_s V_r \\ V_c \in V_g \quad &if \quad V_c > \alpha_g V_r \end{aligned} \tag{7}$$

Where V_c is the current volume of the cell, V_r is the rest volume (as defined above), α_s and α_g are the coefficients that define the extrema of these regions ($\alpha_s \leq \alpha_g$). Often, due to external pressures and environmental space limitations, notwithstanding cell growth, the cell's volume cannot increase and will hence fall in the stop volume region, i.e. the cell ceases to grow. Under this condition, the cell cannot continue its growth until its volume fills the available space.

Mitosis. The present model allows for a growing cell to divide, provided that its volume falls in the growth volume region (see definition above). Key biomechanical aspects of cell proliferation are included in our model. When the cell area (or volume in 3D) is doubled, the axis of cell division is selected, so that the orientation depends on the cell shape, extracellular environment and cell polarization status [62–64]. In a dividing unpolarized cell, this axis, usually perpendicular to the direction in which the cell elongates, causes the cell to split into approximately two equal parts. In a partially polarized cell, however, the axis of cell division is orthogonal to the part of the cell membrane that is in contact with the ECM. Two new daughter nuclei are then placed orthogonal to the axis of cell division, (see Figure 5). This axis must include the center of mass of the nucleus. After the selection of division axis, the model finds the nearest membrane point to this axis, i.e. point P^m_d (Figure 5a). As the structure of the nucleus, during mitosis collapses [65], the nuclear subunits in our model will be eliminated during mitosis, followed by the formation of new nuclear subunits for the daughter cells. In mitosis there are two major mechanical forces that occur. First, during the anaphase stage of mitosis, the shortening of the spindle fibers causes the kinetochores to separate and the chromatids (daughter chromosomes) to be pulled apart and to begin moving toward the poles of the cell [65]. Secondly, during the cytokinesis process, a contractile ring is formed by contractile forces acting upon opposite sides of the cell boundary [65]. This results in the formation of a contractile furrow and causes division of the cell into two daughter cells. In our model, the cell points are divided into two groups, A and B, where the A group consists of membrane points from P^m_d to $P^m_{d+\frac{N}{2}}$ and nucleus points from P^n_d to $P^n_{d+\frac{N}{2}}$ and the remaining points belong to group B, see Figure 5a). To model the first mechanical force, the points of the nucleus in A and B are pulled apart, in an orthogonal direction of axis division with the force f^n_{div}.

$$F^{n,mitosis}_{i,k} = \begin{cases} f^n_{div} & if\ k \in A \\ -f^n_{div} & if\ k \in B \end{cases} \tag{8}$$

During the nucleus separation, the contractile force, f^m_{con}, acts on the boundary points of groups A and B to model the second mechanical force. That is,

$$F^{m,mitosis}_{i,k} = \begin{cases} f^m_{con} & if \quad k\ is\ boundry\ po\text{int}\ A\ or\ B \\ 0 & if \quad k\ is\ boundry\ po\text{int}\ A\ or\ B \end{cases} \tag{9}$$

After the nucleus is divided, i.e. the distance between the center of mass of the nucleus points in groups A and B exceed a certain value, d_{sep}, the cell will be divided into two daughter cells i.e. the subunits which join the boundary points of A and B are eliminated and bind to new first neighbor points in the same group with a new subunit (see Figure 5).

When the area (or volume) of the cell doubles, the number of defining membrane points increases to $\sqrt{2}N_0$, where N_0 is the number of membrane points on the initial cell. After division takes place, each daughter cell will only have $\frac{\sqrt{2}}{2}N_0$ points, and as a result it is possible to simultaneously add $\left(1-\frac{\sqrt{2}}{2}\right)N_0$ points to each cell. To add membrane points, two consecutive points in the membrane are found that have the longest distance and insert a new point between them, and repeat this process until the number of cell points become N_0.

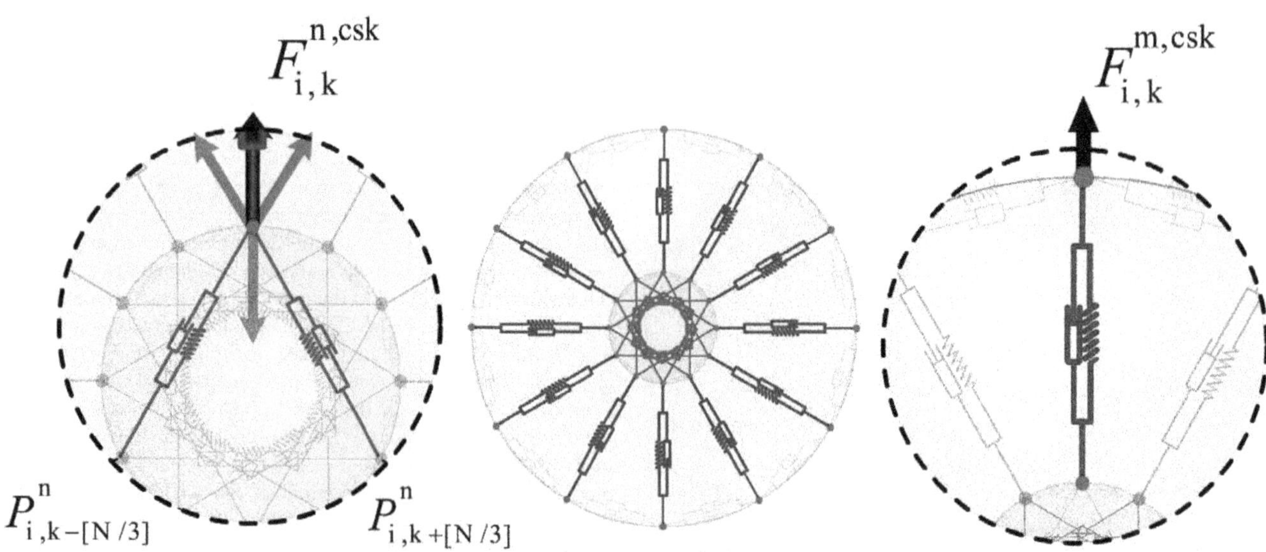

Figure 3. Inner cell structure and forces. The mechanical properties of the cytoskeleton are modeled using Voigt subunits; the spring constants of the model are linear approximations to the elasticity of the inner cell. All springs can be considered subject to a damping force due to the viscosity of the cytoplasm, where linear dash-pots are used to approximate the viscosity of the cytoskeleton. In our model, the cytoskeleton is divided into N uniformly radial distributed parts, each of which is replaced by a Voigt subunit radiating from the nucleus (blue subunits). Each subunit connects two points of the cell and nuclear membrane, which are located at a radial direction from the center of the nucleus. The model also contains N Voigt subunits in the nucleus (red subunits), each of which connect two nuclear membrane points n and n' in which $n'-n$ equal to $[N/3]$, This allows the nucleus to show more resistance to changes in its shape and volume due to exterior pressure. $F^{m,csk}_{i,k}$ is the cytoskeletal force acting on $P^{m}_{i,k}$ and is calculated by Eq. (3). $F^{n,csk}_{i,k}$ is the force acting on $P^{n}_{i,k}$ from the cytoskeleton and nuclear cytoskeleton and is calculated by Eq. (4).

The main phases of cell growth and division are presented in Figure 5b.

Motility. Cell motility is an important biological phenomenon that plays a key role in morphogenesis, metastasis, and wound healing [66]. Cell motility involves the interplay between three different processes, namely, protrusion, adhesion, and contraction. Protrusion occurs during the process of cytoskeletal assembly where the cell front pushes out the cell's leading edge. Next, adhesion occurs with the extracellular environment, whereby the cell establishes adhesion to the surface at the front end and slowly retracts from the back end.

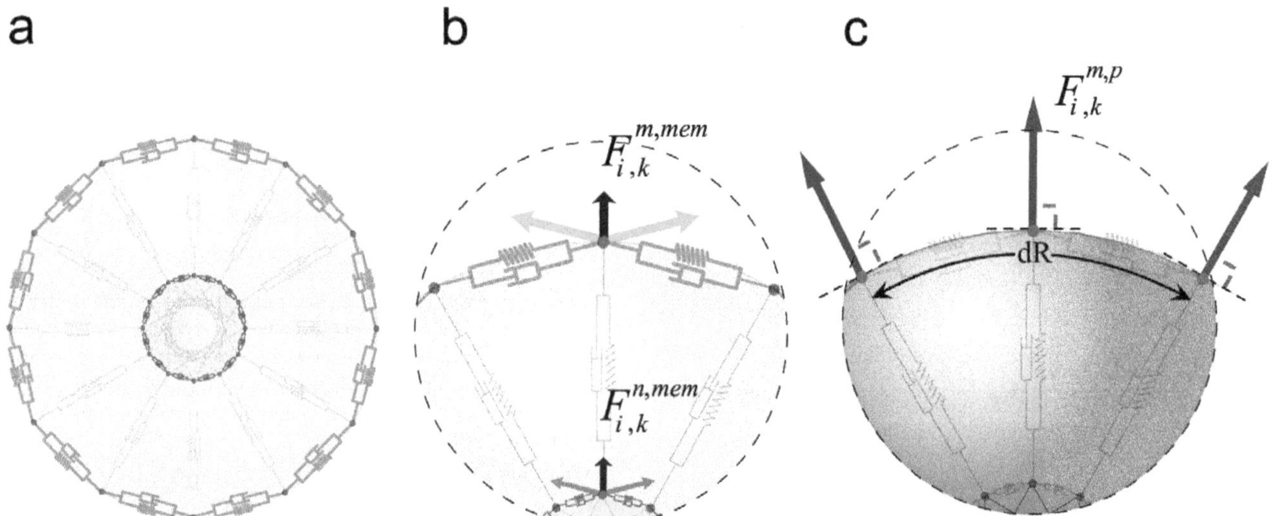

Figure 4. Structure of cell membrane and cytoplasm. a,b) To represent the viscoelasticty of the membrane and cortical cytoskeleton, two consecutive membrane points are connected with a Voigt subunit (green subunits); hence, the model includes N Voigt subunits on the cell membrane and N subunits on the nuclear membrane. The forces acting on each cell from membrane subunits is calculated by Eq. (5); as the figures show, each point is subject to two adjacent subunits. c) An osmotic pressure will act on the membrane. This internal pressure is involved in cell morphology and affects the driving force of cell movement [57–60]. Knowing the persistence lengths of micotubles, and the fact that they appear curved in the cell, it follows therefore, that this filament pushes the membrane outward [39]. Therefore, a pressure field acting upon each point of the cell membrane, representing cytoplasmic pressure with an outward and perpendicular direction to the cell membrane can be defined as $F^{m,p}_{i,j}$ by Eq. (6).

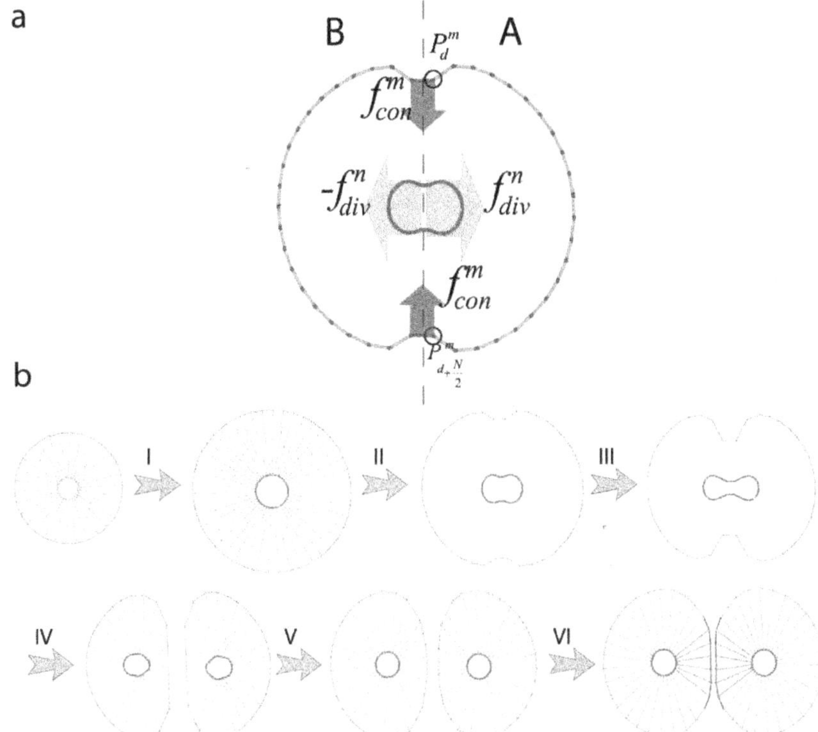

Figure 5. Mitosis and involved forces. a) Several bio-mechanical aspects of cell proliferation are included in our model. First, the cell area (or volume in 3D) is doubled. The axis of cell division is selected (dash-line), in a dividing unpolarized cell, this axis usually is perpendicular to the cell elongation direction in such a way as to split the cell into two approximately equal parts. In a partially polarized cell, however, the axis of cell division is orthogonal to the part of the cell membrane that is in contact with the ECM. Two new daughter nuclei are then placed orthogonal to the axis of cell division. After the selection of division axis, the model finds the nearest membrane point to this axis, i.e. point P_d^m In mitosis there are two major mechanical forces, first in the Anaphase stage of mitosis, shortening the spindle fibers caused by the kinetochores separation, and the chromatids (daughter chromosomes) are pulled apart and begin moving to the cell poles [65]. Second, a contractile ring is formed by contractile forces acting on the opposite sites of the cell boundary in the cytokinesis process [65]. This results in the formation of a contractile furrow and causes division of the cell into two daughter cells. The cell points can therefore be divided into two groups, A and B, where group A consists of membrane points from P_d^m to $P_{d+\frac{N}{2}}^m$ and nucleus points from P_d^n to $P_{d+\frac{N}{2}}^n$ and the remaining points belong to group B. To model the first mechanical force, the points of the nucleus in A and B are pulled apart, in the orthogonal direction to the division axis with force f_{div}^n (Eq.(8)). During the nucleus separation, the contractile force, f_{con}^m, acts on boundary points of A and B groups to model the second mechanical force(Eq. (9)). b) The main phases of cell growth and division. (I) Cell growth. To implement cell growth in the proposed model, the number of membrane points, i.e. the number of viscoelastic compartments, is allowed to increase. When we add two points on each the cell and nuclear membranes, four subunits are added to the system, with the parameters of these new subunits calculated from the average of the first neighbor's homogeneous subunit parameters. With the additional 'growth' point, the circumferential length of the membrane increases in proportion to $\frac{N+1}{N}$. Hence, the rest volume i. e. the volume of the cell when it grows freely without any inner or outer constraint, must increase proportional to $\left(\frac{N+1}{N}\right)^2$. Therefore, the rest length of radial springs is increased in proportion to $\frac{N+1}{N}$. When the area (or volume) of cell doubles, the number of defining membrane points increases to $\sqrt{2}N_0$, where N_0 is the number of membrane points on the initial cell. (II,III) Mitotic process: two types of forces act on points to divide the cell. Due to these forces the cell elongates and prepares for division. (IV) Two new daughter nuclei are then placed orthogonal to the axis of cell division. After the nucleus separates, i.e. the distance between the center of the mass of nuclear points exceeds a certain value, d_{sep}, the cell will divide into two daughter cells, i.e. the subunits which join the boundary points will be eliminated and will bind to a new first neighbor point in the same group with a new subunit. V) After division takes place, each daughter cell will only have $\frac{\sqrt{2}}{2}N_0$ points, and as a result it is possible to simultaneously add $\left(1-\frac{\sqrt{2}}{2}\right)N_0$ points to each cell. To add membrane points, two consecutive points in the membrane are found that have the longest distance and a new point is inserted between them, and this process is repeated until the number of cell points becomes N_0. f) Adhesion of the two daughter cells.

Finally, contraction of the actomyosin filaments causes the rest of the back end of the cell to pull up. These processes cooperate in a spatially heterogeneous structure to generate a complex topology for cell motion and correlation. Coordination between these processes has a significant role on the motility of the cell [66]. To model these three-stages, the cell is first polarized by categorizing the points into two groups, anterior and posterior. The cytoskeletal subunit parameters of these stages will change periodically in a coordinated fashion. In addition, to model the adhesion with a substrate, the drag coefficient for each point is used. These points will also change periodically in coordination with various subunit parameters, as follows:

$$\begin{aligned}
&\left.\begin{aligned} l &= l_{a,0} + sign(\sin(\omega t))l_{a,m} \\ D &= D_{a,0} - sign(\sin(\omega t))D_{a,m} \end{aligned}\right\} \quad \text{if } k \in \text{Anterior Points} \\
&\left.\begin{aligned} l &= l_{p,0} + sign(\sin(\omega t))l_{p,m} \\ D &= D_{p,0} + sign(\sin(\omega t))D_{p,m} \end{aligned}\right\} \quad \text{if } k \in \text{Posterior Points}
\end{aligned} \tag{10}$$

l is the rest length of cytoskeleton subunits spring, the subscript a and p refer to the anterior and posterior region, subscript 0 shows the initial value and subscript m refers to the threshold of parameters in motility, for example $l_{a,m}$ shows the threshold of the spring rest length that is anterior of the crawling cell. ω is the variation frequency of parameters in the posterior and anterior position. D is the drag coefficient of each point (Figure 6) and its value is proportional to the number of adhesions. This idea of relating the number of adhesions to the drag coefficient has been used in other models of cell motility [67–69]. The variation of l represents the protrusion and retraction in the cell that is formed by actamyosin systems.

Apoptosis. The structure and morphology of apoptotic cells show the cell undergoing dramatic changes, including detachment from the neighboring cells, collapse of the cytoskeleton, shrinkage of cell volume and alterations in the cell surface resulting in an irregular bulge in the plasma membrane, called bleb [65]. The process of apoptosis progresses quickly and its products are removed immediately. To model these events, cell adherens junctions first disassemble with the neighboring cells and/or substrates. Then, the rest length of each subunit spring is reduced arbitrarily (five-fold in the current simulations) and the inner pressure of the cell is removed so that the cell collapses and its area gradually reduces until a prescribed minimal value is reached. At this time, the cell is considered to be dead and will be removed from the system. These stages of cell apoptotic death are represented in our model by a gradual reduction in cell area and changes in shape as shown in Figure 7.

Cell polarization. The membrane points are devised in such a way that they can be specified independent of each other. Hence, the properties of each point and its corresponding subunits can be controlled. That is, the points can be categorized into two or more subgroups. By changing their properties independently, apical, basal and lateral regions in our model can be easily defined.

c. ECM

Before the interaction of the cell with its environment can be investigated, the extracellular matrix (ECM), which is a complex structural entity surrounding and supporting cells that are found within mammalian tissue must be modeled. The ECM is often referred to as connective tissue and the cells can connect to the ECM via adhesion receptors. Two methods can be defined for modeling the ECM; in a 2D culture, the ECM or substrate is the area under the cells, hence the cells interact with the ECM by adhesions and adhesions are controlled by a "drag coefficient", so the drag coefficient $D_{i,k}$ can be related to $P_{i,k}$. As mentioned before, referring the drag coefficient to the adhesion intensity is used in previous models such as [62–64], so in the following, if a 2D culture is modeled, the adhesion intensity is equivalent to the drag coefficient. In 3D cultures, our model allows for investigations of a cross section of the real system and the cells immersed in the ECM. In 2D, the contact region of the ECM and cell is a line that surrounds the cell, so an enclosed curve (or ring) can be used for the ECM that surrounds the cells. The ECM is modeled using a chain of subunits connected in series (Figure 8), where each point connects two subunits. These subunits can interact with cell points in the same manner as the interaction of two points of different cells. Depending on the model, the cells are embedded in the outer region of the ECM ring or the inner region. This curve is flexible and the number of its corresponding points can be increased or decreased. The drag coefficient property of each membrane point indicates the interaction of the cell with other cells or with the ECM, which is situated perpendicularly to the cross-sectional region. The model can also incorporate a cellular automata model for the ECM, allowing for the investigation of the diffusion of mobile receptors and signals in the ECM.

d. Environmental effect

Cell-cell and cell-substrate interaction. Each cell can interact with other cells and substrates in two methods, adhesion and repulsive forces due to elasticity (Figure 9).

$$\begin{aligned} F_{i,k}^{cell-cell} &= F_{i,k}^{m,adh} + F_{i,k}^{m,rep} \\ F_{i,k}^{cell-ECM} &= F_{i,k}^{m,adh} + F_{i,k}^{m,rep} - D_{i,k} V_{i,k} \end{aligned} \quad (11)$$

Cells are not often found in isolation, but rather tend to stick to other cells or non-cellular components of their environment. They

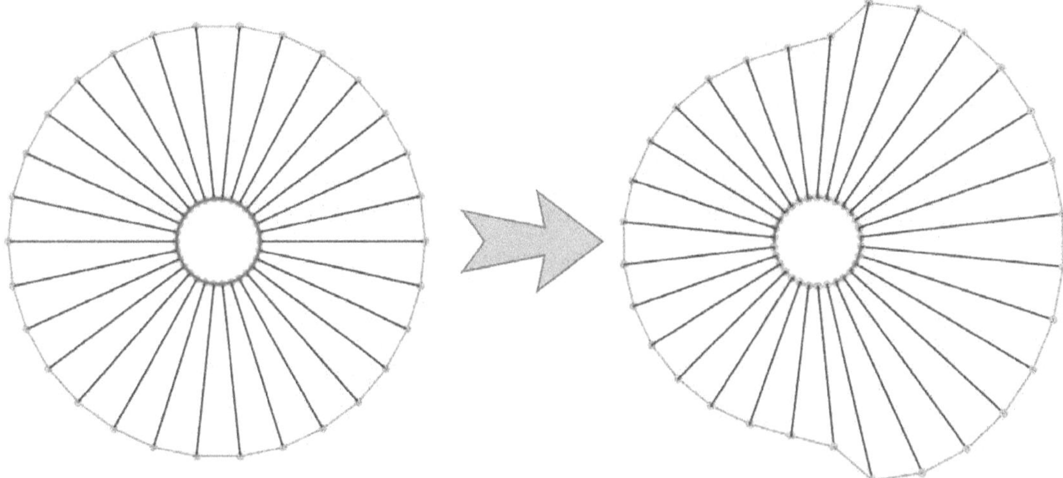

Figure 6. Motility. Cell crawling is generated by the interplay between three different processes, namely, protrusion, adhesion, and contraction. These processes cooperate in a spatially heterogeneous structure to generate a complex topology for cell motion while correlation and coordination between them has a significant role on the motility of the cell [66]. To model these three-stage events, the cell is first polarized by categorizing the points into two groups, the anterior and posterior, where their cytoskeleton subunit parameters will change periodically in a coordinated fashion. In addition to modeling the adhesion with a substrate, the drag coefficient is used for each of the points which will change periodically in coordination with variation of subunit parameters. The method for the variation of the parameters is shown in Eq.(10).

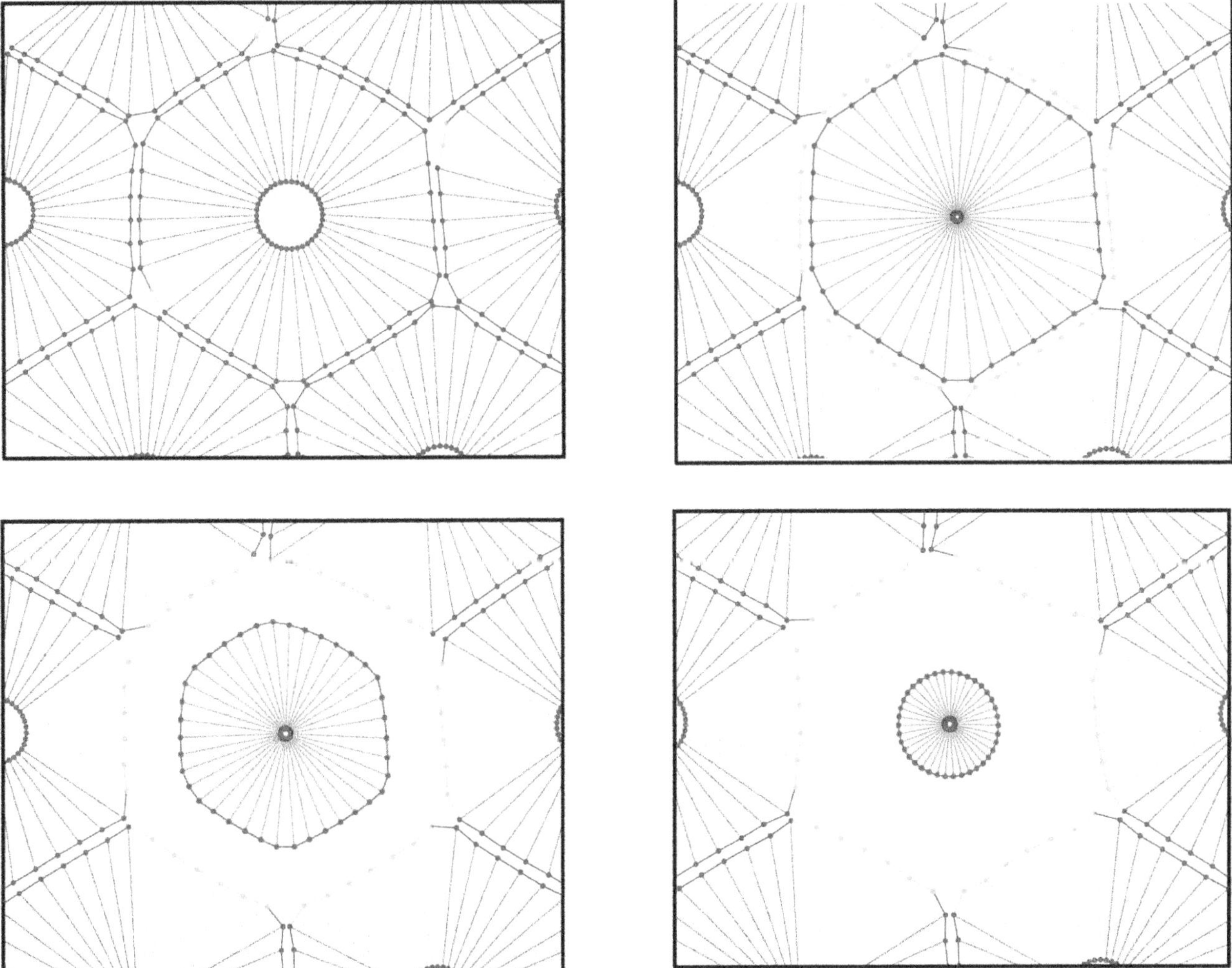

Figure 7. Apoptosis. The structure and morphology of apoptotic cells undergo dramatic changes, including detachment from the neighboring cells, collapse of the cytoskeleton, shrinkage of the cell volume and alternations in the cell surface. Apoptosis progresses quickly and its products are quickly removed. To model these events, cell adherens junctions with their neighboring cells and/or substrate are initially disassembled (top right). Then, the spring constant length of all subunits are reduced arbitrarily and the inner pressure is removed (bottom left), so the cell will collapse and the cell area is gradually reduced until it reaches a prescribed minimal value (bottom right). At this time, the cell is considered to be dead and will be removed from the system.

usually bind directly to one another through cell-surface proteins that form specialized cell-cell junctions. These cell adhesive properties are especially important in epithelial tissues since they constitute barriers between different body compartments.

In our model, all points located on the cell membrane serve as potential sites of cell-cell connections, which can be transformed to either adherent or repulsive forces. Here, simple rules can be considered for the formation of cell adherents and tight junctions that depend only on the cell phenotype and on the distance between neighboring cells, that is whether or not the membrane receptors of one cell fall into the minimum distance, d_0^{adh}, of another cell. Gap junctions and chemical signals are not explicitly included, but it can be assumed that cells are able to communicate and signal information with neighboring cells. Each of the two points from different cells or cell-substrates connect each other with a subunit, if they are within a minimum separation distance of d_0^{adh} (Figure 9a).

For each cell, specific parameters for subunit attachment are assigned, making the adhesion subunit parameters between two cells a function of these parameters. For adhesion between $P_{i,k}^m$ and $P_{j,l}^m$, it can be said:

$$F_{i,k}^{m,adh} = f_{i,k}^{v}(P_{j,l}^m, \bar{B}, \bar{K}, 0)$$
$$\bar{B} = \left(\frac{1}{B_{i,k}^{m,adh}} + \frac{1}{B_{j,l}^{m,adh}} \right)^{-1} \qquad (12)$$
$$\bar{K} = \left(\frac{1}{K_{i,k}^{m,adh}} + \frac{1}{K_{j,l}^{m,adh}} \right)^{-1}$$

Where $B_{i,k}^{m,adh}, K_{i,k}^{m,adh}$ are the attachment subunit parameters of $P_{i,k}^m$ and $B_{j,l}^{m,adh}, K_{j,l}^{m,adh}$ are the attachment subunit parameters of $P_{j,l}^m$. When the cells are pulled apart, they deform, but points remain stuck until a distance $r_{ij} \equiv d_{hys}^{adh} > d_0^{adh}$ at which point their contact ruptures, displaying typical hysteresis behavior. It must be mentioned that sometimes, for example, in apoptosis, the adhesion

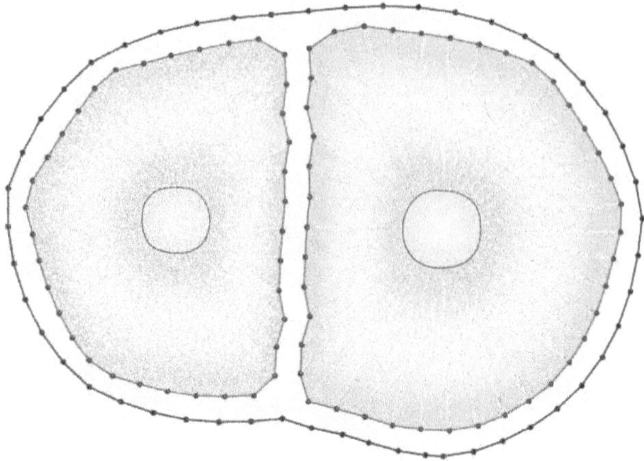

Figure 8. ECM. In 3D culture, our model allows for the investigation of a cross section of the system and the cells that are immersed in ECM. In 2D, the contact region of the ECM and the cell is a line that surrounds the cell; therefore, an enclosed curve (or ring) can be used for the ECM that surrounds the cells (blue curve). The ECM is modeled using a chain of subunits connected in series, where each point connects two subunits (blue curve with red points). These subunits can interact with cell points in a manner similar to the interaction of two points of different cells. This chain is flexible and the number of its corresponding points can be increased or decreased.

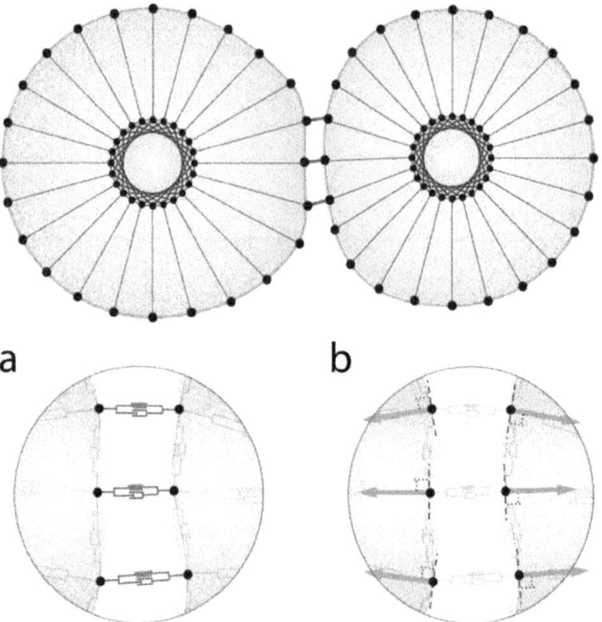

Figure 9. Cell-cell interaction. Each cell can interact with another cell and substrate in two methods, adhesion and/or repulsive forces due to elasticity, as shown in Eq. (11). a) In this model, all points located on the cell membrane serve as potential sites of cell-cell connections. Each two points from different cells or cell-substrates are connected via a Voigt subunit, once they are closer than a determined value of d_0^{adh}. The adhesion subunit parameters between two cells are a function of these parameters, for more detail see Eq. (12). b) The repulsive force acts as a short range force. It is a passive force resulting from the elastic interaction with neighboring cells and acts on each point of the cell, when the distance to the other cell points or substrate is less than $r_{ij} \equiv d_0^{rep} < d_0^{adh}$. The magnitude of the repulsive force is a function of the distance of two surfaces (Eq. (13)) and its direction is perpendicular to the membrane, pointing inward to the inner cell.

can be disrupted unilaterally by one cell without satisfaction of the above condition.

A repulsive force acts as a short range force. It is a passive force resulting from the elastic interaction with neighboring cells and acts on each point of the cell where the distance to the other cell points or substrate falls shorter than $r_{ij} \equiv d_0^{rep} < d_0^{adh}$. The magnitude of the repulsive force is a function of the distance of two surfaces and its direction is perpendicular to the membrane, pointing inward to the inner cell (Figure 9b).

$$F_{i,k}^{m,rep} = \frac{F_0^{rep}}{d_{i,k}^j} \tag{13}$$

Where $d_{i,k}^j$ is the nearest distance between $P_{i,k}^m$ and the membrane surface of j'th cell or ECM.

External field. The cell can be subjected to an external force, such as pulling forces by the surrounding tissue or under certain fields, e.g. electromagnetic fields. This can be represented by adding an external force F^{ext} to each point on the cell membrane.

e. Justification for the use of Voigt elements

It should be noted that although the individual Voigt elements are simple, they combine to form a complex system (Figures 1,2,3 and 8) with dynamics that are beyond the simplicity of individual linear elements. Although our model is composed of a network of linear Voigt elements, the behavior and dynamics of these elements are not linear for several reasons. First, model parameters such as spring constants and viscosity coefficients change dynamically through time based on mechanical and biochemical signaling as well as the state of the cell as previously mentioned. Given that these parameters change dynamically, the elements can no longer be considered linear. Second, during the cell cycle some constant parameters are changed dynamically. For example, in cell growth when a point is added to the membrane, the rest length of radial springs is increased in proportion to $\frac{N+1}{N}$. During apoptosis the parameters change dramatically as previously mentioned, the rest length of each subunit spring is reduced resulting in the cell collapsing and its area gradually decreasing and during motility, the cytoskeletal subunit parameters of these elements will change periodically in a coordinated fashion to generate movement. To further establish the non-linearity and finite-extensibility of elements, the overall number of elements and points changes accordingly during growth and mitosis while during adhesion relevant elements can be created or destroyed based on the distance between two points (on different cells/ECM) which shows that elements are neither linear nor infinitely extensible in all cases. Finally, in the process of developing this model, we felt that the input parameters should best represent those determined through experimental methods. As a result, we selected those established by Coskuna et al. [34] for Voigt elements rather than using arbitrary or speculative parameters for more complex element types. However, the flexibility of this model allows for easy implementation of more complex building blocks such as Maxwell elements, given valid, experimentally derived element parameters.

We acknowledge that the Voigt element is simpler than other element types, however, as our results show; a model based on Voigt elements is capable of reproducing cell behavior. We believe as a rule that as long as a simple model satisfies our interest and can reproduce desired behavior, there is no advantage to increasing model complexity.

Results and Discussion

a. Case studies from relevant biological examples

Monolayer cell culture and effect of adhesion intensity. It is well documented that cell shape, proliferation, and ECM are important aspects of cell culture [70]. The adhesion between cells and ECM can dramatically affect invasion of tumor cells and the quality of the epithelial monolayer of the cell. The first application of our model investigates this phenomenon by simulating a monolayer culture of cells and the exploring the effects of adhesions on tissue formation and morphology. The process began from two cells, which were allowed to reproduce freely while subject to ideal conditions that were suitable for proliferation, without the occurrence of apoptosis.

Typical snapshots of proliferation under two different adhesion intensities are shown in Figure 10. As the figures show, adhesion intensity plays an important role in the morphology of each culture. At low adhesion intensities (low drag coefficients) a filled circular culture can be seen, whereas high adhesion intensities (high drag coefficients) tend to show dendrite morphology, which can be seen frequently in tumors. It is conceivable that this special morphology is due to strong adhesions between cancer cells and the ECM. Our results suggest that increased adherence may lead to decreased culture growth; however, this result is not always supported by experiments. This anomaly may be explained by the fact that our model only incorporates the biomechanical behavior of the cell, whereas there is some signaling pathway that stimulates the growth factors when cells adhere to substrate. Possible methods for incorporating biochemical effects into the model are discussed later in this paper.

To characterize the geometry of the cells in a culture, a form factor, k_f, was introduced [71]:

$$k_f = \rho\sqrt{\frac{\Omega}{n_{cell}}} \tag{14}$$

where Ω is total occupied area, n_{cell} is number of cells, and ρ is cell edge density, which is given by:

$$\rho = \frac{L_b}{\Omega} \tag{15}$$

in which L_b is the sum of the lengths of all internal cell boundaries plus half of the perimeter of the patch; it is assumed that these edges are to be shared between the patch shown and a mirror image patch that adjoins them. Physically, ρ corresponds to the area density of the cell edges. Minimum value of k_f, $\sqrt{\pi}$, occurs when the cell has a circular shape. The value of k_f for cultures with 120 cells against adhesion intensity is shown in Figure 11. This shows a linear relation between k_f and the adhesion intensity, which in turn suggests that the cellular shapes are almost circular at low drag coefficients, and diverge from circular shape as the drag increases.

On the other hand, the epithelial cells in a monolayer appeared as polygonal cells. It also can be seen that the average number of neighbors for any cell is 6, regardless of the value of the drag coefficient.

Growth of epithelial cells and interaction with the ECM. In this simulation, a cross-sectional perspective on cell cultures can be seen where the ECM is a line of points to which cells adhere. These point numbers are dynamic and can change if needed. Most living tissues are typically separated from the exterior by a delimiting interface of epithelial cells. These layers of cells align with the cavities and surfaces of structures throughout the body. Epithelial cells can take any shape and can be classified by their shape or by the function of the cell where they are located. They can take shape as squamous layers or monolayers and these layers can be folded into circular acini or ducts. For example, epithelial cells that are found in the thyroid or cornea of the eye function in aligning fluid-filled lumens [72]. Mature epithelial cells are highly polarized with separate apical and baso-lateral membrane compartments. The basal cell surface is attached to ECM material and in most epithelia the opposite apical surface is free from an apposed extracellular layer. From the histological organization of epithelium, it shows that attachment to the ECM is essential in polarization, and plays an important role in directing the polarity. Observation of epithelial cell growth and morphogenesis in different environments show that morphology *in-vitro* depends on both the structure and composition of the external environment of the cells. The main morphological distinction in 3-D embedded cultures is the formation of cysts, i.e. the stable, self-enclosed monolayers. In suspension cultures, epithelial cells form cysts as well, but the epithelial cells adopt an inverted polarity, laying down basement membranes on the inside of the cyst [1,3–4]. In plane culture, epithelial cells normally constitute a smooth monolayer covering the whole ECM surface like a wrap. Each of these three categories is a representative of the growth of different epithelial cell types *in-vitro*, which have a common morphological scheme [72–73]. This suggests that the presence and relative locations of cells, ECM, and matrix-free (or cell-free) space are very essential for the expected behavior of epithelial cells. Cells plated on a layer of surface culture construct a stable, uniform monolayer as they proliferate (Figure 12a). The axis of division is perpendicular to the ECM, likely related to polarized cells. If a cell detached from the ECM due to the loss of polarity, it will activate the apoptosis pathway. In a different case (see Figure 12b) a hole exists in the ECM, where a cell is located and allowed to attach and proliferate. After polarization it starts to proliferate and creates a stable, lumen-containing cyst, lined by a single layer of epithelial cells. As it can be seen, the ECM is deformed a bit due to the dynamical interaction between the ECM and cells during the growth process. Figure 12c, on the other hand, shows an inverted cyst. A circular ECM is located in a suspended culture, to which a cell attaches and is polarized. Upon completion of proliferation, cells surround the entire surface of the ECM and create inverted cysts, with matrix deposited on the inside of the cyst. If the process is allowed to continue, the cyst will grow further and become larger, corresponding to a bigger ECM. This is due to the fact that the volume of the ECM in our model can freely increase.

Effects of gap in ECM. As a different test case, the effects of gaps in the ECM on the formation of a confluent epithelial monolayer are investigated. The ECM is considered to be rigid and not affected by cells; however, cells still adhere to the ECM and are polarized. Figure 13a shows the final results for various gap sizes. If the gap width is denoted as δ and the radius of a free epithelial cell as R, then it can be seen that cells cannot line the gap for $\delta < 2R$. For $\delta = 2R$ the first cell who comes into contact with a gap will enter it, although due to the pressure of the walls, it would not be able to continue its growth and division, so it fills the entry and blocks the gap. Other cells, accordingly, pass over the gap and again, create a line monolayer. For $\delta = 4R$ cells could not ignore the gap and penetrate it. They continue their proliferation interiorly, however, when they reach the internal right corner, as the forerunning cells are subject to direction change due to the limitation in space, the growth is stopped and the cells are entrapped in the gap. For $\delta > 4R$ the cells can enter and line the gap without any problem. It must be

a

n=2 n=12 n=24

n=36 n=48 n=60

b

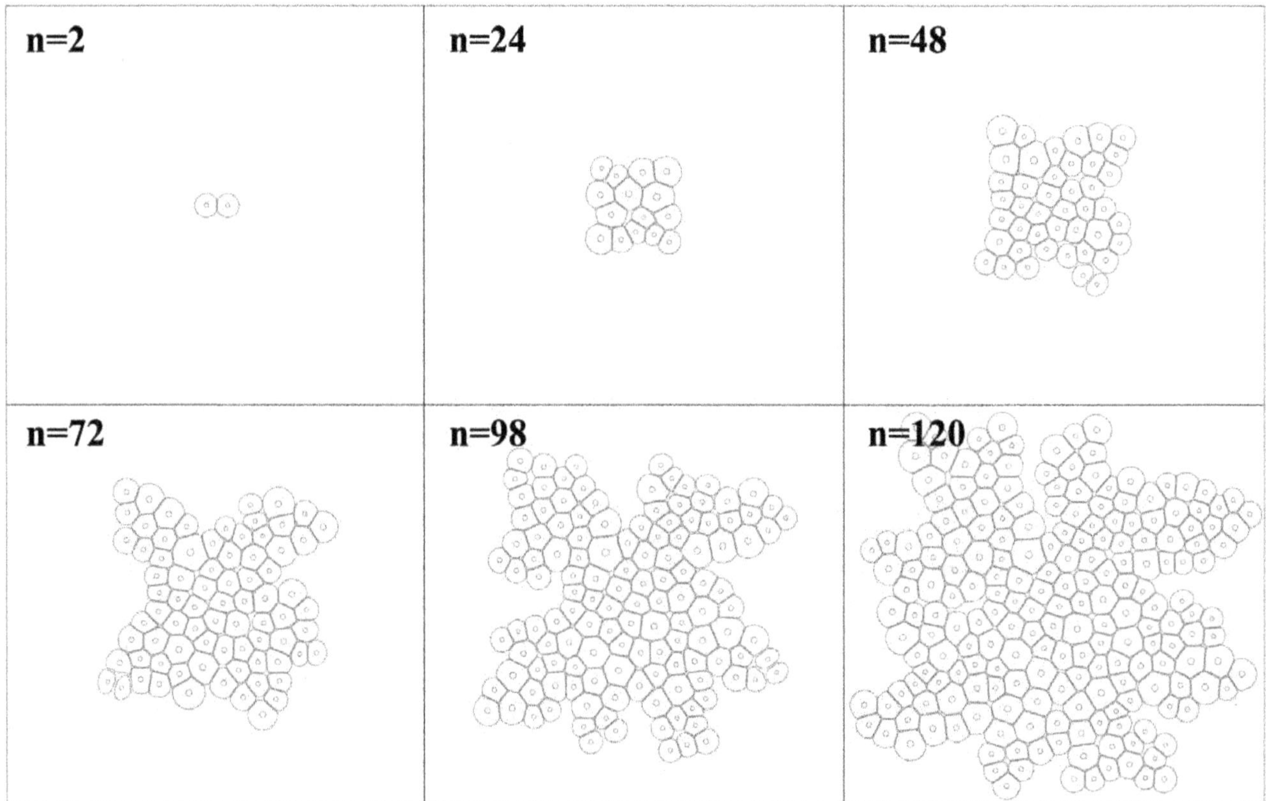

Figure 10. The monolayer culture of cells and the effects of adhesions on tissue formation and morphology. a) In this simulation, D = 0.0001*D0 i.e. low intensity of adhesions. We began from two cells and allowed them to reproduce freely, subject to conditions that are suitable for proliferation without the occurrence of apoptosis. Results show a filled circular culture and fast proliferation. n represents the dimensionless elapsed time. b) D = D0 i.e. high intensity of adhesions. The process began from two cells which were allowed to reproduce freely. The results show dendrite morphology for the culture which can be seen frequently in tumors. It is conceivable that this special morphology is due to strong adhesion between cancer cells and the ECM. The process has a slower proliferation rate than part a. The epithelial cells in a monolayer appear as polygonal cells. It also can be seen that the average number of neighbors for any cell is 6, regardless of the value of the drag coefficient.

mentioned that in all of the above simulations, cells show different behaviors at the corners. The growth rate of cells decreased at the internal corner and increased at the external corner. In addition, at external corners, due to the sudden decrease in contact area, cells detach from the ECM more easily in response to the pressure of neighboring cells. This, in turn, causes the loss of polarity and apoptosis. Figure 13b shows snapshots of the growth process when the gap is equal to $8R$.

Tensegrity and Tissue Morphogenesis. Studies on the mechanisms of epithelial morphogenesis and tubulogenesis have revealed that local changes in ECM structure and its mechanics play essential roles in tissue structure and remodeling. Using the tensegrity-based architecture, a mechanical model of cell structure explains how local changes in ECM mechanics may guide tissue patterning according to that model [47,74]. It has been speculated that up-regulation of the ECM due to local thinning within the ECM can lower any stiffness that may occur. This in turn causes the surrounding cells to apply tractional forces, thereby, causing an increase of forces between the cell-ECM receptors causing changes within cell shape and morphology. Therefore, based on this vision, epithelial cell growth and relocation are restricted to particular groups of cells that adjoin the thinned region. Outward budding occurs when these cells extend and grow. Other cells along the same ECM do not experience this stress and, therefore, remain inactive.

At this stage, an attempt is made to try to model this hypothesis. To do so, a monolayer of epithelial cell is placed on the ECM and

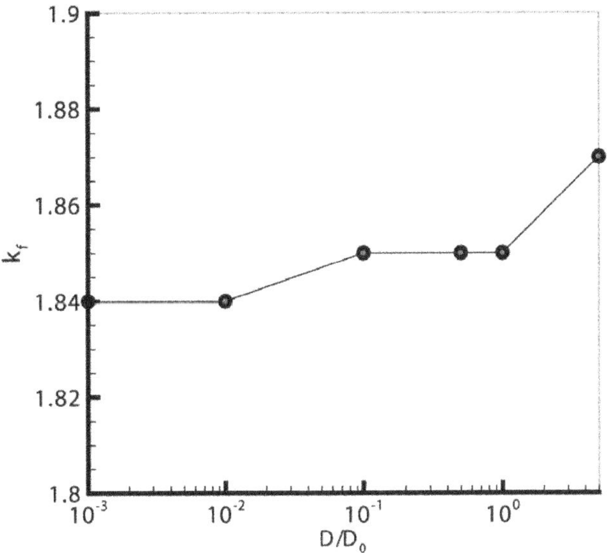

Figure 11. Effect of adhesion intensity on monolayer cell culture properties. The value of k_f for cultures with 120 cells, compared against the adhesion intensity. This graph shows a linear relation between k_f and the adhesion intensity, which in turn suggests that the cellular shapes are almost circular at low drag coefficients, and diverge from being circular as the drag increases.

thinning of the ECM occurs by decreasing the drag coefficient at the center of the ECM (showed in Figure 14 in white). The program runs with two densities of cells, as shown in Figure 14. The cells at this region have localized growth and motility, which drives the ECM downward. As a result, cells find space for more growth and proliferation. Therefore, they continue to drive the ECM further, which finally leads to the creation of a bud. This bud can be the first stage of tubulogenesis. In Figure 14 due to the high density of cells, there is not enough space for the ECM to grow and proliferate, so there is more order and less deformation. But as can be seen in Figure 14b there is proliferation and less symmetry, due to low cell density.

Formation of hollow epithelial acini. The epithelial acini are experimental culture structures that help to explore the detailed mechanism underlying epithelial cancers *in-vitro*, [2,75]. As discussed earlier, well developed epithelial acini are composed of one layer of closely packed epithelial cells covering the hollow lumen. Examples of such cell culture systems that cultivate in vitro in a form of cysts or acini are Madin–Darby canine kidney (MDCK) cells and mammary epithelial MCF-10A cells [1–2]. The details of formation of acinar structures are not completely understood. In general, the mechanism of obtaining an acinar structure is similar in all types of cells. This process begins with a single cell planting itself on the suitable media culture. This pioneer cell starts growth and proliferation to form a small 3-dimensional collection of randomly oriented cells. These cells can be divided in two distinct groups. The first group consists of a surface layer of cells in direct contact with the ECM and the second group is internal cells enclosed entirely by other cells. They do not have any direct contact with the ECM. To continue acini development, cells in the outer layer are polarized and inhibit an asymmetry in an apical-basal surface and become insensitive to proliferative signals. Differentiation of outer cells coincides with the start of the apoptosis pathway of inner cells. As a result, the hollow lumen is formed and the acinar structure remains hollow [2,75]. In this stage, an attempt is made to model self-arrangement of individual eukaryotic cells into a stable hollow acinar structure. In this model, a single cell (Figure 15, n = 1) undergoes several consecutive divisions and gives rise to a small cluster of cells containing two different populations (Figure 15, n = 100–217): the inner cells entirely surrounded by other cells which do not have access to the ECM, and the *outer* cells partially facing the ECM. Further cell proliferation leads to the expansion of the whole cluster. During this stage (Figure 15, n = 150–217) intercalation of outer cells to inner cells (or inward) for preservation of the circular shape of the tumor can be seen. It should be noted that if the adhesion between cells is stronger the process of intercalation is less prevalent. After this stage, when the tumor reaches a certain age, the tumor undregoes further differentiation of outer cells which results in their apical-basal orientation and self-arrangment into one layer of polarized epithelial cells of regular cubical shapes (Figure 15, n = 219). The inner cells are then triggered by polarized cells to enter the apoptosis pathway. As a result, each cell that does not have access to ECM, and is therefore not polarized, will die (Figure 15, n = 219–225). This process then leads to the creation of an inner lumen. Consequently, the proliferation of

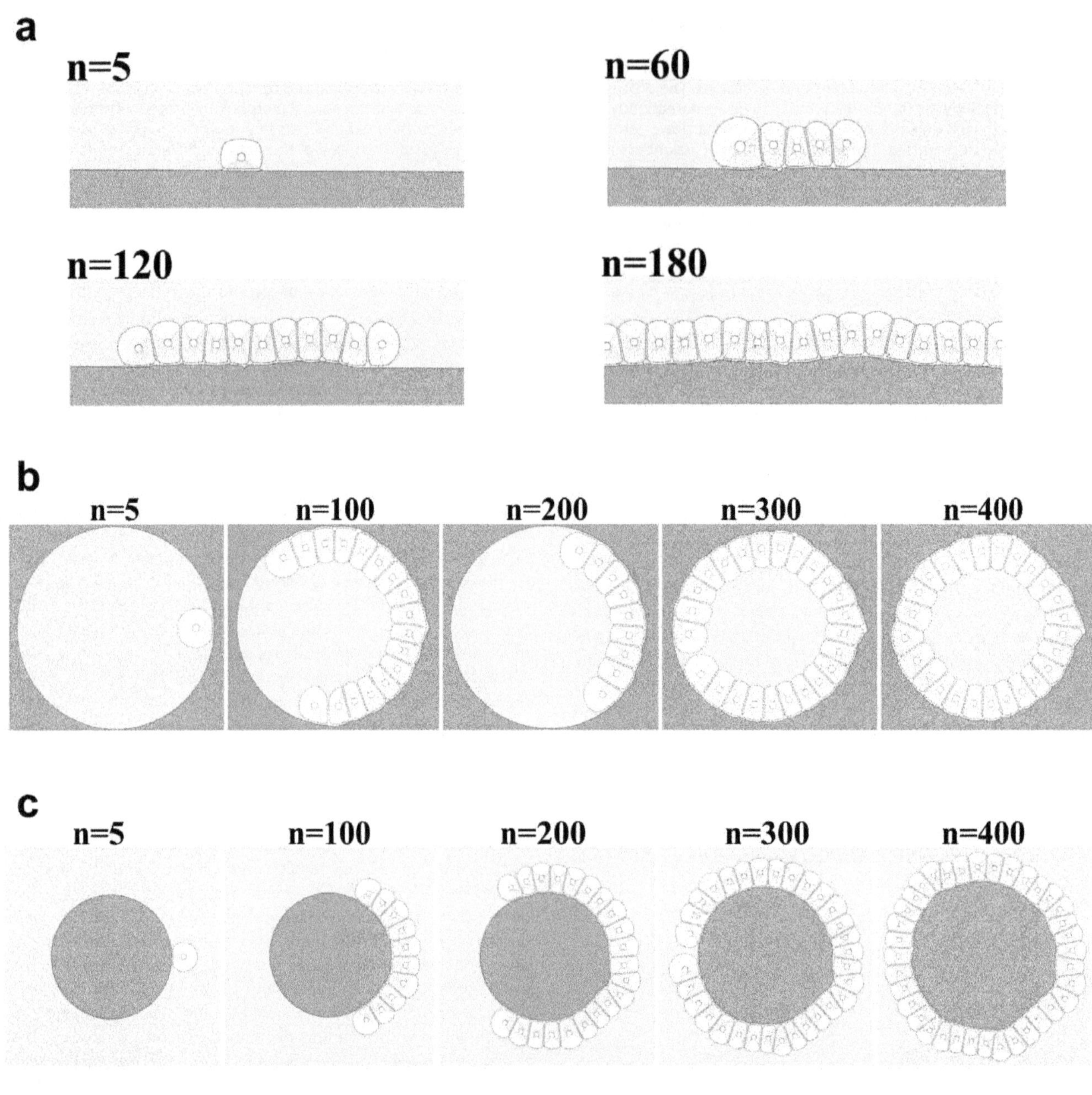

Figure 12. Growth of epithelial cell interacting with the ECM. In this simulation a cross-sectional perspective of cell culture can be seen. Therefore, the ECM is a line of points to which the cells adhere. These points are dynamic and can change if needed. n represents the dimensionless elapsed time. a) Cells plated on a layer of surface culture. As the cell proliferates, a stable, uniform monolayer will be constructed. The axis of division is perpendicular to the ECM, likely related to polarized cells. If a cell detaches from the ECM due to the loss of polarity, it will activate the apoptosis pathway. b) A hole exists in the ECM, where a cell is located for attachment and proliferation. After polarization, the cell starts to proliferate and create a stable, lumen-containing cyst, lined by a single layer of epithelial cells. As it can be seen, the ECM is deformed a bit due to the dynamic interaction between the ECM and cells during the growth process. c) Shows an inverted cyst. A circular ECM is located in a suspended culture, to which a cell is attached and polarized. Upon completion of proliferation, cells surround the entire surface of the ECM and create inverted cysts, with matrix deposited on the inside of the cyst. If the process is allowed to continue, the cyst will grow further and become greater, which corresponds to a bigger ECM. This is because the volume of ECM in our model can freely increase.

polarized cells is suppressed and the final structure stabilizes in the form of a hollow epithelial acinus (Figure 15, n = 250–450). Moreover, the processes of cell proliferation, polarization and apoptosis need to coordinate well in order to maintain the hollow acinar structure in a stable manner. Otherwise overgrowth of the cell may lead to intraductal carcinomas. This coordination shows that this process is very dependent on proper biochemical signaling between cells. The final shape of the tumor is very dependent on the viscosity of the ECM. If the viscosity of the ECM is high enough the tumor attempts to keep a circular morphology. If the viscosity of the ECM is reduced, the tumor deviates from the circular shape.

b. Conclusion

A biomechanical, cell based model was developed that describes both individual cell behavior and cell-environment interaction

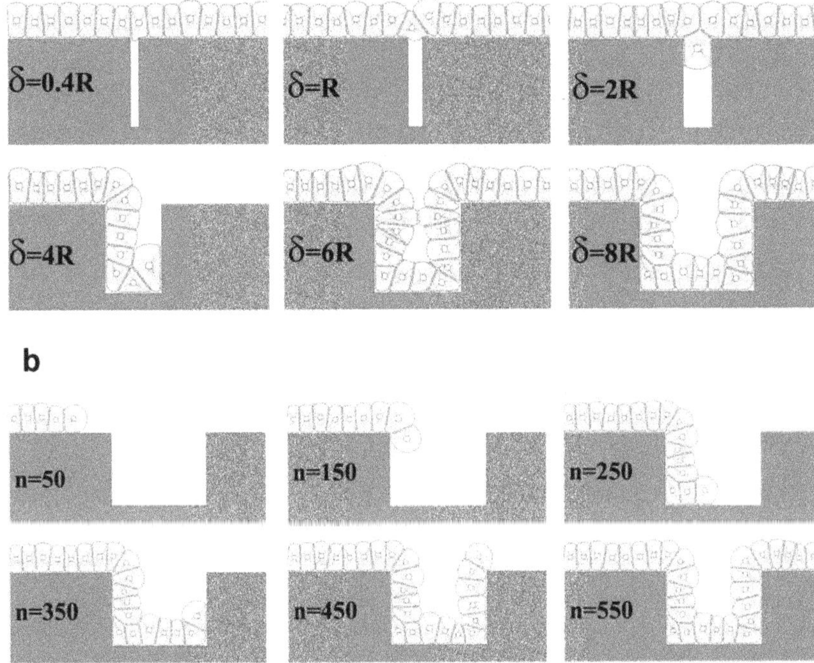

Figure 13. Effects of a gap in ECM surface. ECM is considered to be rigid and not affected by cells; however, cells still adhere to ECM and are polarized. a) Figure shows the final results for various gap sizes. If the gap width is denoted with δ and the radius of a free epithelial cell with R, then it can be seen that cells cannot line the gap for $\delta < 2R$. For $\delta = 2R$ the first cell which meets the gap will enter it, although due to the pressure of the walls it would not be able to continue its growth and division, so it fills the entry and blocks the gap. Other cells pass over the gap and again create a linear monolayer. For $\delta = 2R$ cells cannot ignore the gap and penetrate it. They continue their proliferation into the gap; however, when they reach the internal right corner, because of the limitation in space and the forerunning cells being subject to direction changing, the growth is stopped and the cells are entrapped in the gap. For $\delta > 2R$ the cells can enter the gap without any problem and line it. b) A few snapshots of the growth process when the gap is equal to $8R$. n represents the dimensionless elapsed time. During simulation, cells show differing behaviors at the corners. The growth rate of cells decreases at the internal corner and increases at the external corner. In addition, at external corners, due to the sudden decrease in contact area, cells detach from the ECM more easily in response to the pressure of neighboring cells. This, in turn, leads to loss of polarity and apoptosis.

based on cellular mechanics. The model has the ability to simulate the global and local mechanical characteristics of the single cell. Each cell in this model is an individual unit containing several subcellular elements, such as the plasma membrane, enclosed by viscoelastic elements that play the role of cytoskeleton, and the viscoelastic elements of the cell nucleus. The cell membrane is divided into segments where each segment incorporates the cell's interaction and communication with its environment, such as adherens junctions. These deformable cell models can mimic many aspects of real cells such as growth, cell division, apoptosis and attachment to other cells or ECM. It was shown that these cell models can mimic various topologies of tissue such as cyst or tumor or monolayer. In addition, it was demonstrated that the model is capable to describe such phenomena such as interaction of a culture with a geometrical gap in substrate or buds. This model offers utility to investigate the role of individual cells as a part of tissue and how the property of each individual cell may affect the mechanical and morphological property of the tissue. The model makes it possible to investigate mechanical and physical behavior of different tissue in cell scale in various mechanical conditions. The structure of the model is simple and is based on a small number of parameters, allowing for high performance computing of large cell populations in a reasonable time. One of the important aspects of the model is ability to simultaneously investigate the intra- and extra-cellular biomechanical behavior. By changing the model parameters, it is possible to apply the model to different types of cells and investigate their interaction in different cellular constructs. This model is in the first stage of its life and needs many improvements, for example finding the quantitative parameters for different cell types or improving the inner cell structure such as the nucleus. Most experimental investigations employ a two-dimensional substrate; however, to gain further insight into the behavior of epithelial cells *in-vivo*, we must switch from 2D to a 3D model. With this modification, we can investigate the biomechanical effects in a 3D environment. For this purpose, we must define a 3D cell and rather than a 1D curve for the cell membrane we will have a surface and a network of nodes. Our model can be extended to three dimensional space in a straightforward manner. All equations can be carried over to 3D space without significant changes. A more complex network of nodes and elements may be needed to define the cell structure, but all additional boundary points and forces can be incorporated into the 3D model analogous to methods presented in this paper. The algorithms defining cell processes can also be carried into 3D space with some changes.

One of the biggest challenges in moving from 2D to a 3D model is an increase in the number of total nodes which results in a dramatic increase in the computational cost. For a cell membrane with radius r and N discrete points of length dr we have:

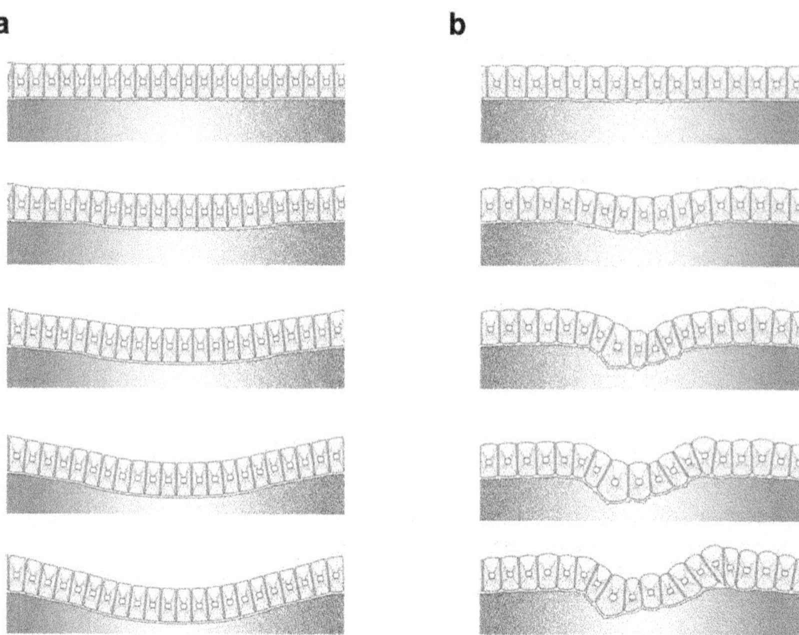

Figure 14. Tensegrity and Tissue morphogenesis. At this stage, an attempt is made to model the tensegrity hypothesis. To do so, a monolayer of epithelial cells is placed on the ECM. This causes the ECM to get thinner, by decreasing the drag coefficient at the center of the ECM (color gradient represents change in drag coefficient). The simulation is run with two densities of cells. The cells at this region have localized growth and motility, which drive the ECM downward. As a result, cells find space for more growth and proliferation. Therefore, they continue to drive the ECM further, which finally leads to the creation of a bud. This bud can be the first stage of tubulogenesis. a) Due to the high density of cells, they do not have enough space to grow and proliferate, so there is more organization and less deformation. b) Shows proliferation and less symmetry due to low cell density.

$$2\pi r = Ndr \Rightarrow r = \frac{Ndr}{2\pi}$$

If we move to a 3D environment where each surface dr^2 contains a single point from the set of points N', the number of points on the surface of the membrane will increase to:

$$N'dr^2 = 4\pi r^2 = 4\pi\left(\frac{Ndr}{2\pi}\right)^2 \Rightarrow \frac{N'}{N} = N$$

The ratio between the number of points in 3D compared to the number of points in 2D will be $\sim N$. Since an additional element (z) is added in 3D, the computational cost will be increased by 50%. Additionally, each point will be connected to 4 other points of the surface rather than only 2 points in 2D and as a result, the computational cost will be increased by a total of $6N$ times. In our case studies, where the initial number of points of each cell was 40, we would expect computational time to increase 240 times that of the original. It should be mentioned that the majority of challenges in transitioning from a 2D model to a 3D model are related to computational obstacles and associated programming techniques rather than biological or physical concepts.

Another major step in developing the model in the future is importing the biochemical aspect of the cell into this model. Cells can respond to a variety of environmental cues in a dynamic environment. These cues can be biochemical or mechanical in nature and can lead to changes in cell function and phenotype, both under normal physiological conditions and in pathological states. Most of the cells are surrounded by a highly complex ECM that is important in maintaining tissue structure but also plays key roles in guiding cell function. Cells bind to the ECM via specific integrin receptors and this binding can directly affect cell function. Furthermore, other signals that a cell receives from its environment are transmitted through and modulated by the ECM. Biochemical signals (e.g., ions, small proteins, or growth factors) must pass through the ECM and in some cases are sequestered and released by the matrix. Mechanical signals (e.g., tensile, compressive forces, or shear forces) are also transmitted by the ECM to the cell via integrin receptors that link the external environment to the cytoplasm and cytoskeleton.

Cell function is regulated by the entirety of the cellular environment, including cell-cell interactions, ECM components, humoral factors, local chemical conditions, and mechanical forces. In vivo and in vitro studies have the advantage that they maintain this complex environment, but the large number of variables that are difficult to control makes it challenging to isolate specific effects in experimental studies. In silico studies have the advantage that treatment variables can be controlled.

The nodes on the membrane can play the role of receptors allowing us to numerically insert chemotactic signals in our model and to use the reaction diffusion system for external signals. With knowledge about the internal biochemical pathway, we can model the biochemical properties of our model. One foreseen challenge in this work is that physical forces play a critical role in cell integrity and development, but little is known regarding how cells convert mechanical signals into biochemical responses [76]. Some molecules like integrins, focal adhesion proteins, and the cytoskeleton in the context of a complex cell structure—when activated by cell binding to the ECM—associate with the skeletal scaffold via the focal adhesion complex. Vinculin is presented as a mechanical coupling protein that contributes to the integrity of the cytoskeleton and cell shape control, and examples are given in literature of how mechanical signals converge into biochemical responses through force-dependent changes in cell geometry and molecular mechanics [77–81].

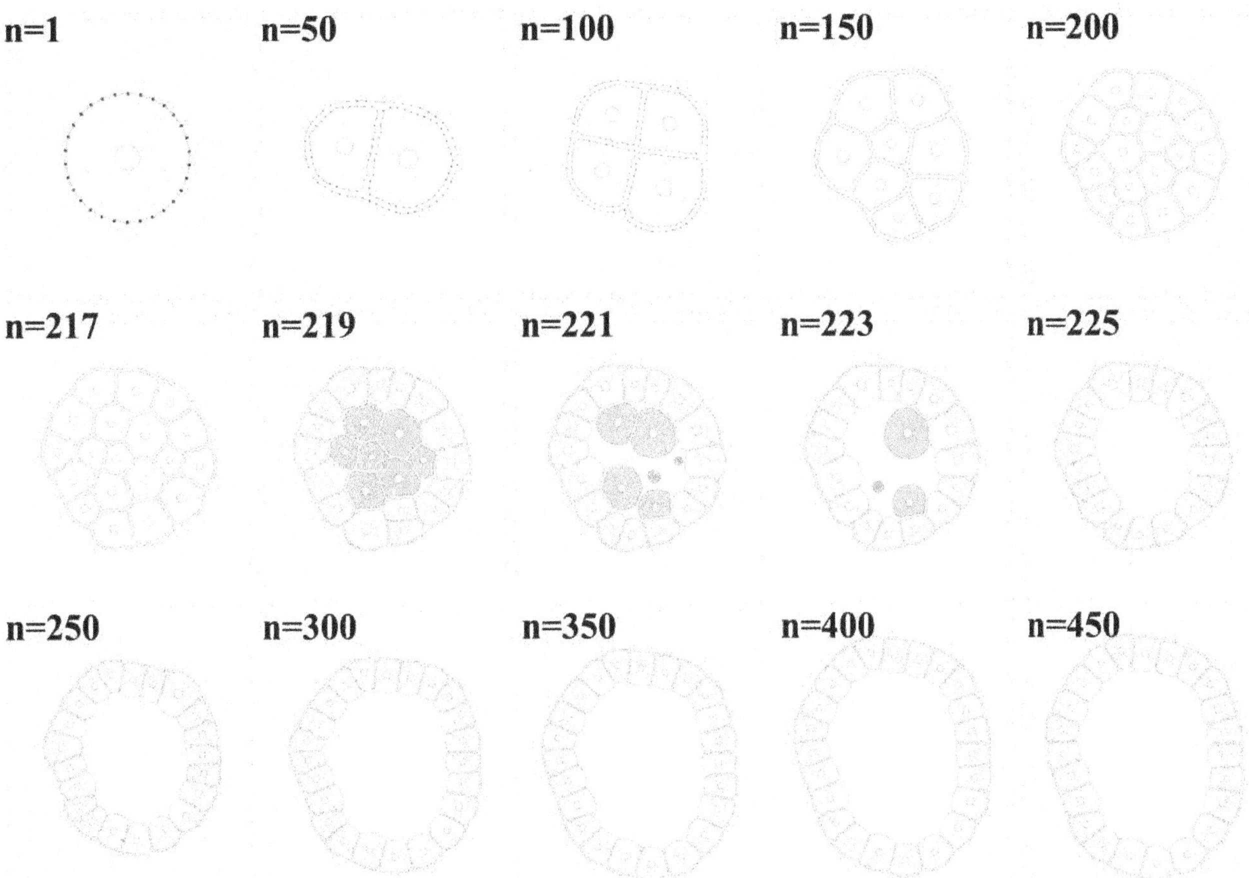

Figure 15. Formation of hollow epithelial acini. This stage shows modeling snapshots of self-arrangement of individual eukaryotic cells into a stable hollow acinar structure. In this model a single cell (n = 1) undergoes several consecutive divisions and gives rise to a small cluster of cells containing two different populations (n = 100–217): the inner cells are entirely surrounded by other cells which do not have access to ECM, and the outer cells partially face the ECM. Further cell proliferation leads to the expansion of the whole cluster. During this stage (n = 150–217) some intercalation of outer cells to the interior for the preservation of the circular shape of the tumor can be seen. As the intensity of adhesion between cells increases, the process of intercalation becomes more difficult. After this stage, when the tumor reaches a certain age, the cell undergoes further differentiation of outer cells and results in their apical-basal orientation and self-arrangement into one layer of polarized epithelial cells of regular cubical shapes (n = 219) and the inner cells are then triggered by polarized cells to enter the process of cell apoptosis. Each cell that does not have access to the ECM and as a result does not get polarized will die (n = 219–225). This process leads to the creation of the inner lumen. Consequently, the proliferation of polarized cells is suppressed and the final structure stabilizes in the form of a hollow epithelial acinus(n = 250–450). Moreover, the processes of cell proliferation, polarization and apoptosis need to be well coordinated in order to maintain the hollow acinar structure in a stable manner; otherwise cell overgrowth may lead to intraductal carcinomas. This coordination shows that this process is very dependent on biochemical signaling between cells. The final shape of the tumor is very dependent on the viscosity of the ECM. If the viscosity of the ECM is high enough (i.e. drag coefficient is high in our model, due to this process trying to move during a minimal distance in energy space), the cell maintains its circular morphology. However, if the viscosity of the ECM is reduced, the cell deviates from the circular shape.

In addition to the discretized approach for modeling the cell object we should use another distinct approach for discretizing the chemotactic signals. For signaling we will use cellular automata (cellular automata can be viewed as spatially extended decentralized system made up of number of individual components and may serve as simple model of complex systems. According to this interpretation, the CA can be traced back to biological modeling especially in reaction diffusion systems). The interaction of two distinct discretized models, i.e. cell and chemotactic signals are very important and require additional effort.

Author Contributions

Conceived and designed the experiments: YJ MRKM. Performed the experiments: YJ. Analyzed the data: YJ MA MRKM. Contributed reagents/materials/analysis tools: YJ MRKM. Wrote the paper: YJ MA MRKM.

References

1. O'Brien LE, Zegers MMP, E.Mostov K (2002) Building epithelial architecture: insights from three-dimensional culture models. Nature Reviews Molecular Cell Biology 3: 7.
2. Debnath J, Brugge JS (2005) Modelling glandular epithelial cancers in three-dimensional cultures. Nature review cancer 5: 14.
3. Wang AZ (1990) Steps in the morphogenesis of a polarized epithelium. I. Uncoupling the roles of cell-cell and cell-substratum contact in establishing plasma membrane polarity in multicellular epithelial (MDCK) cysts. 15 p.
4. Zegers MMP, O'Brien LE, Yu W, Datta A, Mostov KE (2003) Epithelial polarity and tubulogenesis in vitro. Trends in Cell Biology 13: 8.

5. Hogan BLM, Kolodziej PA (2002) Molecular mechanisms of tubulogenesis. Nat Rev Genet 3: 11.
6. Affolter M, Bellusci Sr, Itoh N, Shilo B, Thiery J-P, et al. (2003) Tube or not tube: Remodeling epithelial tissues by branching morphogenesis. Developmental Cell 4: 8.
7. Clark EA, Brugge JS (1995) Integrins and signal transduction pathways: the road taken. Science 268: 7.
8. Ettinger L, Doljanski F (1992) On the generation of form by the continuous interaction between cells and their extracellular matrix. Biol Rev 67: 11.
9. Gumbiner BM (2005) Regulation of cadherin-mediated adhesion in morphogenesis. Nature Reviews Molecular Cell Biology 6: 13.
10. Hagios C, Lochter A, Bissell MJ (1998) Tissue architecture: The ultimate regulator of epithelial function? PhilTrans R Soc Lond B 353: 4.
11. Lecuit T, Lenne P-F (2007) Cell surface mechanics and the control of cell shape, tissue patterns and morphogenesis. Nature Review Molecular Cell Biology 8: 12.
12. Lecuit T (2005) Adhesion remodeling underlying tissue morphogenesis. Trends in Cell Biology 15: 9.
13. Lecuit T, Pilot F (2003) Developmental control of cell morphogenesis: a focus on membrane growth. Nat Cell Biol 5: 6.
14. Anderson ARA (2005) A hybrid mathematical model of solid tumour invasion: the importance of cell adhesion. Mathematical Medicine and Biology 22: 24.
15. Turner S, Sherratt JA (2002) Intercellular adhesion and cancer iInvasion: A discrete simulation using the extended Potts model. Journal of Theoretical Biology 216: 16.
16. Freed LE, Vunjak-Novakovic G (1998) Culture of organized cell communities. Advanced Drug Delivery Reviews 33: 16.
17. Buck CA, Baldwin HS, DeLisser H, Mickanin C, Shen H-M, et al. (1993) Cell adhesion receptors and early mammalian heart development: an overview. Comptes Rendus de l Academie des Sciences Serie iii, Sciences de la Vie 316: 838–859.
18. CHAPLAIN MAJ (1996) Avascular growth, angiogenesis and vascular growth in solid tumours : The mathematical modelling of the stages of tumour development. Mathematical and computer modelling 23: 47–87.
19. Araujo RP, Mcelwain DLS (2004) A history of the study of solid tumour growth: The contribution of mathematical modelling. Bulletin of mathematical biology 66: 43.
20. Dormann S, Deutsch A (2002) Modeling of self-organized avascular tumor growth with a hybrid cellular automaton. In Silico Biology 2: 14.
21. Kansal AR, Torquatob S, Harsh GR, Chiocca EA, Deisboeck TS (2000) Simulated brain tumor growth dynamics using a three-dimensional cellular automaton. Journal of Theoretical Biology 203: 16.
22. Anderson ARA, Pitcarin AW (2003) Application of the Hybrid Discrete-Continuum Technique. In: Alt W, Chaplain M, Griebel M, Lenz J, eds. Polymer and Cell Dynamics Birkhauser. pp 261–279.
23. Düchting W, Ulmer W, Ginsbergl T (1996) Cancer: A challenge for control theory and computer modelling. European Journal of Cancer 32: 10.
24. Ermentrout GB, Edelstein-Keshet L (1993) Cellular Automata Approaches to Biological Modeling. Journal of Theoretical Biology 160: 37.
25. Alber M, Kiskowski M, Glazier J, Jiang Y (2003) On cellular automaton approaches to modeling biological cells. In: Rosenthal J, Gilliam DS, eds. Mathematical Systems Theory in Biology, Communications, Computation and Finance Institute for Mathematics and Its Applications. 1 p.
26. Drasdo D, Kree R, McCaskill J (1995) Monte-carlo approach to tissue-cell populations. Phys Rev E 52: 23.
27. Drasdo D, Hoehme S, Block M (2007) On the role of physics in the growth and pattern formation of multi-cellular systems: What can we learn from individual-cell based models? Journal of Statistical Physics 128: 59.
28. Dallon J, Othmer H (2004) How cellular movement determines the collective force generated by the dictyostelium discoideum slug. J theor Biol 231: 20.
29. Galle J, Loeffler M, Drasdo D (2005) Modelling the effect of deregulated proliferation and apoptosis on the growth dynamics of epithelial cell populations in vitro. Biophys J 88: 4.
30. Newman TJ (2005) Modeling multicellular systems using subcellular elements. Mathematical Biosciences and Engineering 2: 11.
31. Sandersius SA, Newman TJ (2008) Modeling cell rheology with the Subcellular Element Model. Physical Biology.
32. Palsson E, Othmer HG (2000) A model for individual and collective cell movement in Dictyostelium discoideum. PNAS 97: 6.
33. palsson E (2001) A three-dimensional model of cell movement in multicellular systems. Future Generation Computer Systems 17: 18.
34. Coskuna H, Lib Y, Mackey MA (2007) Ameboid cell motility: A model and inverse problem, with an application to live cell imaging data. Journal of Theoretical Biology 244: 11.
35. Rejniak KA (2007) An immersed boundary framework for modelling the growth of individual cells: An application to the early tumour development. Journal of Theoretical Biology 247: 19.
36. Rejniak KA, Anderson ARA (2007) A computational study of the development of epithelial acini: I. Sufficient conditions for the formation of a hollow structure. Bulletin of Mathematical Biology.
37. Rejniak KA, Dillon RH (2007) A single cell-based model of the ductal tumour microarchitecture. Computational and Mathematical Methods in Medicine 8: 9.
38. Rejniak KA, Kliman HJ, Fauci LJ (2004) A computational model of the mechanics of growth of the villous trophoblast bilayer. Bulletin of Mathematical Biology. 34 p.
39. Mofrad MRK, Kamm RD (2006) Cytoskeletal mechanics; Chien S, Saltzman WM, eds. Cambridge: Cambridge University Press. 252 p.
40. Fabry B, Maksym GN, Butler JP, Glogauer M, Navajas D, et al. (2003) Time scale and other invariants of integrative mechanical behavior in living cells. Physical Review E 68: 41914.
41. Gunst SJ, Fredberg JJ (2003) The first three minutes: smooth muscle contraction, cytoskeletal events, and soft glasses Am Physiological Soc. pp 413–425.
42. Yeung A, Evans E (1989) Cortical shell-liquid core model for passive flow of liquid-like spherical cells into micropipets. Biophysical Journal 56: 11.
43. Hochmuth RM, Ting-Beall HP, Beaty BB, Needham D, Tran-Son-Tay R (1993) Viscosity of passive human neutrophils undergoing small deformations. Biophysical Journal 64: 5.
44. Galli C, Guizzardi S, Passeri G, Macaluso GM, Scandroglio R (2005) Life on the wire: on tensegrity and force balance in cells. Acta Bio Med 76: 8.
45. Sultan C, Stamenovic D, Ingber DE (2004) A computational tensegrity model predicts dynamic rheological behaviors in living cells. Annals of Biomedical Engineering 32: 11.
46. Ingber DE (2003) Tensegrity I. Cell structure and hierarchical systems biology. Journal of Cell Science 116: 17.
47. Ingber DE (2003) Tensegrity II. How structural networks influence cellular information processing networks. Journal of Cell Science 116: 12.
48. Cañadas P, Laurent VM, Oddou C, Isabey D, Wendling S (2002) A cellular tensegrity model to analyse the structural viscoelasticity of the cytoskeleton. Journal of Theoretical Biology 218: 19.
49. Wang N, Naruse K, Stamenovic D, Fredberg JJ, Mijailovich SM, et al. (2001) Mechanical behavior in living cells consistent with the tensegrity model. Proceedings of the National Academy of Sciences 98: 7765.
50. Ingber DE, Heidemann SR (2000) Opposing views on tensegrity as a structural framework for understanding cell mechanics. J Appl Physiol 89: 8.
51. Chen CS, Ingber DE (1999) Tensegrity and mechanoregulation: from skeleton to cytoskeleton. Osteoarthritis and Cartilage 7: 14.
52. Castano E, Philimonenko VV, Kahle M, Fukalova J, Kalendova A, et al. (2010) Actin complexes in the cell nucleus: new stones in an old field. Histochem Cell Biol.
53. Ostlund C, Folker ES, Choi JC, Gomes ER, Gundersen GG, et al. (2009) Dynamics and molecular interactions of linker of nucleoskeleton and cytoskeleton (LINC) complex proteins. J Cell Sci 122: 4099–4108.
54. Dahl KN, Ribeiro AJ, Lammerding J (2008) Nuclear shape, mechanics, and mechanotransduction. Circ Res 102: 1307–1318.
55. Wang N, Tytell JD, Ingber DE (2009) Mechanotransduction at a distance: mechanically coupling the extracellular matrix with the nucleus. Nature Reviews Molecular Cell Biology 10: 75–82.
56. Wei C, Lintilhac PM (2003) Loss of stability—a new model for stress relaxation in plant cell walls. Journal of Theoretical Biology 224: 8.
57. Bereiter-Hahn J (1985) Architecture of tissue cells the structural basis which determines shape and locomotion of cells. Acta Biotheoretica 34: 10.
58. Tran-Son-Tay R, Sutera SP, Zahalak GI, Rao PR (1987) Membrane stress and internal pressure in a red blood cell freely suspended in a shear flow. Biophysical Journal 51: 10.
59. Charras GT, Yarrow JC, Horton MA, Mahadevan L, Mitchison TJ (2005) Non-equilibration of hydrostatic pressure in blebbing cells. Nature 435: 5.
60. Yoshida K, Soldati T (2006) Dissection of amoeboid movement into two mechanically distinct modes. Journal of Cell Science 119: 3833.
61. Chandran PL, Mofrad MRK (2010) Averaged implicit hydrodynamic model of semiflexible filaments. Physical Review E 81.
62. Gong Y, Mo C, Fraser SE (2004) Planar cell polarity signalling controls cell division orientation during zebrafish gastrulation. Nature 430: 689–693.
63. Thery M, Jimenez-Dalmaroni A, Racine V, Bornens M, Julicher F (2007) Experimental and theoretical study of mitotic spindle orientation. Nature 447: 493–496.
64. Siegrist SE, Doe CQ (2006) Extrinsic cues orient the cell division axis in Drosophila embryonic neuroblasts. Development 133: 529–536.
65. Lodish H, Berk A, Matsudaira P, Kaiser CA, Krieger M, et al. (2003) Molecular cell biology W.H. Freeman & Company.
66. Bray D (2001) Cell Movements: From Molecules to Motility Garland Publishing.
67. Bottino D, Mogilner A, Roberts T, Stewart M, Oster G (2002) How nematode sperm crawl. Journal of Cell Science 115: 367–384.
68. Mogilner A, Verzi DW (2003) A Simple 1-D Physical Model for the Crawling Nematode Sperm Cell. Journal of Statistical Physics 110: 1169–1189.
69. Flaherty B, McGarry JP, McHugh PE (2007) Mathematical Models of Cell Motility. Cell Biochemistry and Biophysics 49: 14–28.
70. Gruber HE, Hanley Jr. EN (2000) Human disc cells in monolayer vs 3D culture: cell shape, division and matrix formation. BMC Musculoskelet Disord 1: 1.
71. Brodland GW, Chen HH (2000) The mechanics of heterotypic cell aggregates: Insights from computer simulations. Journal of Biomechanical Engineering 122: 402.
72. Hall HG, Farson DA, Bissell MJ (1982) Lumen formation by epithelial cell lines in response to collagen overlay: a morphogenetic model in culture. Proceedings of the National Academy of Sciences of the United States of America 79: 4672.
73. Ojakian GK (2001) Integrin regulation of cell-cell adhesion during epithelial tubule formation. 12 p.
74. Ingber DE (2006) Mechanical control of tissue morphogenesis during embryological development. Int J Dev Biol 50: 12.

75. Debnath J, Mills KR, Collins NL, Reginato MJ, Muthuswamy SK, et al. (2002) The Role of Apoptosis in Creating and Maintaining Luminal Space within Normal and Oncogene-Expressing Mammary Acini. Cell 111: 12.
76. Mofrad M, Kamm R, eds (2009) Cellular Mechanotransduction: Diverse Perspectives from Molecules to Tissues. Cambridge, UK: Cambridge University Press.
77. Lee SE, Kamm RD, Mofrad MRK (2007) Force-induced activation of Talin and its possible role in focal adhesion mechanotransduction. Journal of Biomechanics 40: 2096–2106.
78. Goldmann WH (2002) Mechanical aspects of cell shape regulation and signaling. Cell Biology International 26: 313–318.
79. Vogel V, Sheetz MP (2009) Cell fate regulation by coupling mechanical cycles to biochemical signaling pathways. Current Opinion in Cell Biology.
80. Howard J (2009) Mechanical Signaling in Networks of Motor and Cytoskeletal Proteins. Annual Review of Biophysics 38.
81. Kamm RD, Kaazempur-Mofrad MR (2004) On the Molecular Basis forMechanotransduction. MCB 1: 10.

4

iNOS Ablation Does Not Improve Specific Force of the Extensor Digitorum Longus Muscle in Dystrophin-Deficient mdx4cv Mice

Dejia Li[¤]**, Jin-Hong Shin, Dongsheng Duan***

Department of Molecular Microbiology and Immunology, University of Missouri, Columbia, Missouri, United States of America

Abstract

Nitrosative stress compromises force generation in Duchenne muscular dystrophy (DMD). Both inducible nitric oxide synthase (iNOS) and delocalized neuronal NOS (nNOS) have been implicated. We recently demonstrated that genetic elimination of nNOS significantly enhanced specific muscle forces of the extensor digitorum longus (EDL) muscle of dystrophin-null mdx4cv mice (Li D et al *J. Path.* 223:88–98, 2011). To determine the contribution of iNOS, we generated iNOS deficient mdx4cv mice. Genetic elimination of iNOS did not alter muscle histopathology. Further, the EDL muscle of iNOS/dystrophin DKO mice yielded specific twitch and tetanic forces similar to those of mdx4cv mice. Additional studies suggest iNOS ablation did not augment nNOS expression neither did it result in appreciable change of nitrosative stress markers in muscle. Our results suggest that iNOS may play a minor role in mediating nitrosative stress-associated force reduction in DMD.

Editor: Carlo Gaetano, Istituto Dermopatico dell'Immacolata, Italy

Funding: This work was supported by the National Institutes of Health (AR-49419, DD) and the Muscular Dystrophy Association (DD). The funders had no role in study design, data collection and analysis, decision to publish, or preparation of the manuscript.

Competing Interests: The authors have declared that no competing interests exist.

* E-mail: duand@missouri.edu

¤ Current address: Department of Occupational and Environmental Health, School of Public Health, Wuhan University, Wuhan, Hubei, People's Republic of China

Introduction

Duchenne muscular dystrophy (DMD) is an X-linked lethal muscle disease affecting approximately 1–3 of every 10,000 newborn boys [1]. The primary genetic defect of DMD is dystrophin gene mutation [2]. Dystrophin is a sub-sarcolemmal structural protein essential for muscle cell membrane integrity and signal transduction. In the absence of dystrophin, muscle cells undergo degeneration and necrosis and eventually are replaced by fibrotic and fatty tissues. It is currently not completely clear how the lack of dystrophin leads to this devastating cascade of events. Several mechanisms have been proposed including contraction-induced sarcolemmal rupture, pathogenic calcium overloading, free radical injury, ischemia, inflammation and aberrant signaling (reviewed in [3,4,5]).

Recent studies suggest that inducible nitric oxide synthase (iNOS) may represent a common link among several of these proposed mechanisms [6]. iNOS is a calcium-insensitive NOS [7,8]. Its expression is negligible under normal condition but iNOS is highly up-regulated in inflamed tissues. In dystrophin-deficient mdx mice and DMD patients, iNOS level is markedly elevated in muscle [6,9,10,11]. It is currently not completely clear whether iNOS elevation merely represents an inflammatory signature of muscular dystrophy or it directly contributes to muscle disease in DMD. A recent study by Bellinger et al suggests that iNOS may play an active role in DMD pathogenesis [6].

In normal muscle, the ryanodine receptor (RyR) regulates calcium release from the sarcoplasmic reticulum (SR). When RyR is S-nitrosylated, it becomes leaky. Excessive entry of SR calcium into the cytosol activates calcium-dependent calpain proteases and causes muscle damage and force reduction [12]. Bellinger et al observed a disease-associated RyR S-nitrosylation in the extensor digitorum longus (EDL) muscle of mdx mice. Interestingly, they also found a simultaneous increase of iNOS expression and formation of an iNOS-RyR complex. Based on these findings, the authors proposed that iNOS-mediated RyR S-nitrosylation and subsequent intracellular calcium leaking represent important downstream events in dystrophin-deficient muscular dystrophy. Strategies to reduce iNOS-mediated RyR hypernitrosylation and/or RyR calcium channel leaking may ameliorate DMD [6]. In support of this model, Bellinger et al indeed found that pharmacological inhibition of RyR leaking improved voluntary exercise and EDL muscle specific force in mdx mice [6].

In accordance with these findings, here we hypothesize that genetic elimination of iNOS may improve EDL muscle contractility in dystrophin-null mice, presumably via reduced RyR S-nitrosylation. To test this hypothesis, we crossed the C57Bl/6 (BL6) background iNOS knockout (KO) mice with the BL6 background mdx4cv mice. Progeny mice were genotyped by PCR. After confirming dystrophin and iNOS expression by western blot, we examined the histopathology and contractile profile of the EDL muscle in age-matched male BL6, mdx4cv, iNOS KO and iNOS/dystrophin double knockout (iNOS/Dys DKO) mice. Much to our surprise, ablating iNOS did not reduce histological signs of muscle damage neither did it alter specific muscle forces. BL6 and iNOS KO yielded similar specific twitch and tetanic forces. In mdx4cv and iNOS/Dys DKO mice, specific forces were significantly lower than those of normal. However, there was no significant difference between mdx4cv and iNOS/Dys DKO mice. Interestingly, iNOS/Dys DKO mice appeared slightly more resistant to eccentric contraction-induced injury. To further probe this intriguing finding, we examined nNOS expression and muscle nitrosative stress markers. We did not find evidence of nNOS up-regulation in iNOS-null normal and dystrophic mice. Nitro-tyrosine, total cellular ryanodine receptor 1 (RyR1) and S-nitrosylated RyR1 levels were not altered by iNOS ablation either. Our results suggest that iNOS may be less important than it has been suggested in modulating force generation in dystrophin-deficient muscle.

Materials and Methods

Animals

All animal experiments were approved by the Animal Care and Use Committee of the University of Missouri (#6980) and were in accordance with NIH guidelines. BL6, B6.129P2-Nos2tm1Lau/J (iNOS KO) and (B6Ros.Cg-*Dmdmdx-4Cv*/J (mdx4cv) mice were purchased from The Jackson Laboratory (Bar Harbor, ME). Experimental iNOS/Dys DKO mice were generated by crossing iNOS KO and mdx4cv mice (Figure 1A). The genotype of the iNOS locus was determined using a protocol provided by The Jackson Laboratory (http://jaxmice.jax.org/strain/002609.html). Briefly, two independent PCR reactions were conducted using a common primer (ACATGCAGAATGAGTACCGG) and a wild type allele specific primer (TCAACATCTCCTGGTGGAAC) or a mutant allele specific primer (AATATGCGAAGTGGACC-TCG). The wild type allele yielded a 108 bp band and the mutant allele yielded a 275 bp band (Figure 1B). The mdx4cv genotype was determined by primer competition PCR as we recently reported [13]. The primers include a common primer (GCGCG-GCTTGCCTCTGACCTGTCCTAT), a wild type allele specific primer (GATACGCTGCTTTAATGCCTTTAAGAACAGCT-GCAGAACAGGAGAC) and an mdx4cv allele specific primer (CGGCCAGAACAGCTGCAGAACAGGAGAT). The wild type allele yielded a 141 bp band and the mdx4cv allele yielded a 123 bp band (Figure 1B). The average age of the experimental mice was 9.0±0.7 months (range, 6 to 12 months). Only male mice were used in the study.

Western blot

Whole muscle lysate was obtained from frozen limb muscles [14]. Dystrophin was detected with a monoclonal antibody against the dystrophin C-terminal domain (Dys2, 1:100, clone Dy8/6C5, IgG1; Novocastra, Newcastle, UK). iNOS was detected with a rabbit polyclonal antibody (#482728, 1:1,000, EMD Chemicals, Gibbstown, NJ). nNOS was detected with a rabbit polyclonal antibody against the N-terminal end of nNOS (1:1,000; Upstate, Lake Placid, NY) [14,15,16]. Nitro-tyrosine was detected with a mouse monoclonal antibody (1:1,000; Caymen Chemicals, Ann Arbor, MI) [14]. RyR1 was detected with a mouse monoclonal antibody (1:1000; Affinity Bioreagents, Golden, CO). For total cellular RyR1, the sarcoplasmic reticulum membrane fraction was prepared as described by Saito et al in the presences of 1% protease inhibitor (Roche, Indianapolis, IN) [14,17]. For S-nitrosylated RyR1, the sarcoplasmic reticulum membrane fraction was further purified using a resin-assisted capture method as reported by Forrester et al [14,18].

Rapid blue staining of duplicated gels (Geno Technology, St Louis, MO) was used as loading control for S-nitrosylated RyR1. For all other western blots, membrane was probed with an

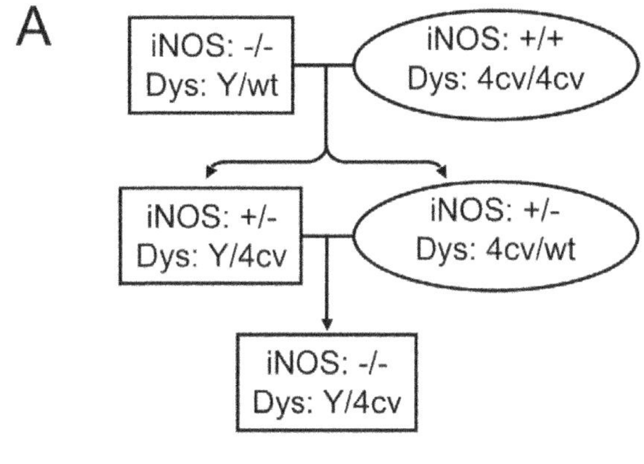

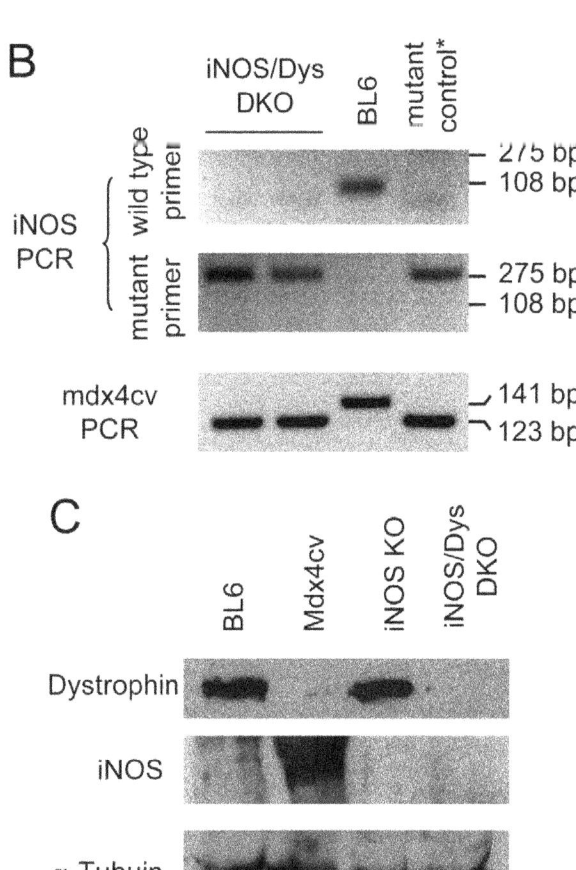

Figure 1. Generation of iNOS/dystrophin double knockout mice. A, Outline of the breeding scheme. Dystrophin and iNOS heterozygous male (Dys, Y/4cv; iNOS, +/−) and female (Dys, wt/4cv; iNOS, +/−) mice were generated by crossing iNOS knockout mice with mdx4cv mice. Crossing among heterozygous mice resulted in iNOS/dystrophin double deficient male mice. Rectangle, male mice; Oval, female mice. **B**, Representative genotyping photomicrographs. Top panel, iNOS PCR. Wild type yields a 108 bp band. Knockout yields a 275 bp band. Bottom panel, mdx4cv PCR. Wild type yields a 141 bp band. Mdx4cv yields a 123 bp band. In iNOS PCR, the mutant control is an iNOS knockout mouse. In mdx4cv PCR, the mutant control is a mdx4cv mouse. The first two lanes show typical results from two independent iNOS/dystrophin double knockout mice. **C**, Representative western blot results. DKO, double knockout; Dys, dystrophin; KO, knockout; wt, wild type.

anti-α-tubulin antibody as the loading control (1:3,000; clone B-5-1-2; Sigma, St Louis, MO).

Histology, immunostaining and nNOS activity staining

Morphological studies were performed in the EDL and tibialis anterior (TA) muscles. Both muscles mainly consist of fast-twitch type II myofibers. Haematoxylin and eosin (HE) staining was used to reveal general histology and centrally nucleated myofibers. Sarcolemmal integrity was assessed with the IgG infiltration assay [14,19,20]. Briefly, an Alex594 conjugated rabbit anti-mouse IgG antibody (1:100; Invitrogen-Molecular Probe, Carlsbad, CA) was applied to 8 μm muscle cross sections. After washing, damaged myofibers were visualized as red color under the Texas red channel with a Nikon E800 fluorescence microscope. Macrophage infiltration was determined by immunohistochemical staining using the Vectastain ABC kit (Vector Laboratories, Burlingame, CA) [21,22]. The murine-specific anti-macrophage antibody (1:500; rat anti-mouse F4/80) was obtained from Caltag Laboratories (Burlingame, CA). Macrophage stained in dark brown color. Fibrosis was examined with Masson trichrome staining according to our published protocol [14,21,23,24]. Fibrous tissue stained in blue color. Enzymatic nNOS activity staining was performed as previously described [14,15,16].

In vitro evaluation of the EDL muscle force

Twitch and tetanic (50, 80, 120, and 150 Hz) forces of the EDL muscle was measured in vitro at 30°C using a 300B dual-mode servomotor transducer (Aurora Scientific, Inc., Aurora, Ontario, Canada). The force data was analyzed using a DMC/DMA software (Aurora Scientific) [25,26,27,28]. Muscle cross-sectional area (CSA) was calculated according to the following equation, CSA = (muscle mass)/(0.44 × Lo × muscle density). 0.44 represents the ratio of muscle fiber length to optimal length for the EDL muscle. Muscle density is 1.06 g/cm^3. The specific force (kN/m^2) was calculated by normalizing the absolute muscle force with the CSA. After tetanic force measurement, the muscle was rested for 10 min and then subjected to eccentric contraction injury according to our previously published protocol [25,26,27,28]. The percentage of force drop following each round of eccentric contraction was recorded.

Statistical analysis

Data are presented as mean ± standard error of mean. Statistical analysis was performed with the SPSS software (SPSS, Chicago, IL). Statistical significance was determined by one-way ANOVA followed by Bonferroni post hoc analysis. Difference was considered significant when $P<0.05$.

Results

Generation of iNOS/Dys DKO mice

To eliminate potential influence of the genetic background, we crossed iNOS KO with mdx4cv mice (Figure 1A). Both strains were on the BL6 background. PCR genotyping revealed the loss of wild type iNOS allele and the presence of iNOS KO allele and mdx4cv mutation in iNOS/Dys DKO mice (Figure 1B) [13]. To further confirm the absence of iNOS and dystrophin in iNOS/Dys DKO mice, we performed western blot (Figure 1C). Dystrophin was detected in BL6 and iNOS KO, but not mdx4cv and iNOS/Dys DKO muscle lysates. BL6 muscle showed nominal iNOS expression [29]. As expected, iNOS level was substantially elevated in mdx4cv muscle but was completely eliminated in iNOS KO and iNOS/Dys DKO muscle (Figure 1C) [10].

Body weight and the anatomic properties of the EDL muscle

Adult male mice (9.0±0.7 months) were used in the study. No significant difference was observed in body weight among BL6, mdx4cv, iNOS KO and iNOS/Dys DKO mice (Table 1). The EDL muscle optimal length did not show significant difference either (Table 1). The EDL muscle weight and cross-sectional area (CSA) were significantly increased in mdx4cv mice (Table 1) [14,28,30]. The EDL muscle of iNOS KO mice had similar weight and CSA to those of BL6 mice [31,32]. Genetic elimination of iNOS significantly reduced the EDL weight and CSA in mdx4cv mice. However, they were still significantly higher than those of normal mice (Table 1).

Characterization of muscle histopathology in iNOS/dystrophin double deficient mice

HE staining was performed to evaluate overall histopathology changes (Figure 2A). BL6 and iNOS null mouse muscles showed uniform myofiber size and peripherally localized myonuclei (Figure 2A top panel). As expected, mdx4cv muscle displayed characteristic dystrophic pathology including variable myofiber size, profound central nucleation and patches of muscle inflammation (Figure 2A middle and bottom panels). Exactly the same histological lesions were seen in iNOS/Dys DKO mouse muscle (Figure 2A middle and bottom panels).

To study sarcolemmal integrity, we performed an in vivo IgG infiltration assay [14,19,27]. While minimal IgG infiltration was seen in BL6 and iNOS KO muscles, we observed profound IgG accumulation in mdx4cv and iNOS/Dys DKO muscles (Figure 2C). We also examined macrophage infiltration by immunohistochemical staining (Figure 2D) and non-specific esterase staining (data not shown). Similar levels of macrophage infiltration were found in mdx4cv and iNOS/Dys DKO muscles. To evaluate fibrosis, we performed Masson trichrome staining. Muscle fibrosis was not seen in BL6 and iNOS KO mice. In both mdx4cv and iNOS/Dys DKO, we observed stripes of blue stained fibrotic tissues (Figure 2E).

iNOS knockout did not alter specific forces of the mdx4cv EDL muscle but resulted in a moderate protection against eccentric contraction-induced force decline

To study the physiological consequences of iNOS ablation on dystrophin-deficient muscle, we measured the specific twitch (1 Hz) force and specific tetanic forces under low (50 Hz), moderate (80 Hz) and high (120 and 150 Hz) stimulation frequencies (Figure 2A and 2B). No significant difference was observed between iNOS KO and BL6 mice. In mdx4cv and iNOS/Dys DKO mice, specific twitch and tetanic forces were significantly reduced. They only reached approximately 50 to 60% of those of

Table 1. Body weight and EDL muscle characterization.

Strain	N	Body Weight (g)	Weight (mg)	Lo (mm)	CSA (mm^2)
BL6	11	39.23±1.97	11.14±0.33	13.06±0.08	1.83±0.05
Mdx4cv	11	37.18±1.41	18.50±0.28 [a]	13.79±0.14	2.88±0.04 [a]
iNOS KO	5	32.93±0.56	12.58±0.41	13.18±0.11	2.05±0.06
iNOS/Dys DKO	4	35.85±0.35	15.85±0.39 [a]	13.71±0.07	2.48±0.05 [a]

[a]Significantly different from all other strains.

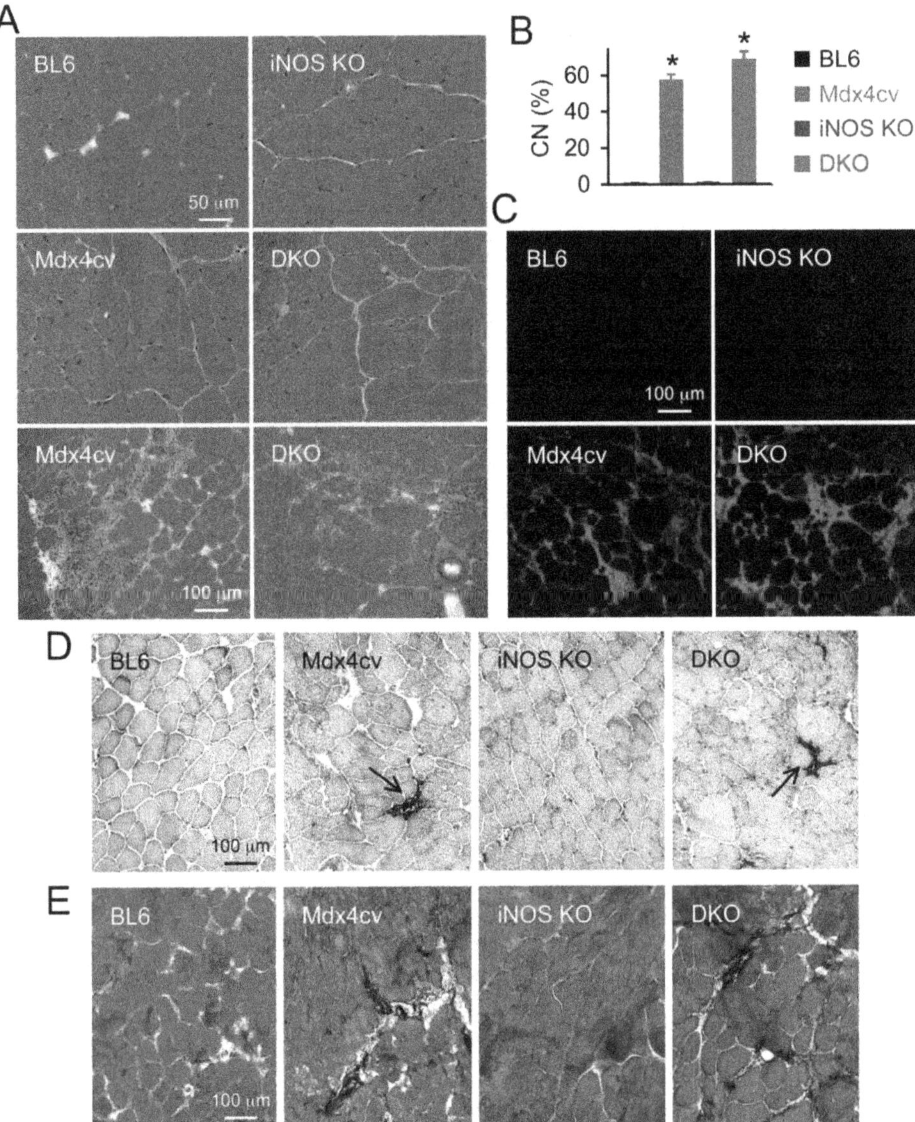

Figure 2. Genetic elimination of iNOS does not reduce limb muscle histopathology in adult mdx4cv mice. A, Representative HE staining photomicrographs. DKO, iNOS/dystrophin double knockout. Scale bar in BL6 image applies to top and middle panels. Middle panel, representative high power photomicrographs revealing central nucleation in mdx4cv and DKO mice; Bottom panel, representative low power photomicrographs showing muscle inflammation in mdx4cv and DKO mice. **B**, Quantification of myofiber with centrally localized nucleus. Asterisk, significantly higher than those of BL6 and iNOS knockout mice but there is no significant difference between mdx4cv and iNOS/Dys DKO mice neither is there a significant difference between BL6 and iNOS knockout mice. **C**, Representative mouse IgG immunostaining photomicrographs. Scale bar applies to all images. There is minimal IgG infiltration in BL6 and iNOS knockout. **D**, Representative histochemical staining of macrophages. Scale bar applies to all images. Arrow, dark brown stained macrophages. **E**, Representative Masson trichrome staining. Stripes of blue stained fibrotic tissues are evident in mdx4cv and iNOS/dystrophin double knockout mice.

normal mice (Figure 3A and B). Although iNOS/Dys DKO mice showed slightly higher numerical values of the specific tetanic forces than those of mdx4cv mice, the difference did not reach statistical significance (Figure 3B).

Next, we examined the force decline profile following repeated cycles of eccentric contraction. iNOS KO and BL6 mice showed similar profiles. In both cases, muscle force was largely preserved over four rounds of eccentric contraction (Figure 3C). Eccentric contraction resulted in significant force loss in both mdx4cv and iNOS/Dys DKO mice. However, the withholding forces of iNOS/Dys DKO mice were constantly higher than those of mdx4cv mice. Statistic significance was reached following two and three rounds of eccentric contraction (Figure 3C).

iNOS ablation did not increase nNOS expression

To determine whether iNOS knockout influences nNOS expression, we performed western blot, nNOS activity staining and nNOS immunofluorescence staining (Figure 4 and data not shown). Consistent with previous reports [33], we did not see a substantial elevation of the total nNOS level in iNOS KO and iNOS/Dys DKO muscle (Figure 4A). Sarcolemmal nNOS expression pattern was not altered either (Figure 4B).

Evaluation of nitrosative stress markers

We recently demonstrated that nNOS ablation reduced nitrosative stress in dystrophin-deficient muscle [14]. To determine whether iNOS knockout resulted in similar benefits, we

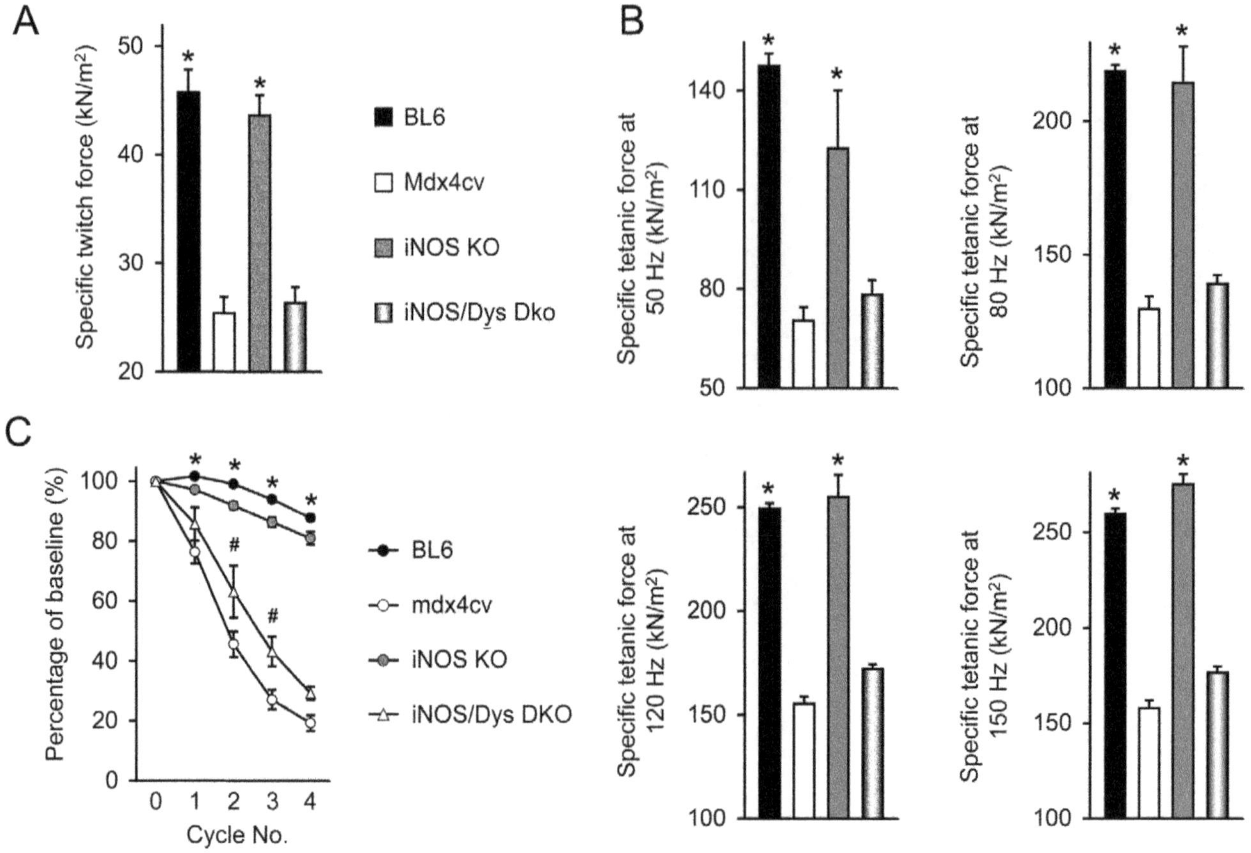

Figure 3. Characterization of EDL muscle contractility in iNOS/dystrophin double knockout mice. A, Specific twitch force. **B**, Specific tetanic forces at 50, 80, 120 and 150 Hz. **C**, Relative force decline following four cycles of eccentric contraction. Sample size, N = 8 for BL10, N = 11 for mdx4cv, N = 5 for iNOS KO, N = 4 for iNOS/Dys DKO. Asterisk, significantly higher than those of mdx4cv and iNOS/Dys DKO mice. However, there is no significant difference between BL6 and iNOS KO mice neither is there a significant difference between mdx4cv and iNOS/Dys DKO mice. Pound sign, value in iNOS/dystrophin double knockout mice is significantly higher than that of mdx4cv mice at the same round of eccentric contraction.

examined nitrotyrosine, total RyR1 and S-nitrosylated RyR1 (Figure 5). In normal mice, neither nNOS knockout nor iNOS knockout changed nitrosative stress markers in muscle (Figure 5) [14]. While nitrosative stress markers were greatly diminished in nNOS/dystrophin double mutant mice [14], minimal differences were noted between mdx4cv and iNOS/Dys DKO mice (Figure 5).

Discussion

Nitrosative stress-mediated RyR S-nitrosylation contributes to force reduction in DMD [6,14]. Reactive nitrogen species derives from nitric oxide (NO), a short-lived, highly reactive molecule [34]. NO is synthesized by NOS. There are several types of NOS including nNOS, iNOS and endothelial NOS. nNOS is the predominant form in normal skeletal muscle [35]. It is anchored at the sarcolemma by collaborative action of dystrophin spectrin-like repeats 16/17 and syntrophin [15]. In the absence of dystrophin, nNOS delocalizes from the sarcolemma to the cytosol and the relative cytosolic NOS activity is substantially increased [14,36,37,38]. As a consequence of pronounced muscle inflammation, iNOS expression is greatly increased in dystrophic muscle (Figure 1C and 2A, D) [6,9,10,11]. To determine which NOS isoform is responsible for pathologic RyR S-nitrosylation and force inhibition, we created two different strains of double

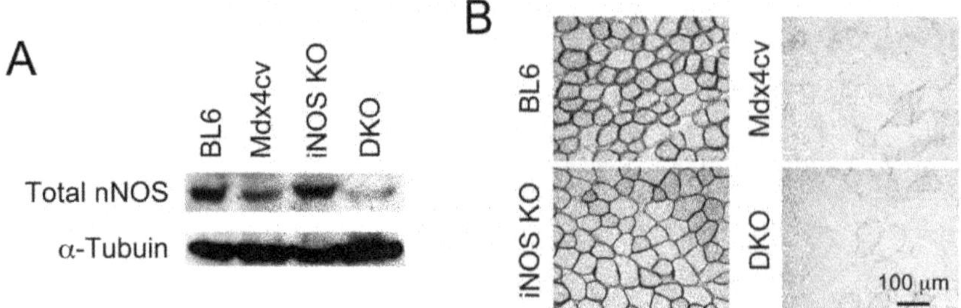

Figure 4. iNOS elimination does not augment nNOS expression. A, Representative western blot of total muscle nNOS. **B**, Representative photomicrographs of nNOS activity staining. Scale bar applies to all images. DKO, iNOS/dystrophin double knockout.

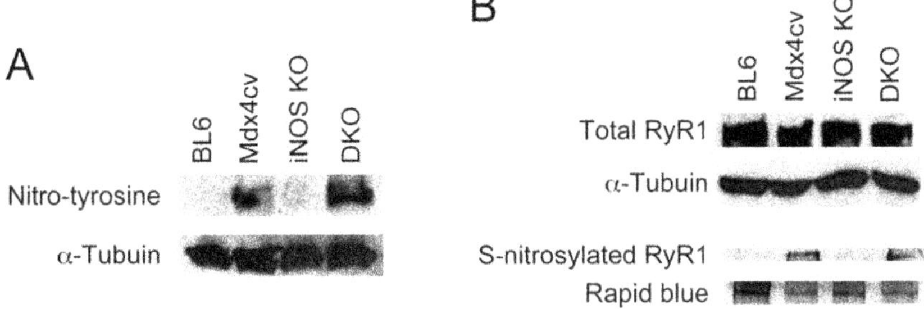

Figure 5. Characterization of nitrosative stress. A, Representative western blot analysis of 3-nitrotyrosine in BL6, mdx4cv, iNOS knockout and iNOS/dystrophin double knockout mice. α-Tubulin was used as the loading control. **B**, Representative western blots for total RyR1 (top panel) and S-nitrosylated RyR1 (bottom panel) in BL6, mdx4cv, iNOS knockout and iNOS/dystrophin double knockout mice. α-Tubulin was used as the loading control for total RyR1. Rapid blue staining was used as the loading control for S-nitrosylated RyR1.

knockout mice (Figure 1) [14]. Both strains are based on dystrophin-null mdx4cv mice. Besides dystrophin deficiency, one strain carries a null mutation in the nNOS gene and the other strain carries a null mutation in the iNOS gene.

In nNOS/dystrophin double null (n-dko) mice, mislocalized cytosolic nNOS is completely removed [14]. At the same time, markers of nitrosative stress (such as nitro-tyrosine and RyR S-nitrosylation) were normalized in n-dko mice. Importantly, specific muscle forces were significantly enhanced [14].

Recently, Villalta et al generated iNOS/dystrophin-double null mice by crossing BL6 background iNOS KO mice with C57Bl/10 background mdx mice [9]. Interestingly, the authors focused their analysis on the soleus muscle, a muscle dominated by slow twitch myofibers. They observed reduced myofiber injury and reduced central nucleation but macrophage density and neutrophil number were not altered in the soleus muscle of iNOS-null mdx mice [9].

To exclude the confounding factor of the genetic background, we generated iNOS/Dys DKO mice in the same genetic background (BL6) (Figure 1). Since DMD preferentially affects fast twitch muscles (such as the EDL and TA muscles) [39,40] and also since our previous studies were performed on the EDL muscle, here we opted to focus our study on the fast twitch muscle. We examined histopathology and also measured specific forces of the EDL muscle (Figures 2 and 3). Based on the findings of Villalta et al [9], we initially thought we should detect substantial reduction of muscle disease in iNOS/Dys DKO mice. Similar to Villalta et al, we did not see a dramatic change in macrophage infiltration (Figure 2D) [9]. However, analysis of multiple aspects of histological lesions (central nucleation, sarcolemmal integrity and muscle fibrosis) did not yield convincing evidence of muscle disease amelioration (Figure 2). According to the model of iNOS-mediated RyR S-nitrosylation [6], we initially expected iNOS/Dys DKO mice to produce significantly higher specific force than mdx4cv mice. Surprisingly, genetic elimination of the iNOS gene did not alter contractility of the EDL muscle in mdx4cv mice (Figure 3). The slight difference in the numerical values of specific tetanic forces was apparently due to the difference in the muscle weight and CSA (Figure 3, Table 1). Additional studies suggest that iNOS ablation did not alter nNOS expression neither did it reduced nitrosative stress markers in iNOS/Dys DKO mice (Figures 4 and 5).

The results from our n-dko mice and iNOS/Dys DKO mice suggest that mislocalized nNOS, rather than elevated iNOS, may play a determining role in nitrosative modification of RyR and force decline in dystrophin-deficient muscle (Figures 3 and 5) [14]. In contrast to nNOS, iNOS activation is not dependent on calcium [7,41,42]. This also seems to fit our model. Considering the fact that resting intracellular calcium concentration is abnormally elevated in DMD muscle [43], it is perceivable that there may exist a positive feedback loop between S-nitrosylated leaky RyR channel and cytosolic nNOS activation. On the other side, the moderate improvement of the eccentric contraction profile of iNOS/Dys DKO mice suggests that elevated iNOS remains a detrimental insult in DMD [9].

Acknowledgments

We thank Keqing Zhang, Yongping Yue and Thomas McDonald for excellent technical assistance.

Author Contributions

Conceived and designed the experiments: DD DL. Performed the experiments: DL JS. Analyzed the data: DD DL JS. Contributed reagents/materials/analysis tools: DD DL JS. Wrote the paper: DD.

References

1. Romitti P, Mathews K, Zamba G, Andrews J, Druschel C, et al. (2009) Prevalence of Duchenne/Becker muscular dystrophy among males aged 5–24 years - four states, 2007. MMWR Morb Mortal Wkly Rep 58: 1119–1122.
2. Kunkel LM (2005) 2004 William Allan Award address. Cloning of the DMD gene. Am J Hum Genet 76: 205–214.
3. Goldstein JA, McNally EM (2010) Mechanisms of muscle weakness in muscular dystrophy. J Gen Physiol 136: 29–34.
4. Petrof BJ (2002) Molecular pathophysiology of myofiber injury in deficiencies of the dystrophin-glycoprotein complex. Am J Phys Med Rehabil 81: S162–174.
5. Batchelor CL, Winder SJ (2006) Sparks, signals and shock absorbers: how dystrophin loss causes muscular dystrophy. Trends Cell Biol 16: 198–205.
6. Bellinger AM, Reiken S, Carlson C, Mongillo M, Liu X, et al. (2009) Hypernitrosylated ryanodine receptor calcium release channels are leaky in dystrophic muscle. Nat Med 15: 325–330.
7. Xie QW, Cho HJ, Calaycay J, Mumford RA, Swiderek KM, et al. (1992) Cloning and characterization of inducible nitric oxide synthase from mouse macrophages. Science 256: 225–228.
8. Nathan C, Xie QW (1994) Nitric oxide synthases: roles, tolls, and controls. Cell 78: 915–918.
9. Villalta SA, Nguyen HX, Deng B, Gotoh T, Tidball JG (2009) Shifts in macrophage phenotypes and macrophage competition for arginine metabolism affect the severity of muscle pathology in muscular dystrophy. Hum Mol Genet 18: 482–496.
10. Louboutin JP, Rouger K, Tinsley JM, Halldorson J, Wilson JM (2001) iNOS expression in dystrophinopathies can be reduced by somatic gene transfer of dystrophin or utrophin. Mol Med 7: 355–364.
11. Bia BL, Cassidy PJ, Young ME, Rafael JA, Leighton B, et al. (1999) Decreased myocardial nNOS, increased iNOS and abnormal ECGs in mouse models of Duchenne muscular dystrophy. J Mol Cell Cardiol 31: 1857–1862.
12. Bellinger AM, Mongillo M, Marks AR (2008) Stressed out: the skeletal muscle ryanodine receptor as a target of stress. J Clin Invest 118: 445–453.

13. Shin J-H, Hakim C, Zhang K, Duan D (2011) Genotyping mdx, mdx3cv and mdx4cv mice by primer competition PCR. Muscle Nerve 43: 283–286.
14. Li D, Yue Y, Lai Y, Hakim CH, Duan D (2011) Nitrosative stress elicited by nNOSmicro delocalization inhibits muscle force in dystrophin-null mice. J Pathol 223: 88–98.
15. Lai Y, Thomas GD, Yue Y, Yang HT, Li D, et al. (2009) Dystrophins carrying spectrin-like repeats 16 and 17 anchor nNOS to the sarcolemma and enhance exercise performance in a mouse model of muscular dystrophy. J Clin Invest 119: 624–635.
16. Li D, Bareja A, Judge L, Yue Y, Lai Y, et al. (2010) Sarcolemmal nNOS anchoring reveals a qualitative difference between dystrophin and utrophin. J Cell Sci 123: 2008–2013.
17. Saito A, Seiler S, Chu A, Fleischer S (1984) Preparation and morphology of sarcoplasmic reticulum terminal cisternae from rabbit skeletal muscle. J Cell Biol 99: 875–885.
18. Forrester MT, Thompson JW, Foster MW, Nogueira L, Moseley MA, et al. (2009) Proteomic analysis of S-nitrosylation and denitrosylation by resin-assisted capture. Nat Biotechnol 27: 557–559.
19. Hainsey TA, Senapati S, Kuhn DE, Rafael JA (2003) Cardiomyopathic features associated with muscular dystrophy are independent of dystrophin absence in cardiovasculature. Neuromuscul Disord 13: 294–302.
20. Amthor H, Egelhof T, McKinnell I, Ladd ME, Janssen I, et al. (2004) Albumin targeting of damaged muscle fibres in the mdx mouse can be monitored by MRI. Neuromuscul Disord 14: 791–796.
21. Smith BF, Yue Y, Woods PR, Kornegay JN, Shin JH, et al. (2011) An intronic LINE-1 element insertion in the dystrophin gene aborts dystrophin expression and results in Duchenne-like muscular dystrophy in the corgi breed. Lab Invest 91: 216–231.
22. Yue Y, Ghosh A, Long C, Bostick B, Smith BF, et al. (2008) A single intravenous injection of adeno-associated virus serotype-9 leads to whole body skeletal muscle transduction in dogs. Mol Ther 16: 1944–1952.
23. Li D, Long C, Yue Y, Duan D (2009) Sub-physiological sarcoglycan expression contributes to compensatory muscle protection in mdx mice. Hum Mol Genet 18: 1209–1220.
24. Bostick B, Yue Y, Long C, Marschalk N, Fine DM, et al. (2009) Cardiac expression of a mini-dystrophin that normalizes skeletal muscle force only partially restores heart function in aged Mdx mice. Mol Ther 17: 253–261.
25. Liu M, Yue Y, Harper SQ, Grange RW, Chamberlain JS, et al. (2005) Adeno-associated virus-mediated microdystrophin expression protects young mdx muscle from contraction-induced injury. Mol Ther 11: 245–256.
26. Lai Y, Yue Y, Liu M, Ghosh A, Engelhardt JF, et al. (2005) Efficient in vivo gene expression by trans-splicing adeno-associated viral vectors. Nat Biotechnol 23: 1435–1439.
27. Yue Y, Liu M, Duan D (2006) C-terminal truncated microdystrophin recruits dystrobrevin and syntrophin to the dystrophin-associated glycoprotein complex and reduces muscular dystrophy in symptomatic utrophin/dystrophin double knock-out mice. Mol Ther 14: 79–87.
28. Li D, Yue Y, Duan D (2008) Preservation of muscle force in mdx3cv mice correlates with low-level expression of a near full-length dystrophin protein. Am J Pathol 172: 1332–1341.
29. Thompson M, Becker L, Bryant D, Williams G, Levin D, et al. (1996) Expression of the inducible nitric oxide synthase gene in diaphragm and skeletal muscle. J Appl Physiol 81: 2415–2420.
30. Li S, Kimura E, Ng R, Fall BM, Meuse L, et al. (2006) A highly functional mini-dystrophin/GFP fusion gene for cell and gene therapy studies of Duchenne muscular dystrophy. Hum Mol Genet 15: 1610–1622.
31. Laubach VE, Shesely EG, Smithies O, Sherman PA (1995) Mice lacking inducible nitric oxide synthase are not resistant to lipopolysaccharide-induced death. Proc Natl Acad Sci U S A 92: 10688–10692.
32. MacMicking JD, Nathan C, Hom G, Chartrain N, Fletcher DS, et al. (1995) Altered responses to bacterial infection and endotoxic shock in mice lacking inducible nitric oxide synthase [published erratum appears in Cell 1995 Jun 30;81(7):following 1170]. Cell 81: 641–650.
33. Perreault M, Marette A (2001) Targeted disruption of inducible nitric oxide synthase protects against obesity-linked insulin resistance in muscle. Nat Med 7: 1138–1143.
34. Jackson MJ, Pye D, Palomero J (2007) The production of reactive oxygen and nitrogen species by skeletal muscle. J Appl Physiol 102: 1664–1670.
35. Stamler JS, Meissner G (2001) Physiology of nitric oxide in skeletal muscle. Physiol Rev 81: 209–237.
36. Brenman JE, Chao DS, Xia H, Aldape K, Bredt DS (1995) Nitric oxide synthase complexed with dystrophin and absent from skeletal muscle sarcolemma in Duchenne muscular dystrophy. Cell 82: 743–752.
37. Chao DS, Gorospe JR, Brenman JE, Rafael JA, Peters MF, et al. (1996) Selective loss of sarcolemmal nitric oxide synthase in Becker muscular dystrophy. J Exp Med 184: 609–618.
38. Thomas GD, Sander M, Lau KS, Huang PL, Stull JT, et al. (1998) Impaired metabolic modulation of alpha-adrenergic vasoconstriction in dystrophin-deficient skeletal muscle. Proc Natl Acad Sci U S A 95: 15090–15095.
39. Webster C, Silberstein L, Hays AP, Blau HM (1988) Fast muscle fibers are preferentially affected in Duchenne muscular dystrophy. Cell 52: 503–513.
40. Moens P, Baatsen PH, Marechal G (1993) Increased susceptibility of EDL muscles from mdx mice to damage induced by contractions with stretch [see comments]. J Muscle Res Cell Motil 14: 446–451.
41. Cho HJ, Xie QW, Calaycay J, Mumford RA, Swiderek KM, et al. (1992) Calmodulin is a subunit of nitric oxide synthase from macrophages. J Exp Med 176: 599–604.
42. Schmidt HH, Pollock JS, Nakane M, Forstermann U, Murad F (1992) Ca2+/calmodulin-regulated nitric oxide synthases. Cell Calcium 13: 427–434.
43. Allen DG, Gervasio OL, Yeung EW, Whitehead NP (2010) Calcium and the damage pathways in muscular dystrophy. Can J Physiol Pharmacol 88: 83–91.

5

Task Dependency of Grip Stiffness—A Study of Human Grip Force and Grip Stiffness Dependency during Two Different Tasks with Same Grip Forces

Hannes Höppner[1]*, Joseph McIntyre[2], Patrick van der Smagt[3]

1 Institute of Robotics and Mechatronics, German Aerospace Center, Wessling, Germany, **2** Centre d'Etudes de la Sensorimotricité, Centre National de la Recherche Scientifique and Université Paris Descartes, Paris, France, **3** Faculty for Informatics, Technische Universität München, Munich, Germany

Abstract

It is widely known that the pinch-grip forces of the human hand are linearly related to the weight of the grasped object. Less is known about the relationship between grip force and grip *stiffness*. We set out to determine variations to these dependencies in different tasks with and without visual feedback. In two different settings, subjects were asked to (a) grasp and hold a stiffness-measuring manipulandum with a predefined grip force, differing from experiment to experiment, or (b) grasp and hold this manipulandum of which we varied the weight between trials in a more natural task. Both situations led to grip forces in comparable ranges. As the measured grip stiffness is the result of muscle and tendon properties, and since muscle/tendon stiffness increases more-or-less linearly as a function of muscle force, we found, as might be predicted, a linear relationship between grip force and grip stiffness. However, the measured stiffness ranges and the increase of stiffness with grip force varied significantly between the two tasks. Furthermore, we found a strong correlation between regression slope and mean stiffness for the force task which we ascribe to a force stiffness curve going through the origin. Based on a biomechanical model, we attributed the difference between both tasks to changes in wrist configuration, rather than to changes in cocontraction. In a new set of experiments where we prevent the wrist from moving by fixing it and resting it on a pedestal, we found subjects exhibiting similar stiffness/force characteristics in both tasks.

Editor: Ramesh Balasubramaniam, University of California Merced, United States of America

Funding: This work has been partially funded by the European Commission's Seventh Framework Programme as part of the projects STIFF under grant no. (FP7-ICT-231576) and The Hand Embodied under grant no. (FP7-ICT-248587). The funders had no role in study design, data collection and analysis, decision to publish, or preparation of the manuscript.

Competing Interests: The authors have declared that no competing interests exist.

* E-mail: hannes.hoeppner@dlr.de

Introduction

A vast body of literature is devoted to the regulation of grip force. Indeed, the force necessary to stably hold an object in our hand is continuously regulated by the CNS [1,2] in a process known as "grip-force/load-force coupling". Already in children at the age of 2, this grip force is regulated depending on an object's weight [3]. Furthermore, the CNS is capable of modulating grip force to account for load forces acting on the hand-held object, such as the inertial forces induced by movement of the arm [4,5], or whole body movement during running [6] and jumping [7].

It has been shown that forces of an uncompensated grip decreases for contracting and increases for expanding objects [8], which evokes the concept of grip *stiffness* (i.e., the change in grip force versus a change in grip aperture) and may play an important role in maintaining grip stability. In a recent study [9] we measured grip stiffness as a function of grip force applied to an object held in a pinch grip. Participants were instructed to perform a force task with visual feedback, i.e., exert a predefined force which could be monitored by displaying the exerted force measured with a load cell. By applying very fast finger position perturbations during grip, we measured the part of stiffness that is related to biomechanics only, known as *passive intrinsic stiffness*, excluding influences from proprioceptive feedback. With these experiments, we demonstrated a linear relationship between grip force and intrinsic grip stiffness contributed by the passive properties of the corresponding muscles. We further showed that this conforms to a model of the pinching hand in which muscle exhibit elastic properties that can be represented by (nonlinear) exponential force-generating elements. A number of studies confirm this finding of a monotonic increase of finger force or torque with stiffness[10–13].

But how do load force, grip force and grip stiffness relate to each other? Can grip stiffness be modulated independent of grip force and if so, would such modulation have functional significance? Furthermore, the way in which we required subjects to apply different grip forces in our previous study (i.e., through visual feedback) was not very natural. What would the stiffnesses be like if a subject would lift an object in a weight task without any feedback about the applied force? Would the stiffnesses measured in the two tasks be comparable? Or would subjects be able to regulate force and stiffness independently?

Two possibilities to decouple grip stiffness and force are acknowledged: either by cocontraction of antagonistic pairs of muscles or by changing the finger/wrist configuration. Carter *et al.* showed that for zero net torque at the interphalangeal joint in the human thumb, joint stiffness highly increases with cocontraction. This demonstrates that net torque or force alone does not determine joint stiffness [13]. Furthermore, wrist flexion and extension causes stretching and shortening of, among others, the corresponding flexor digitorum superficialis and profundus muscles [14], affecting their force/activation relationship as described in the Hill muscle model [15]. This effect can reduce the maximum grip force to 73% of its maximum [16]. Thus, changes in wrist configuration should lead to changes in both grip force and grip stiffness. But even during wrist movements of up to 90°/s, the CNS is able to keep grip force stable [2].

Does the neuromuscular system allow for an active use of these effects on grip stiffness and an independent control of both, force and stiffness? White *et al.* showed that the CNS is able to decouple grip and load force in anticipation of a collision, with a rise in grip force before the expected impact and a peak in grip force around 65 ms after the impact [17]. They hypothesized that the CNS increases the net grip force in order regulate grip stiffness and damping, with the goal of optimizing stability in object manipulation. They did not, however, directly measure grip stiffness. Furthermore, not only might one wish to modulate the grip force on an object to keep it stable in the face of predictable events like a self-generated collision, one might also wish to regulate the stiffness of the grip in anticipation of unexpected perturbations depending on the constraints of a specific task.

In the current study we set out to test for grip stiffness modulation as a function of the natural tendency to increase grip force when lifting increasingly heavy objects [1,2]. We asked human participants to perform the visually-guided force-control task (FT) described above and a task in which they lifted objects of different weight (WT), without any specific instructions or visual feedback about the forces applied to the object in the pinch grip. Given our previous conjecture for the force task:

$$k_{\mathrm{FT}} = -\frac{df_{\mathrm{FT}}}{dx}\Big|_{a=\mathrm{const.}} = m_{\mathrm{FT}} f_{\mathrm{FT}} + n_{\mathrm{FT}} \quad (1)$$

where f is the exerted force, k the stiffness of the pinch grip, x the pinch grip aperture, a the muscle activation and m and n are slope [1/m] and offset [N/m], we can similarly conjecture

$$k_{\mathrm{WT}} = m_{\mathrm{WT}} f_{\mathrm{WT}} + n_{\mathrm{WT}} \quad (2)$$

for the weight task. To compare grip-stiffness/grip-force coupling between these two tasks, we set out to test the following specific hypotheses:

- $\mathbf{H_{0_1}}$: The measured stiffness in both tasks are equal for same grip force, i.e. $k_{\mathrm{FT}}(f) = k_{\mathrm{WT}}(f)$;
- $\mathbf{H_{0_2}}$: The relationship between grip stiffness and grip force are equal for the two tasks, i.e. $m_{\mathrm{FT}} = m_{\mathrm{WT}}$ and $n_{\mathrm{FT}} = n_{\mathrm{WT}}$.

General model of the fingers

In this section we will introduce a general finger model which describes the influence of cocontraction and kinematics on grip stiffness. The model will help us to interpret the measurements. Eq. (3) describes the restoring finger forces f and their relation to the Cartesian stiffness matrix k. This stiffness matrix describes the elastic behaviour caused by a displacement dx of the end point of a finger. Eq. (4) does the same for the finger joint torques T vs. joint stiffness R which is caused by an angular displacement $d\theta$. Finally, Eq. (5) describes the relation between muscle forces F, muscle stiffness matrix M, and muscle elongation dl_{m}:

$$df = -k\,dx, \quad (3)$$

$$dT = -R\,d\theta \quad \text{and} \quad (4)$$

$$dF = -M\,dl_{\mathrm{m}}. \quad (5)$$

ignoretrue The finger and joint velocities are coupled by the Jacobian matrix J, taking into account finger phalanx lengths; while muscle and joint velocities are coupled by the Jacobian matrix μ, which corresponds to muscles moment arms:

$$dx = J\,d\theta \quad \text{and} \quad (6)$$

$$dl_{\mathrm{m}} = \mu\,d\theta \quad (7)$$

ignoretrue from which we can derive that

$$dl_{\mathrm{m}} = J^{-1}\mu\,dx. \quad (8)$$

Note that J and μ are, in fact, functions of θ, but for readability we leave this out in our notation. Eq. (8) couples the finger endpoint and muscle displacements via a ratio of the two Jacobians.

The joint torque is coupled to the Cartesian and muscle force similar to the velocities by the kinematic chain but also by the moment arms represented by the Jacobian matrices:

$$T = J^T f \quad \text{and} \quad (9)$$

$$T = \mu^T F \quad (10)$$

ignoretrue from which we find

$$f = J^{-T}\mu^T F. \quad (11)$$

Again, the endpoint and muscle forces are coupled via a ratio of the two Jacobians. Using these equations and the assumption that the two Jacobians do not change for incremental angular displacements, the relations between the different stiffnesses become

$$R = J^T k J \quad \text{and} \quad (12)$$

$$R = \mu^T M \mu \quad (13)$$

ignoretrue leading to

$$k = J^{-T}\mu^T M \mu J^{-1}. \quad (14)$$

Combining Eqs. (11) and (14) we conclude that, if _f and _k are linearly related, then so are F and M. In words: if the grasp force and Cartesian stiffness are linearly dependent, then this is caused by a linear relationship between the muscle force and muscle stiffness. From these equations we can derive the influence of the two strategies for changing endpoint stiffness and its effects on the stiffness/force characteristic:

Cocontraction will increase the force and stiffness of agonist and antagonist muscles within each finger, while maintaining the same net force f applied by the finger tips. For a given level of co-activation, the operating point on the stiffness/force characteristic of each muscle and each joint will change, but the slope of the stiffness/force characteristic will not be affected. Under the assumption that the kinematic configuration will not be changed due to increased internal forces, cocontraction will lead to an increase in the muscle stiffness M and a proportional increase of the Cartesian stiffness k, without a change of grip force. Thus changing stiffness caused by *cocontraction will affect the offset, but not the slope* of the (linear) grip force–grip stiffness relation. This principle is illustrated in Fig. 1.

From Eq. (14) we can see that a change in the Jacobian by, e.g., changing finger or wrist orientation will have a nonlinear (quadratic) effect on the stiffness/force characteristic and will affect slope and offset.

Note that both strategies will not affect the linear relation between force and stiffness while cocontraction and kinematic orientation remain the same. A change of the slope between the two tasks will indicate an influence caused by a change of the Jacobian rather than by cocontraction. A change of the offset, however, can be caused by either or both. Furthermore, a change in the kinematic configuration possibly predominates effects of cocontraction on the stiffness/force characteristics.

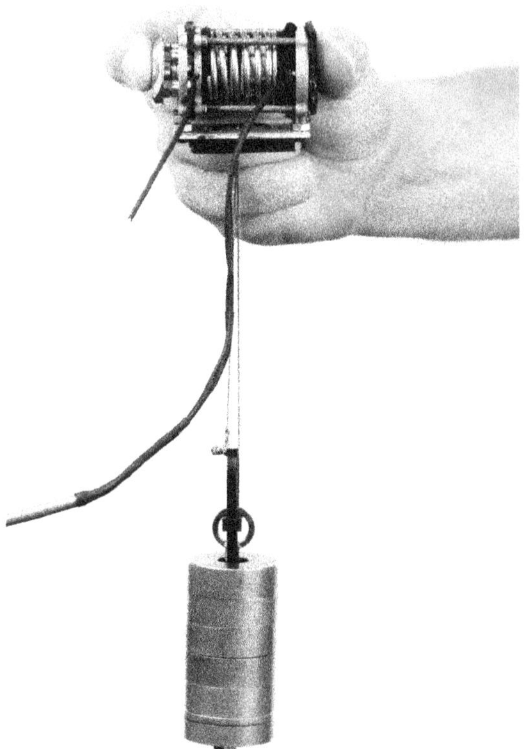

Figure 1. Stiffness change due to cocontraction. Increasing the cocontraction of the corresponding muscles increases the offset in the stiffness/force relationship.

Methods

Device description

The Grasp Perturbator (Fig. 2) used in this experiment was a small cylindrical device with which finger stiffness during pinch grip *in flexion* can be identified. A spring was preloaded by an electromagnet (blue) fixed to a frame (gray) that holds a moving part (red). The grip force was measured with a load cell (black). Note that this device could only apply perturbations in one direction, measuring stiffness of an expanding object. Precise grip force measurement was obtained by guiding the grip force through a button (green) to the load cell. Releasing the spring caused the device to elongate by 7 mm within a few ms. The Perturbator weighed 187 g and its length expanded from 57 to 64 mm when activated. As noted by Van Doren [10], grasp span has a small effect on grip stiffness (stiffness changed only 5% for a change of ± 2 cm in grasp span); we therefore have chosen a fixed Perturbator size. The spring force was 140 N when loaded and 100 N when unloaded, i.e., considerably higher than human pinch-grip force, ensuring identical experimental conditions independent of how firmly the Perturbator was held.

The measurement setup consisted of a host running Windows and a real-time target machine running QNX. The real-time machine ran a Matlab/Simulink model to control the electromagnet and read out the force sensor at 10 kHz. After pressing a release button, the perturbation was applied after a random delay 4 to 7 s. The load cell consisted of a KM10 force sensor and a measurement amplifier GSV-11H (both from ME-Messsysteme GmbH) with a nominal force of 100 N and an overall accuracy of the force signal of 0.1 N were used. We verified that perturbations caused no significant phantom force changes in the device by testing it with known springs. The offset of the measured force signal was calibrated before each trial.

In this study we focused on influences of underlying (bio)mechanical principles, rather than of reflexive feedback, and measured the combination of passive (surrounding tissue and ligaments) and intrinsic stiffness only (stiffness which can be attributed to the active muscle fibres); we refrained from measuring influences of reflexive stiffness. By measuring the grip force with an internal load cell before and shortly after the perturbation—well before the effects of short-latency reflexes—the grip stiffness contributed by the intrinsic properties of the muscles could be identified.

Experimental procedure

A total of 15 healthy right-handed male subjects, age 22–45 years, performed the two experimental protocols, WT and FT, as described below. No subject had a history of neurological disorder

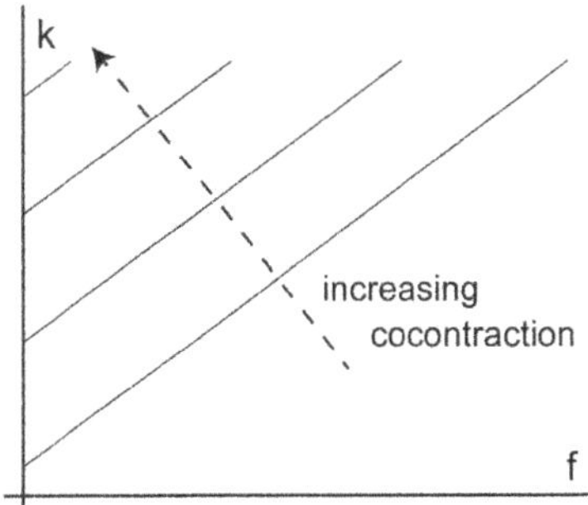

Figure 2. Cross sectional view of the Grasp Perturbator.

nor neuromuscular injury affecting the CNS or the muscles. All subjects gave written consent to the procedures which were conducted partially in accordance with the principles of the Helsinki agreement. Non-conformity concerns the point B-16 of the 59th World Medical Association Declaration of Helsinki, Seoul, October 2008: no physician has supervised the experiment. The collection of subject data was approved by the institutional board for protection of data privacy and by the work council of the German Aerospace Center.

All subjects had previous experience working with the Perturbator and were able to stably hold the device, even after the perturbation. Fully naive subjects would often drop the device during perturbation, leading to useless data because of a missing second static force level.

Ten subjects performed the main experiment in which the arm and wrist were free to move, although subjects were instructed to hold the forearm steady in a horizontal posture. These ten subjects were divided into two groups, counter-balanced as to whether FT or WT was done first (E1 and E2, respectively). To investigate whether changes in the wrist configuration might have an influence on grip stiffness an additional group of 6 subjects (E3) performed the two protocols with the wrist held at a constant orientation with respect to the forearm and with the relaxed arm and wrist supported by a table. We favored fixation over controlling wrist position using optical tracking in order to keep the task natural and to avoid providing visual feedback in the WT. Half of the subjects in E3 (subjects S11, S12, S13) did WT first, the rest FT first. Note that one subject took part in two experiments, and is referred to as S6-1 in E2 and S6-2 in E3. The whole experiment lasted about 90 minutes per subject. No subject reported discomfort during FT, some reported fatigue during WT. Subjects stood throughout the experiment, except for a 10-minute break between FT and WT. We found standing and lifting weights with respect to the WT intuitively more natural than sitting.

Weight Task

In the WT, six different weights of from 0.2, 0.4, 1.2 kg were attached to the Perturbator, and for 10 trials each the subjects had to lift the device off of the table (Fig. 3). The lower arm was requested to be held at approximately a 90 degree angle with the body. There was no visual feedback w.r.t. the grip force to the subject. Once the grasp was stable, the experimenter pressed the button to apply the perturbation between 4 and 7 s later (randomly chosen by the control computer).

Force Task

The procedure of the FT was almost the same as in our previous study [9], except that the subjects lifted and held the Perturbator above the table (as in WT, but with no additional weight attached). The subject received visual feedback about the actual force applied to the Perturbator and was asked to maintain a visually instructed predefined force. Once this force level was reached, the release button was pressed by the experimenter, unknown to the subject, and the perturbation was performed between 4 and 7 s later. Six instructed force levels were randomly presented to each subject, for a total of 10 times per force level.

Since applied grip forces for lifting the weights differed considerably across subjects, we measured the natural grip force when holding the device with different weights—thus leading to different grip forces—and chose 6 different grip force levels to subsequently use for FT. If subjects were instructed to do the FT first, we asked them to lift the Perturbator once with each weight attached before the FT without applying any perturbations. If the WT had to be done first, we used the information of the WT to estimate the required force levels for the FT.

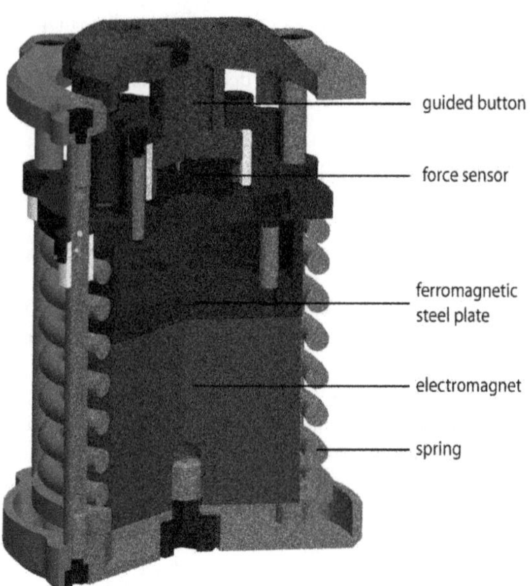

Figure 3. Grasp Perturbator held in a pinch grasp with attached weights.

For both tasks, we preferred experimenter release over automated release because previous experiments revealed increased participant fatigue in the latter case—holding the force level steady for a while, especially at high levels is increasingly difficult and troublesome. Note that the non-rigid coupling between the Perturbator and the additional weight in the WT meant that the inertia of the Perturbator was effectively constant, so that this effect did not have to be accounted for in the data analysis.

Data processing

The force signals were first filtered using a 21-point moving average filter. The time when the electromagnet was released and the time $t_{pert} = 0$ at which the perturbation started (see Fig. 4) varied considerably because the breakdown of the electromagnetic field depends highly on the applied grip forces. We therefore defined t_{pert} as the end of the period T_1, where T_1 was defined as the last 10 ms time interval before t_{peak} having a standard deviation below $5 \cdot 10^{-4}$ N. These numbers were empirically determined and led to stable results. The rise time between start of the perturbation and t_{peak} was on average 3.6 $\pm$ 0.62 ms (SD) and showed no significant correlation with force and weight levels.

The time interval T_1 was used to determine the force level before the perturbation; conversely, we needed to determine a time window T_2 over which the force level *after* perturbation was computed. We defined a second time t_{trust} within which one can ignore effects of fast reflex responses and trust the data to be purely intrinsic, in order to measure tendon- and muscle-based influences only. The mean onset latency of the short-latency reflex is about 30.7 $\pm$ 1.7 ms (SD) for the first dorsal interosseus in the hand [18]. In [19] Allum *et al.* reported a delay of about 20 ms between the onset of the short-latency reflex and first measurable changes in muscle force of stretching triceps surae muscles and releasing tibialis anterior muscles elicited by electrical stimulation. Thus, assuming that this feedback does not have a measurable influence within 40 ms, t_{trust} was allowed to vary downward from

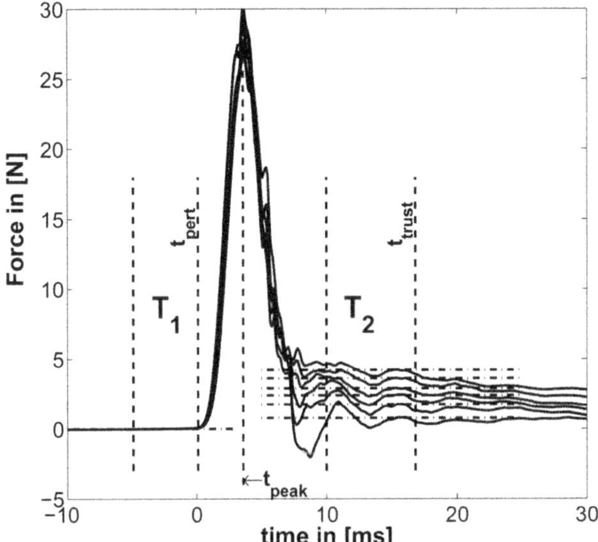

Figure 4. Example for typical Perturbation profile. Force profile before, during, and after a perturbation starting at $t=0$. Additionally, the time windows T_1 and T_2 and the mean of force for six force levels are depicted (mean force $E_{T_1}(f)$ subtracted). The length of T_2 and t_{trust} were found to be optimal at 6.8 and 16.7 ms, respectively.

$t = t_{pert} + 40\text{ms}$ and the duration T_2 was allowed to vary between 5 and 20 ms so as to minimize an objective function.

We decided to use one time window T_2 for all trials with a fixed start and end rather than optimizing either subject-wise or even force level-wise. This avoided comparing different lumped stiffnesses that are affected variously by damping and inertia, even if their influence was expected to be small. Furthermore, we looked at the gradient of the calculated stiffness values normalized by their mean as a kind of measure for stability of the achieved results. The data showed that stable results were achieved if the end of the second time window t_{trust} was at least 4 ms higher than the length of the time window t_{window}. This corresponded to a second time window not intersecting the first and left out the peak of perturbation (see Fig. 4). Thus, T_2 was varied so as to optimize the objective function

$$Z = \frac{1}{n_{sub}} \sum_{i=1}^{n_{sub}} \Big(\frac{1}{n_{level}} \sum_{j=1}^{n_{level}} (\tilde{e}(k_{WT_{ij}}) + \tilde{e}(k_{FT_{ij}}).. + \frac{1}{n_{trial}} \sum_{k=1}^{n_{trial}} (\tilde{e}_{T_2}(f_{WT_{ijk}}) + \tilde{e}_{T_2}(f_{FT_{ijk}})))) \quad (15)$$

using the whole number of trials n_{trial}, levels n_{level} and subjects n_{sub}. We introduce the CSE $\tilde{e}(\cdot) \geq 0$

$$\tilde{e}(\cdot) = \frac{\sigma(\cdot)}{\mu(\cdot)\sqrt{n}}, \quad (16)$$

which combines the coefficient of variation and standard error. The standard error compensates the standard deviation $\sigma(\cdot)$ for sample size n assessing low sample sizes with a higher standard error; the coefficient of variation is a normalized measure of the standard deviation and compensates for the sample mean $\mu(\cdot)$. Since the objective function Eq. (15) mixes data sets of different size and from different dimensions, we had to compensate the standard deviation $\sigma(\cdot)$ for both. $\tilde{e}_{T_2}(f_{FT/WT})$ denotes the CSE of force for each trial within T_2 and $\tilde{e}(k_{FT/WT})$ represents CSE of stiffness values for the different trials, for FT and for WT, respectively. The objective of this optimization was to minimize the oscillations within time interval T_2 and the variation of resulting stiffness values measured under *exactly* the same conditions. Note, that we minimized the variation of stiffness between experiments with identical conditions rather than between different stiffnesses, grip forces, or subjects. The stiffness of each trial was calculated using

$$k = \frac{E_{T_2}(f) - E_{T_1}(f)}{\Delta x}, \quad (17)$$

where $E_{T_{1/2}}(\cdot)$ denotes the average over time intervals $T_{1/2}$. The length of the second time interval T_2 and its end t_{trust} were found to be optimal under named constraints at 6.8 and 16.7 ms, respectively.

Results

Fig. 5, Fig. 6, and Fig. 7 show the results of the experiments for each subject. Each graph depicts the measured stiffness for FT in red and WT in black and their linear regressions as dashed lines. For each force and weight level, the mean values and their SEM in force and stiffness and the mean in force and stiffness used for testing $\mathbf{H_{0_1}}$ are plotted as circles. Additionally, the related R^2 coefficient (values of R^2 close to 1 denote a near-perfect linear regression) for a linear assumption between FT and WT and the two normalized mean inter-subject ratios of stiffness $\Delta k^* = (k_{FT} - k_{WT})/(k_{FT} + k_{WT})$ and linear regression slopes $\Delta m^* = (m_{FT} - m_{WT})/(m_{FT} + m_{WT})$ are depicted. Furthermore, Tables 1 and 2 list the results of the measured stiffnesses and the linear regressions between force and stiffness for each subject in both tasks. Based on these data and regression fits we performed statistical tests of the previously conjectured two hypotheses. For testing these, a fixed level of significance was chosen as $\alpha = 0.05$ for all tests.

Results main experiment—groups E1 and E2

The subjects of groups E1 and E2 were asked to do either FT or WT first with an unconstrained wrist.

$\mathbf{H_{0_1}}$: Equal stiffness for equal grip force ($\mathbf{k_{WT}(f) = k_{FT}(f)}$)

For each subject we tested whether the same stiffness was generated in each task, on average across all grip forces. Since the ranges of grip force differed considerably between the two tasks—especially for subjects doing the FT first (see, e.g., subject S9 in Fig. 6)—we algorithmically adjusted the datasets on a subject-by-subject basis by discarding trials with the highest or lowest grip-force values so as to align the mean grip forces before perturbation in WT vs. FT. We then compared the average stiffness levels. These data were only discarded for testing $\mathbf{H_{0_1}}$. Note that this data adaptation had no qualitative effect on the results (rejection of tested hypothesis or not). Table 1 summarizes the results for each subject in detail; the mean values in force and stiffness are additionally depicted in Fig. 5–6. We tested whether grip stiffness differed for the two tasks by testing if their difference was significantly different from zero, on average across subjects, by performing Student's dependent paired t-test on mean inter-subject stiffness Δk^*, normalized by the sum of k_{WT} and k_{FT} for each subject, for groups E1 and E2. These results (Table 3) indicate that mean stiffness differed significantly ($p<0.05$) with higher stiffness measured in FT, regardless of which task was

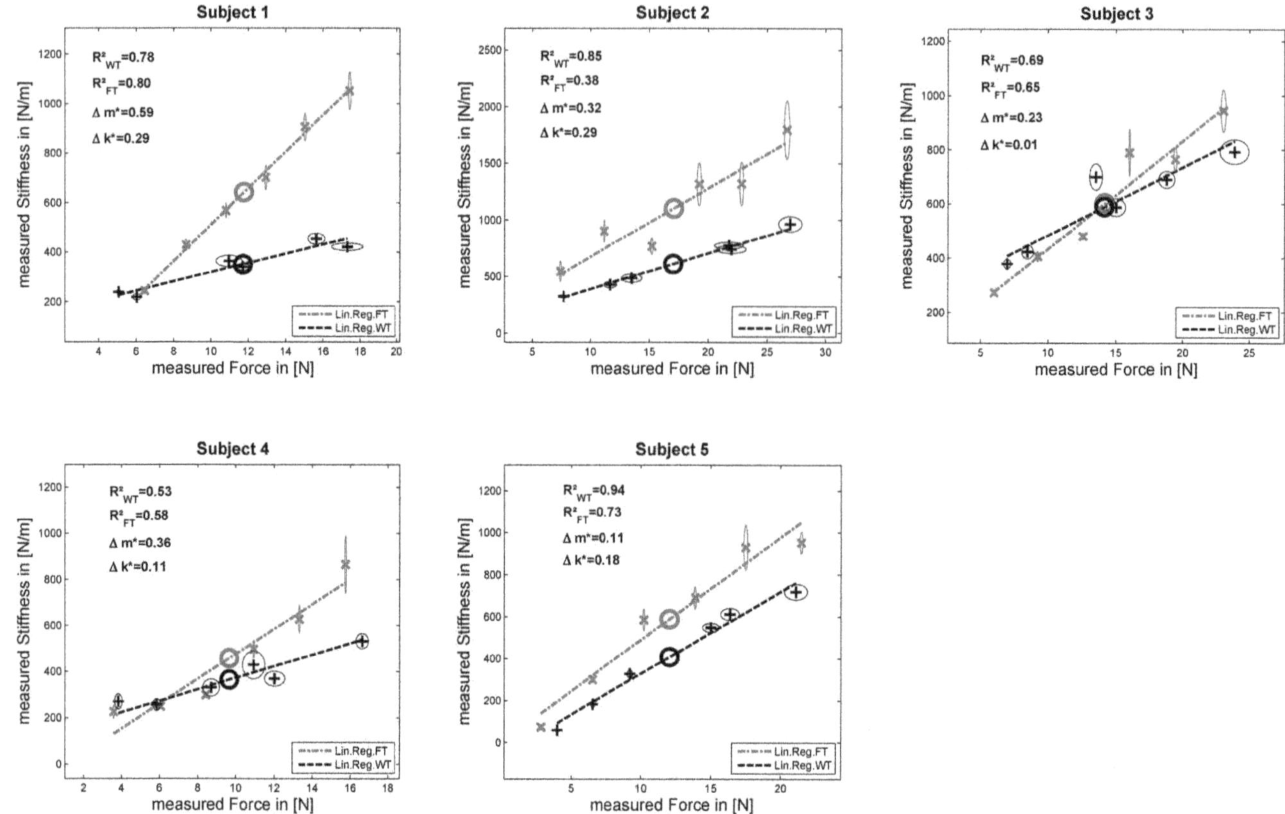

Figure 5. Results Experiment 1. Subjects doing the WT first without a cuff.

performed first by each subject (see Figs. 5 and 6). Furthermore, Table 1 includes results of an F-test for testing if the variances in intra-subject stiffness of both tasks were equal. The results provides evidence that, for all subjects of groups E1 and E2 excluding subject S6-1 and S7, it can be rejected that the variances in intra-subject stiffness were equal (Table 1), even if the tested standard variation was calculated across all data.

H_{0_2}: Equal grip-stiffness/grip-force slopes ($m_{WT} = m_{FT}$) and offsets ($n_{WT} = n_{FT}$)

For each subject and task we did a linear regression between force and stiffness and calculated the slope and offset of the resulting regression (see Table 2 for details). We then tested whether the parameters of the grip-stiffness/grip-force regressions differed between the two tasks, on average across subjects via a dependent paired t-test using the normalized difference of the slopes Δm^* and the mean of the offsets (see Table 4). The results provide evidence that, in general, the slopes in FT differed significantly from WT ($p < 0.05$) with higher slopes in FT, regardless of which task was performed first by each subject. Furthermore, it cannot be rejected that the mean offsets in group E1 or group E2 were equal; conversely, this can be rejected when data from the two groups were combined (E1+E2).

What can we conclude from the above? When holding the weight in the hand, higher muscle activation was required for WT in order to counteract the vertical load. Furthermore, to stabilize the wrist against this vertical load, antagonistic pairs of muscles will have been activated. One might expect a higher measured stiffnesses in comparison to FT, in which no additional weight must be supported. But the opposite was measured: by increasing the load, the stiffness decreased at constant grip force.

One could argue that the higher stiffness in the FT was required to accurately hold a certain force level using cocontraction, while for the WT it was not, because there no visual feedback of force was presented. As we discussed in section "sec:Model," using cocontraction will affect the offset of the stiffness/force relation. Because the results of testing $\mathbf{H_{0_2}}$ provides evidence that the regressed offsets of the two tasks were different, we were interested to know if each of them differed from zero. We found that it can be rejected for the WT across both groups E1 and E2 that the offset listed in Table 2 is equal to the origin (two-tailed t-test; $p < 0.025$), but not for the FT.

We furthermore looked at the correlation between slope and mean intra-subject stiffness across all subjects (no data were discarded; see Table 5). The results indicate that there is a significant correlation between mean stiffness and slope for the FT, which further argues for a stiffness/force relation going through the origin for the FT. As a corollary, the results are consistent with the finding that the stiffness/force curve of a single muscle most likely goes through the origin [20]. Note that the offset of measured stiffness/force characteristic of the antagonistic system at zero net force is not precisely zero because of the *passive* stiffness of surrounding tissues and ligaments in the arm and hand.

Results experiments with fixed wrist—group E3

Given that we found both higher grip stiffness and a higher grip-stiffness/grip-force slope for FT together with an offset in the FT not different from zero and an offset significantly larger than zero for the WT, our results argue strongly for a change in the kinematics as the predominately underlying mechanism rather than a change of cocontraction (see section "sec:Model"). To

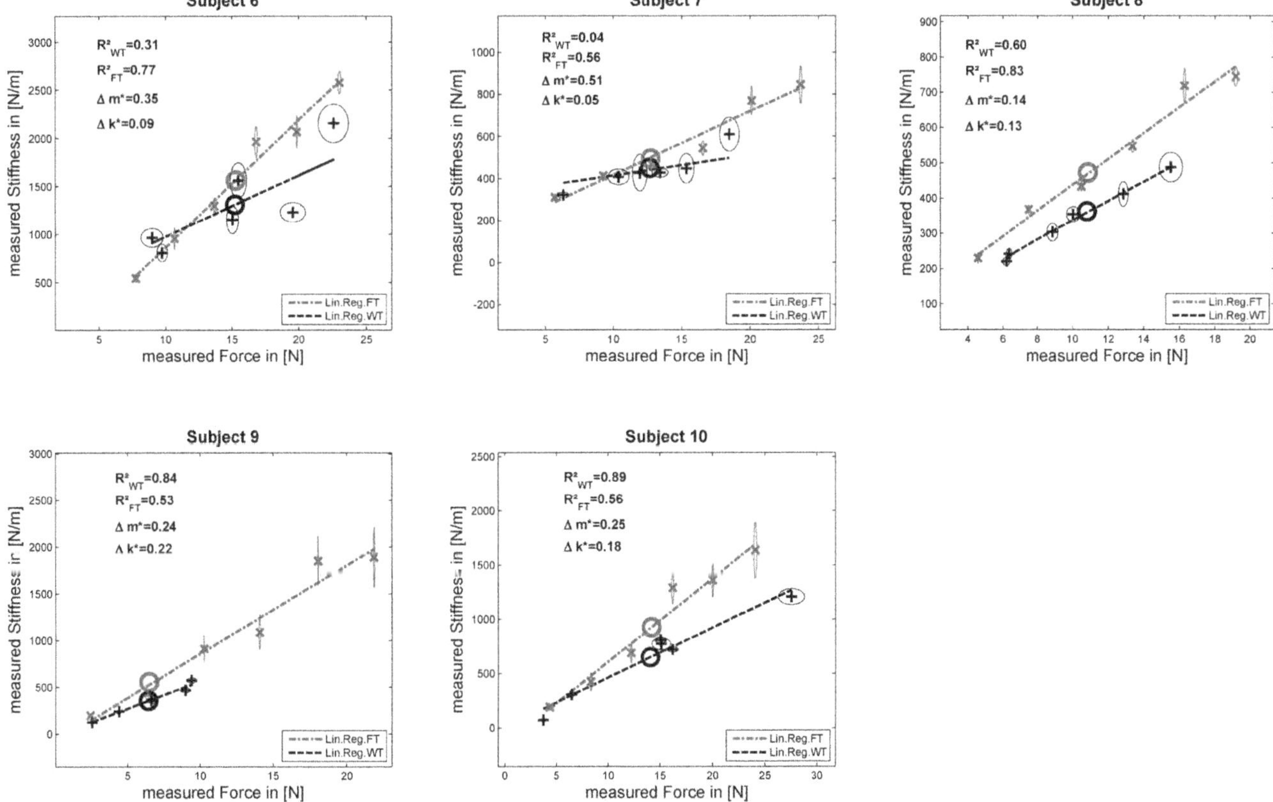

Figure 6. Results Experiment 2. Subjects doing the FT first without a cuff.

further test this hypothesis, subjects in group E3 performed the two tasks with the wrist held in a constant position by a rigid cuff in order to minimize the influence of a change in the kinematics. The cuff used here was made of a thermoplast with a steel plate parallel to the arm axis in order to maximize its stiffness; but still the wrist could be bent within small ranges. In order to prevent subjects from moving their wrist, we additionally rested the arm and hand on a table.

We compared the average stiffness across all grip-force levels, the slope of the grip-stiffness/grip-force relationship and their correlation, the results of which are shown in Table 6. One can see that grip stiffness – grip force relationship, i.e. the slopes and the offsets, differed much less between the two tasks when the wrist was stabilized. Nevertheless, grip stiffness was still higher for FT versus WT. Furthermore, there was a highly significant correlation between mean intra-subject stiffness and the slope of the stiffness/force curve for the WT ($p<0.01$) and FT ($p<0.001$). It cannot be rejected for either task that the mean offset across subjects was equal to zero. Further, the results on testing equal variances in intra-subject stiffness using the F-test provides evidence that, for all subjects of group E3 except 6-2, it cannot be rejected that these variances were equal.

About linearity between force and stiffness

As we initially stated we found a strong linear correlation between force and stiffness during the FT. To close out our description of section "sec:Results" we will further test if linearity was indeed obtained and if it changed between tasks. We used Mandel's technique to test whether a linear or a quadratic model provides a significantly better fit for the relationship between grip stiffness and grip force ([21], p. 165ff). The test compares the standard deviations of the residuals

$$W=\frac{(n-2)s_1^2-(n-3)s_2^2}{s_2^2}, \tag{18}$$

where s_1 and s_2 are the residual standard deviations of a linear and quadratic fit and n the sample size. s_1 and s_2 are computed as

$$s_1=\sqrt{\frac{1}{n-2}\sum_{i=1}^{n}(y_i-\hat{y}_{1_i})^2};\quad s_2=\sqrt{\frac{1}{n-3}\sum_{i=1}^{n}(y_i-\hat{y}_{2_i})^2}, \tag{19}$$

where y_i are the measured and y_{1_i}, y_{2_i} the fitted values. If the linear model is a correct assumption, W will be close to 1; if the quadratic model is a better assumption, the numerator will tend to be larger than the denominator. The Mandel test uses the F-distribution to test for significance: If W is less than or equal to the value of the F-distribution $F(f_1=1;f_2=n-3;\alpha=0.05)$, it can be rejected that a quadratic model provides a considerably better fit to the measured values (f_1 is the number of degrees of freedom of the numerator; f_2 of the denominator).

The results of the Mandel test are listed in Table 2. Note that we also corrected the data for non-normality (see [22], p.78ff for details), because the F-test is very sensitive to non-normally distributed data. Since the results of the Mandel test are identical (rejection or not), we will refrain from a detailed explanation for correction of non-normality. The results listed in Table 2 provide evidence that a linear relationship captures the underlying

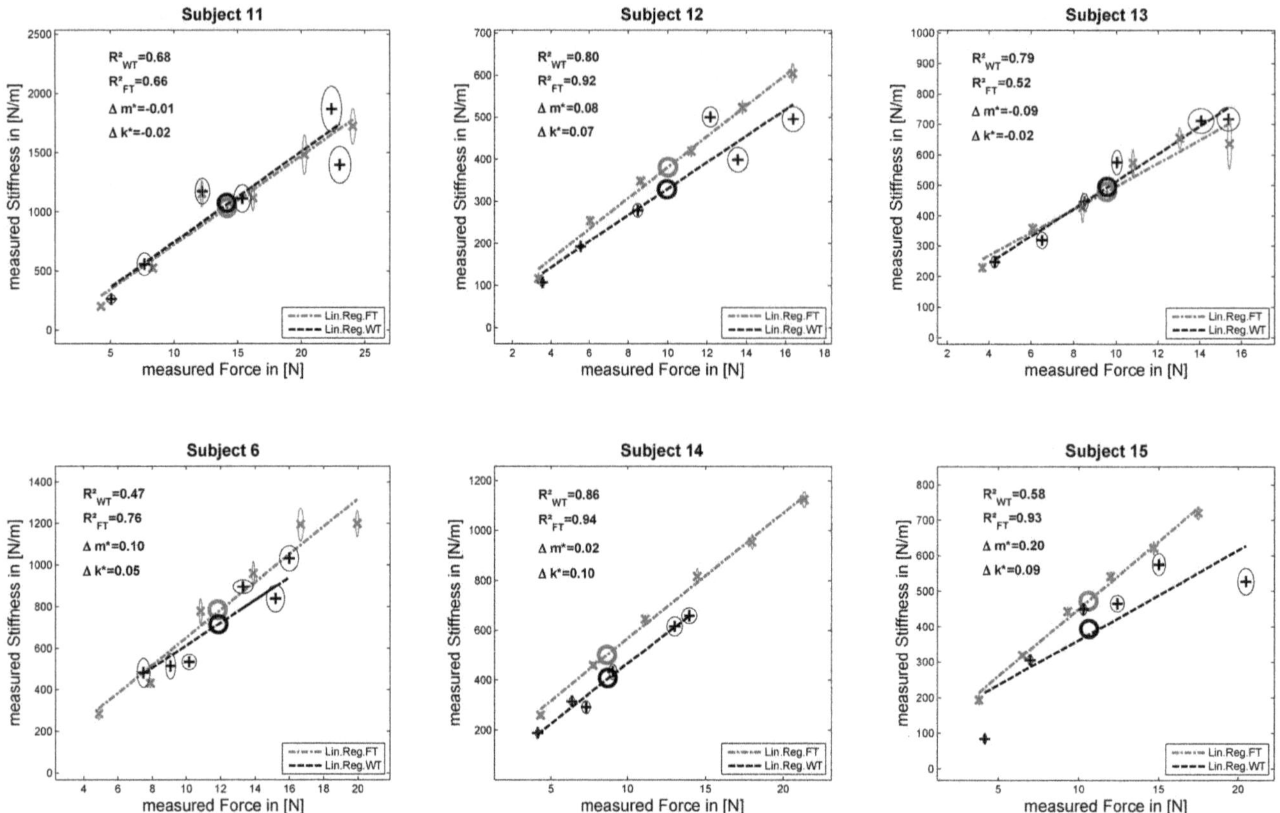

Figure 7. Results Experiment 3. Subjects who performed the experiment with the wrist cuff (WT first: top row, FT first: bottom row).

relationship to a reasonable degree for most of the subjects and tasks, consistent with our findings in [9].

Note the difference between R^2 and the Mandel test for linearity. R^2 indicates the percentage of the variance which can be explained by a (cq.) linear model. Thus, by implication R^2 of a quadratic model is never worse than that of a linear one. The Mandel test compares the difference of both model residuals by taking also the statistical degrees of freedom into account and indicates whether the difference is significant. E.g., the amount of data that can be explained by a linear model for the WT of subject S5 is not bad (93.7%) and indicates a linear relation, but using a quadratic model is significantly better (95.1%).

Discussion and Conclusions

The main result of these experiments is that grip stiffness is regulated independently from grip force, at least to some extent. The conventional assumption that stiffness increases linearly with applied force did hold in all of our experimental conditions, but the parameters of that linear relationship varied according to the task. Mean grip stiffness was considerably higher in FT than in WT, for all subjects of the groups E1 and E2, without any significant differences between early and late trials of single subjects, in much the same way that average grip force varied between static and dynamic grasping of different weights [23], regardless of which task was performed first by each subject. But the slope of the grip stiffness/grip force relationship was also higher for FT. Furthermore, WT stiffness was higher for lower grip forces (compare subjects S1, S3, S4, S6-1, S7 and S10). This is confirmed by the finding that over all subjects of both groups the offsets were significantly higher in the WT ($p<0.025$; one-tailed dependent paired t-test; find the corresponding mean and standard deviation in Table 4). Additionally, the WT offsets were significantly higher than zero, while the FT offsets were not. Together with a strong correlation between slope and mean intra-subject stiffness for the FT, these results portend to a change of finger/wrist configuration as the predominant mechanism underlying this change in the stiffness/force relationship, as opposed to a change in the level of cocontraction of antagonistic muscles of the fingers. We tested this hypothesis with a new set of subjects with their wrist fixed by a cuff and rested on a pedestal so as to maintain the same posture at the wrist. We found that both curves matched in terms of stiffness, slope, and offset and for both tasks a strong correlation between mean intra-subject stiffness and slope was observed. Furthermore, we found variances in intra-subject stiffness matched as well, which also argues in favor of data coming from the same population and thus for similar experimental conditions in both tasks. However, even if not for subjects S11 and S13, the measured mean stiffnesses in the FT were still somewhat higher for the group (see Table 6).

The limitations of our experimental conditions in E3 had to be mentioned as well: fixating the wrist and resting it on a pedestal in order to prevent the wrist from bending reduced activation in WT, possibly leading to lower WT stiffnesses. As we initially explained in section "sec:Model", a change in kinematics possibly predominates effects of cocontraction on the stiffness/force characteristics. Thus, from measurements done within E3 it cannot be excluded, that the difference found in E1 and E2 is a combination of a change in kinematics *and* cocontraction, with subjects using both strategies in the WT simultaneously.

Table 1. Testing $\mathbf{H_{0_1}: k_{WT}(f) = k_{FT}(f)}$.

group	subject	$\overline{k_{WT}}$ [N/m]	$\overline{k_{FT}}$ [N/m]	Δk^*	$\overline{f_{WT}}$ [N]	$\overline{f_{FT}}$ [N]	No. WT	No. FT	F-test [%]
E1	S1	350 ± 99	642 ± 302	0.29	11.7 ± 4.5	11.8 ± 3.7	10%	0%	$9.4e-121$
E1	S2	611 ± 249	1101 ± 648	0.29	17.0 ± 7.3	17.0 ± 6.6	0%	0%	$6.0e-101$
E1	S3	589 ± 160	604 ± 285	0.013	14.2 ± 5.0	14.2 ± 5.6	15%	3.3%	$6.0e-31$
E1	S4	365 ± 151	458 ± 293	0.11	9.7 ± 4.4	9.6 ± 4.2	0%	0%	$8.2e-51$
E1	S5	408 ± 250	588 ± 363	0.18	12.0 ± 6.2	12.0 ± 6.3	0%	0%	0.451
E2	S6-1	1309 ± 622	1565 ± 789	0.089	15.2 ± 5.4	15.2 ± 5.2	0%	0%	6.8
E2	S7	451 ± 197	495 ± 191	0.047	12.7 ± 3.8	12.7 ± 5.1	5.1%	20%	82
E2	S8	362 ± 121	473 ± 189	0.13	10.8 ± 3.3	10.8 ± 4.5	18%	11%	0.201
E2	S9	354 ± 163	557 ± 478	0.22	6.5 ± 2.6	6.5 ± 3.5	0%	48%	$2.5e-101$
E2	S10	649 ± 388	927 ± 693	0.18	14.1 ± 8.0	14.1 ± 6.7	0%	0%	$1.4e-31$
E3	S11	1075 ± 654	1034 ± 625	-0.019	14.1 ± 6.8	14.2 ± 6.8	1.6%	0%	73
E3	S12	329 ± 163	381 ± 172	0.074	9.9 ± 4.7	10.0 ± 4.5	0%	0%	69
E3	S13	495 ± 204	479 ± 211	-0.016	9.6 ± 3.9	9.6 ± 4.0	3.4%	0%	81
E3	S6-2	715 ± 276	785 ± 393	0.047	11.9 ± 3.5	11.9 ± 4.8	0%	6.6%	0.801
E3	S14	408 ± 168	502 ± 197	0.10	8.7 ± 3.0	8.7 ± 3.5	18%	43%	31
E3	S15	394 ± 184	473 ± 184	0.090	10.6 ± 4.7	10.6 ± 4.7	8.3%	11%	99

[1] $\mathbf{H_0}$of the F-test (Variances are equal) is rejected for probability values less than 5%.
The mean and standard deviation of stiffness of both tasks, their normalized difference Δk^*, the percentage of data discarded for this tests and the result of the F-test are listed. Data were discarded such that mean in force of both data sets align.

Furthermore, it should be acknowledged that our results are only valid for expanding objects and thus for the measured stiffness to force characteristics of corresponding musculotendon structure. The measured stiffness to a contracting object might be different and therefore characterizing the reaction as a linear stiffness might not be appropriate. In [10] Van Doren measured grip stiffness by measuring exerted forces of a contracting and expanding handle and used the subtraction of respective forces of both for calculating grip stiffness. But even if the meaning of stiffness measured in this work is different to our estimation, and includes information of an expanding and contracting object (and of reflexes as well), the authors still found a monotonic increase of stiffness with grip force.

Comparing the slopes and the mean stiffness between subjects, one can see that they differed considerably. Some of these large

Table 2. Linear regression and Mandels test for linearity.

group	subject	m_{WT}	m_{FT}	Δm^*	n_{WT}	n_{FT}	R^2_{WT}	R^2_{FT}	M-test WT	M-test FT
E1	S1	19	74	0.59	132	-224	78	80	20	97
E1	S2	31	61	0.32	75	69	85	38	73	24
E1	S3	25	40	0.23	233	37	69	65	40	67
E1	S4	25	54	0.36	123	-60	53	58	7.8	0.611
E1	S5	39	49	0.11	-62	1.6	94	73	0.0151	1.61
E2	S6-1	64	133	0.35	337	-457	31	77	24	50
E2	S7	10	30	0.51	318	117	4.4	56	14	34
E2	S8	27	37	0.14	64	73	60	83	30	65
E2	S9	58	95	0.24	-22	-85	84	53	25	93
E2	S10	46	77	0.25	3.1	-158	89	56	0.161	62
E3	S11	76	75	-0.009	-21	-34	68	66	12	15
E3	S12	31	37	0.08	18	15	80	92	1.71	14
E3	S13	45	38	-0.09	63	117	79	52	13	26
E3	S6-2	55	67	0.10	67	-19	47	76	7.9	1.41
E3	S14	48	50	0.02	-17	65	86	94	77	11
E3	S15	25	38	0.20	109	69	58	93	$5.7e-101$	1.81

[1] For probability values less than 5% it is rejected that a linear relation is as good as a quadratic.
Slope $m_{WT/FT}$ [1/m], their normalized values Δm^*, offset $n_{WT/FT}$ [N/m], the related R^2 [%] coefficient for a linear model and the results of the M-test in [%] are listed.

Table 3. Testing $\mathbf{H_{0_1}}$.

$\frac{k_{FT}-k_{WT}}{k_{FT}+k_{WT}}$	E1	E2	E1+E2
$\bar{x}$	0.18	0.13	0.16
$\sigma^2(x)$	0.12	0.069	0.095
p (two-tailed)	2.9%1	1.3%1	0.058%1

[1] $\mathbf{H_0}$is rejected for probability values less than 5% (paired t-test).
Whereby the two stiffnesses Eqs. (1) and (2) are equal $k_{FT}(f)=k_{WT}(f)$ across subjects. The mean normalized difference of the two stiffnesses Δk^* and its standard deviation (inter-subject variability). Data were discarded such that mean in force of both data sets align.

Table 5. Correlation $\mathbf{r_{WT/FT}}$ between slope and mean intra-subject stiffness and its probability $\mathbf{p_{WT/FT}}$ in % for groups E1 and E2.

$k\sim m$	E1	E2	E1+E2
r_{WT}	24%	57%	59%
r_{FT}	28%	99%	88%
p_{WT}	69%	31%	7.5%
p_{FT}	65%	0.16%1	0.089%1

[1] The correlation is significant.
For probability values less than 5% the correlation is significant. No data were discarded.

differences in inter-subject stiffness could be explained by a difference in grip force, but certainly not everything. Furthermore, for groups E1 and E2, some of the inter-subject variability can be explained by different wrist positions of the subjects. But even within group E3, where the wrist was fixed in one position, the stiffnesses differed considerably between subjects. Measuring planar human arm stiffness, Mussa-Ivaldi [24] reported that qualitative measures such as *shape* and *orientation* of a stiffness ellipse measured at the endpoint are similar over different subjects for different postures, but the quantitative measure *size* is not, and even varies considerably for identical subjects measured on different days.

The force ranges differed considerably between the two tasks, especially for subjects doing FT first. Since we wanted to exclude the influence of which task is done first, we let the subjects of this group only lift each weight once before the FT in order to avoid learning. This leads to a data set of 6 different force levels, while for subjects doing WT first a data set of 60 data points was used to calculate the force levels. Thus, the force ranges between both tasks differed more for the group doing FT first, leading to a larger force range of FT. However, we expect the influence of this difference to be small. Remember that to test $\mathbf{H_{0_1}}$ we only compared data within equal force ranges by discarding extreme values (6.6%) of the data set.

A number of studies have already demonstrated how the finger [25] and wrist [16] can affect fingertip forces and stiffness in the human hand and the idea that one might adjust the configuration of a redundant multi-joint linkage to optimize impedance with respect to the task or to the environment [26,27] has also been proposed. The question which remains to be clarified here is: Are the found differences between the two tasks actively controlled by the CNS? And if yes, why should subjects minimize the influence of the wrist in an FT where they get a visually-presented feedback about variations of the actual grip force?

Table 6. Results of group E3 when the wrist was held in a constant posture by a cuff.

E3	$\frac{k_{FT}-k_{WT}}{k_{FT}+k_{WT}}$	$\frac{m_{FT}-m_{WT}}{m_{FT}+m_{WT}}$	$n_{FT}-n_{WT}$	E3	$k\sim m$
$\bar{x}$	0.046	0.051	−0.91	r_{WT}	92%
$\sigma^2(x)$	0.053	0.099	61	r_{FT}	98%
p (two-tailed)	8.6%	27%	97%	p_{WT}	0.92%2
				p_{FT}	0.091%2

[1] $\mathbf{H_0}$that $k_{FT}=k_{WT}$, $m_{FT}=m_{WT}$ and $n_{FT}=n_{WT}$ is rejected for probability values less than 5% (paired t-test), respectively.
[2] For probability values less than 5% the correlation is significant.
Left table: dependent paired t-test of greater inter-subject grip stiffness, grip-stiffness/grip-force slope and offset for FT versus WT. Right table: Correlation between slope and mean intra-subject stiffness and its probability in %. No data were discarded.

To maximize the efficacy of the visually-guided control loop, one could reasonably strive to minimize the latency between commanded changes in muscle activations and the actual changes of grip force applied at the fingertips. As muscles are constrained by activation dynamics, there is a theoretical limit to the rate of change of muscle force F with respect to time, dF/dt, that a given muscle can produce. The rate of change of force measured at the fingertip would be modulated by the same Jacobian that governs the relationship between muscle force and finger force, and between muscle stiffness and finger stiffness, i.e., $df/dt= J^{-T}\mu^T dF/dt$. Thus, by maximizing the norm of $J^{-T}\mu^T$, one maximizes the ability to rapidly effectuate a change in grip force in response to a visually presented force error. From this point of view, the modulation of grip stiffness observed in our experiments

Table 4. Testing $\mathbf{H_{0_2}}$

$\frac{m_{FT}-m_{WT}}{m_{FT}+m_{WT}}$	E1	E2	E1+E2	$n_{FT}-n_{WT}$	E1	E2	E1+E2
$\bar{x}$	0.32	0.30	0.31	$\bar{x}$	−136	−242	−186
$\sigma^2(x)$	0.18	0.14	0.15	$\sigma^2(x)$	167	319	247
p (two-tailed)	1.6%1	0.88%1	0.012%1	p (two-tailed)	14%	17%	3.9%1

[1] $\mathbf{H_0}$is rejected for probability values less than 5% (paired t-test).
Whereby the two slopes and offsets in Eqs. (1) and (2) are equal $m_{FT}=m_{WT}$ and $n_{FT}=n_{WT}$ across subjects (inter-subject variability). Left table: The mean normalized difference of the two slopes Δm^* and its standard deviation. Left table: The mean difference of the two offsets and its standard deviation. No data were discarded.

is simply a corollary of the real optimization, that of maximizing responsivity to a visual command, rather than an optimization of grip impedance *per se*, to the differences in mechanical constraints between FT and WT. On the other hand, the signal-dependent noise of the corresponding sensors (viz. the Golgi tendon organs) increases with their activation, and will therefore increase its effect on fingertip force. Conclusively, we can only clarify to some extent and not with significance if the found difference is actively optimized or just passively caused by a bent wrist.

All in all, of course static grip stiffness is linearly related to grip force, caused by the exponential stiffness of tendon tissue. But by changing the kinematics of our grip—and thus just changing the force transfer function from muscle to finger—one can actively change the increase of stiffness with force by flexing our wrist and thus change the stability of the grip. In that it is highly relevant that, in our experiments, low stiffness values were obtained when holding objects of different weights rather than exerting a predefined force—a natural task, which we likely have learned to solve at minimal cost.

Acknowledgments

We wish to thank the reviewers, whose competency highly improved the quality of this work, for their constructive and helpful suggestions. The authors confirm all the PLOS ONE policies on sharing data and materials and will make them freely available upon request.

Author Contributions

Conceived and designed the experiments: HH JM PvdS. Performed the experiments: HH. Analyzed the data: HH JM PvdS. Contributed reagents/materials/analysis tools: HH JM PvdS. Wrote the paper: HH JM PvdS. Designed the software used in analysis: HH.

References

1. Edin BB, Westling G, Johannson RS (1992) Independent control of human finger-tip forces at individual digits during precision lifting. The Journal of Physiology 450: 547–564.
2. Johannson RS, Westling G (1984) Roles of glabrous skin receptors and sensorimotor memory in automatic control of precision grip when lifting rougher or more slippery objects. Experimental Brain Research 56: 550–554.
3. Forssberg H, Eliasson A, Kinoshita H, Johansson R, Westling G (1991) Development of human precision grip. i: Basic coordination of force. Experimental Brain Research 85(2): 451–457.
4. Flanagan JR, Wing AM (1993) Modulation of grip force with load force during point-to-point arm movements. Experimental Brain Research 95: 131–143.
5. Flanagan JR, Wing AM (1995) The stability of precision grip forces during cyclic arm movements with a hand-held load. Experimental Brain Research 105: 455–464.
6. Kinoshita H, Kawai S, Ikuta K, Teraoka T (1996) Individual finger forces acting on a grasped object during shaking actions. Ergonomics 39: 243–256.
7. Flanagan JR, Tresilian JR (1994) Grip-load force coupling: A general control strategy for transporting objects. The Journal of Experimental Psychology: Human Perception and Performance 20: 944–957.
8. Zatsiorsky VM, Gao F, Latash ML (2006) Prehension stability: experiments with expanding and contracting handle. J Neurophysiology 95: 2513–29.
9. Höppner H, Lakatos D, Urbanek H, Castellini C, van der Smagt P (2011) The grasp perturbator: Calibrating human grasp stiffness during a graded force task. In: Proc. ICRA|International Conference on Robotics and Automation. pp. 3312–3316. doi:10.1109/ICRA.2011.5980217.
10. Van Doren C (1998) Grasp stiffness as a function of grasp force and finger span. Motor Control 2: 352–378.
11. Hajian AZ, Howe RD (1997) Identification of the mechanical impedance at the human finger tip. Journal of Biomechanical Engineering 119: 109–114.
12. Carter RR, Crago PE, Keith MW (1990) Stiffness regulation by reflex action in the normal human hand. J Neurophysiol 64: 105–18.
13. Carter RR, Crago PE, Gorman PH (1993) Nonlinear stretch reflex interaction during cocontraction. J Neurophysiol 69: 943–52.
14. Brand P, Hollister A (1999) Clinical Mechancis of the Hand. Mosby, 369 pp.
15. Hill AV (1938) The heat of shortening and the dynamic constants of muscle. Proceedings of the Royal Society of London Series B - Biological Sciences 126: 136–195.
16. O'Driscoll SW, Horii E, Ness R, Cahalan TD, Richards RR, et al. (1992) The relationship between wrist position, grasp size, and grip strength. The Journal of Hand Surgery 17: 169–177.
17. White O, Thonnard J, Wing A, Bracewell R, Diedrichsen J, et al. (2011) Grip force regulates hand impedance to optimize object stability in high impact loads. J Neuroscience 189.
18. Tarkka IM, Larsen TA (1986) Short and long latency reflex responses elicited by electrical and mechanical stimulation in human hand muscle. Acta Physiologica Scandinavica 128: 71–76.
19. Allum J, Mauritz K (1984) Compensation for intrinsic muscle stiffness by short-latency reexes in human triceps surae muscles. Journal of Neurophysiology 52: 797–818.
20. Shadmehr R, Arbib M (1992) A mathematical analysis of the force-stiffness characteristics of muscles in control of a single joint system. Biological cybernetics 66: 463–477.
21. Mandel J (1984) The Statistical Analysis of Experimental Data. Courier Dover Publications Inc., 432 pp.
22. de Vaus D (2002) Analyzing Social Science Data: 50 Key Problems in Data Analysis. London: Sage Publications Inc., 402 pp.
23. Zatsiorsky VM, Gao F, Latash ML (2005) Motor control goes beyond physics: differential effects of gravity and inertia on finger forces during manipulation of hand-held objects. Experimental Brain Research 162: 300–308.
24. Mussa-Ivaldi F, Hogan N, Bizzi E (1985) Neural, mechanical, and geometric factors subserving arm posture in humans. The Journal of Neuroscience 5: 2732–2743.
25. Milner T, Franklin D (1998) Characterization of multijoint finger stiffness: dependence on finger posture and force direction. Biomedical Engineering, IEEE Transactions on 45: 1363–1375.
26. Hogan N (1985) The mechanics of multi-joint posture and movement control. Biological Cybernetics 52: 315–331.
27. Rancourt D, Hogan N (2001) Dynamics of pushing. J Mot Behav 33: 351–362.

6

Striatal Pre-Enkephalin Overexpression Improves Huntington's Disease Symptoms in the R6/2 Mouse Model of Huntington's Disease

Stéphanie Bissonnette[1], Mylène Vaillancourt[1], Sébastien S. Hébert[1,2], Guy Drolet[1,2], Pershia Samadi[1,2]*

1 Axe Neurosciences, Centre de recherche du CHU de Québec, CHUL, Québec, Canada, **2** Département de psychiatrie et de neurosciences, Université Laval, Québec, Canada

Abstract

The reduction of pre-enkephalin (pENK) mRNA expression might be an early sign of striatal neuronal dysfunction in Huntington's disease (HD), due to mutated huntingtin protein. Indeed, striatopallidal (pENK-containing) neurodegeneration occurs at earlier stage of the disease, compare to the loss of striatonigral neurons. However, no data are available about the functional role of striatal pENK in HD. According to the neuroprotective properties of opioids that have been recognized recently, the objective of this study was to investigate whether striatal overexpression of pENK at early stage of HD can improve motor dysfunction, and/or reduce striatal neuronal loss in the R6/2 transgenic mouse model of HD. To achieve this goal recombinant adeno-associated-virus (rAAV2)-containing green fluorescence protein (GFP)-pENK was injected bilaterally in the striatum of R6/2 mice at 5 weeks old to overexpress opioid peptide pENK. Striatal injection of rAAV2-GFP was used as a control. Different behavioral tests were carried out before and/or after striatal injections of rAAV2. The animals were euthanized at 10 weeks old. Our results demonstrate that striatal overexpression of pENK had beneficial effects on behavioral symptoms of HD in R6/2 by: delaying the onset of decline in muscular force; reduction of clasping; improvement of fast motor activity, short-term memory and recognition; as well as normalization of anxiety-like behavior. The improvement of behavioral dysfunction in R6/2 mice having received rAAV2-GFP-pENK associated with upregulation of striatal pENK mRNA; the increased level of enkephalin peptide in the striatum, globus pallidus and substantia nigra; as well as the slight increase in the number of striatal neurons compared with other groups of R6/2. Accordingly, we suggest that at early stage of HD upregulation of striatal enkephalin might play a key role at attenuating illness symptoms.

Editor: Philipp J. Kahle, Hertie Institute for Clinical Brain Research and German Center for Neurodegenerative Diseases, Germany

Funding: This work was supported by start-up grant from CHUQ, and faculty of medicine at Laval University to PS. The funders had no role in study design, data collection and analysis, decision to publish, or preparation of the manuscript.

Competing Interests: The authors have declared that no competing interests exist.

* E-mail: Pershia.samadi@fmed.ulaval.ca

Introduction

Huntington's disease (HD) is a dominant inherited neurodegenerative disease characterized by motor, cognitive and psychiatric symptoms including depression, weight loss and dementia. The disease is caused by a CAG trinucleotide expansion in the exon 1 of the huntingtin gene, which is translated into polyglutamine in the N-terminal region of HD protein [1,2]. When the number of CAG repeats is more than 36, mutant huntingtin aggregates in the nuclei and can disrupt transcriptional factors leading to neurodegeneration [3]. Although the mutated huntingtin protein is expressed ubiquitously throughout the brain, the most striking neurodegenerative changes are first observed preferentially in striatal medium spiny neurons [4–6]. However, the reason of this early vulnerability is not yet well known.

The opioid system which is directly involved in many physiological effects, such as analgesia, reward, learning, memory and mood [7] is mainly present in the basal ganglia. The striatum, the input structure of the basal ganglia, and the site of interaction between dopamine (DA) and glutamate, is among the brain regions with the highest levels of opioid receptors (μ, δ, κ) and opioid peptides pre-enkephalin (pENK) and pre-dynorphin (pDYN), the precursors of enkephalin and dynorphin, respectively [8,9]. Evidence gathered from neurochemical and pharmacological studies point to an important role of opioid peptides in the balanced and/or coordinated activity of the striatal output pathways in pathological conditions such as Parkinson's disease [10–13]. Moreover, the neuroprotective properties of opioids have been recognized recently [14]. Activation of δ opioid receptors (δORs) has been shown to have neuroprotective effect against cerebral ischemia in rats [15–18]. In addition, opioid-mediated signaling is implicated in cell survival [19–21], and in protection of motor networks during perinatal ischemia [22]. *In vitro* and *in vivo* enhanced survival of DAergic neurons after neurotoxin exposure [21], and even neuroprotection against mitochondrial respiratory chain injury [23] have also been demonstrated. Other studies provided evidence of higher survival of intrastriatal grafted DAergic neurons treated with an enkephalin analog in a rodent model of PD [24].

Interestingly, an early sign of neuronal dysfunction in HD is the reduction of pENK mRNA expression due to mutated huntingtin protein [25–27]. Indeed, GABAergic striatopallidal (pENK-containing) neurons are more vulnerable to neurodegeneration and their loss has been seen at earlier stage of disease, even at presymptomatic stage, compared to the loss of striatonigral (pDYN-containing) neurons [25–27]. The pENK mRNA expression is reduced in surviving neurons at presymptomatic stage of HD [26–28]. However, no data are available about the role of striatal pENK in the basal ganglia motor circuit in HD. The objective of our investigation was to identify whether striatal pENK up-regulation can improve behavioral dysfunction in transgenic mice model of HD, and/or reduce or delay striatal neuronal loss. Among the transgenic mouse models, the R6/2 line is considered as a mainstay of HD research because of its rapid and reproducible progression of HD-like symptomatology including: progressive striatal neuronal loss; decline in weight gain and muscular force from 9 weeks of age; onset of abnormal dystonic limb movement (clasping) at 4 weeks; reduction in fast activity as early as 6 weeks indicating that movement speed appears to be a more sensitive measure of decline in locomotor activity compared with distance traveled alone; deficits in motor performance and coordination as early as 6 weeks; and cognitive decline [29–31]. In this study, we used *in vivo* novel technology using viral vector gene transfer to overexpress pENK in striatal neurons of the transgenic R6/2 mouse model of HD. Our results provide the first evidence that striatal overexpression of pENK has beneficial effects in the improvement of behavioral dysfunction in R6/2 mouse model of HD, as manifested by delay in decline of limb muscular force, reduction of abnormal clasping movement, increase of fast motor activity, normalization of anxiety-like behavior, and alleviation of different cognitive performances. The observed behavioral improvement has not been accompanied by the rescue of decline in striatal volume. However, a slight improvement of striatal neuronal number was observed five weeks following pENK gene delivery compared with other groups of R6/2.

Materials and Methods

Viral vector construction

The construction of rAAV2-GFP-pENK and rAAV2-GFP (control) plasmids, and the generation of adeno-associated viruses (AAVs, serotype 2/2), was carried out at Gene Transfer Vector Core, University of Iowa (www.uiowa.edu/gene/). Briefly, the full-length cDNA sequence of rat pENK (Y07503) was subcloned into the *ClaI* and *XhoI* sites of the pFBAAVmU6mcsIRESeGFP plasmid. Positive clones were verified by sequencing, and pENK (and eGFP) expression was validated in cells. The virus was then generated and purified as previously described [32,33].

Animals

The experiments were performed using male mutant gene carrier (R6/2) and wild type (WT) mice from the same breeding colony (B6CBATg(HDexon1)62Gpb/3J) maintained at the animal care facility in accordance with the standards of the Canadian Council on Animal Care. The breeders, males and ovary-transplanted females, were from the same strain, obtained from a line maintained at The Jackson Laboratory (Bar Harbor, ME, USA) involving a C57BL/6 and CBA background. The genotype and CAG repeat lengths expressed by offspring was determined by Laragen (Culver City, CA, USA). The number of CAG repeats in transgenic mice was 115–125. All animal experiments were accomplished under the guidelines of the Canadian Guide for the Care and Use of Laboratory Animals, and all procedures were approved by the Institutional Animal Care Committee of Laval University. Mice were weighed once a week. All behavioral protocols were performed during the light phase at the same time of the day.

Experimental design

The study involved a wild type (WT) group and R6/2 littermates carrying mutant huntingtin protein. The latter were randomized into 3 groups: Intact R6/2 mice which received no treatment, R6/2 mice having received striatal rAAV2-GFP (GFP), or rAAV2-GFP-pENK. All striatal injections were performed at 5 weeks of age. The mice were euthanized at 10 weeks and the brains were processed for post-mortem experiments.

Stereotaxic injection of adeno-associated virus

Following anesthesia with ketamine (100 mg/kg, intraperitoneally; ip) and xylazine (10-mg/kg, ip), the head of 5 weeks old R6/2 mice was fixed in a stereotaxic frame (Kopf Instruments, CA, USA). Bilateral injection of rAAV2-GFP as a control or rAAV2-GFP-pENK was made directly into the striatum at coordinate relative to bregma: anterior/posterior 0.62 mm, lateral/medial 1.8 mm, and 3.5 mm ventral to the dura mater [34]. Microinjections were performed using a 5 µl Hamilton syringe with a 30 gauge bevel needle. A total injection volume of 3 µl was delivered to the striatum in each hemisphere with an infusion rate of 0.1 µl/min. After injection, the needle remained in place for an additional 10 minutes to allow the diffusion of rAAV2- vectors and then it was slowly withdrawn.

Behavioral characterization

Grip Strength. The muscular force of experimental mice was weekly evaluated using the Grip Strength from week 4 of age. The apparatus (Columbus Instruments, Columbus, OH, USA) can measure the peak tension (T-PK) exerted instinctively by a mouse as the examiner attempts to pull it off from a wire mesh grid by gently dragging at the base of the tail [30]. The device provides a digital readout of maximal force generated, expressed in grams (g). During each weekly observation, a given mouse underwent 7 successive trials, with 5 to 10 seconds-intertrial intervals on the table. The mean T-PK of at least 5 successful trials, produced by all limbs was calculated and analyzed.

All behavioral apparatus were cleaned out with 70% ethanol after each test for each mouse. The observer was blind to genotype and treatment for all behavioral assessments.

Clasping Score. Clasping behavior was evaluated and scored as a semi-quantitative measure of limb dystonia [30]. Limb movements were videotaped when mice were suspended by the tail at a height of at least 30 cm for 20 seconds, followed by a brief touchdown and a subsequent suspension for another 20 seconds. Clasping was defined as a retraction of a limb towards the body and rated by an observer unaware of experimental groups. The extent of clasping at each limb was graded as follows: None = 0; mild = 0.25, when the fore- or hind- limb retracted toward the midline but did not reach the midline and the contraction was not sustained; moderate = 0.5, a high amplitude limb traction to or beyond the midline, but not sustained; severe and constant = 0.75, a high amplitude limb retraction sustained for more than 15 seconds. Fore- and hind- limbs clasping behavior was summed for each animal for a maximal clasping score of 3. The scores from the two tail suspension trials were then averaged and recorded.

Open field. Spontaneous locomotor activity of mice was examined weekly in an open field (50×50 cm square), from 4 weeks of age, using a video tracking system (Videotrack, Viewpoint Life Sciences, Montreal, Canada) with infrared backlighting [30,35]. The system is able to analyse locomotor activity into different velocities as follows: slow movements (< 5 cm/sec); moderate movements (between 5-20 cm/sec); or fast movements (> 20 cm/sec). Total distance traveled by the animal during the 2 hours testing period, as well as the duration and distance covered at each velocity were measured. Locomotor activities were monitored continuously over the testing period, with output intervals of 3 minutes. A habituation session of 10 minutes preceded the locomotor activity monitoring when mouse was placed in the open field.

Elevated plus maze. The elevated-plus-maze was used to evaluate anxiety-like behaviors in experimental animals. The apparatus consisted of two open arms (each 44 cm×10 cm) and two closed arms of the same dimensions that extended from a common central platform (10 cm×10 cm). The maze was raised 90 cm above the floor under normal ambient overhead lighting conditions. Video-tracking system (ANY-MAZE, Stoelting) was used for the behavioral assessment in elevated plus maze. Mice at 8 weeks old were placed individually in the center square facing an open arm and allowed to explore the maze for 5 min. An arm entry was counted when all four paws were inside the arm. Exit from an arm was defined as when both forepaws left that arm. The time spent in the closed and open arms, the number of entries into the open and closed arms was tracked. Percent of time spent in open arm (time spent in the open arms as a proportion of time spent in all four arms) and percent of entries to open arm (entries to open arm as a proportion of total entries to all four arms) were used for analyses.

Barnes maze. Memory and learning were also evaluated using the Barnes maze [36,37]. The maze consists of a circular platform (92 cm diameter) surrounded by 20 holes (5 cm diameter, equidistant), one providing an escape. The mouse was placed in a dark chamber in the center of the maze and aversive stimuli subsequently activated (bright light and noise). Prior to the first trial, each mouse was introduced to an adaptation period on day 1, in which it was conducted to the target hole allowing the escape box for 1 min. In the acquisition phase, mouse was subjected to 4 trials per day with an inter-trial interval of 20 min for four consecutive days. Each trial ended when the mouse entered the goal escape tunnel or for a maximum of 3 minutes. The reference memory phase or probe trials were conducted on the 5th day and 12th day following the first trials in order to test short- and long-term retention memory, respectively. During the probe trials, the escape route was removed and replaced with a standard hole through which the animal could not enter. The mouse was tested during a 90 seconds period. The time required to find the target hole was recorded as the primary latency using the ANY-MAZE video tracking system. Spatial cues with distinct shapes were placed around the maze and kept constant throughout the experiment.

Novel object recognition. Mice either at 4 or 9 weeks of age were used for the novel object recognition test. The test was carried out in the same experimental apparatus as described for open field. In order to investigate novel object recognition in mice at 9 weeks of life, an experimentally naïve batch of mice, including all experimental groups was introduced. During training, two identical objects were introduced to mice and they were allowed to explore them for 5 minutes. The objects were cleaned with ethanol 70% between trials to minimize olfactory cues. The first recognition test carried out one hour after the training. In this first trial which lasted for 5 minutes one of the objects were substituted for a novel one (new) while the other remained unchanged (familiar). The second trial was performed 24 hours after training in which the novel object was again replaced with a novel object of a different shape and the animal was allowed to explore them during 5 minutes. Movements were recorded by video-tracking system (ANY-MAZE, Stoelting). Results are expressed in percent of the time to visit the new object, defined as the time spent exploring the new object/total time exploring new plus familiar objects.

Tissue Preparation for post-mortem analyses

Five weeks after rAAV2- injections (i.e. at the end of week 10), animals were deeply anaesthetized, perfused transcardially with RNAse free 0.9% heparinized saline followed by 4% paraformaldehyde in phosphate buffer and then decapitated. Brains were extracted, postfixed in 4% PFA for 48 hours, and passed sequentially through 15% and 30% phosphate buffered sucrose solutions. Brains were then cut into 40 μm coronal sections using a freezing microtome and free-floating sections were collected serially in 6 vials containing phosphate-buffered saline (0.1M PBS, pH 7.4).

Immunofluorescence

In order to verify the site of injections, brain sections were submitted to GFP-DAPI double immunofluorescence staining and investigated under a fluorescent microscope. One set of brain sections from each animal were blocked in PBS containing 5% bovine serum albumin (BSA) and 0.3% Triton X-100 for 30 min. The sections were then incubated overnight at 4°C with the primary antibody, rabbit anti-GFP (1:1000; Invitrogen) in PBS containing 2% BSA and 0.1% Triton X-100. Following 3 washes in PBS, fluorescent rabbit secondary antiserum (Alexa Fluor 488, 1:500; Invitrogen) was added at room temperature for one hour, followed by DAPI (1:1000, Invitrogen) staining for 5 minutes. After last wash in PBS, the sections were mounted and then coverslipped with PermaFluor™ Aqueous Mounting Medium (Thermo Scientific).

In situ hybridization

One set of brain sections from each animal were processed for *in situ* hybridizations under RNAase-free conditions. The sections were hybridized with [^{35}S]UTP radiolabelled cRNA probes for detection of pENK mRNAs. The pENK probe (935 bp, from nucleotide −104 to 830) was generated from the linearized rat cDNA contained in pSP64 (antisense) and pSP65 (sense) plasmids [38]. The pENK cDNA template was linearized with *Eco*RI restriction enzyme, and the antisense probe was synthesized with [^{35}S]UTP and T7 RNA polymerase [39].

Briefly, hybridization technique was performed as follows: after short fixation of 5 minutes in 4% PFA/PBS, free-floating sections were washed in PBS and incubated for 10 minutes in proteinase K/PBS, followed by second fixation in 4% PFA/PBS during 10 minutes. After washing with PBS and ddH2O, sections were incubated for 10 minutes in 0.25% acetic anhydride in 2% triethanolamine, and then washed in saline-sodium citrate (SSC) for 5 minutes. *In situ* hybridization was done at 58°C overnight in a standard hybridization buffer containing 50% formamide as previously described [30,40]. Following stringency washes, sections were mounted onto Superfrost plus slides, air-dried and dehydrated during 2 minutes in 30%, 60%, and 100% ethanol. The slide-mounted tissue sections were then air-dried and exposed to radioactive sensitive films (Kodak, Biomax MR, New Haven, CT), together with ^{14}C standard slides (American Radiolabeled Chemicals, Inc., St Louis), during 21 to 24 hours at room temperature. Films were scanned and analysis of striatum (divided in four subregions along a medial-lateral and dorso-ventral axis) was performed using public domain National Institutes of Health image analysis software (NIH ImageJ, Bethesda, MD), normalizing optical density using the corpus callosum as a reference for background activity.

Immunohistochemistry

One set of coronal brain sections were submitted to NeuN immunostaining. Following incubation in $NaBH_4$ (0.5% w/v) for 20 minutes, the sections were incubated in TBS solution containing 0.5% Triton X-100 and 0.03% H_2O_2 during 30 minutes. Sections were then blocked in solution containing 10% bovine serum albumin (BSA), 0.3% Triton X-100, and 5% normal goat serum (NGS) in TBS for 30 min at room temperature. Sections were then probed for 48 to 72 hours at 4°C with mouse NeuN monoclonal antibody (Invitrogen) diluted to 1:500 in TBS solution containing 2% BSA, 0.1% Triton X-100, and 2% NGS. They were then placed for 1 hour at room temperature in a solution containing biotinylated goat anti-mouse IgG (1:400, Jackson immune-research) and subsequently incubated in the TBS solution containing avidin–biotin peroxidase complex (Vectastain Elite ABC Kit; Vector Laboratories, Burlington, ON), for 1 hour at room temperature. All steps were followed by appropriate washes in TBS. Finally, the reaction was developed in 3,3′-diaminobenzidine tetrahydrochloride (DAB) solution (Sigma, St. Louis, MO) and 0.1% of 30% hydrogen peroxide (Sigma, St. Louis, MO) at room temperature. Following the DAB reaction, sections were mounted out of distilled water onto slides, air-dried, counterstained with 0.1% cresyl violet (Sigma, St. Louis, MO) (Nissl stain), dehydrated in ascending grades of ethanol, cleaned in xylene, and coverslipped with DPX (BDH Laboratories Supply), and kept until stereological quantification.

Enkephalin immunohistochemistry on free floating brain sections has also been used to estimate the intensity of enkephalin immunoreactivity in the striatum and the density of enkephalin containing striatal fibers [41], using rabbit leucine-enkephalin antibody (Immunostar, 1:10000) and biotinylated donkey anti-rabbit IgG (1:2000, Jackson immune-research). The reaction was developed in DAB solution and 0.1% of 30% hydrogen peroxide as described above. The sections were then mounted on slides, air-dried, and after dehydration in ascending grades of ethanol, they were cleaned in xylene, and coverslipped with DPX. Image analysis of enkephalin immunoreactivity at striatal levels, globus pallidus (GP) and substantia nigra (SN) was performed using public domain National Institutes of Health image analysis software (NIH ImageJ, Bethesda, MD). Optical densities were normalized to the respective white matter (e.g. corpus callosum, internal capsule as a reference for background activity) on each section.

Stereology

Unbiased stereology was carried out on NeuN-Nissl stained coronal sections using the Stereo Investigator program (Microbrightfield, USA; V6) and a Nikon Eclipse 80i microscope equipped with a motorized XYZ stage. The optical fractionator was used to obtain unbiased estimates of the total number of neurons. The striatum was delineated according to defined boundaries [30,42] using a stereotaxic atlas of the mouse brain [34]. Briefly, the selection includes levels throughout the striatum including regularly spaced sections caudal and rostral to the decussation of the anterior commissure. The dorsal, medial and lateral limits of the striatum are well defined [34]. Ventrally, the striatum interfaces with the amygdala and substantia innominata in its postcommissural part and with the nucleus accumbens in its precommissural division. The ventral limit of the striatum at the postcommissural part is well delineated on NeuN-Nissl stains. However, the ventral limit of the striatum at its precommissural part is an arbitrary interface. At the precommissural levels analyzed, we therefore delimit the dorsal striatum from the nucleus accumbens with a line that extends from above the ventral most part of the lateral ventricle medially, to the tapered external capsule laterally, at an angle of 25–30° below the axial plane. Section thickness was assessed and neuronal counts were performed under oil immersion using a 60× Plan Apo objective lens (1.40/0.17 DIC N2). The Cavalieri method was used to measure the striatal volume. The systemic random sampling grid size was 500×500 μm and the optical fractionator brick size was 80×80 μm. Neurons were defined as NeuN positive profiles measuring at least 5 μm in diameter. Glial cells are distinct as Nissl positive cells with diameter less than 7 μm, or Nissl positive cells with diameter more than 7 μm, light violet staining, and irregular shape as probable activated glia. The investigator was blind to the mouse treatment.

Statistical analyses

Statistical analysis of data in behavioral and post-mortem experiments between WT and different groups of R6/2 mice were carried out by two-way or one-way analysis of variance (ANOVA) followed by *post hoc* analysis using Bonferroni and Dunn test (Stat-View, Abacus Corporation, Baltimore, MD, USA). Data are presented as a mean ± SEM. A *p*-value <0.01 was considered to be significant for all Bonferroni and Dunn *post hoc* analysis.

Results

The site of injections

Representative images of the site of injection of rAAV2- in the striatum, revealed by GFP-DAPI double labeling, compared to the schematic of the mouse brain (adapted from the atlas of Franklin and Paxinos, 2008), are presented in Figure 1.

It should be noted that only mice with proper injection site were included in analysis.

Striatal pENK mRNA expression

Representative autoradiograms of striatal pENK mRNA (*in situ* hybridization), compared to the schematic of the mouse brain are presented in Figure 1.Two-way ANOVA detected significant difference between different groups in the expression of striatal pENK mRNA, without any difference between right and left striatum [$F(\text{treatment})_{3,31} = 29.42$, $p<0.0001$; $F(\text{right vs. left})_{1,31} = 0.11$, $p = 0.73$, and $F(\text{treatment} \times \text{right vs. left})_{3,31} = 0.10$, $p = 0.96$] [R6/2: intact (n = 5), GFP- (n = 4), pENK (n = 5); WT: (n = 5)] (Fig. 2A, B). *Post hoc* analysis indicated that pENK mRNA expression was significantly increased in the striatum of R6/2 mice having received rAAV2-pENK compared with GFP-injected and intact R6/2 mice ($p<0.0001$ and $p<0.002$, respectively). Further analysis in each hemisphere noted significant difference in different striatal subregions between different groups in the right [lateral: $p = 0.0002$; medial: $p = 0.0002$; dorsal: $p = 0.0005$; ventral: $p<0.0001$], and left [lateral: $p = 0.0001$; medial: $p = 0.0007$; dorsal: $p = 0.0004$; ventral: $p<0.0001$] hemispheres. Although pENK mRNA is increased in lateral striatum of pENK-injected R6/2 mice compared with GPF group but this difference did not reach significance (right and left: $p>0.01$). The level of pENK mRNA in lateral striatum of WT mice was higher than different groups of R6/2 mice at right (intact: $p = 0.0004$, GFP: $p<0.0001$, pENK: $p = 0.002$) and left (intact: $p = 0.0001$, GFP: $p<0.0001$, pENK: $p = 0.0001$) hemispheres (Fig. 2A, B). At medial and dorsal subregions of the striatum, concentration of pENK mRNA was higher in mice having striatal overexpression of pENK compared with intact and GFP-injected R6/2 mice at right [medial (intact: $p = 0.0004$, GFP: $p = 0.002$); dorsal (intact: $p = 0.009$, GFP: $p = 0.001$)] and left [medial (intact: $p = 0.007$, GFP: $p = 0.0007$); dorsal (intact: $p = 0.01$, GFP: $p = 0.001$)] hemispheres. Interesting-

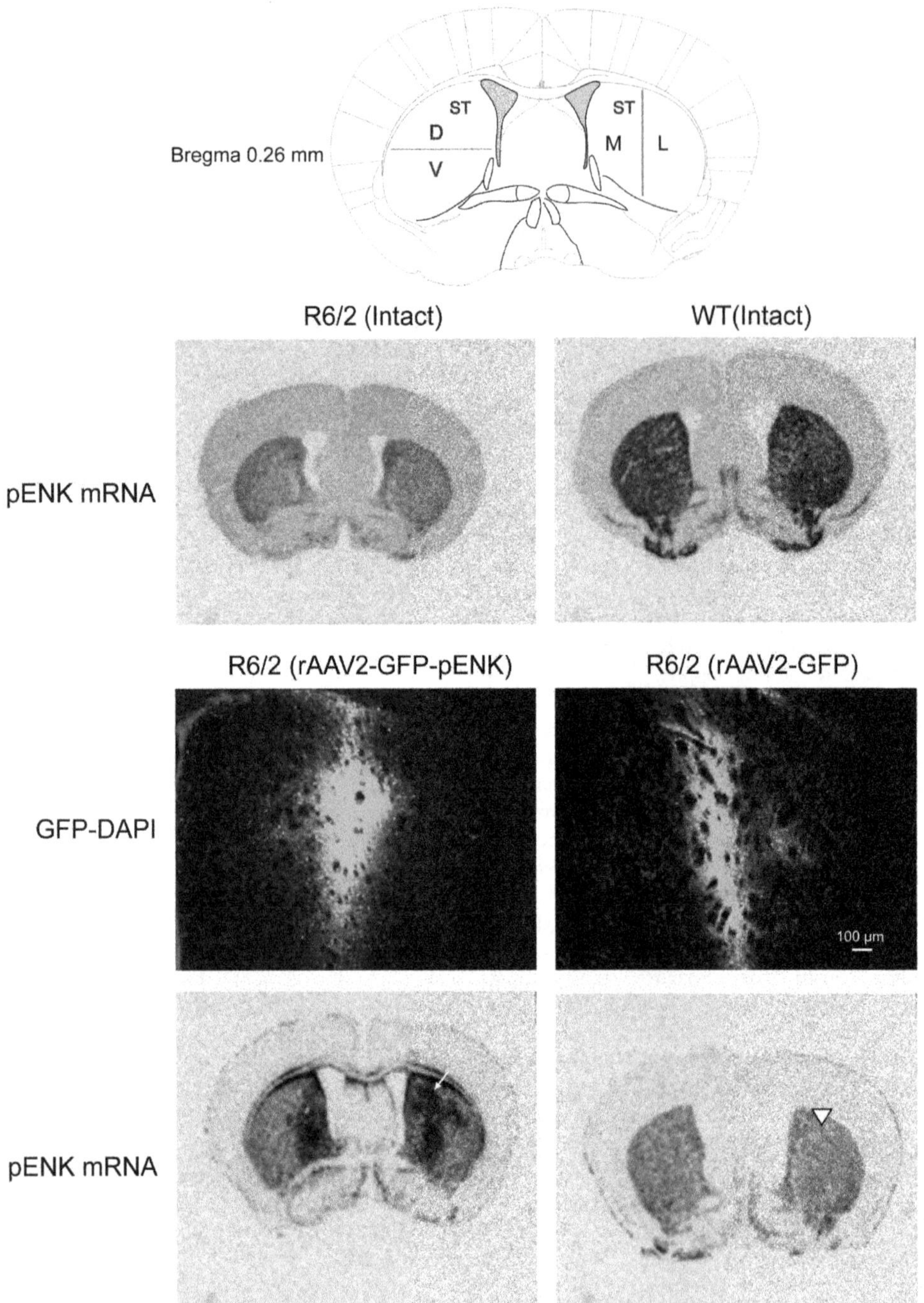

Figure 1. Representative images of the site of injection of rAAV2- in the striatum, revealed by GFP-DAPI double labeling, as well as representative autoradiograms of striatal pENK mRNA (*in situ* hybridization), compared to the schematic of the mouse brain (adapted from the atlas of Franklin and Paxinos, 2008). Arrow indicates the site of injection of rAAV2-GFP-pENK which corresponds to the overexpression of striatal pENK mRNA. Arrowhead indicates the site of injection of rAAV2-GFP without any changes in the expression of striatal pENK mRNA.

ly, no difference for the level of pENK mRNA was detected between WT and pENK-injected R6/2 mice at medial and dorsal striatum at right and left hemispheres. However, in WT mice pENK mRNA at medial and dorsal striatal subregions was higher than intact and GFP-injected R6/2 mice at right [medial (intact: $p = 0.0009$, GFP: $p = 0.0001$); dorsal (intact: $p = 0.001$, GFP: $p = 0.0002$)] and left [medial (intact: $p = 0.004$, GFP: $p = 0.0004$); dorsal (intact: $p = 0.001$, GFP: $p = 0.0002$)] hemispheres. No difference was observed between intact and GFP-injected R6/2 mice at medial and dorsal striatal subregions at right and left hemispheres (Fig. 2A, B). pENK mRNA is also increased in ventral striatal region of pENK-injected R6/2 mice compared with GPF- injected mice (right: $p = 0.005$; left: $p = 0.006$), but this increase did not reach significance compared with intact R6/2 group. In WT mice the concentration of pENK mRNA in ventral part of the striatum was higher than different R6/2 groups at right (intact: $p = 0.0002$, GFP: $p < 0.0001$, pENK: $p = 0.005$) and left (intact: $p = 0.0004$, GFP: $p < 0.0001$, pENK: $p = 0.002$) hemispheres (Fig. 2A, B).

Behavioral characterization

Behavioral assessments began at week 4, one week prior to the striatal delivery of rAAV2- (on week 5) to ensure that the behavioral alterations possibly observed in following weeks were not due to pre-existing differences among groups. In order to avoid the confounding effects of a given test on the performance of mice in another, the timing of the tests were carefully selected. Specially, Barnes maze and Novel object preference tests were carried out at least one week apart.

Weight gain

The animals were weighed once weekly and the average weight in each week was compared among groups. Significant differences were noted when different groups of mice were compared at different ages [$F(\text{groups})_{3,241} = 17.84$, $p < 0.0001$; $F(\text{age})_{6,241} = 17.37$, $p < 0.0001$, and $F(\text{groups} \times \text{age})_{18,241} = 2.01$, $p = 0.009$] [R6/2: intact (n = 11), GFP- (n = 4), pENK (n = 6); WT: (n = 17)]. *Post hoc* analysis showed a significant difference between: WT mice compared to the intact ($p < 0.0001$), GFP- ($p < 0.0001$), and pENK- ($p = 0.0002$) injected R6/2 groups; as well as pENK- R6/2 mice compared to GFP- injected group ($p = 0.01$). Further analysis demonstrated that the weight in all experimental groups was similar at 4 weeks of age ($p = 0.64$), however WT mice gained more weight over time compared to R6/2 groups (Fig. 3A). Moreover, striatal injection of rAAV2-GFP further accelerated the disturbance in weight gain of R6/2 mice over time, such that in these mice the failure in weight gain started from 8 weeks of age ($p = 0.01$ vs. WT), while weight gain was impaired in intact R6/2 mice from week 9 ($p = 0.001$ vs. WT). Interestingly, the decline in weight gain was delayed until week 10 in pENK- R6/2 mice compared to WT ($p = 0.0002$) (Fig. 3A).

Grip strength

The muscle force exerted by all limbs to grasp grid mesh was measured using Grip Strength. Tension peak (T-PK) forces were recorded and compared as a criterion for animal muscular strength. T-PK generated when mice held the wire grid mesh using all limbs was significantly different between groups at different ages [$F(\text{groups})_{3,241} = 23.08$, $P < 0.0001$; $F(\text{age})_{6,241} = 12.95$, $P < 0.0001$, and $F(\text{groups} \times \text{age})_{18,241} = 2.54$, $p = 0.0007$] [R6/2: intact (n = 13), GFP- (n = 4), pENK (n = 6); WT: (n = 17)]. *Post hoc* analysis noted greater muscular force in WT mice compared to intact ($p < 0.0001$), GFP- ($p < 0.0001$), and pENK- ($p = 0.005$) injected R6/2 mice. It is interesting to note that impaired grip strength was even more pronounced in GFP group than intact ($p = 0.01$), and pENK- ($p = 0.0001$) injected R6/2 groups. As illustrated in Figure 2B, one-way ANOVA followed by Bonferroni *post hoc* test detected a progressive impairment in muscular force of all limbs in all studied ages from week 6 to 10 in GFP-injected R6/2 group compared to WT ($p = 0.01$; $p < 0.0001$, respectively). Although GFP-injected R6/2 mice had an overall worse performance than intact R6/2 mice, but this difference did not reach significance at any ages. Compared with WT mice, the decline in all limbs force in intact R6/2 mice emerged at weeks 9 and 10 ($p = 0.005$ and $p < 0.0001$, respectively) (Fig. 3B). Interestingly, striatal overexpression of pENK had a beneficial impact on the muscular force of R6/2 mice by delaying the onset of decline in all limbs force. Indeed, the difference between pENK-injected R6/2 mice and WT was reached significant level only at week 10 ($p = 0.0001$). Moreover, the improvement of T-PK produced by all limbs in pENK-injected R6/2 mice was significant at weeks 6 and 7 compared with GFP-injected group ($p = 0.002$, $p = 0.01$, respectively), and at week 6 compared with intact R6/2 mice ($p = 0.005$) (Fig. 3B).

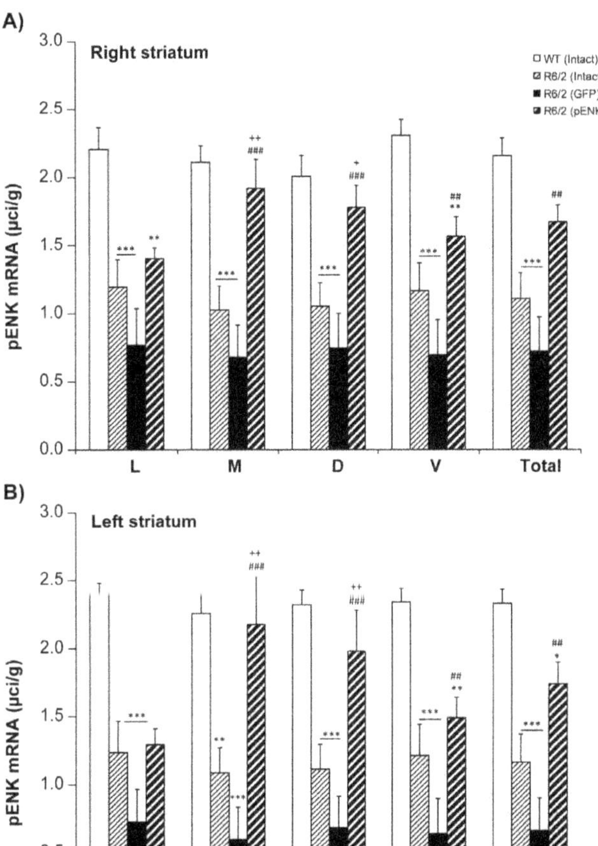

Figure 2. pENK mRNA expression in the striatum of different groups of R6/2 and WT mice. The level of pENK mRNA was increased in right (A) and left (B) striatum (total) of R6/2 mice having received striatal injection of rAAV2-pENK compared with intact and GFP-injected R6/2 mice. Moreover, upregulation of pENK mRNA was evident in all striatal subregions of pENK-injected mice compared with GFP-injected R6/2. The increased expression of pENK mRNA was more pronounced in medial and dorsal parts of the striatum. Indeed, in the medial and dorsal striatum no difference was observed between pENK-injected R6/2 mice and WT. L: lateral; M: medial; D: dorsal; V: ventral regions of the striatum. Data are presented as mean ± SEM. ** $p < 0.005$, *** $p < 0.0005$ vs. WT; ## $p < 0.005$, ### $p < 0.0005$ vs. R6/2 (GFP). + $p < 0.05$, ++ $p < 0.005$, +++ $p < 0.0005$ vs. intact R6/2.

Clasping phenotype

Clasping was scored as a dystonic movement illustrated by the abnormal retraction of limbs toward the body. Two way ANOVA showed a difference for involuntary clasping scores between different groups of mice at different ages [$F(\text{groups})_{3,204} = 66.52$, $P < 0.0001$; $F(\text{age})_{6,204} = 12.61$, $p < 0.0001$, and $F(\text{groups} \times \text{age})_{18,204} = 3.63$, $p < 0.0001$] [R6/2: intact (n = 8), GFP- (n = 4), pENK (n = 6); WT: (n = 15)]. *Post hoc* analysis noted a difference between WT and each of R6/2 groups ($p < 0.0001$). In addition, clasping score was different between pENK-injected R6/2 mice compared with intact ($p = 0.01$), and GFP- ($p = 0.0002$) mice. Further analysis using one way ANOVA followed by

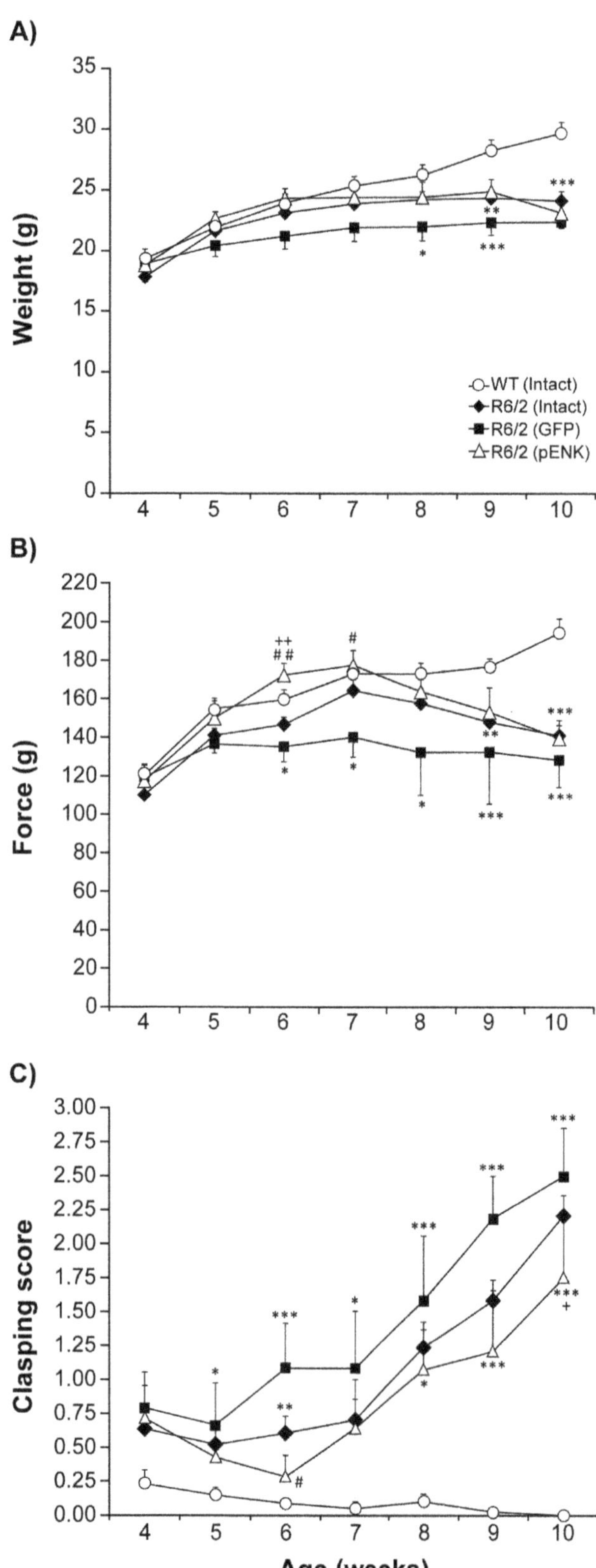

Figure 3. Weight, muscular force, and abnormal clasping movement of different groups of R6/2 mice and WT at different ages. At week 10, all groups of R6/2 mice displayed significantly lower weights compared to their WT counterparts. However, the failure in weight gain started sooner in R6/2 mice having received striatal rAAV2-GFP compared with pENK-injected mice. Interestingly, the decline in weight gain was delayed until week 10 in pENK- R6/2 mice compared to WT (A). The muscle force was recorded for all for- and hind- limbs as tension-peak (T-PK) to grasp grid mesh, using Grip Strength. GFP-injected R6/2 mice had an overall worse performance than other R6/2 mice. However, striatal overexpression of pENK improved the muscular force of R6/2 mice and delayed considerably the onset of decline in all limbs force (B). Higher clasping score was observed in GFP-injected R6/2 mice at different ages. However, striatal overexpression of pENK delayed the onset of this abnormal movement until week 8 compared with WT. Moreover, clasping score in pENK-injected R6/2 mice was less than GFP- injected group at 6-old-week (C). Data are presented as mean ± SEM. ** $p<0.01$, and *** $p<0.0001$ vs. WT; + $p<0.01$ vs. R6/2 (Intact); # $p<0.01$, ## $p<0.01$, ### $p<0.005$ vs. R6/2 (GFP).

Bonferroni *post hoc* test showed that clasping in intact and GFP-injected R6/2 mice was higher than WT littermates from week 5 ($p=0.01$) and then progressively increased with age until week 10 ($p<0.0001$) (Fig. 3C). Interestingly, the highest expression of abnormal clasping movement was observed in GFP-injected R6/2 mice at different ages (Fig. 3C). However, overexpression of pENK in the striatum delayed the onset of this abnormal movement until week 8 compared with WT ($p=0.01$). Moreover, the improvement of clasping movement in pENK-injected R6/2 mice was evident at weeks 6 compared with GFP-injected group ($p=0.01$), and at 10 weeks old compared with intact R6/2 mice ($p=0.01$) (Fig. 3C).

Locomotor activity in open field

Total distance travelled. When the total distance traveled during 2 hours was analyzed in terms of groups and age, a significant difference was observed between different groups of mice as well as their interaction [$F(\text{groups})_{3,258}=49.73$, $p<0.0001$; $F(\text{age})_{6,258}=1.33$, $p=0.24$, and $F(\text{groups}\times\text{age})_{18,258}=3.95$, $p<0.0001$] [R6/2: intact (n = 14 to 10), GFP- (n = 5 to 4), pENK (n = 6); WT: (n = 17)]. *Post hoc* analysis noted a difference between WT and each of R6/2 groups ($p<0.0001$). Further analysis showed that the total distance travelled during two hours was not different between different groups at weeks 4 and 5 ($F_{3,38}=0.09$, $p=0.97$; $F_{3,38}=0.07$, $p=0.98$, respectively) (Fig. 4A). However, a significant difference was observed between R6/2 mice and aged-matched WT mice from weeks 6 to 10 ($F_{3,38}=2.92$, $p=0.04$; $F_{3,31}=22.72$, $p<0.0001$, respectively). The reduction of distance travelled by intact R6/2 mice emerged at week 6 compared to WT control ($P=0.007$) and was sustained in all ages. The total distance travelled during two hours was also reduced from weeks 7 to 10 in R6/2 mice receiving either rAAV2-GFP ($p=0.0002$, $p<0.0001$) or rAAV2-GFP-pENK ($p=0.008$, $p<0.0001$) compared to age-matched WT mice. There was no difference among the R6/2 mice in various groups (Fig. 4A).

Distance travelled and time elapsed at various movement velocities. As movement with various velocities is differently affected in R6/2 mouse model of HD [30], different movement speeds were compared between different groups of mice.

A comparison of total distance traveled during fast activity from weeks 6 to 10 (as % of aged-matched WT) revealed a significant difference between different groups of R6/2 mice ($F_{2,22}=4.73$, $p=0.01$) (Fig. 4B). Indeed, *post hoc* analysis showed an improvement of fast activity in pENK-injected R6/2 mice (54% of WT) compared with GFP-injected group (14% of WT) ($p=0.007$). While the distance traveled during moderate (Fig. 4C) and slow (Fig. 4D) activity was higher in pENK-injected (59% and 88% of WT) compared with GFP- (36%, 69% of WT) and intact (44%, 77% of WT) R6/2 mice, however this difference did not reach significance ($F_{2,22}=1.70$, $p=0.21$ and $F_{2,22}=2.00$, $p=0.16$, respectively).

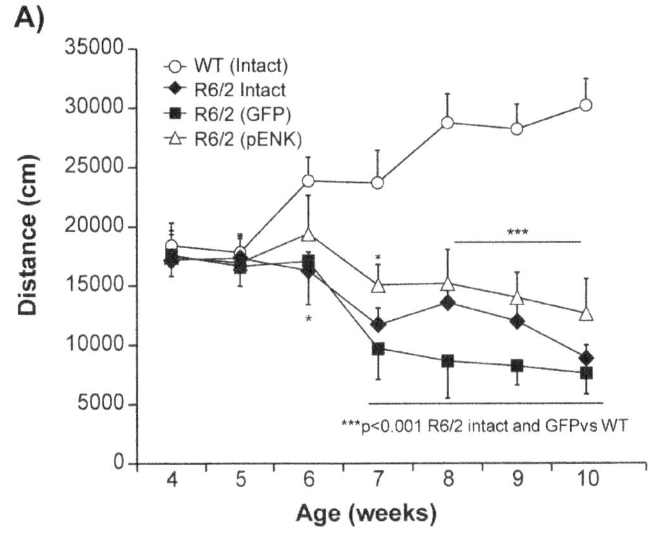

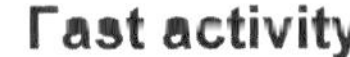

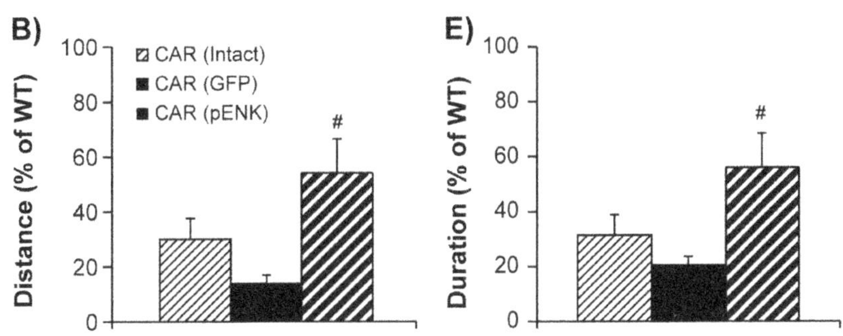

Moderate activity

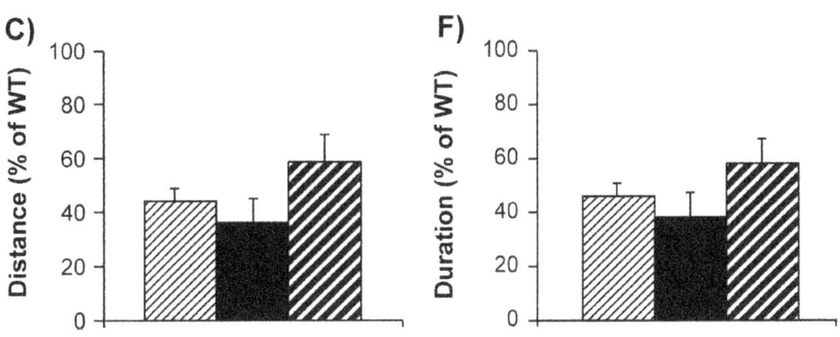

Slow activity

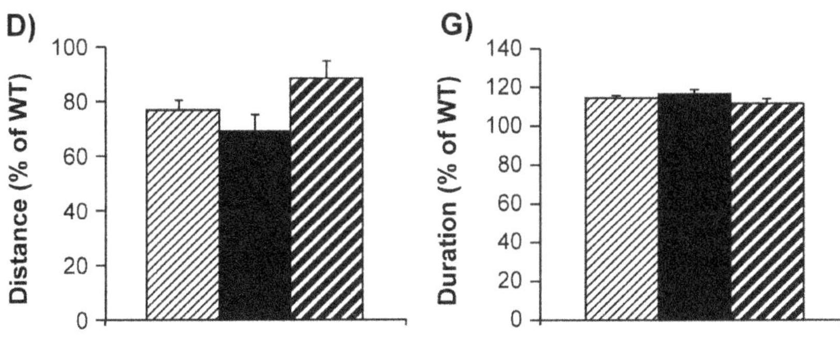

Figure 4. Spontaneous locomotor activity, distance travelled, and duration spent at various movement velocities in different groups of R6/2 mice compared with WT. The total distance traveled by mice in open field, during 2 hours, was reduced in different groups of R6/2 mice compared with WT (A). However, the reduction of locomotor activity was more pronounced in GFP-injected group. The distance (B) and duration of time (E) spent in fast speed was higher in pENK-injected compared with GFP-injected R6/2 mice. While the distance and duration of time spent in moderate speed (C, F) and slow speed (D, G) tended to be higher in pENK-injected R6/2 compared with other R6/2 groups, however this difference did not reach significance. Data are presented as mean ± SEM. * p<0.01, *** p<0.001 vs. WT; # p<0.01 vs. R6/2 (GFP).

The duration of time spent in fast speed (percent of aged-matched WT group) was significantly different between various groups of R6/2 mice ($F_{2,22} = 3.88$, $p = 0.03$). From weeks 6 to 10, R6/2 mice having received striatal rAAV2-GFP-pENK spent significantly longer time in fast activity (56% of WT) compared with rAAV2-GFP (21% of WT) R6/2 mice ($p = 0.01$) (Fig. 4E). While pENK-injected R6/2 mice (58% of WT) spent more time in moderate velocity than GFP- (38% of WT) and intact (46% of WT) groups (Fig. 4F), however this difference did not reach significance ($F_{2,22} = 1.21$, $p = 0.32$). No difference in time moving at slow velocity, from weeks 6 to 10, was observed between pENK-injected (112% of WT), GFP-injected (117% of WT), and intact (115% of WT) R6/2 mice ($F_{2,22} = 1.09$, p = 0.35) (Fig. 4G).

Elevated plus maze

The elevated plus maze was employed to assess the anxiety in different groups of R6/2 mice (Intact: n = 14; GFP: n = 4; pENK: n = 6) compared with WT (n = 17) at 8 weeks old (3 weeks after striatal rAAV2- injections). Statistical analysis detected a significant difference between various groups for percentage of entries ($F_{3,37} = 37.55$, $p<0.0001$) (Fig. 5A) and proportion of time ($F_{3,37} = 38.36$, $p<0.0001$) (Fig. 5B) spent in the open arm. Interestingly, irrespective of their treatments, all R6/2 mice (intact, GFP- and pENK-injected) made significantly more percentage of entries onto the open arm, and spent more proportion of time in the open arm compared with their WT littermates (intact and GFP groups $P<0.0001$, pENK $p = 0.0002$) (Figs. 5A,B), suggestive of a lower level of anxiety in R6/2 genotype. Of importance, striatal pENK overexpression induced a noticeable reduction in proportions of entries and elapsed time in the open arms compared with intact age-matched R6/2 mice (respectively $p = 0.008$ and $p = 0.002$) (Figs. 5A,B). In addition, the percentage of entries and the proportion of time spent in the closed arms was exactly the reverse of what was seen for the open arms (Figs. 5A,B).

Barnes maze

The Barnes maze test was initiated at week 7 to examine the striatum-dependent memory and learning. Following four days of training, two probe trials were performed on days 5th and 12th to test short- and long-term retention memory. During the course of the training (days 1 to 4), all mice learned to find the target hole as indicated by a progressive reduction in primary latencies. No difference was detected in the latency times to find the target hole over the training period among the experimental groups ($F_{3,27} = 1.47$, $p = 0.25$) [R6/2: intact (n = 7), GFP- (n = 4), pENK (n = 6); WT: (n = 14)] (Fig. 5C). However, a significant difference was observed between different groups for latency to find target hole on days 5th and 12th [$F(\text{groups})_{3,54} = 12.39$, $p<0.0001$; $F(\text{probe})_{1,53} = 0.46$, $p = 0.50$, and $F(\text{groups} \times \text{probe})_{3,54} = 0.91$, $p = 0.44$]. Further analysis on probe day 5th noted a significant difference in primary latency among the groups ($F_{3,27} = 4.53$, $p = 0.01$) (Fig. 5D). Indeed, intact R6/2 mice spent longer time to reach the target hole than their WT counterparts but this difference did not reach significance ($p>0.01$). Of great note, striatal injection of rAAV2-GFP further worsened the maze performance in probe day 5th compared to WT ($p = 0.002$). Interestingly, striatal pENK overexpression corrected the short memory disturbance seen in R6/2 mice ($p = 0.48$ vs. WT) (Fig. 5D). In probe day 12th, there was a significant difference in primary latency to find the target hole among groups ($F_{3,27} = 9.85$, $p = 0.0001$). At day 12th, intact and GFP-injected R6/2 mice showed disturbance in long-term memory compared with WT ($p = 0.0003$). Unlike its action in short-term memory, nonetheless, striatal pENK overexpression failed to provide a beneficial effect in long-term retention test ($p = 0.002$ vs. WT) (Fig. 5D).

Novel object recognition task

This cognitive test was performed to assess the memory function by means of preference for a novel object in different experimental groups. Different groups were tested at week 4 (before manipulation) and week 9 (4 weeks after rAAV2- injections in the striatum). At 4 weeks of age, R6/2 showed similar exploratory behavior to WT in training session as well as in 1 hour and 24 hours retention trials (data not shown). Moreover, at 9 weeks of age, during the training session, no preference was seen for two identical objects among different experimental groups ($F_{3,19} = 0.82$, $p = 0.50$). However, a significant difference was detected between different groups of mice for exploring a new object in retention trials at 1 or 24 hours [$F(\text{groups})_{3,38} = 5.95$, $p = 0.002$; $F(\text{hours})_{1,38} = 0.69$, $P = 0.41$, and $F(\text{groups} \times \text{hours})_{3,38} = 1.19$, $p = 0.33$]. Further analysis detected a significant difference between various groups of [R6/2: intact (n = 6), GFP- (n = 3), pENK (n = 3); WT: (n = 12)] in 1 hour retention test ($F_{3,19} = 5.24$, $p = 0.003$). At this age (week 9), intact R6/2 mice spent a significantly less time exploring the novel object compared to WT ($P = 0.008$). GFP-injected R6/2 mice also displayed a recognition deficit compared with WT and pENK-injected animals ($p = 0.001$ and $p = 0.01$, respectively) (Fig. 5E). In addition, GFP- R6/2 mice tended to show less preference toward novel object than the intact R6/2 but this difference did not reach the significance level. In sharp contrast, novel object recognition was significantly improved in R6/2 mice receiving striatal rAAV2-GFP-pENK injection compared to GFP-injected R6/2 mice. It appears that striatal pENK overexpression efficiently rescues recognition function in R6/2 mice as there was no difference in novel object discrimination between the latter and their WT littermates ($p = 0.49$) (Fig. 5E). The novel object exploration time did not vary among experimental groups at 24 hours retention test ($F_{3,19} = 1.40$, $p = 0.27$) (Fig. 5E).

Enkephalin intensity in the striatum and striatal fibers

Representative images of immunohistochemistry against enkephalin in the striatum, GP and SN in different groups of R6/2 and WT mice [R6/2: intact (n = 8), GFP- (n = 4), pENK (n = 5); WT: (n = 7)] are presented in Figure 6A. Two-way ANOVA detected significant difference in enkephalin density at dorsal, lateral and total striatum between different groups [dorsal: $F(\text{treatment})_{3,40} = 5.27$, $P<0.004$; lateral: $F(\text{treatment})_{3,40} = 5.00$, $p<0.004$: total: $F(\text{treatment})_{3,40} = 3.85$, $p<0.01$], while the difference between right and left striatum and the interaction for treatment ×right vs. left hemisphere was not significant (Fig. 6B).

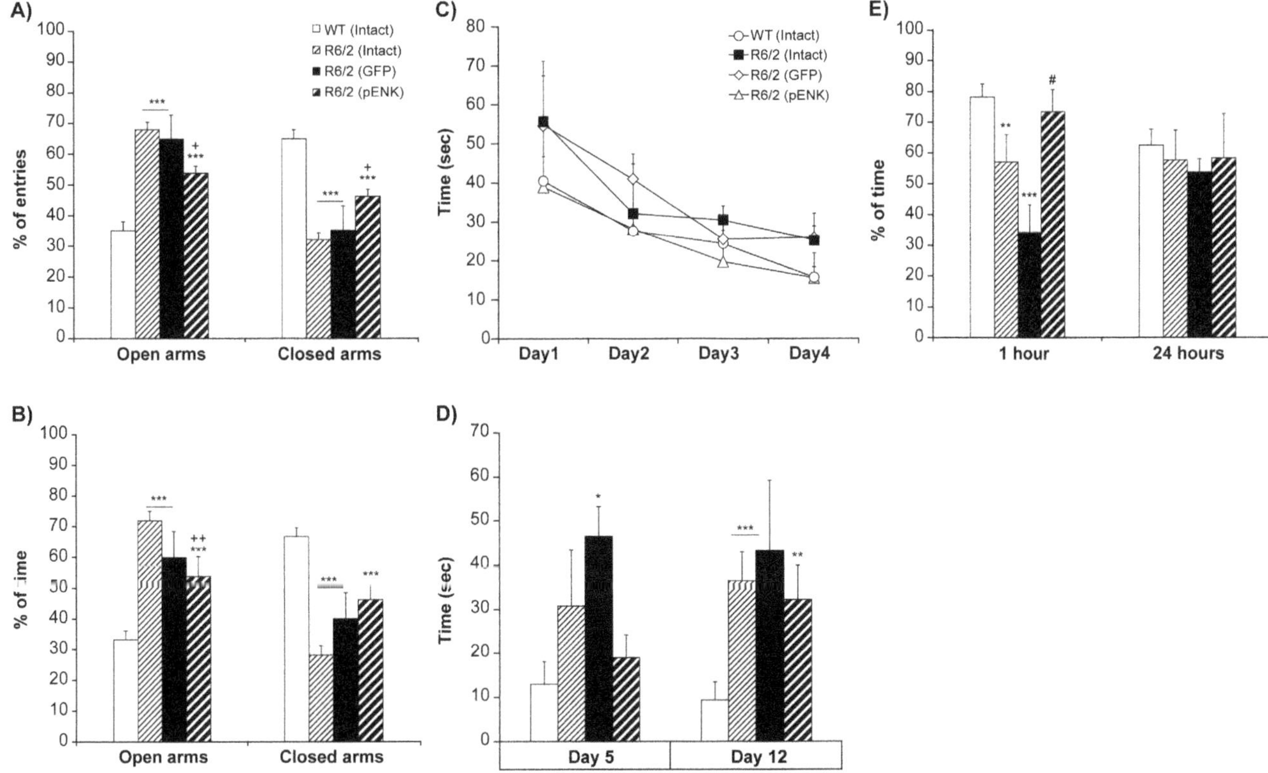

Figure 5. Elevated plus maze, Barnes maze, and Novel object recognition test in different groups of R6/2 and WT mice. Entry and time spent in open and closed arms of elevated plus maze (A, B): At week 8 of age, all R6/2 mice showed more percentage of entries (A), and spent more time in the open arm (B) compared with WT. In R6/2 mice having striatal overexpression of pENK, a reduction in percent of entries (A) and percent of time elapsed (B) in the open arms was observed compared with intact age-matched R6/2 mice. The percentage of entries and the proportion of time spent in the closed arms was exactly the reverse of what was seen for the open arms. Data are presented as mean percent of entries or mean percent of time spent in the open or closed arms / time spent in all four arms ± SEM. *** $p<0.0005$ vs. WT; + $p<0.01$, ++ $p<0.005$ vs. R6/2 (Intact). Learning and memory in Barnes maze (C, D) and Novel object recognition test (E): In Barnes maze performance, started at week 7 of age, no difference was observed in latency to find escape hole between different groups during trial days (C). At probe day 5th (D), R6/2 mice having striatal injection of rAAV2-GFP showed increased latency to find target hole compared to WT and pENK-injected R6/2 mice. Whereas no difference was detected between pENK-injected R6/2 mice and WT, while intact R6/2 mice tended to spent longer time to reach the target hole compared with WT counterparts. At probe day 12th (D), the time latency to find target hole was higher in all groups of R6/2 than WT. Novel object recognition test, at week 9, showed that in 1 hour retention test (E), intact R6/2 mice spent less time to explore the novel object compared to WT. Less preference toward novel object was even more pronounced in GFP-injected R6/2 mice compared with WT and pENK-injected group. Interestingly, recognition of novel object was considerably improved in R6/2 mice having striatal overexpression of pENK. Data are presented as percent of the time spent exploring the new object/ total time exploring new and familiar objects ± SEM. * $p<0.01$, ** $p<0.005$, *** $p<0.0005$ vs. WT; + $p<0.01$, ++ $p<0.005$ vs. R6/2 (Intact); # $p<0.01$ vs. R6/2 (GFP).

Post hoc analysis indicated that enkephalin intensity was significantly increased in the dorsal and lateral striatum of R6/2 mice having received rAAV2-pENK compared with GFP-injected and intact R6/2 mice (dorsal: $p=0.0005$ and $p=0.004$; lateral: $p=0.0006$ and $p=0.006$, respectively). Moreover, the level of enkephalin density was higher in total striatum compared with R6/2 (intact) ($p=0.004$) (Fig. 6B). Although the density of enkephalin positive fibers in GP of pENK-injected R6/2 mice was higher than other groups of mice, but this difference did not reach significance (Fig. 6C). As the GP receives ENK-containing neurons from the striatum we suggest that the immunoreactivity chromogenbased has already reached saturation level in mice having striatal overexpression of pENK, and that's why despite the higher level of ENK in GP of pENK-injected animals this difference did not reach significance. Interestingly, the density of enkephalin positive fibers was different in the SN of different treated groups [F(treatment)$_{3,40}$ = 14.24, $p<0.0001$; F(right vs. left)$_{1,40}=0.44$, $p=0.51$, and F(treatment ×right vs. left)$_{3,40}=0.37$, $p=0.77$]. Importantly, *Post hoc* analysis detected higher density of enkephalin positive fibers in the SN of R6/2 mice having striatal overexpression of pENK, not only compared with R6/2 intact and GFP-injected groups ($p<0.0001$, +52.2%, +57.2%, respectively), but also compared with WT ($p<0.0001$,) +47.2%) (Fig. 6C).

Stereological analyses

Unbiased stereological counts using optical fractionator method has been used to investigate the changes in the number of striatal neurons and glia, as well as striatal volume of different groups of R6/2 mice compared with WT. Indeed, in agreement with other studies [30,31], our results confirmed the presence of striatal neuronal loss in R6/2 transgenic mouse model of HD, revealed by a difference for the number of NeuN positive neurons between various experimental groups ($F_{3,17}=7.30$, $p=0.002$) [R6/2: intact (n = 5), GFP- (n = 4), pENK (n = 6); WT: (n = 6)]. *Post hoc* analysis showed a higher number of NeuN positive neurons in the striatum of 10 weeks old WT mice compared with those from intact

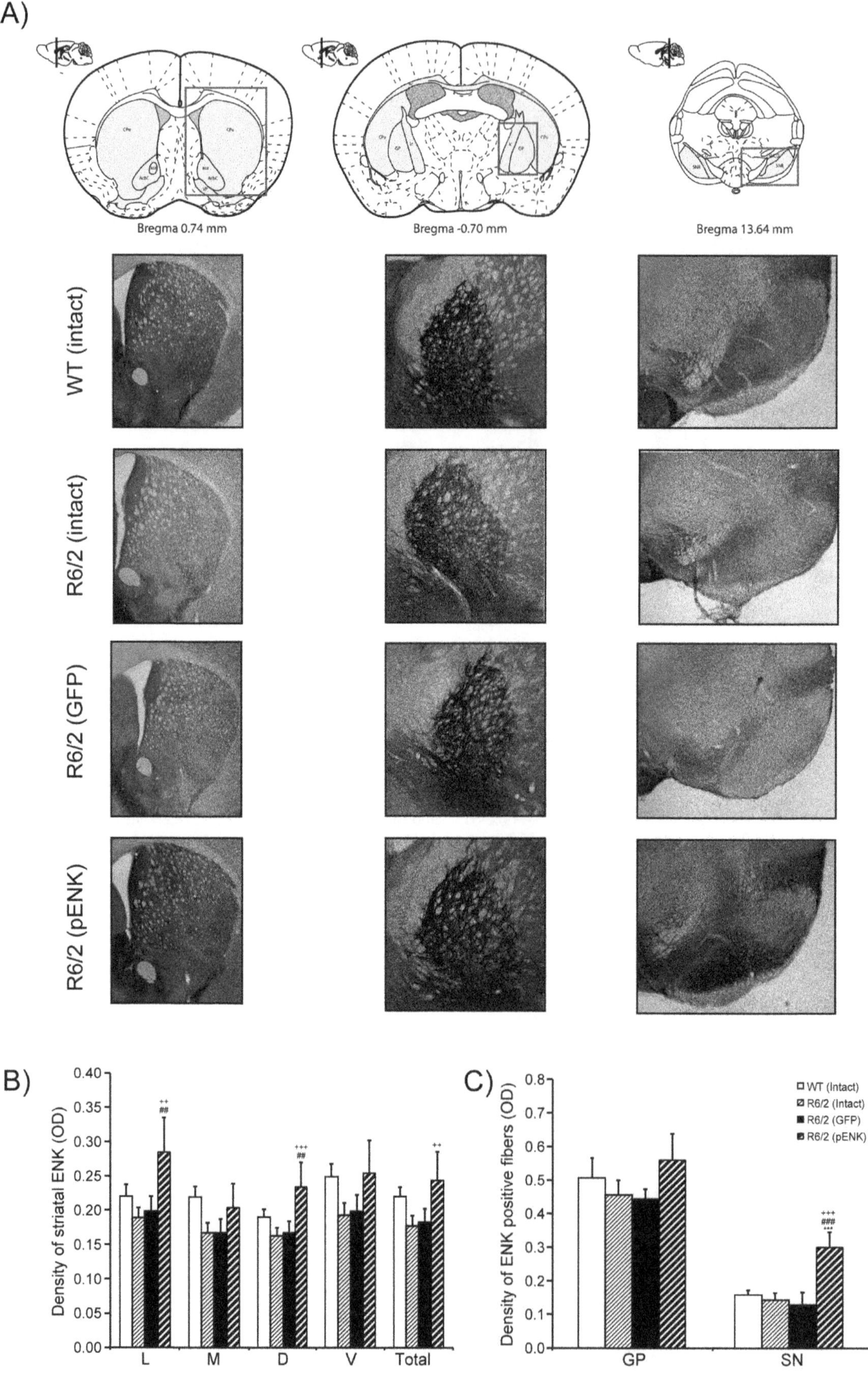
A)
Bregma 0.74 mm
Bregma -0.70 mm
Bregma 13.64 mm
WT (intact)
R6/2 (intact)
R6/2 (GFP)
R6/2 (pENK)
B)
Density of striatal ENK (OD)
L
M
D
V
Total
C)
Density of ENK positive fibers (OD)
GP
SN
WT (Intact)
R6/2 (Intact)
R6/2 (GFP)
R6/2 (pENK)

Figure 6. Enkephalin immunoreactivity in the striatum, globus pallidus and substantia nigra of different groups of R6/2 and WT. Representative images of immunohistochemistry against enkephalin in the striatum, GP and SN in different groups (A). The density of enkephalin positive neurons was increased in the total striatum of pENK-injected R6/2 mice compared with intact R6/2 mice. Moreover, the increased density of enkephalin in the lateral and dorsal subregions of the striatum was higher in pENK-treated group compared with intact and GFP-injected R6/2 mice (B). No significant difference was observed for the density of enkephalin positive fibers in the GP between different groups; however, the density of enkephalin positive fibers was importantly increased in the SN of R6/2 mice having striatal overexpression of pENK (C). L: lateral; M: medial; D: dorsal; V: ventral regions of the striatum; GP: globus pallidus; SN: substantia nigra. Data are presented as mean ± SEM. **** p<0.0001 vs. WT; ## p<0.005, ####p<0.0001 vs. R6/2 (GFP). ++ p<0.005, +++ p<0.0005, ++++ p<0.0001 vs. intact R6/2.

($p = 0.0007$, 71% of WT), and GFP-injected ($p = 0.001$, 72% of WT) R6/2 mice. Nevertheless, this difference did not reach significance when WT mice were compared with pENK-injected R6/2 mice ($p > 0.01$, 85% of WT) (Fig. 7A). In addition, at 10 weeks old, a difference was noted in the number of glial cells between different groups ($F_{3,17} = 3.12$, $p > 0.01$) when all Nissl positive cells were taking into account. *Post hoc* analysis indicated that the number of glial cells was higher in WT compared with intact R6/2 mice ($P = 0.01$, 78% of WT). However, no change was observed in the number of Nissl positive cells between WT and GFP- or pENK-injected R6/2 mice ($p > 0.01$) (Fig. 7B). Moreover, the volume of the striatum was significantly different between various groups of mice at 10 weeks old ($F_{3,17} = 50.48$, $p < 0.0001$). In fact, in all groups of R6/2 mice the volume of the striatum was smaller than age-matched WT ($p < 0.0001$) (Fig. 7C).

Discussion

In the present study, we investigated whether striatal overexpression of pENK can reduce or delay behavioral dysfunction and/or striatal neuronal loss in R6/2 transgenic mouse model of HD. Our results, to our knowledge are the first to show that increased enkephalin transmission in the striatum could delay the progression of behavioral symptoms of HD in R6/2 mouse model by: a) improvement and delaying the onset of decline in grip strength which is one of the behavioral dysfunction in R6/2 mouse model of HD due to progressive loss in muscular force [30,31]; b) reduction of clasping as an abnormal dystonic movement which is present in this mouse model and its severity increases with age [30,31]; c) improvement of fast motor activity which is reduced considerably, more than moderate and slow activities, in R6/2 mice [30]; d) reduction of the percentages of entries and time spent in the open arms which is usually more elevated in R6/2 mice compared with WT [43]; e) improvement of short-term memory and recognition function which is altered in all mouse models of HD [29,44], as well as in HD patients even before the onset of motor symptoms [45]. It is also important to note that the surgery by itself (e.g. decreased of food consumption after surgery) might be the cause of worsening HD-like symptoms in GFP-injected R6/2 mice, even compared to R6/2 intact. Interestingly, striatal pENK overexpression could overcome and delay the effect of surgery in weight loss, as well as decline in different behavioral functions compared to GFP-injected mice. At 10 weeks old, pENK striatal overexpression had also slight beneficial effect on striatal neuronal number compared with other groups of R6/2.

Striatal pENK overexpression, density of enkephalin in the striatum, and behavioral symptoms in R6/2 mice

An important question that could be raised here is how pENK overexpression in the striatum could have beneficial effects on HD symptoms in the R6/2 mouse model of HD? One of the first neurodegenerative changes in HD is the loss of striatal medium spiny neurons with the preferential and earlier degeneration of striatopallidal neurons containing opioid peptide enkephalin [26,46]. This concept is reinforced by data suggesting that striatal neurons containing enkephalin receive more glutamatergic cortical inputs and are more directly affected by cortical activity [46,47], despite the more abundant expression of huntingtin in striatonigral projection neurons [48]. The effect of excitatory glutamatergic inputs to the striatum can be regulated by presynaptic receptors on corticostriatal terminals [46]. Nevertheless in HD, cellular pathology induced by mutant huntingtin in the presynaptic terminals might result in an increased release of glutamate [46,49]. Indeed, the primary proposed cellular mechanism underlying degeneration of medium spiny neurons is the overactivity of corticostriatal glutamate transmission [46,49–51]. Therefore, plausible approaches to reduce the glutamate release from corticostriatal terminals might be relevant in the treatment of HD. Accordingly, surgical lesions of the corticostriatal pathways, administration of glutamate release inhibitors or glutamate transporter upregulators, increased striatal neuronal survival and improved behavioral and biochemical phenotypes in R6/2 mice [52–55]. Interestingly, it was shown that the main action of enkephalin on striatal neurons, mainly through δ opioid receptors (δORs), is to provide the presynaptic inhibition of corticostriatal excitatory synaptic input [56,57]. Therefore, we suggest that reduction of corticostriatal signalling *via* activation of presynaptic δORs through enkephalin released from striatal collaterals [58], might play an important role at delaying or attenuating motor dysfunction (e.g. locomotor activity, abnormal clasping, muscular force) in R6/2 mice having striatal overexpression of pENK. Indeed, this suggestion corroborates with our results concerning the increased density of striatal enkephalin in pENK-injected R6/2 mice.

Striatum has also a crucial role not only in the control of movement but also in instrumental learning [59], working memory and reversal learning [60]. In HD, cognitive deficits are even detectable prior to motor dysfunction, first in memory functions and then in executive functions [29,44]. Interestingly, deficits in recognition memory and spatial memory induced by mutant huntingtin may be caused, at least in part, by protein kinase-A (PKA) over-activation [61]. It was shown that cAMP signaling cascade is increased in the striatum of R6 mice [62], and PKA substrates are hyper-phosphorylated in the striatum of mouse models of HD at pre-symptomatic stages [63]. Since one of the actions of enkephalin at the cellular level is inhibition of adenylate cyclase and reduction of intracellular cAMP level and signaling cascade [9,64], therefore, it is possible to speculate that striatal pENK overexpression *via* activation of opioid receptors and reduction of cAMP level and/or PKA activity could play a role in the improvement of cognitive symptoms (e.g. short-term memory and recognition) observed in pENK-injected R6/2 mice.

Imbalance in Ca^{++} homeostasis and regulation have been implicated in the pathogenesis of many neurodegenerative diseases including HD. Importantly, striatal neurons are particularly vulnerable to excessive Ca^{++} influx [29,65–67] while, the increased expression of a calmodulin fragment which normalizes intracellular Ca^{++} release improved motor function, weight loss and neuropathology in the R6/2 mouse model of HD [68]. In accordance with the inhibitory effect of opioids on Ca^{++} influx

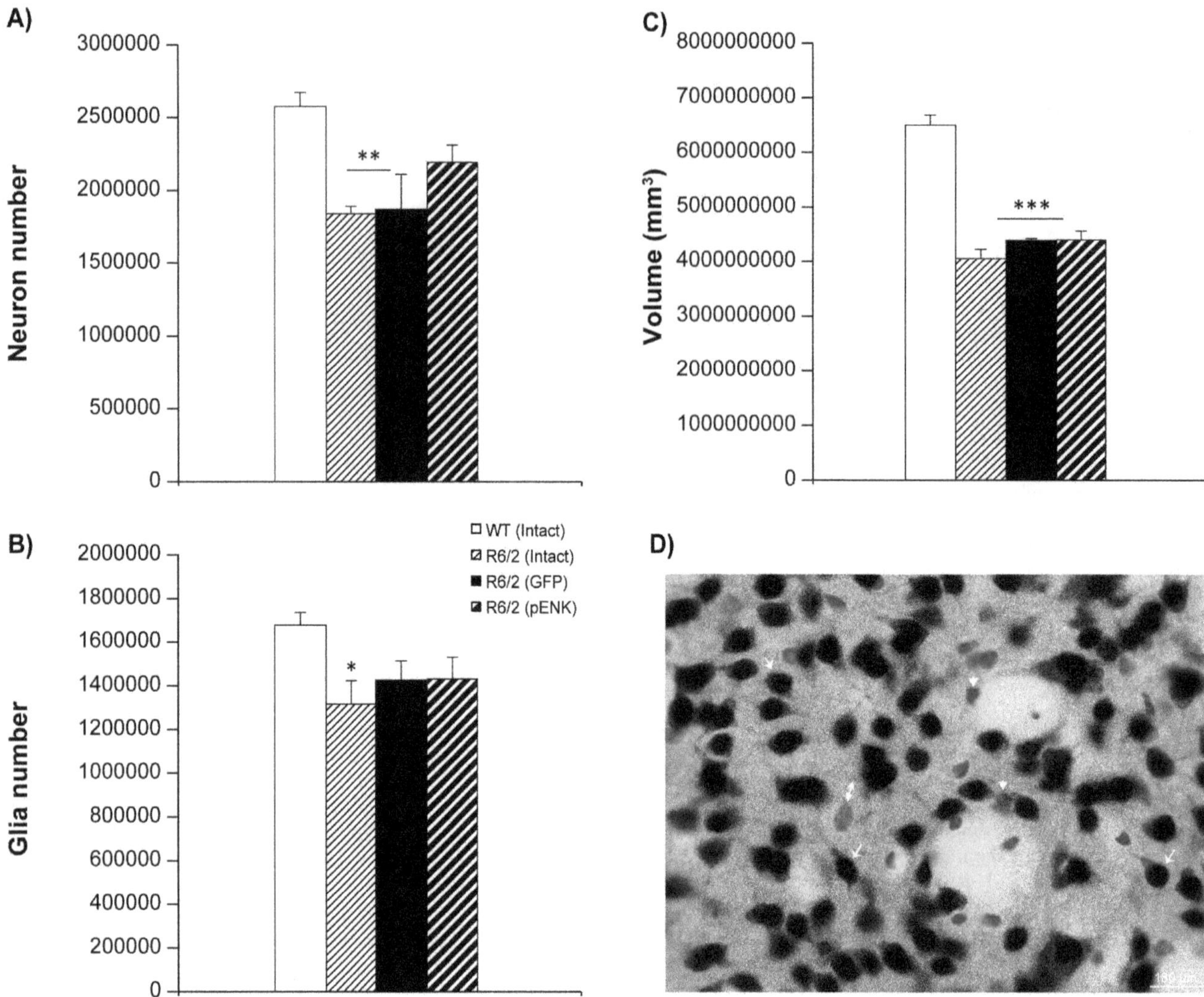

Figure 7. Morphological changes in the striatum of different groups of R6/2 mice and WT at week 10 of age. Unbiased stereology revealed that the total number of striatal NeuN positive neurons (A) was reduced in the striatum of intact and GFP-injected R6/2 mice compared with WT. However, this difference did not reach significance when WT mice were compared with pENK-injected R6/2 mice. The number of glial cells was higher in WT compared with intact R6/2 mice (B). The volume of the striatum was reduced in all groups of R6/2 mice compared with WT (C). Representative coronal brain sections stained with NeuN-Nissl for unbiased stereology (D); arrow: NeuN positive (neuron), arrowhead: Nissl positive (glia, <7 μm), and two headed arrows: Nissl positive (glia, >7 μm). Data are presented as mean ± SEM. * $p<0.01$, ** $p<0.001$, *** $p<0.0001$ vs. WT.

[64], we suggest that overexpression of striatal enkephalin *via* inhibition of Ca^{++} currents could also play a role in the improvement of behavioral dysfunction in the R6/2 mouse model of HD.

Striatal pENK overexpression, density of enkephalin in striatal fibers and behavioral symptoms in R6/2 mice

Several studies revealed that altered activity of the GP is responsible for at least a part of the cognitive and motor symptoms of HD [69–71]. Indeed, endogenous metabolic marker, cytochrome oxidase (COX) histochemistry, showed an increased neuronal metabolic activity in the GP of transgenic rat model of HD [72]. Further studies also provide evidence that GP deep brain stimulation (DBS) has the potential to improve both motor and cognitive symptoms in transgenic rat model of HD [73,74]. Within the GP both presynaptic and postsynaptic μ and δ opioid receptors are present [8]. Moreover, all GP projection neurons have local collateral axons [75] that may strongly inhibit GP neurons because they terminate on the perikarya and proximal dendrites of GP neurons [76]. As enkephalin expression is substantially reduced in the striatum and external pallidum of HD brain [25], we may also suggest that higher density of enkephalin positive fibers in GP of pENK-injected R6/2 mice, could maintain the inhibitory function of the GP through activation of presynaptic opioid receptors on collateral terminals and could then contribute to the improvement of behavioral symptoms in this group.

Interestingly, the density of enkephalin positive fibers in SN of pENK-injected R6/2 mice was significantly higher, two folds, than all other groups. Driving ectopic expression of enkephalin in a nucleus which normally does not receive enkephalinergic projections is not directly 'fixing' the neurochemical abnormality that is observed in HD. However, such ectopic expression allow us to propose that the increased level of enkephalin in SN of R6/2 mice having pENK overexpression, through activation of opioid receptors on striatonigral terminals may participate to the presynaptic inhibition of GABA-mediated transmission in substantia nigra reticulata (SNr) [77,78] and be involved in the improvement of behavioral dysfunction, more especially abnormal clasping movement. Moreover, we may also suggest that in pENK-injected R6/2 mice, enkephalin-induced presynaptic activation of μ, δ and κ opioid receptors on subthalamic nucleus (STN) efferent [8,79] by inhibition of excitatory neurotransmission in SNr might reduce the activity of SNr and could then contribute to disinhibition of thalamus and consequently to the improvement of behavioral symptoms in this group.

Striatal pENK overexpression and striatal morphology

According to the particular vulnerability of striatal neurons to excessive Ca^{++} [29,65–67], and the inhibitory effect of enkephalin on Ca^{++} influx [64], we expected that overexpression of striatal enkephalin *via* activation of opioid receptors and subsequent inhibition of Ca^{++} currents could also delay striatal neurons from degeneration in the R6/2 mouse model of HD. As the number of striatal neurons tended to be higher in pENK-injected mice compared to other groups of R6/2 and no difference was observed between pENK-injected R6/2 mice and WT, we may also propose that striatal pENK overexpression could delay striatal atrophy but could not prevent it at 10 weeks of age. However, striatal pENK overexpression had no beneficial effect on the decline in striatal volume of R6/2 mice. This can be explained in part by the atrophy of corticostriatal afferents which may contribute to the reduction of striatal volume. Indeed, the decline in striatal volume, starting as early as week 6, precedes striatal neuronal loss [30], parallel to the reduction of brain-derived neurotrophic factor (BDNF, trophic factor essential for neuronal survival) in different cortical areas from week 4 or 6 [30]. Therefore, we suggest that at early stage of the disease, striatal enkephalin could play a role in the reduction of excitotoxicity. Nevertheless, based on downregulation of transcription of several important neuronal genes [80–82] and further disease progression (atrophy of corticostriatal afferents and the progressive neurodegeneration of striatonigral dynorphin-containing neurons at later stage of disease), the level of opioid receptors might also be gradually downregulated, and the positive effect of enkephalin on striatal neuron morphology may eventually fail. Indeed, the reduction of striatal opioid receptor binding (20% to 40%) was shown in HD patients [83]. This proposition is in agreement with gradual decline in beneficial effect of striatal pENK overexpression on some behavioral symptoms in R6/2 from week 9 of age.

Conclusion

We suggest that in HD, striatal enkephalin system at early stage of disease might play a role at attenuating illness symptoms *via*: a) the presynaptic inhibition of the corticostriatal glutamatergic input by opioid receptors activation, more specifically δORs; b) the inhibitory effect of opioid receptors on Ca^{++} influx; c) the reduction of cAMP signaling cascade.

The results of this study might open new horizon to investigate the cellular and molecular mechanisms by which enkephalin modulates motor response and signalling in HD, and may also contribute to the development of new therapeutical strategies and the gain in the quality of life in HD patients.

Acknowledgments

The authors would like to thank Dr. Emmanuel Planel for having supplied the Barnes maze.

Author Contributions

Conceived and designed the experiments: PS. Performed the experiments: SB MV. Analyzed the data: SB PS. Contributed reagents/materials/analysis tools: SSH GD PS. Wrote the paper: PS. Revised the paper: SSH GD PS.

References

1. The Huntington's Disease Collaborative Research Group (1993) A novel gene containing a trinucleotide repeat that is expanded and unstable on Huntington's disease chromosomes. Cell 72: 971–983.
2. Ross CA (1995) When more is less: pathogenesis of glutamine repeat neurodegenerative diseases. Neuron 15: 493–496.
3. Saudou F, Finkbeiner S, Devys D, Greenberg ME (1998) Huntingtin acts in the nucleus to induce apoptosis but death does not correlate with the formation of intranuclear inclusions. Cell 95: 55–66.
4. Li SH, Schilling G, Young WS, Li XJ, Margolis RL et al. (1993) Huntington's disease gene (IT15) is widely expressed in human and rat tissues. Neuron 11: 985–993.
5. Fusco FR, Chen Q, Lamoreaux WJ, Figueredo-Cardenas G, Jiao Y et al. (1999) Cellular localization of huntingtin in striatal and cortical neurons in rats: lack of correlation with neuronal vulnerability in Huntington's disease. J Neurosci 19: 1189–1202.
6. Reiner A, Albin RL, Anderson KD, D'Amato CJ, Penney JB et al. (1988) Differential loss of striatal projection neurons in Huntington disease. Proc Natl Acad Sci U S A 85: 5733–5737.
7. Bodnar RJ (2009) Endogenous opiates and behavior: 2008. Peptides 30: 2432–2479.
8. Peckys D, Landwehrmeyer GB (1999) Expression of mu, kappa, and delta opioid receptor messenger RNA in the human CNS: a 33P in situ hybridization study. Neuroscience 88: 1093–1135.
9. Williams JT, Christie MJ, Manzoni O (2001) Cellular and synaptic adaptations mediating opioid dependence. Physiol Rev 81: 299–343.
10. Bezard E, Ravenscroft P, Gross CE, Crossman AR, Brotchie JM (2001) Upregulation of striatal preproenkephalin gene expression occurs before the appearance of parkinsonian signs in 1-methyl-4-phenyl- 1,2,3,6-tetrahydropyridine monkeys. Neurobiol Dis 8: 343–350.
11. Bezard E, Gross CE, Brotchie JM (2003) Presymptomatic compensation in Parkinson's disease is not dopamine-mediated. Trends Neurosci 26: 215–221.
12. Samadi P, Gregoire L, Hadj TA, Di Paolo T, Rouillard C et al. (2005) Naltrexone in the short-term decreases antiparkinsonian response to l-Dopa and in the long-term increases dyskinesias in drug-naive parkinsonian monkeys. Neuropharmacology 49: 165–173.
13. Samadi P, Bedard PJ, Rouillard C (2006) Opioids and motor complications in Parkinson's disease. Trends Pharmacol Sci 27: 512–517.
14. Barry U, Zuo Z (2005) Opioids: old drugs for potential new applications. Curr Pharm Des 11: 1343–1350.
15. Yang Y, Xia X, Zhang Y, Wang Q, Li L et al. (2009) delta-Opioid receptor activation attenuates oxidative injury in the ischemic rat brain. BMC Biol 7: 55.
16. Su DS, Wang ZH, Zheng YJ, Zhao YH, Wang XR (2007) Dose-dependent neuroprotection of delta opioid peptide [D-Ala2, D-Leu5] enkephalin in neuronal death and retarded behavior induced by forebrain ischemia in rats. Neurosci Lett 423: 113–117.
17. Ma MC, Qian H, Ghassemi F, Zhao P, Xia Y (2005) Oxygen-sensitive {delta}-opioid receptor-regulated survival and death signals: novel insights into neuronal preconditioning and protection. J Biol Chem 280: 16208–16218.
18. Wang S, Duan Y, Su D, Li W, Tan J et al. (2011) Delta opioid peptide [D-Ala2, D-Leu5] enkephalin (DADLE) triggers postconditioning against transient forebrain ischemia. Eur J Pharmacol 658: 140–144.
19. Qin L, Liu Y, Qian X, Hong JS, Block ML (2005) Microglial NADPH oxidase mediates leucine enkephalin dopaminergic neuroprotection. Ann N Y Acad Sci 1053: 107–120.
20. Polakiewicz RD, Schieferl SM, Gingras AC, Sonenberg N, Comb MJ (1998) mu-Opioid receptor activates signaling pathways implicated in cell survival and translational control. J Biol Chem 273: 23534–23541.
21. Borlongan CV, Su TP, Wang Y (2000) Treatment with delta opioid peptide enhances in vitro and in vivo survival of rat dopaminergic neurons. Neuroreport 11: 923–926.
22. Johnson SM, Turner SM (2010) Protecting motor networks during perinatal ischemia: the case for delta-opioid receptors. Ann N Y Acad Sci 1198: 260–270.
23. Zhu M, Li MW, Tian XS, Ou XM, Zhu CQ et al. (2009) Neuroprotective role of delta-opioid receptors against mitochondrial respiratory chain injury. Brain Res 1252: 183–191.

24. Borlongan CV, Su TP, Wang Y (2001) Delta opioid peptide augments functional effects and intrastriatal graft survival of rat fetal ventral mesencephalic cells. Cell Transplant 10: 53–58.
25. Menalled L, Zanjani H, MacKenzie L, Koppel A, Carpenter E et al. (2000) Decrease in striatal enkephalin mRNA in mouse models of Huntington's disease. Exp Neurol 162: 328–342.
26. Sun Z, Del Mar N, Meade C, Goldowitz D, Reiner A (2002) Differential changes in striatal projection neurons in R6/2 transgenic mice for Huntington's disease. Neurobiol Dis 11: 369–385.
27. Albin RL, Qin Y, Young AB, Penney JB, Chesselet MF (1991) Preproenkephalin messenger RNA-containing neurons in striatum of patients with symptomatic and presymptomatic Huntington's disease: an in situ hybridization study. Ann Neurol 30: 542–549.
28. Deng YP, Albin RL, Penney JB, Young AB, Anderson KD et al. (2004) Differential loss of striatal projection systems in Huntington's disease: a quantitative immunohistochemical study. J Chem Neuroanat 27: 143–164.
29. Crook ZR, Housman D (2011) Huntington's Disease: Can Mice Lead the Way to Treatment? Neuron 69: 423–435.
30. Samadi P, Boutet A, Rymar VV, Rawal K, Maheux J et al. (2013) Relationship between BDNF expression in major striatal afferents, striatum morphology and motor behavior in the R6/2 mouse model of Huntington's disease. Genes Brain Behav 12: 108–124.
31. Stack EC, Kubilus JK, Smith K, Cormier K, Del Signore SJ et al. (2005) Chronology of behavioral symptoms and neuropathological sequela in R6/2 Huntington's disease transgenic mice. J Comp Neurol 490: 354–370.
32. He TC, Zhou S, da Costa LT, Yu J, Kinzler KW et al. (1998) A simplified system for generating recombinant adenoviruses. Proc Natl Acad Sci U S A 95: 2509–2514.
33. Zolotukhin S, Potter M, Zolotukhin I, Sakai Y, Loiler S et al. (2002) Production and purification of serotype 1, 2, and 5 recombinant adeno-associated viral vectors. Methods 28: 158–167.
34. Franklin KBJ, Paxinos G (2008) The mouse brain in stereotaxic coordinates.
35. Bailoo JD, Bohlen MO, Wahlsten D (2010) The precision of video and photocell tracking systems and the elimination of tracking errors with infrared backlighting. J Neurosci Methods 188: 45–52.
36. Mathis C, Bott JB, Candusso MP, Simonin F, Cassel JC (2011) Impaired striatum-dependent behavior in GASP-1-knock-out mice. Genes Brain Behav 10: 299–308.
37. Drouin-Ouellet J, LeBel M, Filali M, Cicchetti F (2012) MyD88 deficiency results in both cognitive and motor impairments in mice. Brain Behav Immun 26: 880–885.
38. Yoshikawa K, Williams C, Sabol SL (1984) Rat brain preproenkephalin mRNA. cDNA cloning, primary structure, and distribution in the central nervous system. J Biol Chem 259: 14301–14308.
39. Poulin JF, Berube P, Laforest S, Drolet G (2013) Enkephalin knockdown in the central amygdala nucleus reduces unconditioned fear and anxiety. Eur J Neurosci. 10.1111/ejn.12134 [doi]
40. Beaudry G, Langlois MC, Weppe I, Rouillard C, Levesque D (2000) Contrasting patterns and cellular specificity of transcriptional regulation of the nuclear receptor nerve growth factor-inducible B by haloperidol and clozapine in the rat forebrain. J Neurochem 75: 1694–1702.
41. Baydyuk M, Russell T, Liao GY, Zang K, An JJ et al. (2011) TrkB receptor controls striatal formation by regulating the number of newborn striatal neurons. Proc Natl Acad Sci U S A 108: 1669–1674.
42. Sadikot AF, Sasseville R (1997) Neurogenesis in the mammalian neostriatum and nucleus accumbens: parvalbumin-immunoreactive GABAergic interneurons. J Comp Neurol 389: 193–211.
43. File SE, Mahal A, Mangiarini L, Bates GP (1998) Striking changes in anxiety in Huntington's disease transgenic mice. Brain Res 805: 234–240.
44. Van Raamsdonk JM, Pearson J, Slow EJ, Hossain SM, Leavitt BR et al. (2005) Cognitive dysfunction precedes neuropathology and motor abnormalities in the YAC128 mouse model of Huntington's disease. J Neurosci 25: 4169–4180.
45. Lemiere J, Decruyenaere M, Evers-Kiebooms G, Vandenbussche E, Dom R (2004) Cognitive changes in patients with Huntington's disease (HD) and asymptomatic carriers of the HD mutation—a longitudinal follow-up study. J Neurol 251: 935–942.
46. Cepeda C, Wu N, Andre VM, Cummings DM, Levine MS (2007) The corticostriatal pathway in Huntington's disease. Prog Neurobiol 81: 253–271.
47. Lei W, Jiao Y, Del Mar N, Reiner A (2004) Evidence for differential cortical input to direct pathway versus indirect pathway striatal projection neurons in rats. J Neurosci 24: 8289–8299.
48. Fusco FR, Martorana A, De MZ, Viscomi MT, Sancesario G et al. (2003) Huntingtin distribution among striatal output neurons of normal rat brain. Neurosci Lett 339: 53–56.
49. Milnerwood AJ, Raymond LA (2007) Corticostriatal synaptic function in mouse models of Huntington's disease: early effects of huntingtin repeat length and protein load. J Physiol 585: 817–831.
50. Andre VM, Cepeda C, Levine MS (2010) Dopamine and glutamate in Huntington's disease: A balancing act. CNS Neurosci Ther 16: 163–178.
51. Milnerwood AJ, Gladding CM, Pouladi MA, Kaufman AM, Hines RM et al. (2010) Early increase in extrasynaptic NMDA receptor signaling and expression contributes to phenotype onset in Huntington's disease mice. Neuron 65: 178–190.
52. Miller BR, Dorner JL, Shou M, Sari Y, Barton SJ et al. (2008) Up-regulation of GLT1 expression increases glutamate uptake and attenuates the Huntington's disease phenotype in the R6/2 mouse. Neuroscience 153: 329–337.
53. Schiefer J, Landwehrmeyer GB, Luesse HG, Sprunken A, Puls C et al. (2002) Riluzole prolongs survival time and alters nuclear inclusion formation in a transgenic mouse model of Huntington's disease. Mov Disord 17: 748–757.
54. Schiefer J, Sprunken A, Puls C, Luesse HG, Milkereit A et al. (2004) The metabotropic glutamate receptor 5 antagonist MPEP and the mGluR2 agonist LY379268 modify disease progression in a transgenic mouse model of Huntington's disease. Brain Res 1019: 246–254.
55. Stack EC, Dedeoglu A, Smith KM, Cormier K, Kubilus JK et al. (2007) Neuroprotective effects of synaptic modulation in Huntington's disease R6/2 mice. J Neurosci 27: 12908–12915.
56. Jiang ZG, North RA (1992) Pre- and postsynaptic inhibition by opioids in rat striatum. J Neurosci 12: 356–361.
57. Wang H, Pickel VM (2001) Preferential cytoplasmic localization of delta-opioid receptors in rat striatal patches: comparison with plasmalemmal mu-opioid receptors. J Neurosci 21: 3242–3250.
58. Parent A, Sato F, Wu Y, Gauthier J, Levesque M et al. (2000) Organization of the basal ganglia: the importance of axonal collateralization. Trends Neurosci 23: S20–S27.
59. Yin HH, Knowlton BJ (2004) Contributions of striatal subregions to place and response learning. Learn Mem 11: 459–463.
60. Wei CJ, Singer P, Coelho J, Boison D, Feldon J et al. (2011) Selective inactivation of adenosine A(2A) receptors in striatal neurons enhances working memory and reversal learning. Learn Mem 18: 459–474.
61. Giralt A, Saavedra A, Carreton O, Xifro X, Alberch J et al. (2011) Increased PKA signaling disrupts recognition memory and spatial memory: role in Huntington's disease. Hum Mol Genet 20: 4232–4247.
62. Ariano MA, Aronin N, Difiglia M, Tagle DA, Sibley DR et al. (2002) Striatal neurochemical changes in transgenic models of Huntington's disease. J Neurosci Res 68: 716–729.
63. Torres-Peraza JF, Giralt A, Garcia-Martinez JM, Pedrosa E, Canals JM et al. (2008) Disruption of striatal glutamatergic transmission induced by mutant huntingtin involves remodeling of both postsynaptic density and NMDA receptor signaling. Neurobiol Dis 29: 409–421.
64. Waldhoer M, Bartlett SE, Whistler JL (2004) Opioid receptors. Annu Rev Biochem 73: 953–990.
65. Chan CS, Gertler TS, Surmeier DJ (2009) Calcium homeostasis, selective vulnerability and Parkinson's disease. Trends Neurosci 32: 249–256.
66. Day M, Wang Z, Ding J, An X, Ingham CA et al. (2006) Selective elimination of glutamatergic synapses on striatopallidal neurons in Parkinson disease models. Nat Neurosci 9: 251–259.
67. Mosharov EV, Larsen KE, Kanter E, Phillips KA, Wilson K et al. (2009) Interplay between cytosolic dopamine, calcium, and alpha-synuclein causes selective death of substantia nigra neurons. Neuron 62: 218–229.
68. Dai Y, Dudek NL, Li Q, Fowler SC, Muma NA (2009) Striatal expression of a calmodulin fragment improved motor function, weight loss, and neuropathology in the R6/2 mouse model of Huntington's disease. J Neurosci 29: 11550–11559.
69. Ayalon L, Doron R, Weiner I, Joel D (2004) Amelioration of behavioral deficits in a rat model of Huntington's disease by an excitotoxic lesion to the globus pallidus. Exp Neurol 186: 46–58.
70. Reiner A (2004) Can lesions of GPe correct HD deficits? Exp Neurol 186: 1–5.
71. Beal MF, Ferrante RJ (2004) Experimental therapeutics in transgenic mouse models of Huntington's disease. Nat Rev Neurosci 5: 373–384.
72. Vlamings R, Benazzouz A, Chetrit J, Janssen ML, Kozan R et al. (2012) Metabolic and electrophysiological changes in the basal ganglia of transgenic Huntington's disease rats. Neurobiol Dis 48: 488–494.
73. Temel Y, Cao C, Vlamings R, Blokland A, Ozen H et al. (2006) Motor and cognitive improvement by deep brain stimulation in a transgenic rat model of Huntington's disease. Neurosci Lett 406: 138–141.
74. Tan SK, Vlamings R, Lim L, Sesia T, Janssen ML et al. (2010) Experimental deep brain stimulation in animal models. Neurosurgery 67: 1073–1079.
75. Nambu A, Llinas R (1997) Morphology of globus pallidus neurons: its correlation with electrophysiology in guinea pig brain slices. J Comp Neurol 377: 85–94.
76. Ogura M, Kita H (2000) Dynorphin exerts both postsynaptic and presynaptic effects in the Globus pallidus of the rat. J Neurophysiol 83: 3366–3376.
77. Abou-Khalil B, Young AB, Penney JB (1984) Evidence for the presynaptic localization of opiate binding sites on striatal efferent fibers. Brain Res 323: 21–29.
78. Tokuno H, Chiken S, Kametani K, Moriizumi T (2002) Efferent projections from the striatal patch compartment: anterograde degeneration after selective ablation of neurons expressing mu-opioid receptor in rats. Neurosci Lett 332: 5–8.
79. Delfs JM, Kong H, Mestek A, Chen Y, Yu L et al. (1994) Expression of mu opioid receptor mRNA in rat brain: an in situ hybridization study at the single cell level. J Comp Neurol 345: 46–68.
80. Zhai W, Jeong H, Cui L, Krainc D, Tjian R (2005) In vitro analysis of huntingtin-mediated transcriptional repression reveals multiple transcription factor targets. Cell 123: 1241–1253.
81. Bruce AW, Donaldson IJ, Wood IC, Yerbury SA, Sadowski MI et al. (2004) Genome-wide analysis of repressor element 1 silencing transcription factor/

neuron-restrictive silencing factor (REST/NRSF) target genes. Proc Natl Acad Sci U S A 101: 10458–10463.

82. Rigamonti D, Bolognini D, Mutti C, Zuccato C, Tartari M et al. (2007) Loss of huntingtin function complemented by small molecules acting as repressor element 1/neuron restrictive silencer element silencer modulators. J Biol Chem 282: 24554–24562.

83. Weeks RA, Cunningham VJ, Piccini P, Waters S, Harding AE et al. (1997) 11C-diprenorphine binding in Huntington's disease: a comparison of region of interest analysis with statistical parametric mapping. J Cereb Blood Flow Metab 17: 943–949.

Trajectory Adjustments Underlying Task-Specific Intermittent Force Behaviors and Muscular Rhythms

Yi-Ching Chen[1,2], Yen-Ting Lin[3], Chien-Ting Huang[4], Chia-Li Shih[5], Zong-Ru Yang[4], Ing-Shiou Hwang[4,5]*

1 School of Physical Therapy, Chung Shan Medical University, Taichung City, Taiwan, **2** Physical Therapy Room, Chung Shan Medical University Hospital, Taichung City, Taiwan, **3** Physical Education Office, Asian University, Taichung City, Taiwan, **4** Institute of Allied Health Sciences, College of Medicine, National Cheng Kung University, Tainan City, Taiwan, **5** Department of Physical Therapy, College of Medicine, National Cheng Kung University, Tainan City, Taiwan

Abstract

Force intermittency is one of the major causes of motor variability. Focusing on the dynamics of force intermittency, this study was undertaken to investigate how force trajectory is fine-tuned for static and dynamic force-tracking of a comparable physical load. Twenty-two healthy adults performed two unilateral resistance protocols (static force-tracking at 75% maximal effort and dynamic force-tracking in the range of 50%–100% maximal effort) using the left hand. The electromyographic activity and force profile of the designated hand were monitored. Gripping force was off-line decomposed into a primary movement spectrally identical to the target motion and a force intermittency profile containing numerous force pulses. The results showed that dynamic force-tracking exhibited greater intermittency amplitude and force pulse but a smaller amplitude ratio of primary movement to force intermittency than static force-tracking. Multi-scale entropy analysis revealed that force intermittency during dynamic force-tracking was more complex on a low time scale but more regular on a high time scale than that of static force-tracking. Together with task-dependent force intermittency properties, dynamic force-tracking exhibited a smaller 8–12 Hz muscular oscillation but a more potentiated muscular oscillation at 35–50 Hz than static force-tracking. In conclusion, force intermittency reflects differing trajectory controls for static and dynamic force-tracking. The target goal of dynamic tracking is achieved through trajectory adjustments that are more intricate and more frequent than those of static tracking, pertaining to differing organizations and functioning of muscular oscillations in the alpha and gamma bands.

Editor: Kelvin E. Jones, University of Alberta, Canada

Funding: This research was supported by a grant from the National Science Council, R.O.C. (http://web1.nsc.gov.tw/mp.aspx?mp = 7), under Grant No. NSC-101-2410-H-040-017. The funders had no role in study design, data collection and analysis, decision to publish, or preparation of the manuscript.

Competing Interests: The authors have declared that no competing interests exist.

* E-mail: ishwang@mail.ncku.edu.tw

Introduction

Visuomotor tracking is a critical function of the motor system. However, intrinsic trajectory control is affected by variations in the state of the motor system [1,2], since motor responses are not strictly smooth. A larger size of force variability greatly drifts the force output away from an intended priori standard. The complexity of force variability is another dimension of force variability [3,4], typically indexed with entropy measures [3,5] to characterize the degree of fluctuation predictability over a force data stream [6,7]. The size and the complexity of force variability of a visuomotor task can be differently organized. For instance, tracking with visual feedback is more accurate and has a smaller size but a greater complexity of force variability than tracking without visual feedback [1,3,8]. An increase in force complexity is related to engagement of trajectory adjustments using on-line sensory inputs, rather than to task degradation [1,9]. One of the major sources of force or kinematic variability comes from sampled feedback processes of the visuomotor system [10,11] for enhancing the stability of the visuomotor system against long feedback delays [10,12]. However, sampled feedback brings about movement intermittency, as manifested with discrete blocks of pulse-like elements in movement trajectory. Movement intermittency becomes less evident in pursuit of a predictable target [13,14] or removal of visual feedback [10]. Both kinematic and force profiles exhibit intermittency, which is related to internal coding of the planned trajectory and error correction [14,15].

Exertion level is a key factor of force variability underlying progressive recruitment of fast-twitch motor units [16] and variations in code rating [17]. On account of an exertion-dependent increase in force variability [18,19], precise control of force is far more difficult at a higher force range than at a lower force range. Force stability at a higher force range presumably relies on task-dependent variations in code rating in that motor units are largely recruited [20]. As movement accuracy at large force output is insufficient for precision tasks, force scaling at a higher force range is often overlooked. Little attention has been paid to contrasting force variability properties between static and dynamic force-tracking at relatively high exertion levels. It is apparent that static and dynamic force-tracking challenge the visuomotor system to different extents, including visual information load [21], proprioceptive inputs [22], target constraints to produce the criterion force [23], and so on.

The present study sought to contrast the size and complexity of force intermittent behaviors between static and dynamic force-tracking at relatively high exertion levels of equivalent physical loads. Because of the different time and target constraints, we expected intermittent force behavior and the scaling property of individual force pulse for the two force-tracking tasks to be task-dependent. Another focus of this study was to explain the task-dependent intermittent force behavior with oscillatory activities in the working muscle. It was hypothesized that, in comparison to static force-tracking, dynamic force-tracking would lead to larger force intermittency and a smaller amplitude ratio of the a priori standard of intended pursuit relative to force intermittency, greater complexity and spectral dispersion of the force intermittency profile, and greater force pulse metrics with different statistical properties. In addition, muscular oscillations during static and dynamic force-tracking were differently organized with respect to tracking protocols. Our observations on force intermittency dynamics and muscular oscillations extend previous work to gain better insight into how force trajectories are planned to satisfy differing task needs.

Methods

Ethics Statement

The research project was approved by an authorized institutional human research review board (Chung Shan Medical University Hospital Institutional Review Board, CSMUH IRB), and all subjects signed informed consents before the experiment, conforming to the Declaration of Helsinki.

Subjects

Twenty-two male subjects (mean: 21.6±1.2 years) from a local community and a university participated in this study. All of the subjects were self-reported as being right-handed, and none of them had symptoms or signs of neuromuscular diseases.

Experiment Procedures

This study employed two unilateral resistance protocols of gripping, static and dynamic force-tracking. Each protocol consisted of three trials of 20 seconds, which were randomly completed by our participants with inter-trial periods of rest of at least 3 minutes. The subject sat on a chair with the left arm hanging naturally by the trunk and gripped a hand dynamometer (sensitivity: 0.01 N, bandwidth: DC–1 kHz, Model 9810P, Aikoh, Japan) connected to an analog amplifier (Model: PS-30A-1, Entran, UK). The force output and the target curve were displayed on a computer monitor to guide the force exertion of the force-tracking maneuver. Before the experiment, all subjects first performed 3 maximal voluntary contractions (MVC) of 3 seconds, separated by 3-minute pauses. The mean of the maximal force for the 3 MVCs was defined as the peak gripping force. During static force-tracking, the subjects needed to produce a constant force of 75% of peak gripping force with the aid of visual feedback. Dynamic force-tracking required the subjects to exert a load-varying isometric force to couple a 0.5 Hz sinusoidal target wave in the range of 50%–100% of peak gripping force. The target signal moved vertically in a range of 7.2° of visual angle (i.e., 3.6° above and 3.6° below the eye level on the screen), and visual feedback gain in terms of visual angle per MVC was identical for static and dynamic force-tracking. Muscle activity of the left flexor digitorum superficialis (FDS) was recorded by surface electromyography. A bipolar surface electrode unit (1.1 cm in diameter, gain = 365, CMRR = 102 dB, Imoed Inc., USA) was placed at an oblique angle approximately 4 cm above the wrist on the palpable muscle mass. All signals were sampled at 1 kHz by an analog-to-digital converter with 16-bit resolution (DAQ Card-6024E; National Instruments Inc., Austin, TX, USA), controlled by a custom program on a Labview platform (Labview v.8.5, National Instruments Inc., Austin, TX, USA).

Data Processing

The size and complexity of the force intermittency profile. Gripping force was down-sampled to 100 Hz in off-line analysis and then conditioned with a low-pass filter (cut-off frequency: 6 Hz) [24]. Mean gripping forces of an experimental trial for both force-tracking paradigms were determined. Then force output of the tracking tasks was dichotomized into two different force components, primary movement and force intermittency profile, akin to the algorithms proposed by Roitmen et al. (2004) and Selen et al. (2006) [25,26]. In brief, the primary movement was a smooth and deterministic force component of the force-tracking task, spectrally identical to the target rate. Also, the primary movement approximated target movement in amplitude. Therefore, the primary movement symbolizes the a priori standard of intended pursuit to couple the target signal. On the other hand, the force intermittency profile was a stochastic force component that contributed to force variability. The force intermittency profile was irregular, containing a number of individual force pulses (Fig. 1A). Recent studies have validated that force pulses are not noises, but part of an additive accuracy control to remedy tracking deviations from the target trajectory [26,27]. The dichotomy of gripping force was helpful to specify structural changes in the force intermittency profile (force variability) and to differentiate task effects on deterministic and stochastic force components for static and dynamic tracking. For the static force-tracking, the primary movement was a force level of 75% MVC. The force intermittency profile of static force-tracking could be obtained by removing the linear trend of the force time series (Fig. 1A, left). For the dynamic task, the primary movement was a 0.5 Hz sinusoidal wave with amplitude roughly in the range of 50%–100% MVC. The force intermittency profile of dynamic force-tracking was obtained by conditioning the force output with a zero-phasing notch filter that passes all frequencies except for a target rate at 0.5 Hz (Fig. 1A, right). The transfer function of the notch filter was $H(Z) = b_0 \frac{(1-e^{j\omega_0}z^{-1})(1-e^{-j\omega_0}z^{-1})}{(1-re^{j\omega_0}z^{-1})(1-re^{-j\omega_0}z^{-1})}$, $r = .9975$, $\omega_0 = \pi/360$. Subtracting the force intermittency profile from the dynamic force output gave the sinusoidal component of the target rate in the gripping force, previously described as the primary movement for the dynamic task.

Root mean square (RMS) was applied to the primary movement and the force intermittency profile to calculate the amplitudes of the two force components. The RMS of the force intermittency profile symbolized the size of force variability. The amplitude ratio of the primary movement to force intermittency ($R_{PM/FI}$) was defined as the RMS of the primary movement divided by the RMS of the force intermittency profile. Spectral distribution of the force intermittency profile was estimated with the Welch method and a fast Fourier transform with a spectral resolution of 0.1 Hz. Mean frequency and spectral dispersion (spectral ranges between the 10th and 90th percentiles of the power spectra) were determined from the force intermittency spectral profile. The complexity of the force intermittency profile (i.e., the complexity of force variability) was quantified with multi-scale entropy (MSE) to reveal a sample entropy (SampEn) curve across different time scales (Appendix S1) [6,28]. Each time scale represented 10 ms for the sampling rate of 100 Hz. MSE areas under the time scales 1–25 (or 10–250 ms) and 26–60 (or 260–600 ms) were empirically determined to measure the complexity of the force intermittency profile on short and high time scales, respectively. The MSE area of the overall time scale of 1–60 was the sum of MSE areas under the time scales 1–25 and 26–60. A higher MSE area indicated a noisier structure with greater signal complexity.

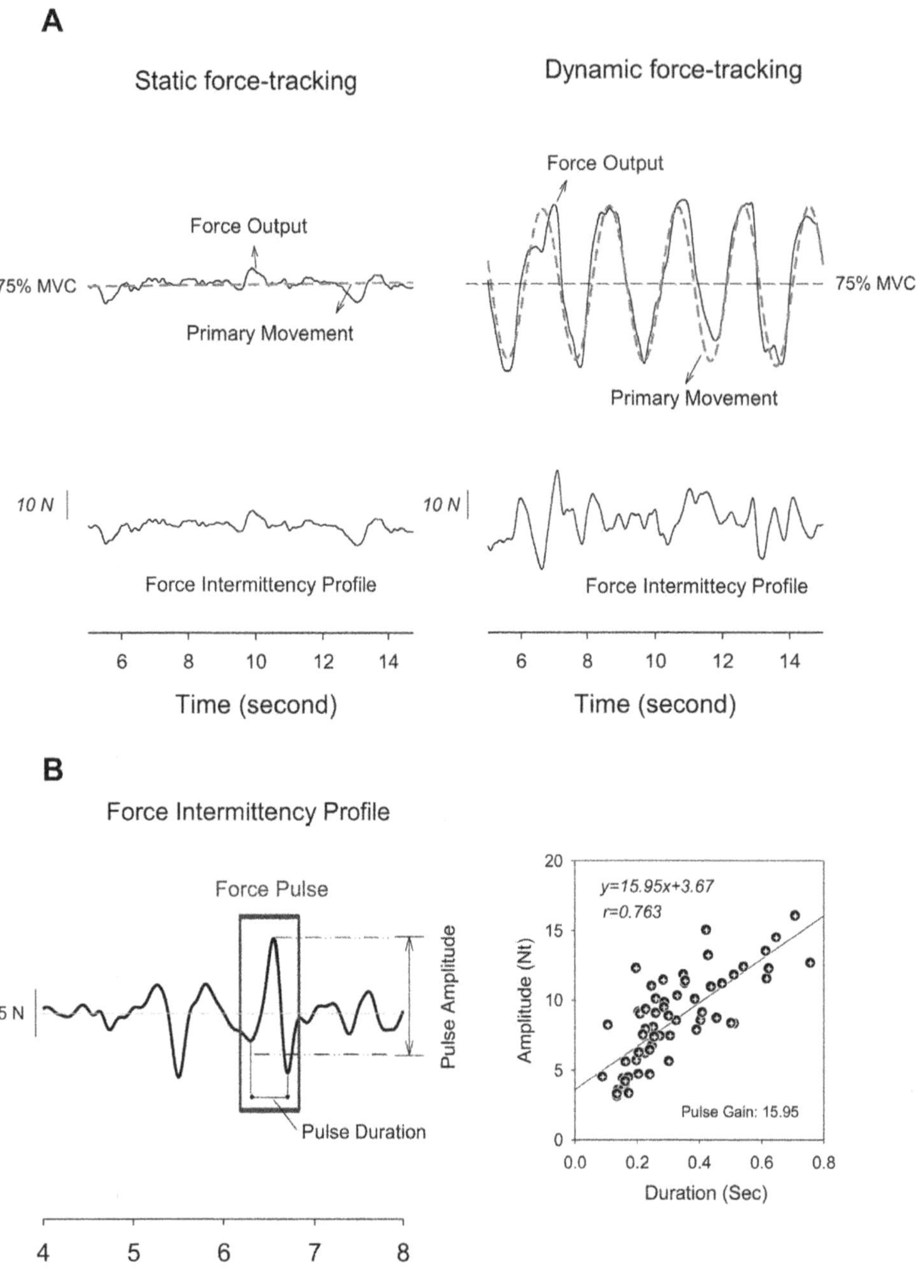

Figure 1. Illustrative examples of force intermittency profile, primary movement, and force pulse. (A) Feature extraction of force intermittency profile and primary movements from force outputs of static and dynamic force-tracking. (B) Representative force intermittency profile during dynamic and static tasks.

Force pulse variables. Individual force pulses in a force intermittency profile were identified afterwards. Local peak in the force intermittency profile was defined as a force pulse, and a force intermittency profile contained many force pulses. Amplitude of each force pulse was the difference between a local maximum and the average value of the two nearest minima (Fig. 1B, left) [24,25]. The pulse duration was the time between two successive local minima in the force intermittency profile. For each subject, we characterized the pulse amplitude and duration of each pulse in a force intermittency profile during static and dynamic force-tracking and then calculated the probability distribution of pulse amplitude and pulse duration to get mean pulse amplitude and mean pulse duration. Linear regression between the pulse duration and pulse amplitude in a force intermittency profile provided a duration-amplitude regression slope, or pulse gain (Fig 1B, right) [24,25]. Force pulse gain of the three experiment trials during static and dynamic force-tracking was averaged across the subjects.

EMG variables. EMG of the FDS muscles were conditioned with band-pass filters (pass band for EMG: 1~400 Hz). The amplitude of the EMG of the FDS muscles for the entire period of a trial was represented with RMS. The EMG data after band-pass filtering were rectified for spectral analysis [29]. Rectification of

Table 1. The contrast of amplitude variables of the primary movement and force intermittency between static and dynamic tracking.

Amplitude variable[1]	Static	Dynamic	*Statistics*
RMS_PM (N) [3]	126.23±4.97	124.19±4.36	
RMS_FI (N) [4]	3.49±0.32	5.68±0.26***	Λ =0.032, *P*=.000 [2]
$R_{PM/FI}$ [5]	48.01±3.49†††	22.52±0.51	

[1]Values were presented as mean ± se.
[2]Post-hoc for static force-tracking vs. dynamic force-tracking (***: Dynamic > Static, *P*<.001; †††: Static > Dynamic, *P*<.001).
[3]RMS_PM: root mean square of primary movement.
[4]RMS_FI: root mean square of force intermittency profile.
[5]$R_{PM/FI}$ denotes amplitude ratio of the primary movement to force intermittency.

surface EMG is believed to enhance the spectral peaks that symbolize common oscillatory inputs or the mean firing rate of an active muscle [30,31,32]. The power spectra of the both un-rectified and rectified EMG signals were computed using Welch's method. A Hanning window with a window length of 1.6 seconds and an overlap of 0.4 seconds was used. Spectral resolution was 0.244 Hz. The spectral profile of rectified EMG of the three trials was averaged and then normalized with the mean spectral amplitude to reduce population variability. We obtained mean spectral peaks in the alpha (8–12 Hz), and gamma (35–50 Hz) bands from three tracking trials during static and dynamic force-tracking. All signal processing was completed using Matlab (Mathworks Inc., Natick, MA, USA).

Statistical Analysis. For each subject, all force and EMG variables of the three trials were averaged for the static and dynamic force-tracking tasks. A paired t-test was used to compare the mean gripping force between static and dynamic force-tracking. Hotelling's T^2 test was used to contrast the population means of force intermittency properties between static and dynamic force-tracking, including the amplitude parameter of force intermittency (RMS values of primary movement/force intermittency and $R_{PM/FI}$), spectral parameters of force intermittency (mean frequency and spectral dispersion), complexity of force intermittency (MSE areas in short, long, and overall time scales), scaling of force pulses (pulse amplitude, pulse duration, and pulse gain), and EMG variables (alpha peak and gamma peak, and RMS) of the FDS muscle. Post-hoc analysis was conducted for all Hotelling's T^2 tests with Bonferroni correction to determine the significance levels for multiple comparisons. For both tracking conditions, the correlation between the force amplitude variables (RMS_PM, RMS_FI, and $R_{PM/FI}$) and standardized amplitude of spectral peaks was examined with Pearson's correlation. Likewise, the correlation between the force intermittency complexity (MSE areas in low and high time scales) and standardized amplitude of spectral peaks was also examined with Pearson's correlation. The levels of significance for the determination of differences were 0.05. All statistical analyses were completed with the statistical package for Social Sciences (SPSS) for Windows v. 15.0 (SPSS Inc., USA).

Results

Basic Force Characteristics

The results of paired t statistics suggested an insignificant protocol effect on mean gripping force between dynamic force-tracking (128.79±6.05 N) and static force-tracking (130.89±6.11 N) (t_{21} = −1.471, *P*=0.156), which validated that the physical work of the two loaded paradigms was very similar.

Force Intermittency Properties and Force Pulse Metrics

Table 1 contrasts the mean amplitudes for the primary movement (PM) and force intermittency (FI) profile between static and dynamic tracking. Hotelling's T^2 suggested a significant protocol effect on RMS values of the primary movement and force intermittency profile, as well as the amplitude ratio of $R_{PM/FI}$ (Wilks' Λ =032, *P*<.001). Post-hoc analysis revealed that the RMS value of the force intermittency profile during dynamic force-tracking was greater than that during static force-tracking (*P*<.001), whereas the RMS value of the primary movement did not differ between the two force-tracking conditions (*P*=.301). Static force-tracking exhibited a greater $R_{PM/FI}$ (48.01±3.49) than did dynamic force-tracking (22.52±0.51) (*P*<.001). Figure 2A shows the power spectra of force intermittency between static and dynamic force-tracking for all subjects. The mean frequency and spectral dispersion of the force intermittency profile differed with force-tracking mode (Wilks' Λ = .035, *P*<.001), with greater mean frequency and spectral dispersion for dynamic force-tracking (*P*<.001) (Fig. 2B). Figure 3A shows the results of MSE analysis and pooled SampEn curves across different time scales for static and dynamic tracking. Dynamic force-tracking appeared to exhibit a larger SampEn in the low time scale 1–25 but a smaller SampEn in the high time scale 26–60 than those of static force-tracking. Hotelling's T^2 and post-hoc analysis were consistent with that observation (Wilks' Λ =.106, *P*<.001). Dynamic force-tracking had a larger MES area (59.7±0.3) under the time scale 1–25 than did static force-tracking (57.9±0.3) (*P*=.001), but an opposite trend was noted for the MES area under the time scale 26–60 (Dynamic: 68.8±0.5; Static: 75.6±0.5) (*P*<.001) (Fig. 3B). The MES area of the overall time scale 1–60 for dynamic tracking (128.6±0.6) was significantly lower than that for static force-tracking (133.6±0.7) (*P*<.001) (Fig. 3B), because of a more potent effect on the deceasing trend of the MES area in the high time scale.

The fundamental element in the force intermittency profile was the force pulse, the scaling parameters of which were examined between static and dynamic force-tracking (Table 2). Hotelling's T^2 statistics showed that the pulse variables differed with tracking protocol (Wilks' Λ =.135, *P*<.001). Post-hoc analysis suggested that the pulse amplitude of dynamic force-tracking (9.88±.53 N) was larger than that of static force-tracking (3.30±.35 N) (*P*<.001). Dynamic force-tracking exhibited a longer pulse duration (.448±.007 sec) than did static force-tracking (.378±.110 sec) (*P*<.001). The pulse gain (amplitude-duration regression slope) of dynamic force-tracking (26.59±1.39 N/sec) was significantly greater than that of static force-tracking (11.78±1.17 N/sec) (*P*<.001).

EMG Variables and Muscular Oscillations

Figure 4A contrasts the pooled spectral profiles of un-rectified/rectified EMG of the FDS muscle between static and dynamic force-tracking. Both EMG spectral profiles exhibited two prominent spectral peaks in 8–12 Hz and 35–50 Hz. Hotelling's T^2 statistics showed that EMG spectral variables varied with force-tracking protocol (Un-rectified EMG: Wilks' Λ =.722, *P*=.039; Rectified EMG: Wilks' Λ =.496, *P*=.003) (Fig. 4B). For rectified EMG, post-hoc analysis further revealed that static force-tracking (normalized spectral amplitude: 3.30±0.34) had a greater alpha spectral peak (8–12 Hz) than dynamic force-tracking (2.27±0.15) (*P*=.009). Conversely, the dynamic task (standardized amplitude:

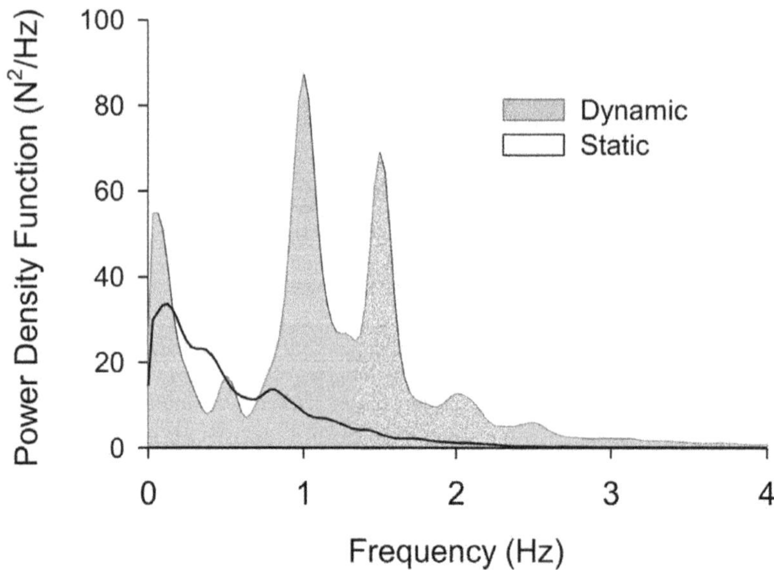

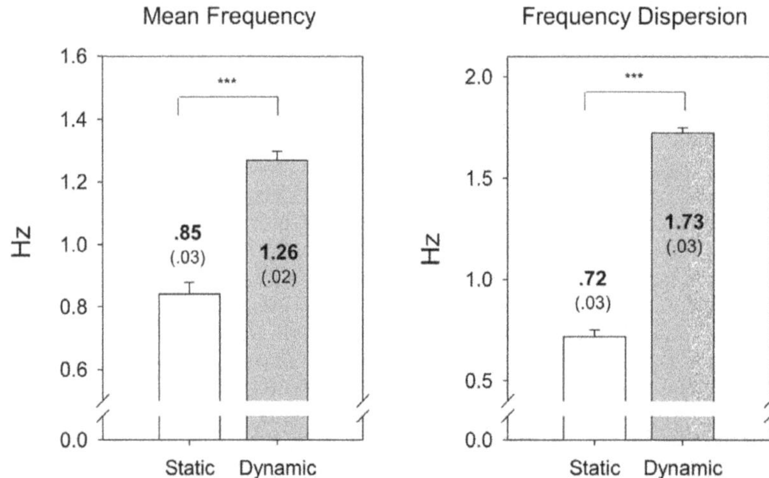

Figure 2. Contrast of spectral features of force intermittency profile between static and dynamic force-tracking. (A) Pooled spectral distributions of force intermittency profile during static and dynamic force-tracking, (B) population means of mean frequency and spectral dispersion for force intermittency profiles (Post-hoc test: ***: Dynamic > Static, P<.001).

1.86±0.19) exhibited a larger gamma rhythm (35–50 Hz) than the static task (standardized amplitude: 1.42±0.07) (P=.011). Variations in standardized spectral peaks in the alpha and gamma bands between static and dynamic gripping for un-rectified EMG were similar to those of rectified EMG. Static gripping resulted in a greater alpha peak but a smaller gamma peak (alpha: 0.45±0.10; gamma: 2.20±0.13) than dynamic gripping (alpha: 0.24±0.03; gamma: 2.77±0.27) (P<.05). However, the EMG RMS of the FDS muscle was not significantly different between dynamic (0.065±0.005 mV) and static force-tracking (0.064±0.005 mV) (P=.829).

Table 3 shows relationships between the force intermittency variables and muscular oscillations for static and dynamic force-tracking. For static force-tracking, the standardized amplitude of the 8–12 Hz spectral peak was not significantly related to any force intermittency variables (P>.05). For dynamic force-tracking, the standardized amplitude of 35–50 Hz spectral peak was also correlated negatively and positively with force intermittency amplitude (P<.05) and the amplitude ratio of $R_{PM/FI}$ (P<.001), respectively. However, the standardized amplitude of the 8–12 Hz spectral peak was independent of any force variables (P>.05), though the muscular oscillation was significantly suppressed in comparison with that during static force-tracking.

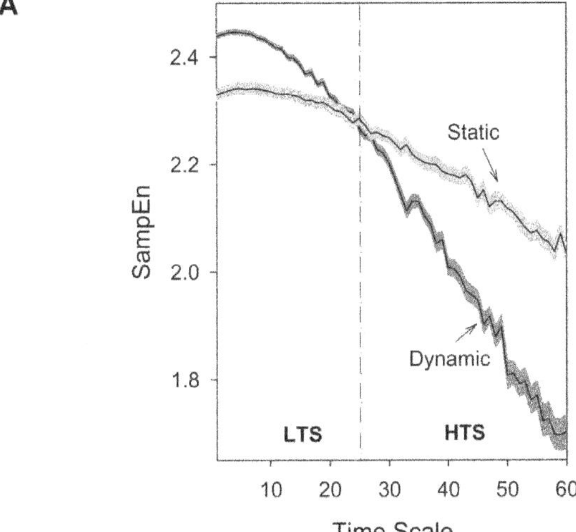

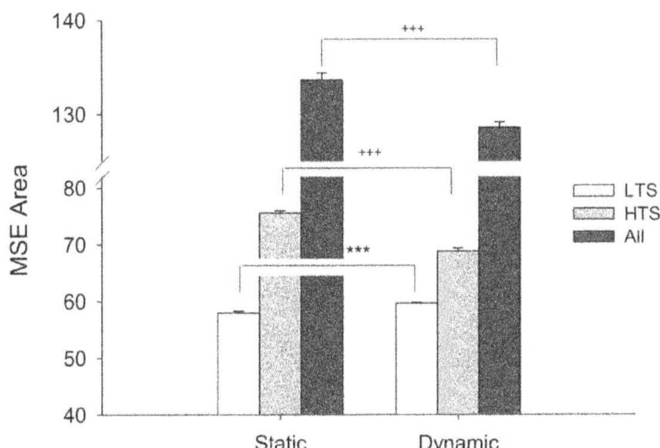

Figure 3. Contrasts of pooled complexity measures of force intermittency profile between static and dynamic force-tracking. (A) Sample entropy (SampEn) versus time scales, (B) Multi-scale entropy area (MSE area) for the low time scale of 1–25 (LTS), high time scale of 26–60 (HTS), and overall time scale of 1–60 (All). Each time scale represents 10 ms due to the sampling rate of 100 Hz. (Post-hoc test: ***: Dynamic > Static, $P \leq .001$; †††: Static > Dynamic, $P < .001$).

Discussion

The present study first revealed that the size and complexity of force intermittency as well as muscular oscillation were organized with the target goal of the force-tracking tasks. The dynamic force-tracking brought about a greater size of force intermittency with higher and wider spectral dispersion than did static force-tracking. In comparison with static tracking, dynamic tracking exhibited a greater complexity of force intermittency in the low time scale but, conversely, a greater regularity of force intermittency in the high time scale. Concurrent with task-dependent scaling of force intermittency, dynamic force-tracking exhibited a more potentiated 35–50 Hz muscular oscillation but a smaller 8–12 Hz muscular oscillation than did static force-tracking. In light of the force intermittency and muscular rhythm, there exist strategic differences in force regulation between dynamic and static force-tracking of a comparable load along with an underlying greater cognitive challenge for repetitive transient force changes during dynamic force-tracking.

Trajectory Optimization and Task-dependent Force Intermittency Properties

In this study, force output during a tracking maneuver was dichotomized into two force components, the smooth primary movement and the force intermittency profile. Contrary to a primary movement that signifies a priori standard preprogrammed in pursuit of a visual target [24,25,27], the force intermittency profile reflects an error-correction strategy in an attempt to remedy deviations during goal-directed movement. Under the framework of sampled movement control [10,11,12], force pulses in a force intermittency profile are centrally-scalable, superimposed onto the primary movement to tune a force trajectory [24,26,27]. Since dynamic tracking produced larger force intermittency and a smaller $R_{PM/FI}$ ratio than did static force-tracking (Table 1), dynamic force-tracking weighs more heavily on the error-correction process, entailing more intensive integration of proprioceptive and visual inputs than does static tracking [33]. Also, corrective adjustments to dynamic force-tracking were more frequent in order to generate motor commands in shorter time scales, on account of the higher number of high-frequency components with greater spectral dispersion in the force intermittency profile (Figs. 2A, 2B). Irrespective of static and dynamic tracking, force intermittency had a spectral range under 2 Hz, consistent with the Vaillancourt et al. (2002) [34], who reported a 0–2 Hz dominant frequency in force output during static continuous isometric contraction with low and high visual gains. Interestingly, force intermittency during dynamic force-tracking appeared to oscillate at harmonics of the target rates (primarily 1.0 Hz, 1.5 Hz, and 2 Hz). It is speculated that the subjects recurrently updated the trajectory control at particular rates, which have been noted to code kinematic properties of repetitive hand movement in the cortico-cerebello-cortical loop [35,36].

Although the complexity of force intermittency is typically characterized with approximate entropy [5,7,37] or uni-scale SampEn [23], this study adopted a new complexity measure with the use of multi-scale entropy (MSE). The methodological advantage of using MSE is that it allows assessment of SampEn across multiple time scales on the basis of multiple coarse-grained sequences and long-range temporal correlations, such that MSE accounts for time-dependent complexity and the presence of memory effects in physiological data [6,28]. In the low time scale 1–25, dynamic force-tracking exhibited a greater force intermittency complexity (larger

Table 2. The contrast of force pulse variables between static and dynamic tracking.

Force pulse variable[1]	Static	Dynamic	*Statistics*
Mean Amplitude (N)	3.30±.35	9.88±.53***	
Mean Duration (Sec)	.378±.011	.448±.007***	Λ = 0.135, $P = .000$ [2]
Pulse Gain[3] (N/Sec)	11.78±1.17	26.59±1.39***	

[1]Values were presented as mean ± se.
[2]Post-hoc for static force-tracking vs. dynamic force-tracking (***: Dynamic > Static, $P < .001$).
[3]Pulse gain also denotes amplitude-duration slope of force pulse.

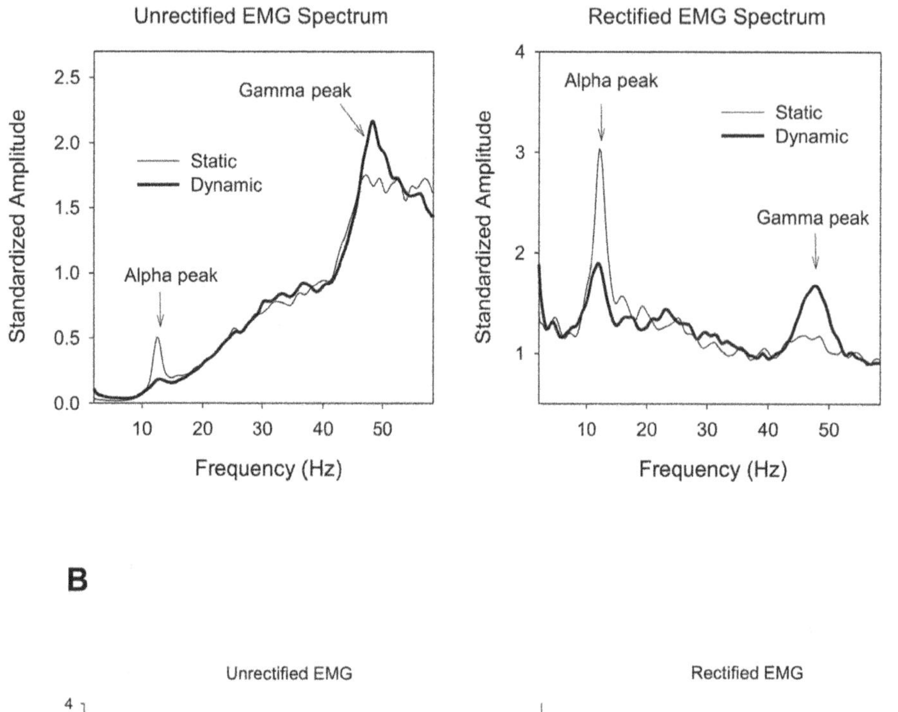

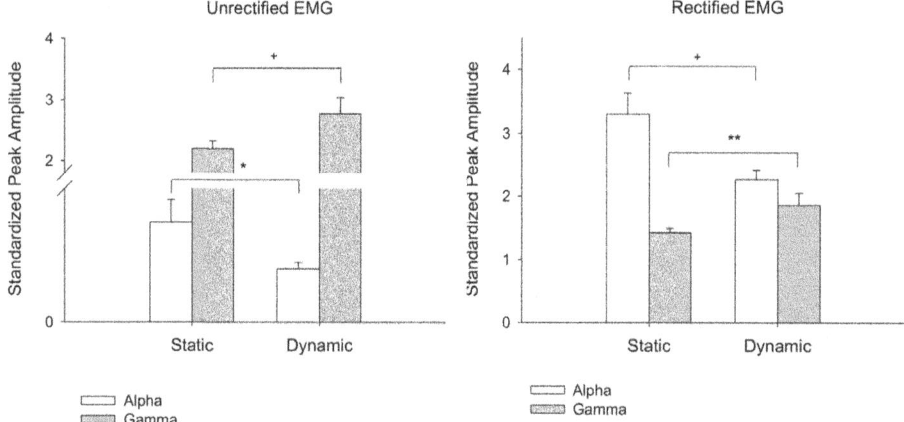

Figure 4. Contrasts of spectral features of the EMG between static and dynamic force-tracking. (A) Pooled spectral profiles of un-rectified and rectified EMG, (B) The means and standard errors of standardized amplitude for 8–12 Hz and 35–50 Hz spectral peaks. (Post-hoc test: *: Dynamic $>$ Static, $P<.05$; ††: Static $>$ Dynamic, $P<.01$; †: Static $>$ Dynamic, $P<.05$).

MSE area) than did static force-tracking (Figs. 3A, 3B), physically in accordance with the wider spectral spreads in high frequency of the force intermittency profile. Dynamic force-tracking in the shorter time scale was more informative, probably because the force tracking system adapted the required force output to multiple changing sensory inputs from the periphery to remedy tracking deviations in a short interval [33]. However, force intermittency of dynamic force-tracking in the high time scale 26–60 were conversely more regular (smaller MSE area) than those of static force-tracking (Figs. 3A, 3B). Since the target cycle of 0.5 Hz for dynamic force-tracking was 500 ms, it was very likely that the force intermittency data in the former half of the target cycle shared some stochastic properties with the latter half of the target cycle. Therefore, the force intermittency sequence after the course-gaining process with a window length exceeding half of the target cycle (time scale = 25) presented memory effects with higher possibility of predictability (lower SampEn curve) than did the force intermittency sequence in the static condition. This scenario suggests that fine-tuning of force trajectory during dynamic tracking was rhythmically encoded in every half a target cycle. The trajectory corrective mode for time-to-valley force and time-to-peak force during dynamic force-tracking could be analogous. Because the effect of SampEn in the high time scale on complexity measures overpowered that in the low time scale, the overall MSE area of dynamic force-tracking was still lower than that of static force-tracking (Fig. 3B). This observation on overall MSE area can explain a more regular movement trajectory for

Table 3. Pearson's correlation coefficients between force intermittency characteristics and muscular oscillations.

	Static	Dynamic	
(n = 22)	Alpha	Alpha	Gamma
$RMS_{\_PM}$[1]	r = −.336, P = .126	r = −.289, P = .192	r = −.223, P = .319
$RMS_{\_FI}$[2]	r = −.365, P = .095	r = −.208, P = .354	r = −.426, P = .048* [7]
$R_{PM/FI}$[3]	r = .382, P = .079	r = −.381, P = .081	r = .654, P = .001** [7]
$MSE_{\_LTS}$[4]	r = .052, P = .189	r = .282, P = .204	r = .295, P = .183
$MSE_{\_HTS}$[5]	r = .118, P = .602	r = −.104, P = .645	r = .057, P = .800
$MSE_{\_All}$[6]	r = .088, P = .698	r = −.031, P = .892	r = .089, P = .695

[1]$RMS_{\_PM}$ represents root mean square of primary movement.
[2]$RMS_{\_FI}$ represents root mean square of force intermittency profile.
[3]$R_{PM/FI}$ represents amplitude ration of primary movement relative to force intermittency profile.
[4]$MSE_{\_LTS}$ represents multi-scale entropy area of low time scale 1–25.
[5]$MSE_{\_HTS}$ represents multi-scale entropy area of high time scale 26–60.
[6]$MSE_{\_All}$ represents multi-scale entropy area of overall time scale 1–60.
[7]The shaded area indicates a significant level of correlation coefficient. (*: $P<.05$; **: $P<.005$).

tracking a periodically-moving target [5,23]. Like force intermittency properties, force pulse metrics were differently organized with target accuracy constraints. Dynamic tracking exhibited greater pulse amplitude and pulse duration than did static tracking (Table 2). In addition, to keep in line with a rhythmic target movement, the central nervous system had to multiply pulse gain (or scaling amplitude-duration slope) during dynamic tracking (Table 2). Therefore, the dynamic target goal was accomplished by additive accuracy control that preferentially increased the gain of spatial scaling of force pulse more than the gain of temporal scaling of force pulse. A similar change in scaling amplitude-duration slope of kinematic submovement was reported, when tracking speed progressively increased during circular manual tracking [24,25].

Oscillatory Muscular Activity and Task-dependent Trajectory Adjustments

The variations in force intermittency property for the static and dynamic force-tracking pertained to differing organization of muscular oscillations at 8–12 Hz and 35–50 Hz in the FDS muscle (Fig. 4A). Research has shown that muscular oscillations in the EMG spectral peaks are related to grouped motor unit firing rates, especially enhanced EMG rectification that suppresses EMG spectral features related to the motor unit action potential shape (higher-frequency components) [31,38]. Although we did not directly measure the EEG-EMG piper rhythm (EMG-EEG coherence), it is likely that the muscular oscillations at 8–12 Hz and 35–50 Hz were physiological tremor [39,40] and the gamma band of the EMG piper rhythm [1,41], respectively. They could be the peripheral parts of EEG-EMG piper rhythm serving to regulate motor unit firing during force tracking maneuvers. For dynamic force-tracking, the most noteworthy finding was the potentiation of the low gamma band of the EMG piper rhythm (Fig. 4B). In fact, oscillatory muscle activity in 35–50 Hz is in line with converging evidence that the gamma band in corticomuscular coherence presents during phasic movement [1,42] and repetitive isotonic contraction [43]. The occurrence of gamma synchrony is thought to be of functional relevance when a motor task entails temporal modulation in movement patterns with global alertness to integrate sensory-motor information [1,42,44]. Our observation adds to this hypothesis by showing a significant negative correlation between 35–50 Hz muscular oscillation and force intermittency amplitude (Table 3). Hence, we may well argue that the gamma EMG piper rhythm is specified for fine-tuning force trajectory during dynamic tracking. The more gamma EMG piper rhythm associates with the lesser corrective attempts and the greater priori standard of tracking maneuver relative to force intermittency ($R_{PM/FI}$). In addition, we noted a significant suppression of alpha muscular oscillation during dynamic force-tracking, as compared with that of static tracking (Fig. 4B). Iyer et al. [45] also reported a roughly 12 Hz motor unit discharge during static and quasi-sinusoidal isometric contraction at the same mean force level. However, what is still not completely clear is the role of 8–12 Hz muscular oscillatory activity in the shift of tracking mode in this study.

In this study, muscular rhythm was assessed with spectral peaks of surface EMG. EMG rectification is a prevailing approach prior to calculating corticomuscular coherence for maximizing information about the grouped firing rate frequencies of active motor units [30–32]. However, some researchers argue against the appropriateness of the pre-processing procedure, as rectified EMG does not necessarily enhance the peak detection of corticomuscular coherence and may produce inconsistent coherence spectra in some cases [46,47]. Regarding this methodological controversy, we also validated our observations with spectral analysis using raw EMG. Two prominent spectral peaks were consistently noted in the spectral profiles of raw and rectified EMG, with similar parametric changes in standardized peak amplitude with respect contraction mode. In addition, we did not observe a significant EMG oscillation in the beta range (13–21 Hz) in either profile during static force-gripping, though previous studies have shown that the beta EMG-EEG piper rhythm is critical to maintaining force stability during sustained isometric contraction [1,29,42]. Physically, an evident EMG-EEG coherence in the beta band just represents a relatively high degree of an in-phase oscillation at 13–21 Hz for both EEG and EMG signals; however, it does not mean a prominent beta oscillation as compared to other spectral ingredients in the EMG signal. Despite this fact, future work is still needed to find cortical control over the task-specific scaling of force intermittency force-tracking of different patterns, on account of the functional interactions between cortical and spinal oscillatory networks.

Conclusions

In light of characteristic differences in the primary movement and force intermittency, we noted that neuro-mechanic control of force trajectory for static and dynamic force-tracking at a relatively high exertion level was task-dependent. Dynamic force-tracking exhibits a greater amount of force intermittency, with higher spectral components and greater complexity in the low time scale than that of static force-tracking. The target goal of dynamic force-tracking is achieved through frequent and vast trajectory adjustments, underlying intricate short-term and similar error-correction processes over half a target cycle. Unlike during static force-tracking, alpha muscular oscillation is markedly suppressed during dynamic force-tracking. The emergence of gamma muscular oscillation during dynamic force-tracking is likely to be responsible for the scaling of force intermittency and force trajectory adjustments. At a relatively high exertion level, modulations of muscular oscillation and force intermittency properties agree with the theoretical postulation that internal force coding to stabilize movement trajectory differs vastly with target constraints.

Author Contributions

Conceived and designed the experiments: YCC ISH. Performed the experiments: YTL CLS. Analyzed the data: YCC YTL. Contributed reagents/materials/analysis tools: CTH ZRY. Wrote the paper: YCC ISH.

References

1. Andrykiewicz A, Patino L, Naranjo JR, Witte M, Hepp-Reymond MC, et al. (2007) Corticomuscular synchronization with small and large dynamic force output. BMC Neurosci 8: 101.
2. Slifkin AB, Newell KM (1999) Noise, information transmission, and force variability. J Exp Psychol Hum Percept Perform 25: 837–851.
3. Jordan K, Newell KM (2004) Task goal and grip force dynamics. Exp Brain Res 156: 451–457.
4. Sosnoff JJ, Valantine AD, Newell KM (2006) Independence between the amount and structure of variability at low force levels. Neurosci Lett 392: 165–169.
5. Hong SL, Newell KM (2008) Motor entropy in response to task demands and environmental information. Chaos 18: 033131.
6. Costa M, Goldberger AL, Peng CK (2002) Multiscale entropy analysis of complex physiologic time series. Phys Rev Lett 89: 068102.
7. Pincus SM (2001) Assessing serial irregularity and its implications for health. Ann N Y Acad Sci 954: 245–267.
8. Baweja HS, Patel BK, Martinkewiz JD, Vu J, Christou EA (2009) Removal of visual feedback alters muscle activity and reduces force variability during constant isometric contractions. Exp Brain Res 197: 35–47.
9. Kuznetsov NA, Riley MA (2010) Spatial resolution of visual feedback affects variability and structure of isometric force. Neurosci Lett 470: 121–125.
10. Miall RC, Weir DJ, Stein JF (1986) Manual tracking of visual targets by trained monkeys. Behav Brain Res 20: 185–201.
11. Navas F, Stark L (1968). Sampling or intermittency in hand control system dynamics. Biophys J 8: 252–302.
12. Miall RC, Weir DJ, Stein JF (1993) Intermittency in human manual tracking tasks. J Mot Behav 25: 53–63.
13. Sosnoff JJ, Newell KM (2005) Intermittency of visual information and the frequency of rhythmical force production. J Mot Behav 37: 325–334.
14. Slifkin AB, Vaillancourt DE, Newell KM (2000) Intermittency in the control of continuous force production. J Neurophysiol 84: 1708–1718.
15. Walker N, Philbin DA, Fisk AD (1997) Age-related differences in movement control: adjusting force intermittency structure to optimize performance. J Gerontol B Psychol Sci Soc Sci 52: P40–52.
16. Henneman E (1957) Relation between size of neurons and their susceptibility to discharge. Science 126: 1345–1347.
17. Negro F, Holobar A, Farina D (2009) Fluctuations in isometric muscle force can be described by one linear projection of low-frequency components of motor unit discharge rates. J Physiol 587: 5925–38.
18. Jones KE, Hamilton AF, Wolpert DM (2002) Sources of signal-dependent noise during isometric force production. J Neurophysiol 88: 1533–1544.
19. Bedrov YA, Dick OE, Romanov SP (2007) Role of signal-dependent noise during maintenance of isometric force. Biosystems 89: 50–57.
20. Erim Z, De Luca CJ, Mineo K, Aoki T (1996) Rank-ordered regulation of motor units. Muscle Nerve 19: 563–573.
21. Hong SL, Newell KM (2008) Visual information gain and the regulation of constant force levels. Exp Brain Res 189: 61–69.
22. Prochazka A, Gillard D, Bennett DJ (1997) Implications of positive feedback in the control of movement. J Neurophysiol 77: 3237–3251.
23. Svendsen JH, Samani A, Mayntzhusen K, Madeleine P (2011) Muscle coordination and force variability during static and dynamic tracking tasks. Hum Mov Sci 30: 1039–1051.
24. Pasalar S, Roitman AV, Ebner TJ (2005) Effects of speeds and force fields on force intermittencys during circular manual tracking in humans. Exp Brain Res 163: 214–225.
25. Roitman AV, Massaquoi SG, Takahashi K, Ebner TJ (2004) Kinematic analysis of manual tracking in monkeys: characterization of movement intermittencies during a circular tracking task. J Neurophysiol 91: 901–911.
26. Selen LP, van Dieën JH, Beek PJ (2006) Impedance modulation and feedback corrections in tracking targets of variable size and frequency. J Neurophysiol 96: 2750–2759.
27. Selen LP, Franklin DW, Wolpert DM (2009) Impedance control reduces instability that arises from motor noise. J Neurosci 29: 12606–12616.
28. Costa M, Priplata AA, Lipsitz LA, Wu Z, Huang NE, et al. (2007) Noise and poise: Enhancement of postural complexity in the elderly with a stochastic-resonance-based therapy. Europhys Lett 77: 68008.
29. Kilner JM, Baker SN, Salenius S, Hari R, Lemon RN (2000) Human cortical muscle coherence is directly related to specific motor parameters. J Neurosci 20: 8838–8845.
30. Boonstra TW, Breakspear M (2012) Neural mechanisms of intermuscular coherence: implications for the rectification of surface electromyography. J Neurophysiol 107: 796–807.
31. Myers LJ, Lowery M, O'Malley M, Vaughan CL, Heneghan C, et al. (2003) Rectification and non-linear pre-processing of EMG signals for cortico-muscular analysis. J Neurosci Methods 124: 157–165.
32. Stegeman DF, van de Ven WJ, van Elswijk GA, Oostenveld R, Kleine BU (2010) The alpha-motoneuron pool as transmitter of rhythmicities in cortical motor drive. Clin Neurophysiol 121: 1633–1642.
33. Huang CT, Hwang IS (2012) Eye-hand synergy and intermittent behaviors during target-directed tracking with visual and non-visual information. PLoS One 7: e51417.
34. Vaillancourt DE, Larsson L, Newell KM (2002) Time-dependent structure in the discharge rate of human motor units. Clin Neurophysiol 113: 1325–1338.
35. Bourguignon M, De Tiège X, de Beeck MO, Van Bogaert P, Goldman S, et al. (2012) Primary motor cortex and cerebellum are coupled with the kinematics of observed hand movements. Neuroimage 66C: 500–507.
36. Liu J, Perdoni C, He B (2011) Hand movement decoding by phase-locking low frequency EEG signals. Conf Proc IEEE Eng Med Biol Soc 2011: 6335–6338.
37. Hu X, Newell KM (2012) Force and time gain interact to nonlinearly scale adaptive visual-motor isometric force control. Exp Brain Res 221: 191–203.
38. Yao W, Fuglevand RJ, Enoka RM (2000) Motor-unit synchronization increases EMG amplitude and decreases force steadiness of simulated contractions. J Neurophysiol 83: 441–452.
39. Hwang IS, Yang ZR, Huang CT, Guo MC (2009) Reorganization of multidigit physiological tremors after repetitive contractions of a single finger. J Appl Physiol 106: 966–974.
40. Elble RJ, Randall JE (1976) Motor-unit activity responsible for 8- to 12-Hz component of human physiological finger tremor. J Neurophysiol 39: 370–383.
41. Schoffelen JM, Poort J, Oostenveld R, Fries P (2011) Selective movement preparation is subserved by selective increases in corticomuscular gamma-band coherence. J Neurosci 31: 6750–6758.
42. Omlor W, Patino L, Hepp-Reymond MC, Kristeva R (2007) Gamma-range corticomuscular coherence during dynamic force output. Neuroimage 34: 1191–1198.
43. Muthukumaraswamy SD (2010) Functional properties of human primary motor cortex gamma oscillations. J Neurophysiol 104: 2873–2885.
44. Gwin JT, Ferris DP (2012) Beta- and gamma-range human lower limb corticomuscular coherence. Front Hum Neurosci 6: 258.
45. Iyer MB, Christakos CN, Ghez C (1994) Coherent modulations of human motor unit discharges during quasi-sinusoidal isometric muscle contractions. Neurosci Lett 170: 94–98.
46. Neto OP, Christou EA (2010) Rectification of the EMG signal impairs the identification of oscillatory input to the muscle. J Neurophysiol 103: 1093–1103.
47. McClelland VM, Cvetkovic Z, Mills KR (2012) Rectification of the EMG is an unnecessary and inappropriate step in the calculation of corticomuscular coherence. J Neurosci Methods 205(1): 190–201.

8

Muscle Damage and Its Relationship with Muscle Fatigue During a Half-Iron Triathlon

Juan Del Coso*, **Cristina González-Millán, Juan José Salinero, Javier Abián-Vicén, Lidón Soriano, Sergio Garde, Benito Pérez-González**

Exercise Physiology Laboratory, Camilo José Cela University, Madrid, Spain

Abstract

Background: To investigate the cause/s of muscle fatigue experienced during a half-iron distance triathlon.

Methodology/Principal Findings: We recruited 25 trained triathletes (36±7 yr; 75.1±9.8 kg) for the study. Before and just after the race, jump height and leg muscle power output were measured during a countermovement jump on a force platform to determine leg muscle fatigue. Body weight, handgrip maximal force and blood and urine samples were also obtained before and after the race. Blood myoglobin and creatine kinase concentrations were determined as markers of muscle damage.

Results: Jump height (from 30.3±5.0 to 23.4±6.4 cm; $P<0.05$) and leg power output (from 25.6±2.9 to 20.7±4.6 W · kg^{-1}; $P<0.05$) were significantly reduced after the race. However, handgrip maximal force was unaffected by the race (430±59 to 430±62 N). Mean dehydration after the race was 2.3±1.2% with high inter-individual variability in the responses. Blood myoglobin and creatine kinase concentration increased to 516±248 µg · L^{-1} and 442±204 U · L^{-1}, respectively ($P<0.05$) after the race. Pre- to post-race jump change did not correlate with dehydration (r = 0.16; $P>0.05$) but significantly correlated with myoglobin concentration (r = 0.65; $P<0.001$) and creatine kinase concentration (r = 0.54; $P<0.001$).

Conclusions/significance: During a half-iron distance triathlon, the capacity of leg muscles to produce force was notably diminished while arm muscle force output remained unaffected. Leg muscle fatigue was correlated with blood markers of muscle damage suggesting that muscle breakdown is one of the most relevant sources of muscle fatigue during a triathlon.

Editor: David F. Wieczorek, University of Cincinnati College of Medicine, United States of America

Funding: The authors have no support or funding to report.

Competing Interests: The authors have declared that no competing interests exist.

* E-mail: jdelcoso@ucjc.edu

Introduction

The triathlon is an endurance sport activity that combines phases of swimming, cycling and running. Although the most renowned distance for a triathlon race is the full distance (also known as Iron distance), shorter triathlon races (e.g. Olympic or half-iron distances) have become popular since they are more accessible to amateur and recreational athletes. Independent of the distance, the triathlon is one of the most fatiguing exercise activities since it combines long duration (from 1 h 50 min in the Olympic distance to more than 14 hours in the Ironman distance) with high exercise intensity [1]. However, only a small number of studies have been geared to determine the muscle fatigue experienced by triathletes. Margaritis et al. [2] found a decreased capacity to generate force in the knee extensor and flexor muscles after a half-iron triathlon. Similarly, Suzuky et al. [3] found that jump height during squat and countermovement jumps (CMJ) significantly decreased after an Iron triathlon along with a reduction in the maximal isometric strength of the knee extensors. Thus, it seems apparent that muscle performance is diminished after a triathlon race, but its origin remains elusive.

According to Jeukendrup [1], dehydration and carbohydrate depletion are the most likely causes of fatigue during a triathlon race. Dehydration alone [4] or in combination with hyperthermia [5,6] may lessen maximal isometric strength production. Thus, drinking during exercise to avoid dehydration and hyperthermia should be a primary goal for triathletes, especially to avoid a body mass loss superior to 2% [7]. However, it has been found that triathletes do not dehydrate excessively and that the body mass loss experienced during the triathlon is mostly due to reduced fat and skeletal muscle mass [8,9]. In addition, it has been found that the dehydration level does not correlate with total race time in a triple iron triathlon [10]. According to these studies, triathletes seem well informed about the necessity of rehydrating during exercise, diminishing the deleterious effects of dehydration during a triathlon.

During exercise, an insufficient supply of glucose may result in hypoglycemia and consequently muscle fatigue. For this reason, several investigations have established that the ingestion of carbohydrates improves endurance capacity by maintaining blood glucose content [11,12]. Carbohydrate ingestion also helps to maintain muscle force production and central nervous system (CNS) activation during prolonged exercise [13]. In triathlon male athletes, it has been found that race finishing time was inversely related to carbohydrate intake during the race, although this relation was not found in females [14]. Since the rate of exogenous carbohydrate oxidation is close to1 g/min, a carbohydrate intake of ~60 g/hour has been suggested [15]. Therefore, the intake of carbohydrates during a triathlon to preserve the homeostasis of blood glucose is a crucial factor for avoiding muscle fatigue.

A reduction in plasma sodium concentration below 135 mmol · L^{-1}, mainly as a result of excessive fluid consumption, has been previously reported in triathletes [9,16]. This electrolyte imbalance is considered as a serious medical problem during ultra-distance events [1] since it is associated with weakness and mental confusion. Even coma and death may occur with sodium concentrations below 126 mmol · L^{-1}. However, the association between the decrease in plasma sodium content and muscle fatigue has not been previously established in triathletes. During prolonged cycling in the heat, Coso et al. [5] found that the ingestion of rehydrating drinks with low sodium content reduced plasma sodium concentration and worsened the maintenance of isometric muscle strength. This negative effect on muscle strength was present even when plasma sodium was not lower than 137 mmol · L^{-1}, so the reduction in sodium concentration may affect muscle performance with values higher than those typically related with hyponatremia.

Another factor that could affect muscle fatigue in the triathlon is myofibril damage, mainly produced during the running leg. Swimming and cycling are activities that produce minor muscle damage in the involved muscles. However, running is a weight-bearing activity that includes concentric and eccentric actions in the leg muscles. In a recent study, it has been found that urinary myoglobin concentration (a marker of muscle breakdown) correlates with leg muscle power reduction after a marathon [17], although other blood markers of muscle damage do not correlate with muscle fatigue after a triathlon [2]. The purpose of this study was to investigate the cause/s of muscle fatigue which ensues during a half-iron distance triathlon. We hypothesized that the source of muscle fatigue will be multifactorial, with dehydration, hypoglycemia, electrolyte imbalance and muscle damage as the main factors responsible for muscle force loss during a half-iron triathlon.

Methods

Subjects

Thirty one triathletes volunteered to participate in this investigation. However, six of these participants failed to complete the triathlon race and their records were excluded from the study. Thus, this investigation includes data from 25 healthy and well-trained triathletes. All the participants had previous experience of at least 3 yrs and had trained for ~2 h · day^{-1}, 4–5 days · week-1 during the previous year. In addition, the participants had completed at least one prior triathlon in the half-iron distance. The characteristics of the participants are summarized in Table 1. Participants completed a short questionnaire on training status and medical history. Potential participants with a history of muscle disorder, cardiac or kidney disease or those taking medications were excluded.

Ethics Statement

Participants were fully informed of any risks and discomforts associated with the experiments before giving their informed written consent to participate. The study was approved by the Camilo Jose Cela Ethics Committee in accordance with the latest version of the Declaration of Helsinki.

Table 1. Morphological characteristics of the participants and their performance in the Half-Ironman triathlon race. Data are mean±SD and ranges for 25 healthy triathletes.

	Mean ± SD	Range
Age (yr)	35.7±6.5	25–54
Height (cm)	178±7	160–191
Weight (kg)	75.1±9.8	58.4–92.5
Body fat (%)	8.6±3.9	3.4–16.0
Half-iron triathlons completed	17±22	1–97
Total race time	5:12:20±00:34:59	04:05:55–06:08:06
2.0 km swim time	00:33:52–00:04:11	00:27:13–00:42:33
90 km cycle time	02:44:53–00:18:37	02:11:16–03:17:07
Half-marathon time	01:49:01–00:27:23	01:26:43-02:19:53

Experimental Protocol

One to three days before the race, participants underwent a physical examination to ensure that they were in good health. Ninety-to-sixty minutes before the race, participants arrived at a zone close to the start line to assess pre-exercise variables. Participants voided and a urine sample was obtained to determine urine specific gravity (U_{sg}) and other urinary variables. Participants' body fat composition and pre-race body water content were then calculated using bioimpedance (BC-418, Tanita, Japan). After that, a 22-G catheter was inserted into an antecubital vein and a 7 mL blood sample was drawn. Next, participants completed a 10 min warm-up consisting of dynamic exercises and practice jumps. After that, participants performed two countermovement vertical jumps for maximal height on a force platform (Quattrojump, Kistler, Switzerland). Handgrip maximal force production in both hands was measured by using a handgrip dynamometer (Grip-D, Takei, Japan). Finally, participants were weighed in their competition clothes (±50 g scale; Radwag, Poland) and headed to the start line to participate in a half-iron distance triathlon.

The race consisted of 1.9 km of swimming, 75 km of cycling (1100 m of net increase in altitude) and 21.1 km of running. The triathlon was held in June 2011 in the surrounding area of a city located at 975 m altitude. Mean±SD (range) dry temperature during the event was 22.3±6.9°C (13–30°C) with a relative humidity of 72.8±8.0% (65–85%). Water temperature during the swim section was 19±1°C. No instructions about pace, drinking or feeding during the race were given to the participants to avoid any influence of this investigation on their habitual routines during the race. So, participants drank and consumed food *ad libitum* and swam, cycled and ran at their own pace. Performance times for the swimming, cycling and running phases and the total time are shown in Table 1.

Within 3 min of the end of the race, participants went to a finish area and performed two countermovement vertical jumps (see below). Post-race body weight and body water content were then recorded with the same devices and clothes used for the pre-race measurement. Participants were instructed to avoid drinking from the finish line till the post-race weighing and an experimenter assured compliance. Then, participants rested for five minutes and a venous blood sample was obtained using the procedures described previously. After that, subjects were provided with fluid (water and sports drinks) to promote urine production. Thirty to 60 minutes after the race, a representative sample of the first post-race void was collected in a sterile container. After that, participants finished their participation in the study. The dehydration level attained during the race was calculated as percent reduction in body weight (pre-to post-race), assuming that body mass changes was produced by a reduction in participants' water content. Similarly, we calculated the reduction in body water content using pre and post-race body water measurements by bioimpedance.

Maximal countermovement jump

Before and just after the race, participants performed two maximal countermovement jumps on a force platform (Quattro-jump, Kistler, Switzerland) to assess changes in jump height and leg power production. For this measurement, participants began stationary in an upright position with their weight evenly distributed over both feet. Each participant placed their hands on their waist in order to remove the influence of the arms on the jump. On command, the participant flexed their knees and jumped as high as possible while maintaining the hands on the waist and landed with both feet. After 1 min rest, the counter-movement jump was repeated. Leg muscle power output during the impulse phase (concentric part of the jump) and jump height were determined as previously described [17].

Blood samples

A portion of each blood sample (2 mL) was introduced into a tube with EDTA and blood glucose concentration (Accu-chek, Spain), hemoglobin concentration and hematocrit were determined within the same day. Changes in blood volume and plasma volume from rest were calculated with the equations outlined by Dill and Costill [18]. Red blood cell, white blood cell and platelet counts were determined by using an automated blood counter. The remaining blood (5 mL) was allowed to clot and serum was separated by centrifugation (10 min at 5000 g) and frozen at −80°C until the day of analysis. On a later day, the serum portion was analyzed for sodium, potassium and chloride concentrations (Nova 16, NovaBiomedical, Spain). In addition, myoglobin, creatine kinase (CK) and lactate dehydrogenase (LDH) concentrations were measured as blood markers of muscle damage.

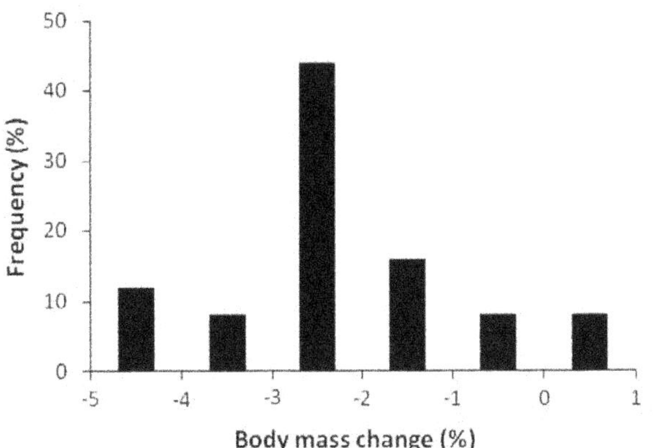

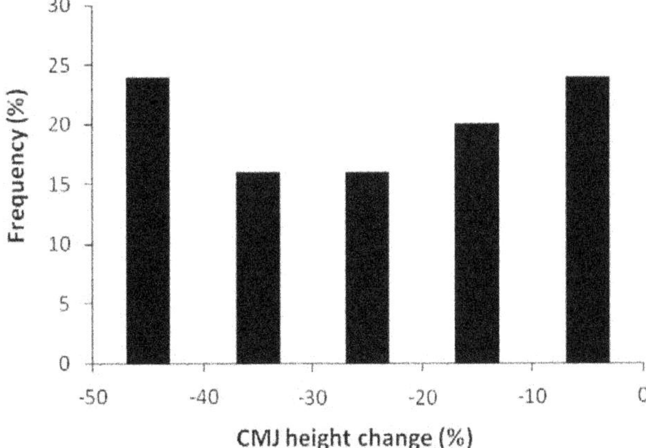

Figure 1. Body mass and jump height changes after a half-iron distance triathlon. Data are frequencies for 25 experienced triathletes.

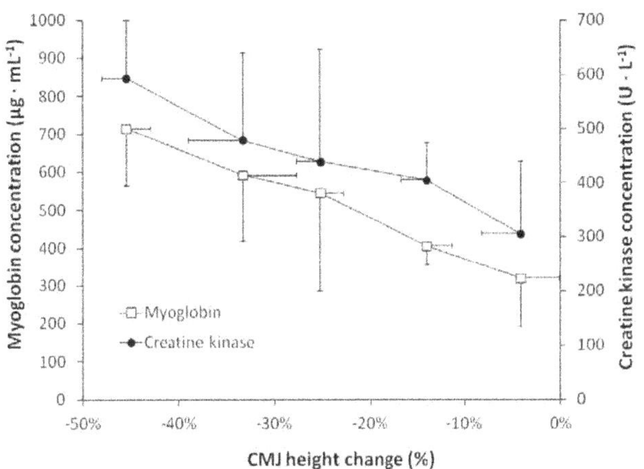

Figure 2. Associations among jump height loss and blood markers of muscle damage. Relationship between the changes in jump height (x-axis) and serum myoglobin concentration (y-axis 1) and serum creatine kinase concentration (y-axis 2) after a half-iron distance triathlon. Data mean ± SD for 25 experienced triathletes grouped by their jump height loss after race.

Urine samples

Pre and post-race urine samples were immediately analyzed (within 2 hours) for specific gravity (Usg), pH, protein, glucose, ketones and bilirubin concentrations. We also determined the presence of leukocytes and erythrocytes in the urine using reactive strips (Combur Test, Roche, Switzerland). For these measurements, the strip was dipped in the urine sample and the excess was wiped off with a clean absorbent paper. Then, the test strip was placed on the tray of a photometer (Urisys 1100, Roche Switzerland) and the aforementioned variables were measured after 1 min of incubation. After each ten sample batch, the photometer was calibrated with control strips provided by the manufacturer.

Statistical Analysis

Data are presented as mean ± SD. Initially, we tested the normality of each variable with the Shapiro-Wilk test. Changes in the variables from pre to post-race were analyzed with Student's t test for paired samples. To simplify the presentation of data, participants were grouped by their change in jump height using 10% intervals. Urine variables were presented by the frequency of subjects that presented a determined value. We used Pearson's correlation to assess the association between two variables. The significance level was set at $P<0.05$. We also performed a multiple regression analysis in a stepwise interactive mode, based on previous investigations [19] aiming to assess the influence of the measured variables on the muscle fatigue experienced during a half-iron triathlon (i.e., CMJ height loss).

For this calculation, the measured variables in the study were included based on their correlation with the residual ($P<0.1$) and their intercorrelation with variables already in the equation. The regression equation produced was accepted at a significance level of $P<0.01$. The degree of variance on CMJ height loss explained by means of each parameter was calculated using regression coefficients. Using the standardized regression coefficients, the relative contribution of the different variables to the variance explained was calculated as follows:

$$Parnal\ contribution\ r^2 = \left(\frac{[standardized\ regression\ coefficient\ for\ parameter]/}{\Sigma[of\ all\ standardized\ regression\ coefficients\ inequation]} \right) \times r^2.$$

Finally, the r^2values were adjusted for the number of cases and the number of parameters in the analysis. This statistical analysis was performed using the SPSS v.18 software package (SPSS Inc., USA).

Results

Dehydration and body water change

After the race, most participants had reduced their pre-exercise body mass (from 75.2±9.6 to 73.3±9.5 kg; $P<0.05$) with a mean dehydration of 2.3±1.2%. However, the dehydration attained after the race was diverse among individuals (Figure 1A). Most participants (44% of the total) reduced their body mass between 2 and 3% while only 12% of participants dehydrated more than 4% (peak dehydration was 4.3%). On the contrary, 8% of the triathletes slightly increased their body weight with a maximal gain of 0.3%. Body water followed a similar pattern (from 48.8±5.4 kg before the race to 46.5±5.5 kg after the race; $P<0.05$) with a mean body water deficit of 4.2±2.1%. The dehydration level attained during the race and the body water deficit were significantly correlated ($r=0.71$; $P<0.05$). However, there was no significant correlation between dehydration and CMJ height change ($r=-0.16$; $P=0.44$) or body water loss and CMJ height change ($r=-0.01$; $P=0.96$).

Countermovement jump height and handgrip force

Before the race, mean CMJ jump height was 30.3±5.0 cm and mean power output during the concentric phase of the jump was 25.6±2.9 W kg^{-1}. After the race, CMJ jump height (23.4±6.4 cm; $P<0.05$) and jump power output (20.7±4.6 W/kg; $P<0.05$) were significantly reduced by 23±16% and 19±15%, respectively. Although all participants reduced their CMJ jump from pre-exercise values, there was an elevated inter-individual variability in the responses (Figure 1B). On the contrary, handgrip maximal force production in the dominant (from 438±57 N pre-exercise to 436±65 N after the race; $P=0.85$) and non-dominant hand (from 422 N±63 pre-exercise to 423±59 N after the race; $P=0.77$) was unaffected after the triathlon race.

Blood responses

From pre-race values, blood volume and plasma volume were significantly reduced by 2.9±3.0% and 4.3±3.0%, respectively ($P<0.05$). The changes in the remaining blood variables are shown in Table 2. As a consequence of plasma volume reduction, hemoglobin and hematocrit concentration increased after the race ($P<0.05$). Post-exercise platelet count increased by 15±9% ($P<0.05$), leukocyte count by 200±9% ($P<0.05$) while erythrocytes remained unchanged. Post-race blood glucose concentration increased by 15±5 mg · dL^{-1} in comparison to pre-race values ($P<0.05$). While sodium and chloride concentrations were significantly reduced after the race ($P<0.05$), and potassium concentration slightly increased ($P<0.05$). Finally, the concentrations of all the blood markers of muscle damage showed varying increases, from pre to post race ($P<0.05$). There was a negative correlation between the CMJ jump height change and post-race myoglobin concentration ($r=-0.65$; $P<0.001$) and post-race creatine kinase concentration ($r=-0.54$; $P<0.001$; Figure 2), but this correlation was not significant with the LDH concentration ($r=0.01$; $P=0.96$).

Urinary responses

Before the race, all the twenty five triathletes had U_{sg} below 1.020. Although U_{sg} values significantly increased from pre-to post-race (Table 3; $P<0.05$), only 2 participants (8% of the sample) exceeded 1.020 after the race. The half-iron triathlon increased the urinary concentration of erythrocytes, leukocytes, proteins and ketones by varying amounts ($P<0.05$). On the contrary, urine pH and bilirubin concentration remained unchanged after the race.

Discussion

The aim of this investigation was to determine the sources of muscle fatigue experienced by triathletes during a half-iron distance race. According to previous investigations, dehydration, hypoglycemia, electrolyte imbalance and muscle damage are probable factors affecting muscle force output in the triathlon. In the present investigation, we measured all these variables before and after a half-iron race and performed a multiple regression analysis to determine the influence of each variable on the pre-post race change in CMJ height. The main outcomes were: (a) body mass loss (Figure 1A) and body water deficit after the race were moderate and these variables were modestly correlated with jump height loss; (b) blood glucose content increased while serum sodium and chloride concentrations decreased after the race (Table 2), although their values were far from constituting a serious electrolyte imbalance; (c) blood markers of muscle damage strongly correlated with jump height loss (Figure 2), suggesting

Table 2. Blood responses before (Pre) and after (Post) a half-iron triathlon race. Data are mean ± SD for 25 triathletes.

Variable (units)	Pre	Post	P value
Hemoglobin (g · dL^{-1})	14.7±0.8	15.2±0.9	<0.05
Hematocrit (%)	45.4±2.4	46.3±2.4	<0.05
Erythrocytes (10^9 · L^{-1})	4926±310	4898±351	NS
Leukocytes (10^9 · L^{-1})	5.5±1.0	16.1±2.5	<0.05
Platelets (10^9 · L^{-1})	249±36	286±46	<±0.05
Glucose (mmol · L^{-1})	5.1±0.7	6.3±1.6	<0.05
Sodium (mmol · L^{-1})	141.4±1.6	140.4±1.9	<0.05
Potassium (mmol · L^{-1})	4.5±0.2	4.7±0.7	<0.05
Chloride (mmol · L^{-1})	101.2±2.0	98.3±2.4	<0.05
Myoglobin (μg · L^{-1})	14±17	516±248	<0.05
Creatine kinase (U · L^{-1})	145±72	442±204	<0.05
LDH (U · L^{-1})	298±66	598±252	<0.05

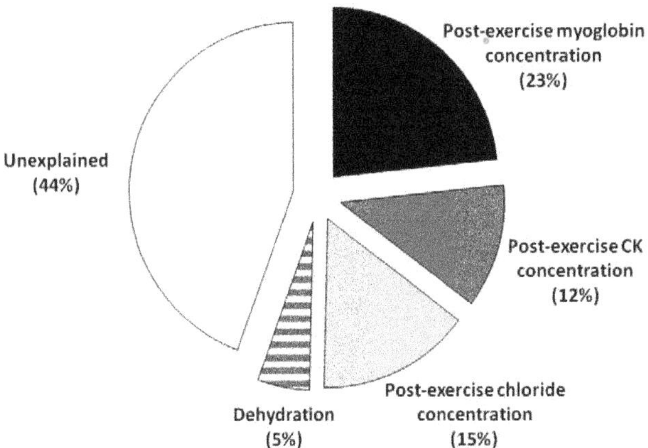

Figure 3. Amount of variance explained (adjusted r2) for CMJ height loss after the half-iron triathlon. The best regression equation includes blood variables (post-exercise myoglobin, creatine kinase and chloride concentrations) and the dehydration attained after the race. The remaining portion represents the unexplained variance.

that muscle breakdown is one of the primary causes of muscle fatigue during a triathlon. With all these data, we have explained 56% of the variance in muscle fatigue which ensued during a half-iron triathlon (Figure 3).

All the triathletes that participated in this study experienced a reduction in jump height and leg power production after the race, a clear sign of muscle fatigue as found previously [3]. However, the individual responses for jump height change were diverse (Figure 1B). The explanation for the variance in muscle fatigue responses after the triathlon race is presented in Figure 3. Pre-to-post race change in jump height depended on the post-exercise blood myoglobin concentration (23%), the post-exercise blood chloride concentration (15%), the post-exercise blood CK concentration (12%) and dehydration (5%). With this model we can determine which factors modulate muscle fatigue during a triathlon race. Nonetheless, there is still a high proportion of muscle fatigue variability that remains unexplained with our experimental design, which warrants further investigation.

According to the multifactorial analysis, 35% of jump height loss experienced by the triathletes is explained by means of blood markers of muscle damage (i.e., myoglobin and CK). Although we did not measure CK isoforms (e.g. MM, BB and MB) to differentiate the origin of muscle breakdown, we assume that the largest part of the CK increase found in the post-race blood samples was from skeletal muscle. As presented in Figure 2, those triathletes with a higher reduction in jump height were the ones with a higher concentration of myoglobin and CK after the race. These data suggest that muscle breakdown produced in the triathlon is one of the primary factors for muscle fatigue in triathletes. While there is no study that has reported moderate-to-severe muscle damage after swimming or cycling, the references to muscle damage after endurance running are abundant [20,21,22]. The continuous foot strikes during the running leg demand concentric and eccentric actions of the leg muscles and can damage muscle fibers [23].

During an iron triathlon, Margaritis et al. [2] did not find an association between blood CK concentration and the reduction in knee extensor and flexor muscle force production during several days after the race. These authors concluded that blood markers of muscle damage cannot be used to predict the magnitude of the muscle function impairment during the triathlon. In contrast, Coso et al. [17] found a relationship between the myoglobin concentration in the first urine after a marathon race and leg muscle power reduction, concluding that muscle damage is a good predictor of leg muscle fatigue after running. The present investigation also indicates that muscle damage, estimated by blood myoglobin and CK concentrations, is the main factor affecting muscle fatigue in triathletes. Thus, the strategies to diminish the extent of muscle fatigue in triathletes should include the avoidance of muscle damage.

A dehydration level above 2% has been repeatedly related to muscle force loss during endurance exercise events [7] and it has been proposed as one of the main factors responsible for fatigue during triathlon events [1]. In the present study, however, the variance in CMJ height loss explained by means of dehydration was only 5% (Figure 3) which suggests that the influence of dehydration on muscle fatigue during the triathlon was minor. Although dehydration was present in most triathletes, the levels attained by the majority of triathletes were moderate (mean 2.3±1.2%). Thirty two percent of the sample dehydrated less than 2%, 52% of the participants dehydrated between 2 and 4% and the remaining 12% dehydrated more than 4% (Figure 1A). The poor association between dehydration and the loss of CMJ height indicates that the triathletes with higher levels of dehydration did not loss more jump height than the ones with better rehydration during the race. We assume that the proper drinking behavior showed by most triathletes in this study reduced the influence of dehydration on the muscle fatigue.

The concurrence of sodium loss by sweating and the high intake of water or low-sodium drinks during long distance triathlon causes some triathletes to present hyponatremia (<135 mmol $\cdot$ L^{-1}; [9,16]). This electrolyte imbalance has been related to clinical complications in exercise medicine, since its symptoms include weakness, fainting or even death. However, blood sodium concentration may also play an important role in the preservation of muscle function during exercise. Vrijens and Reher [24] reported a relationship between decreased blood sodium concentration and time to fatigue during a prolonged cycling event. Similarly, Coso et al. [5] found a relationship between sodium deficit and muscle fatigue during prolonged cycling even with a mean sodium concentration above 137 mmol $\cdot$ L^{-1}. In the present investigation, blood sodium concentration decreased from 141 to 140 mmol $\cdot$ L^{-1} but this variable was not correlated with CMJ height loss (r = 0.02; P = 0.92). In contrast, blood chloride content changed from 101 to 98 mmol $\cdot$ L^{-1} and post-exercise values significantly correlated with CMJ height loss (r = 0.34; P<0.05). It has been found that intramuscular sodium and chloride contents remain unchanged after prolonged exercise that produces profuse

Table 3. Urinary responses before (Pre) and after (Post) a half-iron triathlon race. Data are mean±SD for 25 triathletes.

Variable (units)	Pre	Post	P value
U_{sg}	1.012±0.006	1.018±0.006	<0.05
pH	6.2±1.1	6.1±1.2	0.84
Erythrocytes (U $\cdot$ μL^{-1})	1.4±0.3	18.3±51.5	<0.05
Leukocytes (U $\cdot$ μL^{-1})	0.0±0.0	7.3±11.6	<0.05
Proteins (mg $\cdot$ dL^{-1})	3.0±3.3	89.6±134.9	<0.05
Ketones (mg $\cdot$ dL^{-1})	0.2±1.0	24.4±39.9	<0.05
Bilirubin (mg $\cdot$ dL^{-1})	0.2±0.6	0.2±0.4	0.71

sweating while the excitability of the muscle cell membrane is unaffected. Although lacking a clear explanation, maintaining blood electrolyte concentration during exercise may help to preserve muscle function.

During exercise of ~1 hour of duration, glucose supply for the skeletal muscle comes from glycogen stores in the muscle and liver. If the exercise bout is of long duration (>1 hour), main glycogen stores deplete and blood borne glucose is also used as the energy substrate, threatening blood glucose homeostasis [25]. It has been found that hypoglycemia attenuates the activation of the CNS and hence reduces the capacity to generate force in the active muscle [13]. For this reason, the reduction in blood glucose concentration has been proposed as a source of muscle fatigue during the triathlon [1]. When blood glucose is maintained by ingesting carbohydrates during exercise, muscle force and CNS activation are better preserved [13]. Interestingly, participants in this investigation increased by 0.8±0.5 mmol · L^{-1} the blood glucose concentration from pre-to-post exercise (Table 2), as has been previously found in other athletes participating in endurance events [26]. Although we did not record carbohydrate ingestion during the race, previous studies have found that triathletes have appropriate rates of carbohydrate intake, especially during the cycling leg [14] According to our data, blood glucose concentration was well maintained in triathletes, reducing the influence of hypoglycemia as a source of fatigue during a half-iron race.

Several studies have reported that muscle force production is ameliorated in hyperthermic individuals with or without dehydration [6,27,28]. During prolonged cycling in the heat that produced hyperthermia, Nybo and Nielsen [27] reported a reduction in both leg and arm force production, despite arm muscles not being involved during the cycling activity. These authors suggested that hyperthermia produces a central effect that affects muscle function in both active and non active muscles, although different outcomes have been found in another analogous study [29]. In the present investigation we did not assess body temperature, but during an iron triathlon with an environmental temperature similar to the present investigation (23.3 *vs* 22.3°C), mean core temperature in triathletes was only 38.1°C [30]. In addition, while leg muscle power and jump height were reduced after the race, handgrip force remained unchanged from pre-to-post exercise, contrary to the results reported by Nybo and Nielsen. The maintenance of arm force while leg force was reduced disagrees with the existence of hyperthermia and its effects on CNS activation.

Exercise, particularly high-intensity and endurance activities produce several urinary abnormalities. Hematuria is one of the most commonly found abnormalities after sports activity [31] and it is present with a higher frequency in weight-bearing exercise activities (running *vs* cycling; [32]). Others studies have reported that hematuria is present in 20-to-50% of marathon finishers [33,34]. The present study found that erythrocyte concentration increased from 1.4±0.3 to 18.3±51.5 U · μL^{-1} in the first urine after the triathlon. In addition, the prevalence of hematuria increased from 0 to 36% after the race, with one participant above 250 U · μL^{-1}. Although there was no incidence of kidney complications after the race, these data suggest the necessity of obtaining an exercise history when urinary abnormalities are present in triathletes.

In summary, during a half-iron triathlon in a temperate environment, leg muscle function was significantly impaired while muscle force in the upper extremities remained unchanged. Furthermore, the source of leg muscle fatigue experienced by triathletes was diverse and depended on several factors. Post-exercise myoglobin and creatine kinase concentrations correlated with CMJ height loss after the race, indicating that muscle fiber damage is one of the key factors for muscle fatigue in the triathlon. In contrast, dehydration and blood glucose concentration had a minor role in muscle fatigue mainly due to appropriate rehydrating and feeding during the race. Strategies to lessen muscle fatigue during triathlon events should comprise a reduction in muscle damage.

Acknowledgments

The authors wish to thank the subjects for their invaluable contribution to the study. In addition, we are very grateful to the Organization of Ecotrimad for their contribution to the study.

Author Contributions

Conceived and designed the experiments: JC CGM JJS JAV LS SG BPG. Performed the experiments: JC CGM JJS JAV LS SG BPG. Analyzed the data: JC JJS JAV LS. Contributed reagents/materials/analysis tools: JC CGM JJS JAV LS SG BPG. Wrote the paper: JC.

References

1. Jeukendrup AE, Jentjens RL, Moseley L (2005) Nutritional considerations in triathlon. Sports Med 35: 163–181.
2. Margaritis I, Tessier F, Verdera F, Bermon S, Marconnet P (1999) Muscle enzyme release does not predict muscle function impairment after triathlon. J Sports Med Phys Fitness 39: 133–139.
3. Suzuki K, Peake J, Nosaka K, Okutsu M, Abbiss CR, et al. (2006) Changes in markers of muscle damage, inflammation and HSP70 after an Ironman Triathlon race. Eur J Appl Physiol 98: 525–534.
4. Judelson DA, Maresh CM, Anderson JM, Armstrong LE, Casa DJ, et al. (2007) Hydration and muscular performance: does fluid balance affect strength, power and high-intensity endurance? Sports Med 37: 907–921.
5. Coso JD, Estevez E, Baquero RA, Mora-Rodriguez R (2008) Anaerobic performance when rehydrating with water or commercially available sports drinks during prolonged exercise in the heat. Appl Physiol Nutr Metab 33: 290–298.
6. Coso JD, Hamouti N, Estevez E, Mora-Rodriguez R (2011) Reproducibility of two electrical stimulation techniques to assess neuromuscular fatigue. Eur J Sport Sci 11.
7. Sawka MN, Burke LM, Eichner ER, Maughan RJ, Montain SJ, et al. (2007) American College of Sports Medicine position stand. Exercise and fluid replacement. Med Sci Sports Exerc 39: 377–390.
8. Knechtle B, Knechtle P, Rosemann T, Oliver S (2010) A Triple Iron triathlon leads to a decrease in total body mass but not to dehydration. Res Q Exerc Sport 81: 319–327.
9. Speedy DB, Noakes TD, Kimber NE, Rogers IR, Thompson JM, et al. (2001) Fluid balance during and after an ironman triathlon. Clin J Sport Med 11: 44–50.
10. Knechtle B, Duff B, Amtmann G, Kohler G (2008) An ultratriathlon leads to a decrease of body fat and skeletal muscle mass–the Triple Iron Triathlon Austria 2006. Res Sports Med 16: 97–110.
11. Jeukendrup A, Brouns F, Wagenmakers AJ, Saris WH (1997) Carbohydrate-electrolyte feedings improve 1 h time trial cycling performance. Int J Sports Med 18: 125–129.
12. Coggan AR, Coyle EF (1987) Reversal of fatigue during prolonged exercise by carbohydrate infusion or ingestion. J Appl Physiol 63: 2388–2395.
13. Nybo L (2003) CNS fatigue and prolonged exercise: effect of glucose supplementation. Med Sci Sports Exerc 35: 589–594.
14. Kimber NE, Ross JJ, Mason SL, Speedy DB (2002) Energy balance during an ironman triathlon in male and female triathletes. Int J Sport Nutr Exerc Metab 12: 47–62.
15. Jeukendrup AE, Jentjens R (2000) Oxidation of carbohydrate feedings during prolonged exercise: current thoughts, guidelines and directions for future research. Sports Med 29: 407–424.
16. Speedy DB, Rogers IR, Noakes TD, Wright S, Thompson JM, et al. (2000) Exercise-induced hyponatremia in ultradistance triathletes is caused by inappropriate fluid retention. Clin J Sport Med 10: 272–278.
17. Coso JD, Salinero JJ, Abián-Vicen J, González-Millán C, Garde S, et al. (2012) Dehydration or rhabdomyolysis to predict muscle fatigue during a marathon in the heat? Annual conferece of the Spanish Olympic Committee In press.
18. Dill DB, Costill DL (1974) Calculation of percentage changes in volumes of blood, plasma, and red cells in dehydration. J Appl Physiol 37: 247–248.
19. Coso JD, Hamouti N, Ortega JF, Fernandez-Elias VE, Mora-Rodriguez R (2011) Relevance of individual characteristics for thermoregulation during exercise in a hot-dry environment. Eur J Appl Physiol 111: 2173–2181.

20. Schiff HB, MacSearraigh ET, Kallmeyer JC (1978) Myoglobinuria, rhabdomyolysis and marathon running. Q J Med 47: 463–472.
21. Smith JE, Garbutt G, Lopes P, Pedoe DT (2004) Effects of prolonged strenuous exercise (marathon running) on biochemical and haematological markers used in the investigation of patients in the emergency department. Br J Sports Med 38: 292–294.
22. Clarkson PM, Hubal MJ (2002) Exercise-induced muscle damage in humans. Am J Phys Med Rehabil 81: S52–69.
23. Friden J, Sjostrom M, Ekblom B (1983) Myofibrillar damage following intense eccentric exercise in man. Int J Sports Med 4: 170–176.
24. Vrijens DM, Rehrer NJ (1999) Sodium-free fluid ingestion decreases plasma sodium during exercise in the heat. J Appl Physiol 86: 1847–1851.
25. Coyle EF, Coggan AR, Hemmert MK, Ivy JL (1986) Muscle glycogen utilization during prolonged strenuous exercise when fed carbohydrate. J Appl Physiol 61: 165–172.
26. Millet GY, Tomazin K, Verges S, Vincent C, Bonnefoy R, et al. (2011) Neuromuscular consequences of an extreme mountain ultra-marathon. PLoS One 6: e17059.
27. Nybo L, Nielsen B (2001) Hyperthermia and central fatigue during prolonged exercise in humans. J Appl Physiol 91: 1055–1060.
28. Coso J, Estevez E, Mora-Rodriguez R (2008) Caffeine effects on short-term performance during prolonged exercise in the heat. Med Sci Sports Exerc 40: 744–751.
29. Saboisky J, Marino FE, Kay D, Cannon J (2003) Exercise heat stress does not reduce central activation to non-exercised human skeletal muscle. Exp Physiol 88: 783–790.
30. Laursen PB, Suriano R, Quod MJ, Lee H, Abbiss CR, et al. (2006) Core temperature and hydration status during an Ironman triathlon. Br J Sports Med 40: 320–325; discussion 325.
31. Abarbanel J, Benet AE, Lask D, Kimche D (1990) Sports hematuria. J Urol 143: 887–890.
32. McInnis MD, Newhouse IJ, von Duvillard SP, Thayer R (1998) The effect of exercise intensity on hematuria in healthy male runners. Eur J Appl Physiol Occup Physiol 79: 99–105.
33. Gur H, Kucukoglu S, Surmen E, Muftuoglu A (1994) Effects of age, training background and duration of running on abnormal urinary findings after a half-marathon race. Br J Sports Med 28: 61–62.
34. Reid RI, Hosking DH, Ramsey EW (1987) Haematuria following a marathon run: source and significance. Br J Urol 59: 133–136.

9

An Inverse Finite Element Method for Determining the Tissue Compressibility of Human Left Ventricular Wall during the Cardiac Cycle

Abdallah I. Hassaballah[1,2*], Mohsen A. Hassan[1,2,3], Azizi N. Mardi[1,2], Mohd Hamdi[1,2]

1 Department of Mechanical Engineering, Faculty of Engineering, University of Malaya, Kuala Lumpur, Malaysia, **2** Center of Advanced Manufacturing & Material processing, Faculty of Engineering, University of Malaya, Kuala Lumpur, Malaysia, **3** Department of Mechanical Engineering, Faculty of Engineering, Assiut University, Assiut, Egypt

Abstract

The determination of the myocardium's tissue properties is important in constructing functional finite element (FE) models of the human heart. To obtain accurate properties especially for functional modeling of a heart, tissue properties have to be determined in vivo. At present, there are only few in vivo methods that can be applied to characterize the internal myocardium tissue mechanics. This work introduced and evaluated an FE inverse method to determine the myocardial tissue compressibility. Specifically, it combined an inverse FE method with the experimentally-measured left ventricular (LV) internal cavity pressure and volume versus time curves. Results indicated that the FE inverse method showed good correlation between LV repolarization and the variations in the myocardium tissue bulk modulus K (K = 1/compressibility), as well as provided an ability to describe in vivo human myocardium material behavior. The myocardium bulk modulus can be effectively used as a diagnostic tool of the heart ejection fraction. The model developed is proved to be robust and efficient. It offers a new perspective and means to the study of living-myocardium tissue properties, as it shows the variation of the bulk modulus throughout the cardiac cycle.

Editor: Wolfgang Rudolf Bauer, University Hospital of Würzburg, Germany

Funding: This work was supported by the High Impact Research (HIR) Grant (HIR-MOHE-D000001-16001) from the Ministry of Higher Education, Malaysia. The funders had no role in study design, data collection and analysis, decision to publish, or preparation of the manuscript.

Competing Interests: The authors have declared that no competing interests exist.

* E-mail: abdallahhassaballah@yahoo.com

Introduction

One of the tools that can potentially lead to the early detection of human heart failures is the understanding of the mechanical behavior of the human left ventricle (LV) in normal and diseased states. This leads to continuous interest in the determination of the material properties of myocardium through the mechanical testing of excised strips of myocardium. These strips under prescribed homogeneous loading conditions give stress-strain relationships. Originally, these tests were done uniaxially but more recently, biaxial tests were also performed. Uniaxial test is used to define passive stress-strain relationships in the fiber direction [1]. It is very useful test in determining the general characteristics of the behavior of cardiac tissue in both healthy and diseased states, but is not sufficient to provide a unique description of three-dimensional (3D) constitutive behavior of the myocardium. Due to the incompressibility of cardiac tissue, biaxial tests can be used to determine certain multidimensional stress-strain relationships for the fiber and cross-fiber [2]. Despite the frequent assumption that human myocardial tissue is incompressible, the fact remains: all myocardial tissues have some degree of compressibility. Furthermore, the issue of the compressibility of myocardium tissue is raised due to the systolic intra- and extra-vascular blood displacements [3]. As a result of the previously mentioned fact, it is clear that the myocardium tissue compressibility changes during the cardiac cycle.

The information embodied in the myocardial tissue bulk modulus adds further insight to the mechanical nature of the soft tissue. Bulk modulus is very important as a standalone parameter, and as additional information to the shear/Young's modulus. Precise values of the myocardium bulk modulus are especially required to improve the accuracy of finite element (FE) simulation for the modeling of the human heart. In the last several decades, publications related to cardiac modeling have handled the myocardial bulk modulus in many different approaches. The published values of myocardial bulk modulus recorded by researchers who were interested in simulating the performance of the LV during the diastolic phase are quite small, for instance 28 kPa [4] and 160 kPa [5]. This may be attributed to small changes in ventricular wall volume. Some studies evaluated the bulk modulus under the assumption that during the rapid filling phase, the volume change of the ventricular wall should be less than 10%. Additionally, relatively high values of bulk modulus were used by researchers who analyzed the systolic phase, for example 380 kPa [6], 600 kPa [7], and 25 MPa [8]. Using high values for bulk modulus during systolic phase are due to the systolic intra- and extra-vascular blood displacements that give rise to the compressibility of the tissue. Mean constant value of myocardial bulk modulus was assumed during each cardiac phase.

Despite the widespread use of uniaxial and biaxial tests for determining the myocardium characteristics, there are four major problems that arise from these kinds of studies [9,10]:

1. Tests were carried out on non-human tissue, and as a result may not be directly applicable to humans.
2. The properties may not be directly applicable to FE models of the heart due to heterogeneous behavior of the myocardium.
3. The mechanical properties of myocardium changed drastically immediately after death.
4. The variation in the values of the mechanical properties according to the experimental loading conditions.

All the above limitations lead researchers to find different ways to run their experiments without having to excise samples of myocardium. Hence, a group of researchers moved to use Magnetic Resonance Imaging (MRI) and FE or mathematical methods to determine the mechanical properties *in vivo* [11,12], while others applied the scanning acoustic microscope with high frequency ultrasound to measure the bulk modulus and describe the mechanical properties of the myocardium [13]. However, most bulk modulus experimental values obtained from these studies are very high (≈3 GPa), and cannot be used directly to FE modeling. To overcome these shortcomings, the FE approach is suggested to determine, *in vivo,* the myocardial tissue bulk modulus during the cardiac cycle.

Usually, FE analysis can be done directly once the input parameters such as LV geometry, LV internal cavity pressure and the myocardium tissue properties are known. Once the model is constructed, the desired outputs such as deformation behavior, LV cavity volume, LV wall stresses and strains can be predicted from the model. However, it is not uncommon in reality that some or all of the output values are known from experiments beforehand, while some of the input parameters still need to be determined. This requires the FE analysis to be done in an inverse way, where iteration of FE simulation is performed to find the material properties that give the best fit between the computed and experimentally measured LV internal cavity volumes. An inverse FE approach is a complex engineering process that can determine the unknown causes of known consequences. This approach has the advantage that the determination of the dynamic properties is measured non-invasively [14–17].

A novel method combining the experimentally measured LV pressure-volume curves and an inverse FE method is proposed to determine myocardial bulk modulus. The main purpose of this research is to develop an inverse FE procedure with ANSYS® computer code for the determination of the bulk modulus of human LV during cardiac cycle. The proposed inverse technique is based on published experimental measured LV pressure-volume curves. By using these outputs of published LV experimental data, the bulk modulus versus time curve is traced through inverse technique. Based on the obtained results, the repeated changes of myocardium tissue bulk modulus in the LV wall during cardiac cycle result in a highly efficient global function of the normal heart. Therefore, the myocardium bulk modulus can be effectively used as a diagnostic tool of the heart ejection fraction.

Methods

2.1 Left Ventricle Geometry and FE Model

An inverse FE model was adopted to evaluate the LV tissue compressibility during cardiac cycle. 3D-FE model was built to simulate the deformation mechanics of the LV using ANSYS® commercial software. To simplify the analysis, FE simulation model was represented by an ellipsoid, truncated at two-thirds of the major axis including two sets of fibers (myocardial fibers bound by a mesh of collagen fibers), which were attached to each other to form a spatial network. The geometric parameters and dimensions of the LV model in the initial undeformed configuration (at hypothetical zero pressure applied inside the LV cavity) are shown in Figure 1. The wall thickness of the LV model, in the reference unstressed state, was divided into seven equal thickness layers. Figure 2A shows the initial shape of a typical FE mesh used for the present computations, while Figure 2B shows the end-diastolic deformed shape of the FE mesh. The wall of LV model was discretized with 20-node hexahedral element; with the exception of the apical region which was meshed using 10-node tetrahedral element. The current FE mesh consisted of 22,080 total number of elements and 29,777 nodes. This discretization of the current LV model was sufficient and any further mesh refinement showed very little improvement [18]. The LV blood cavity was modeled by the hydrostatic fluid 3D solid element; this element is well suited for calculating fluid (blood) volume and pressure for coupled problems involving fluid-solid interaction. Hydrostatic fluid elements were overlaid on the faces of 3D solid element enclosing the fluid volume. Figure 2C shows the section view in the FE mesh in order to clarify the shape of the elements used for modeling the LV internal cavity. The hydrostatic fluid element was defined by nine nodes; eight nodes on the internal surface of LV cavity (endocardium) and the remaining ninth node at the base center, which is also called "the pressure node". This pressure node was used to define the LV pressure which was assumed to be uniform through the LV cavity; the predefined value of pressure was automatically moved to the centroid of the fluid volume. In all FE computations the LV cavity and LV wall volumes were kept constant at 50 ml and 73.6 ml respectively. The circumference of the LV internal cavity was divided into 48 equally spaced divisions, i.e. 48 elements along the circumferential direction.

Two separate parallel sets of 3D fiber network; contractile muscle fibers bundles (myofibers) bound by a mesh of collagen fibers were embedded within continuum 3D solid element to reproduce the globally anisotropic behavior of cardiac tissue. Computationally, these fibers were modeled as layers of uniformly spaced reinforcement bars (rebar) within the continuum 3D elements; each layer was set to be parallel to two of the isoparametric directions in the element's local coordinate system.

The collagen fibers were arranged in the radial direction, while the myofibers orientation changed with position within the LV wall. The 3D reinforcing element was used to simulate both myofiber and collagen fiber. The continuum 3D element is suitable for simulating reinforcing fibers with arbitrary orientations and used to model the myofiber force. The force was restricted in the direction of the fiber only (uniaxial fiber tension). The reinforcing element was firmly attached to its base element, i.e. no relative movement between the reinforcing element and the base was allowed. FE computations were conducted with myofibers and collagen fibers volume fractions of 0.7 and 0.015, respectively [19,20].

2.2 LV Myofiber Architecture

The human muscle fibers oriented at different angles throughout the ventricle wall in the form of sheets that are separated by a complex structure of cleavage surfaces (see Figure 3) [21–23]. The myofibers could be fully described by two inclination projection angles; the helix angle (β) and the transverse angle (η) in the two perpendicular planes. The transmural distribution of helix angle (β) varies in a linear manner through wall thickness from the lowest negative value at the epicardium to the highest positive

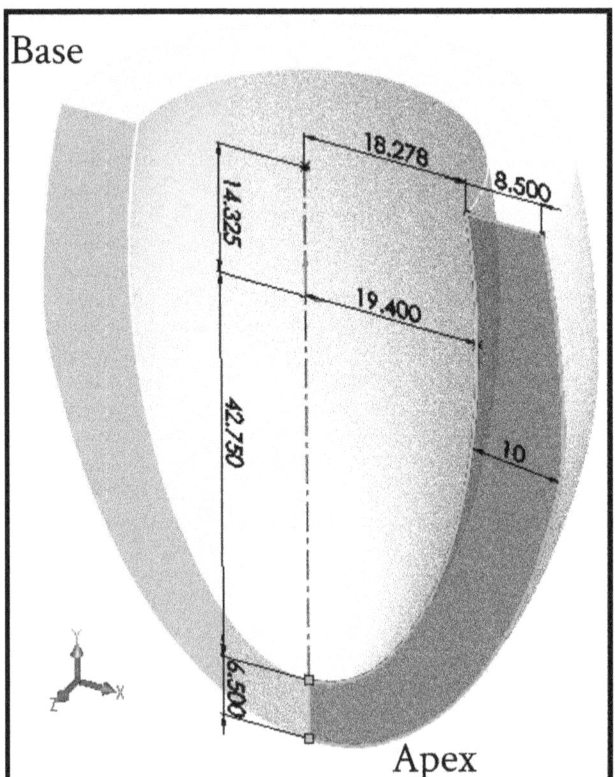

Figure 1. Geometric parameters of the thick-walled ellipsoid truncates at two thirds of major axis used to simulate LV model (for clarification half solid model presented).

value at the endocardium, while the transverse angle (η) varies in a linear manner through along the longitudinal axis of the LV from the lowest negative value at the apex to the highest positive value at the base [24,25,21,26,27]. The corresponding variations of the fiber helix angles (β) through the eight regions are as follows (see Figure 4); septum-basal region (−60° : +40°), anterior-basal region (−40° : +60°), lateral-basal region (−20° : +50°), posterior-basal region (−20° : +60°), septum-apical region (−50° : +40°), anterior-apical region (−20° : +60°), lateral-apical region (−20° : +50°), and posterior-apical region (−20° : +60°) vary smoothly across the LV wall thickness from a negative angle at epicardium to positive angle at endocardium respectively [28].

The distribution of transverse angle (η) was taken as a variable value in a linear manner from +15° at the base to the circumferential direction (η = 0°) in the equatorial region to −15° at the apex [24]. Meanwhile, the collagen fibers were arranged in the radial directions.

2.3 Loading and Boundary Conditions

To demonstrate the performance of the proposed FE model, LV pressure versus time curve for a healthy human heart was used (see Figure 5). This case was adapted from the experimental measurements carried out by Hall [29]. The LV pressure versus time curve given in Figure 5 represents the FE model with applied loads, while the accompanying LV internal cavity volume were adopted as the FE model target values.

The external surface of the heart is affected by the surrounding organs (lungs, ribcage and diaphragm). In order to simulate the boundary conditions imposed by these surrounding organs and tissues, an elastic foundation 3D structural surface effect element with a stiffness K_f = 0.02 kPa was used [4,30]. Due to the lack of information about the influence of the surrounding organs and tissue on the deformation of the heart, a uniform elastic foundation was assumed.

To prevent rigid body motion of the model, degrees of freedom for all nodes at the base were suppressed in the longitudinal direction (UY = 0). To avoid possible excessive deformations of FE mesh elements, the pressure node was fixed laterally (UX = UZ = 0) (see Figure 2).

2.4 Myocardium Active and Passive Material Properties

The LV pressure response to its changing volume during ejection phase relies on the active elastance property activated by the muscle action. During systolic phase, the muscle generate adequate contractile force (muscle active force) to provide sufficient LV pressure to open the aortic valve, and pump an appropriate volume of blood [31]. At the beginning of the isovolumic contraction, the LV internal cavity pressure increases rapidly until the peak pressure and consequently the muscle contraction force continually increase, to sustain increasing LV pressures. Both the LV pressure and muscle contraction force increased simultaneously until its peak. During cardiac cycle the LV wall is subjected to dual forces; the active force generated by the myocardium muscles and the force generated by the blood pressure in the LV cavity. The active muscle force is not only governed by the myocardium passive properties but also depend mainly on myocardium active elastance operating throughout the cardiac cycle.

In this study we suggest a simple method to calculate the active myofiber elastance properties by taking into consideration that the maximum value of myofiber Young's modulus does not exceed 0.5 MPa [32,33]. The active myofiber elastic properties during cardiac cycle can be simply calculated by multiplying the LV pressure value (given in Figure 5) with constant value that equals to 29.5, i.e. the value of active myofiber Young's modulus depending linearly on the intracavital pressure. This constant value is equal to 0.5 (maximum myofiber Young's modulus) divided by the maximum value of LV pressure. The computation of active myofiber Young's modulus based on the above calculated constant represents the hypothesis of the present study. Figure 6 shows the calculated active myofiber Young's modulus versus time during one cardiac cycle. The time dependent calculated values of active myofiber Young's modulus is applied on the FE model in order to calculate the contraction force in the myocardial wall.

The myocardium tissue (matrix) was represented as an isotropic, slightly compressible hyperelastic material with relatively soft properties. The Ogden model with two parameters was used in the present study and having the following parameters; μ_1 = 0.22 MPa, μ_2 = 0.11 MPa, α_1 = 11.77 and α_2 = 14.34 [34]. The tissue bulk modulus K of the LV model was tuned so that the simulation behaves in accordance with the measured pressure vs. volume curve (patient-specific datasets).

The collagen fiber behavior was represented by isotropic linear elastic with large displacements, to simulate the large strains occurring in the collagen fiber during LV filling. Collagen properties are as follows; the Young's modulus (E) = 50 kPa, Poisson's ratio (**ν**) = 0.49, and density (**ρ**) = 1000 kg/m^3 [35].

2.5 Solution Procedures and Inverse Identification of Myocardium Tissue Compressibility

Figure 7 shows the inverse FE computation sequence procedures for the evaluation of the myocardial bulk modulus. The myocardium tissue bulk modulus satisfying the required output was inversely identified. The LV pressure versus time curve (see

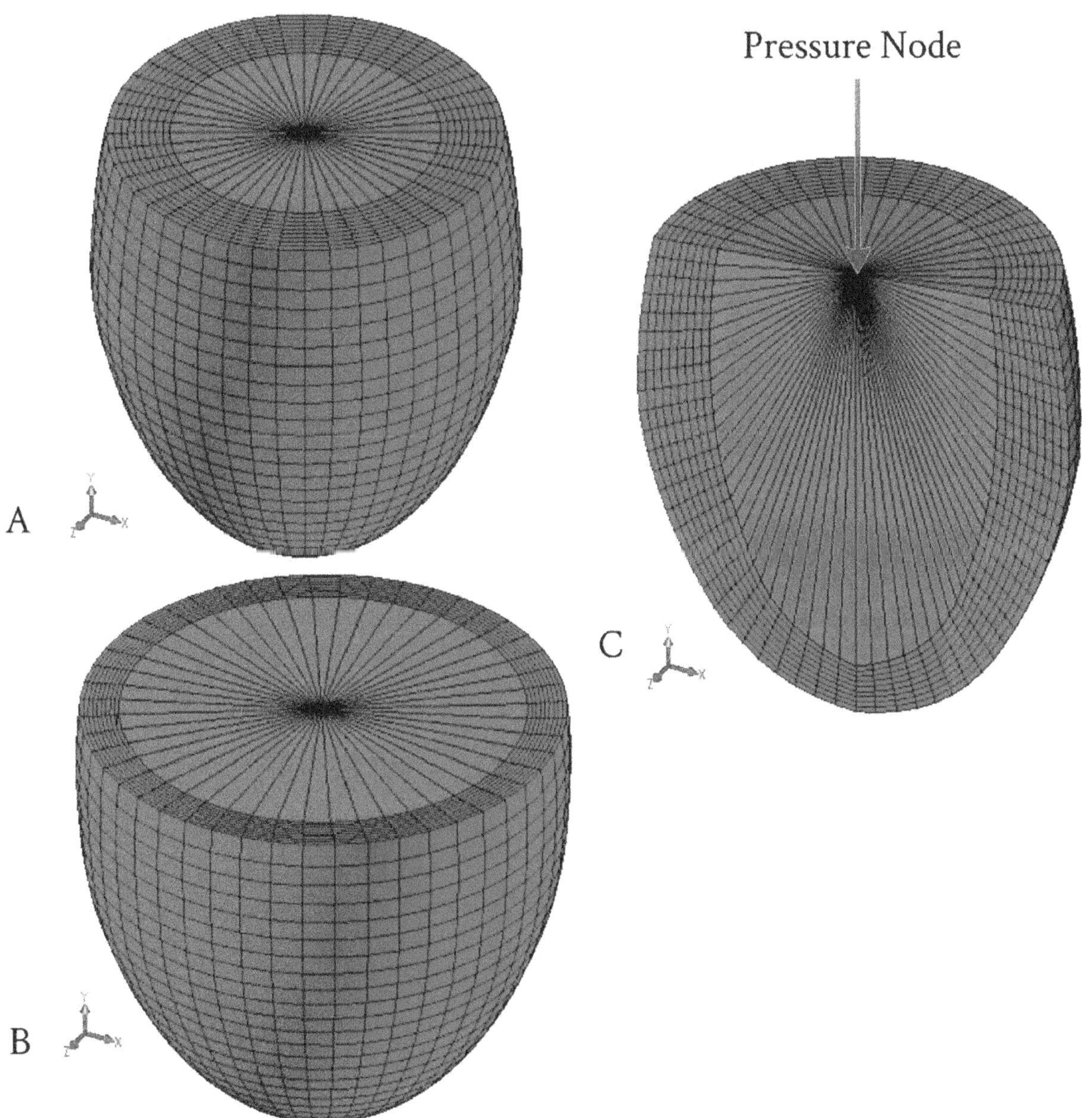

Figure 2. The left ventricular FE mesh. (A) Initial shape of the FE mesh; (B) Deformed shape of the FE mesh at the LV end-diastolic; and (C) Section view in the FE mesh to declare the elements used to simulated the LV cavity.

Figure 5) as the inputs were applied on the internal surface of LV cavity (endocardium) via the pressure node of the hydrostatic fluid element (see Figure 2C). The other passive material properties of myocardium tissue (see item 2.4) were fixed as material constants. The calculated active myofiber Young's modulus (see Figure 6) was used to simulate the muscle active contraction force generated through the LV wall during the cardiac cycle.

An initial guess value of tissue compressibility for the myocardium was then applied and by successive computations this was refined until the calculated LV cavity volume matched the measured volume. Iterative FE computation for the LV cavity volume during the cardiac cycle was carried out. At the end of each computation step, the predicted LV cavity volume of the FE model was compared to the measured value. The computation ended if the relative error between the computed and measured values $\leq 1\%$. For this calculation, the total computation time for each run was taken about 1000 s using PC Intel Core i7 (2.93 GHz with RAM 2.00 GB). At the start of all FE computations the LV wall initially was assumed to be stress free (LV cavity pressure equals zero).

2.6 FE Model Merits and Limitations

A new FE inverse model is presented that features the ability to determine the myocardial tissue bulk modulus during cardiac cycle. Other advantages of the proposed method include:

1. Slightly compressible hyperelastic tissue properties.
2. Realistic boundary conditions based on MRI observations.
3. Myofibers orientation simulated based on the obtained data from MRI.

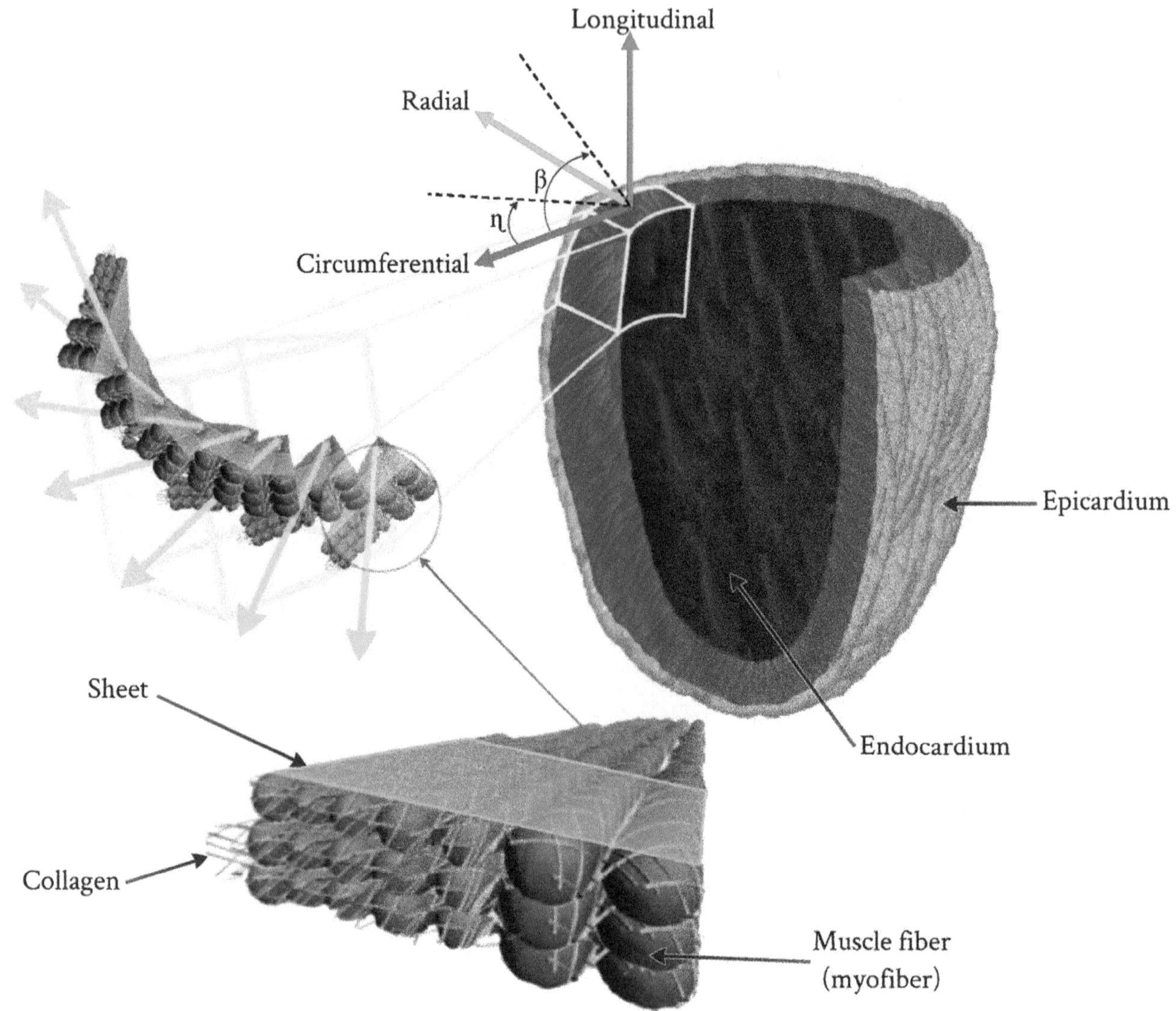

Figure 3. Resprentation of fibers in the LV and the local myocardial coordinate system.

4. The effect of interaction between blood and the internal cavity of LV wall.
5. The effect of surrounding organs and tissues on the deformation of the heart.

However, this model is limited in a number of important ways, including:

1. Simplified geometry for the LV.
2. An incomplete understanding of some heart diseases.
3. The model's inability to study effects of electrical activation, blood flow, porous medium, and cardiac metabolism.
4. The used measured data taken for a healthy human heart "ideal proband".
5. More realistic tissue mechanical properties of LV are still needed.

These limitations and weaknesses can be used as the bases in future model improvements.

Results and Discussion

3.1 Volume Variations of LV Cavity During One Cardiac Cycle

Figure 8 shows the comparison between the predicted FE and experimentally measured LV cavity volumes. The LV cavity volumes increased rapidly from 110 ml to 130 ml (end diastolic volume EDV = 130 ml), shortly after the beginning of atrial systole phase through time = 0.1 sec. Then, LV cavity volume remained constant during the isovolumic contraction phase until time = 0.21 sec. After that, a sudden decrease in LV cavity volume can be seen at the onset of the rapid ejection phase until time = 0.3 sec, followed by a slight decrease during the reduced ejection phase until time = 0.43 sec, at the end systolic phase. The size of LV cavity volume at the moment was equal to that at the end systolic volume (ESV = 50 ml). The LV cavity volume remained constant during the isovolumic relaxation phase until time = 0.5 sec, followed by a rapid increase during the rapid filling phase until time of 0.65 sec. Finally, the LV volume slightly

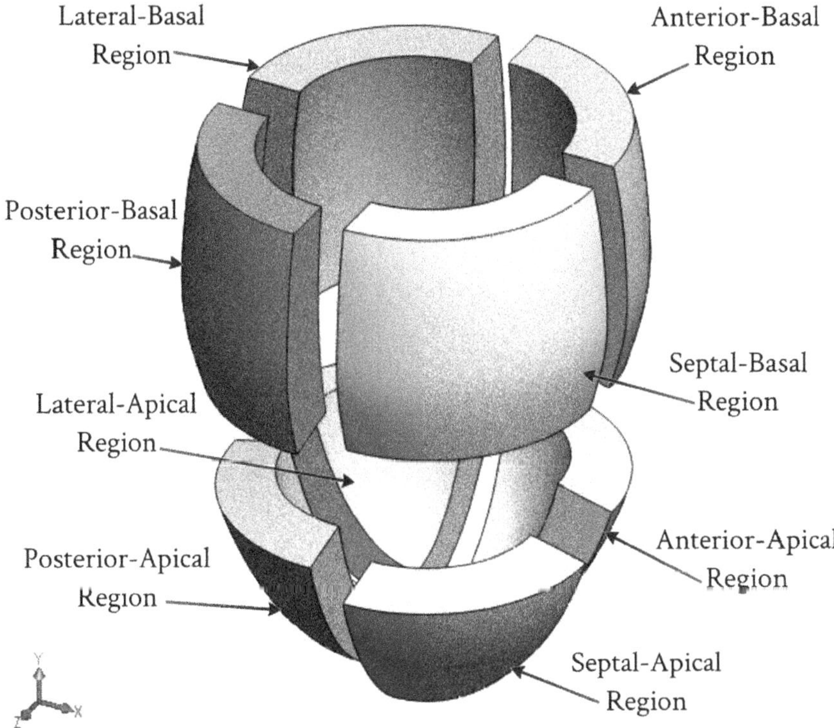

Figure 4. Eight regions of the LV that are used for clarification the helix angle (β).

increased during the reduced filling phase up to the end of cardiac cycle.

The LV cavity volume was locally adapted in response to several stimuli, such as systole phase (isovolumic contraction and ejection) and diastole phase (isovolumic relaxation, rapid filling, reduced filling and atrial contraction). Comparing the present simulation results of LV cavity volumes with corresponding values reported in groups of normal healthy subjects in previous studies [36–39], it was found that the present model can accurately predict the change in the LV cavity volume during the cardiac cycle. It can also be found that the various events (cardiac cycle phases) can be sharply defined. It should be noted that most of those studies ignored the effect of atrial systole on LV volume while others failed to accurately represent all cardiac cycle phases precisely isovolumetric contraction and isovolumetric relaxation.

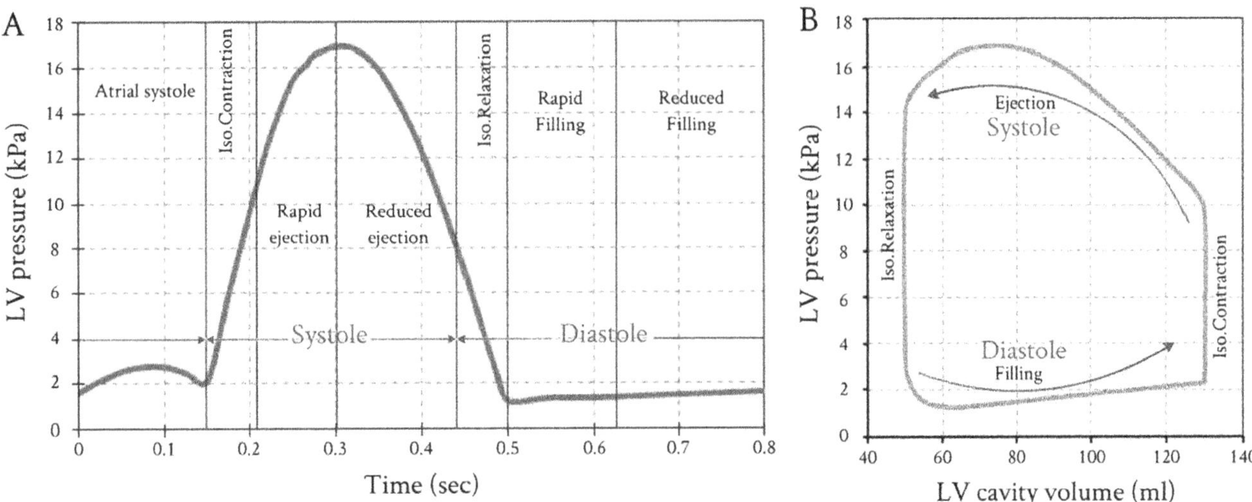

Figure 5. Variations of LV pressure and volume vs. time throughout one cardiac cycle. (A) Measured LV pressures started from atrial systole; and (B) Accompanied PVR loop with stroke volume (SV) 80 ml, LV peak pressure 16.93 kPa, and ejection fraction (E_f)61.55%. (The LV pressure data obtained from published measurements by Hall, 2011 [29]).

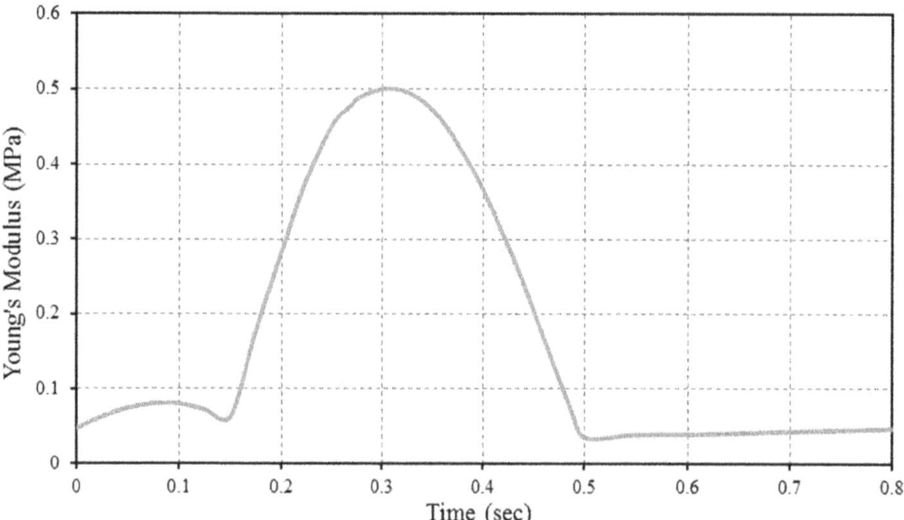

Figure 6. Calculated active myofiber Young's modulus (myocardial stiffness) during one cardiac cycle.

3.2 Variations of Tissue Compressibility during One Cardiac Cycle

During cardiac cycle, the myocardium wall tissue is exposed to successive active contraction and relaxation in consequence of depolarization and repolarization, respectively. Due to heart beating and LV pressure dynamics response, a significant amount of energy can be expended to compress the heart wall, essentially squeezing the myocardium cells closer together.

Figure 9 shows the FE results for the myocardium tissue compressibility variations during one cardiac cycle. It can be noticed that the myocardium tissue is nearly incompressible during a short period of time about 0.16 sec throughout the cardiac cycle (approximately not exceeding 20% of total cardiac cycle time). The tissue showed incompressible behavior during the reduced ejection and isovolumic relaxation phases. The myocardium tissue incompressibility is a common notion used in numerical simulations and analytical studies [40–43]. This is mainly for the purpose of simplifying the analytical formulations and the interpretation of experimental data.

From Figure 9, it can be noticed that myocardium tissue compressibility decreased rapidly at the beginning of the rapid ejection phase. After that, myocardium tissue compressibility increased gradually at the rapid filling phase and remained nearly constant during reduced filling, followed by further increase during the atrial systole (increased about 30% of the maximum of tissue compressibility). Increasing of myocardium tissue compressibility leads to LV wall growth and remodeling. The ability of the present FE model to simulate the observations of growth and remodeling consistent with the previous theoretical study obtained by Kroon et al. [40] and also with the empirical observations using diffusion tensor MRI carried out by Teske et al. [44]. The difference between the maximum myocardium tissue compressibility is 3 kPa^{-1} and its minimum value ($\approx$ 0 kPa^{-1}) can be used as a good index for the normal ventricular function. The decrease in this value means abnormal cardiac function occurrences, maybe due to myocardial infarction or heart dysfunction. The myocardium tissue compressibility increased with decreasing in the contractile force of the ventricles. This lead to an increase in LV cavity size which means that the heart cannot pump blood efficiently and structural alterations of the myocardium (i.e. heart is enlarged and the heart's pumping ability is impaired). Hence, the myocardial tissue compressibility should be considered if myocardial performance, myocardial deformation and heart wall stresses, response time, is critical.

Like many biological tissues, myocardium tissue is able to adapt to changes in mechanical load through growth (change in mass) and remodeling (change in tissue properties) [40]. This hypothesis has confirmed by the results obtained using the present FE model. The LV wall volume was locally adapted (change in tissue compressibility) in response to several stimuli, such as early systolic fiber stretch, fiber shortening during ejection, and contractility.

3.3 Variations of Bulk Modulus during One Cardiac Cycle

Figure 10B shows the FE results for the variations of myocardium bulk modulus during one cardiac cycle. Great variations in the values of the myocardium bulk modulus occurred during the rapid ejection and isovolumic relaxation phases. The myocardium bulk modulus reached to its maximum value at end of ejection and began to decline at the beginning of isovolumic relaxation, i.e. the tissue of LV wall was stiffened by contraction and softened by relaxation. It can be noticed that the myocardium bulk modulus increased exponentially during ejection phase till its peak value, then followed by a linear decrease during isovolumic relaxation phase (i.e. the myofibrils return to their original length). The peak value of bulk modulus occurred at 0.43 sec and the duration time for bulk modulus changes from 0.3 sec to 0.5 sec.

With regard to the timing, the computed duration times for bulk modulus changes were compared to the electrocardiogram (ECG) during one cardiac cycle (see Figure 10C). It can be noticed that the duration times for the onset and ending of LV repolarization marked by T wave (on surface ECG) agree very well with the onset and ending duration times of bulk modulus changes (see Figure 10C). Also, it can be noticed that the onset and ending times of LV repolarization from 0.3 sec to 0.5 sec are sharply defined. Actually, the electrical signals were not included in the present FE analysis, but their impacts are included in the present FE model by introducing the myofiber active elastance. From Figure 10A–C, it can be noticed that there is a good correlation (synchronization) between the instantaneous variation of myocar-

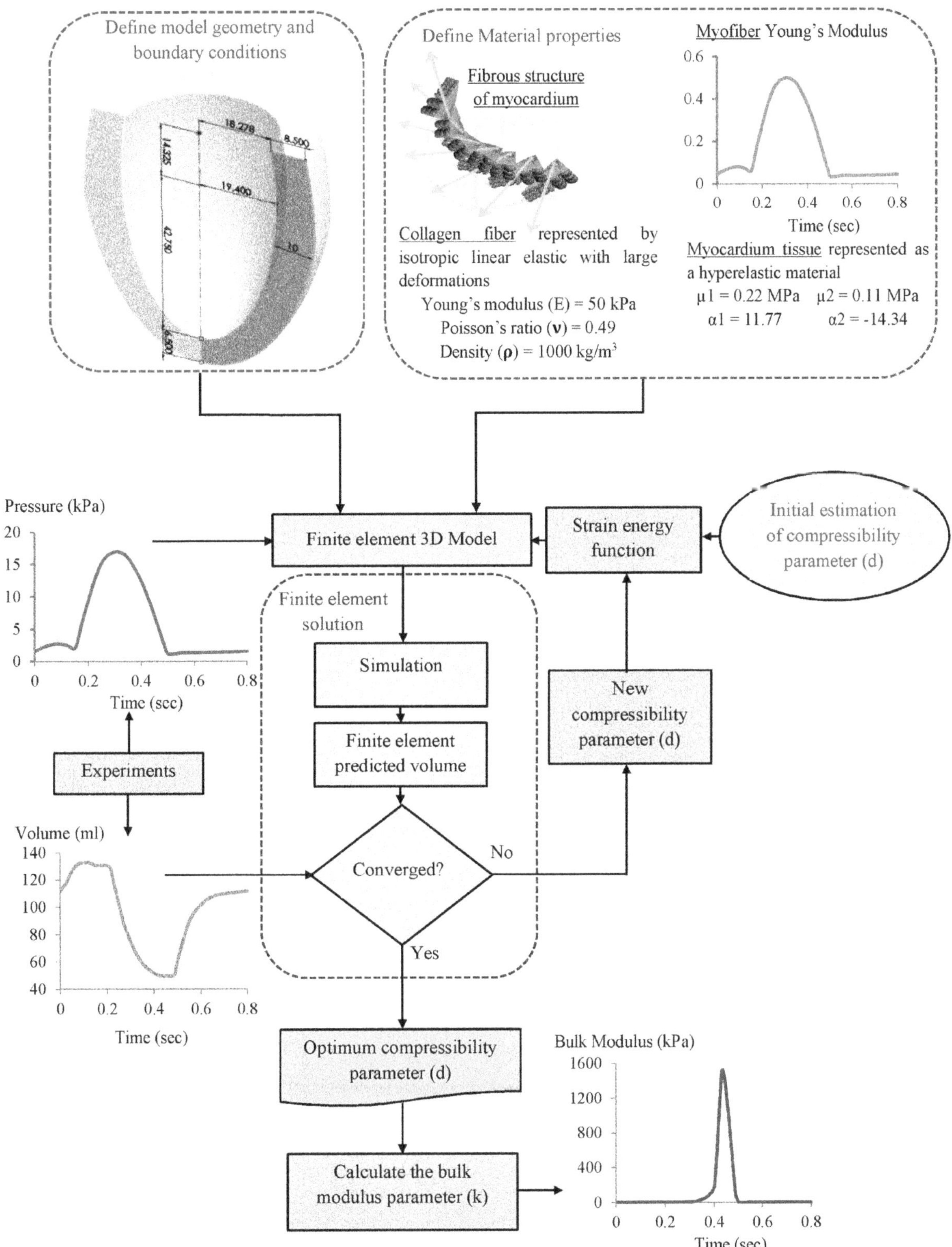

Figure 7. Flowchart of the inverse FE computation sequences for the LV tissue compressibility identification.

dium tissue bulk modulus and the onset and ending of LV repolarization (T wave).

The bulk modulus for myocardium tissue predicted by the current FE model is considerably less than the experimental values measured by Masugata et al. [45]. This is potentially a result of the bulk modulus for myocardium tissue changed drastically immediately after death. Also, there are challenges in the proper acquisition of human myocardium tissue samples and protocols for

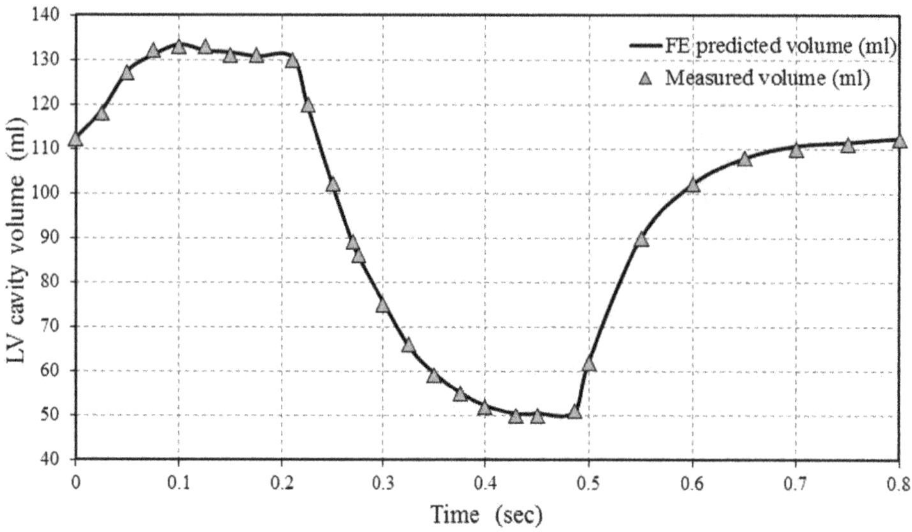

Figure 8. Comparison between the FE predicted LV cavity volume and experimentally measured data.

appropriate experimentation. Diversity of results can also be explained by the differences in the FE models simulation and experimental conditions or the choice of model parameters.

In conclusion, it was concluded that cyclic variation of bulk modulus as predicted by FE model exists during the cardiac cycle with the myocardium tissue being stiffer in systole than it is in diastole. Such behaviors was observed in the experimentally measured shear stiffness for normal myocardium throughout the cardiac cycle using Magnetic Resonance Elastography (MRE) by Kolipaka et al. [46].

3.4 Comparison between Predicted FE Bulk Modulus and Ejection Fraction

The predicted myocardium bulk modulus (K) and ejection fraction (E_f) were compared. Four different LV pressure-volume diagrams with different sets of physiological conditions were used, see Figure 11A, B. The initial LV cavity volumes of the used models were 50 ml, 50 ml, 65 ml, and 70 ml for Model_1, Model_2, Model_3, and Model_4 respectively, while the LV wall thickness was kept constant as described in Figure 1. Figure 11C shows the variations of the predicted myocardium bulk modulus during one cardiac cycle. It can noticed that a discrepancy among the peak values of myocardium bulk moduli exists; 1500 kPa, 2855 kPa, 4760 kPa, and 8000 kPa, which correspond ejection fractions of 61.5% [29], 58.3% [47], 56.3% [48] and 53.6% [49] respectively.

Figure 12 shows the variations of the maximum bulk modulus versus ejection fraction. It is clear that the ejection fraction increased with decreasing peak values of myocardium bulk modulus. Such decrease (i.e. increases of myocardial tissue compressibility) caused an increase of myocardial contraction, which led to an increase of heart ejection fraction. Further study is still required to verify the correlation among the myocardium tissue bulk modulus as a marker for heart function, strain and

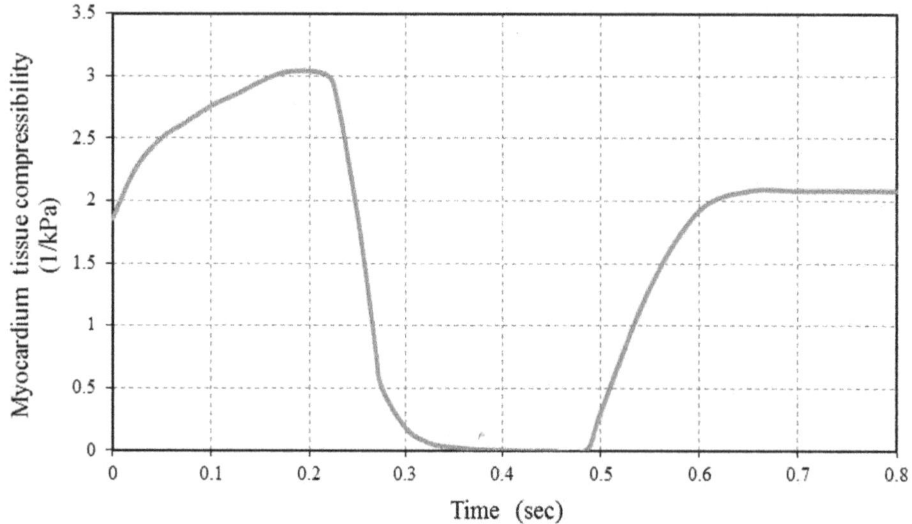

Figure 9. FE computed myocardial tissue compressibility during one cardiac cycle vs. time.

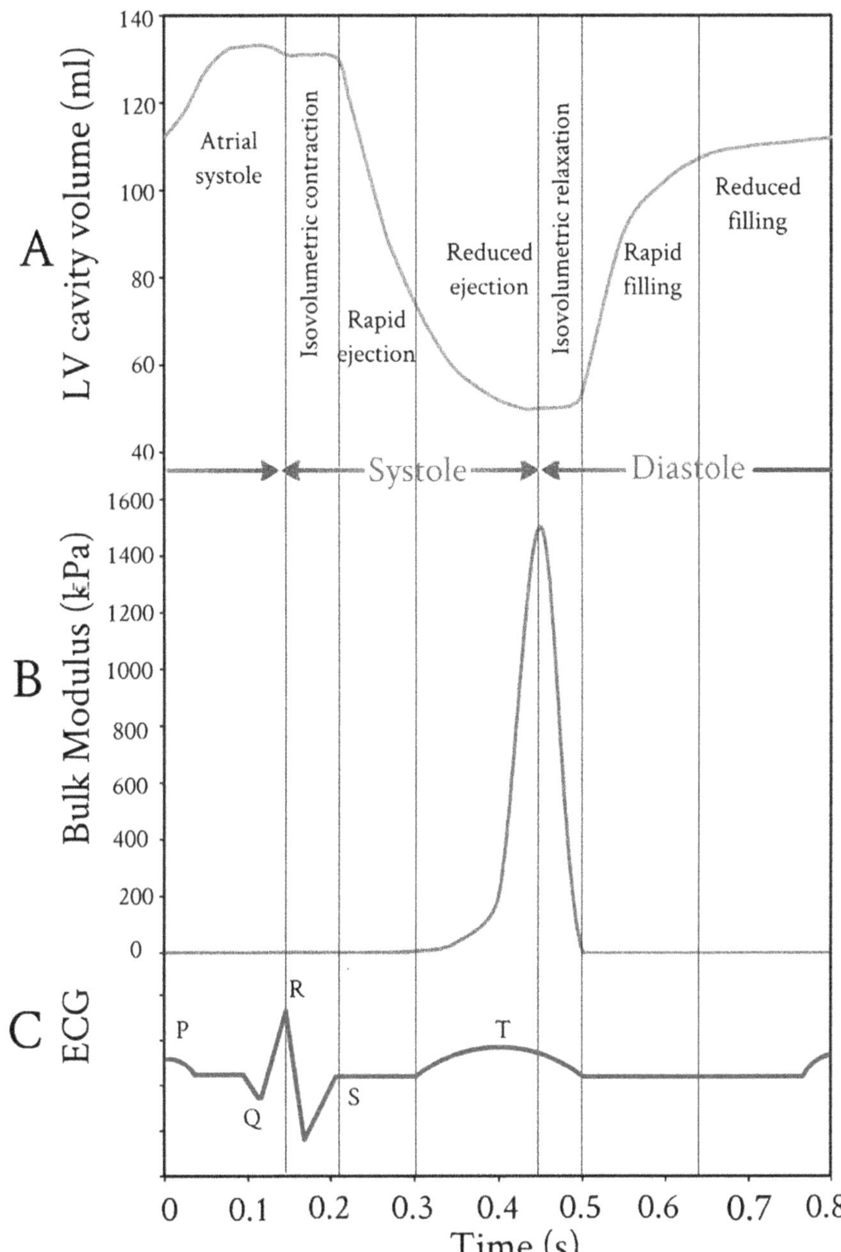

Figure 10. Variations of LV cavity volume, tissue bulk's modulus, and electrocardiogram vs. time throughout one cardiac cycle. (A) FE computed LV cavity ventricular volume; (B) FE computed myocardium tissue bulk's modulus; and (C) Accompanied electrocardiogram (ECG).

strain rate. Finally, the above results confirm the hypothesis, in the computing the active myofiber Young's modulus and the usage of inverse FE analysis for the determination of myocardium tissue bulk modulus.

Conclusions

A novel method combining FE inverse model and LV pressure-volume diagrams was developed to determine the myocardial tissue bulk modulus. The human LV wall (for simplicity) modeled as a thick-walled ellipsoid truncated at two thirds of major axis with spatial myofiber angle distribution was used. The ellipsoidal geometry has been chosen to model the human LV, as it is close to the real anatomical shape, and yet quite simple. The myocardial bulk modulus of different LV pressure-volume diagrams (with four different sets of physiological conditions; stroke volume, LV maximum pressure and ejection fraction), was determined. Based on the results and discussion presented in the preceding section, the following conclusions can be drawn:

1. The myocardium bulk modulus can be used as a diagnostic tool (clinical indicator) of the heart ejection fraction.
2. Our results show that the present FE model is sensitive to the overall cardiac function parameters expressed in terms of LV pressure-volume variations during cardiac cycle and ejection fraction.

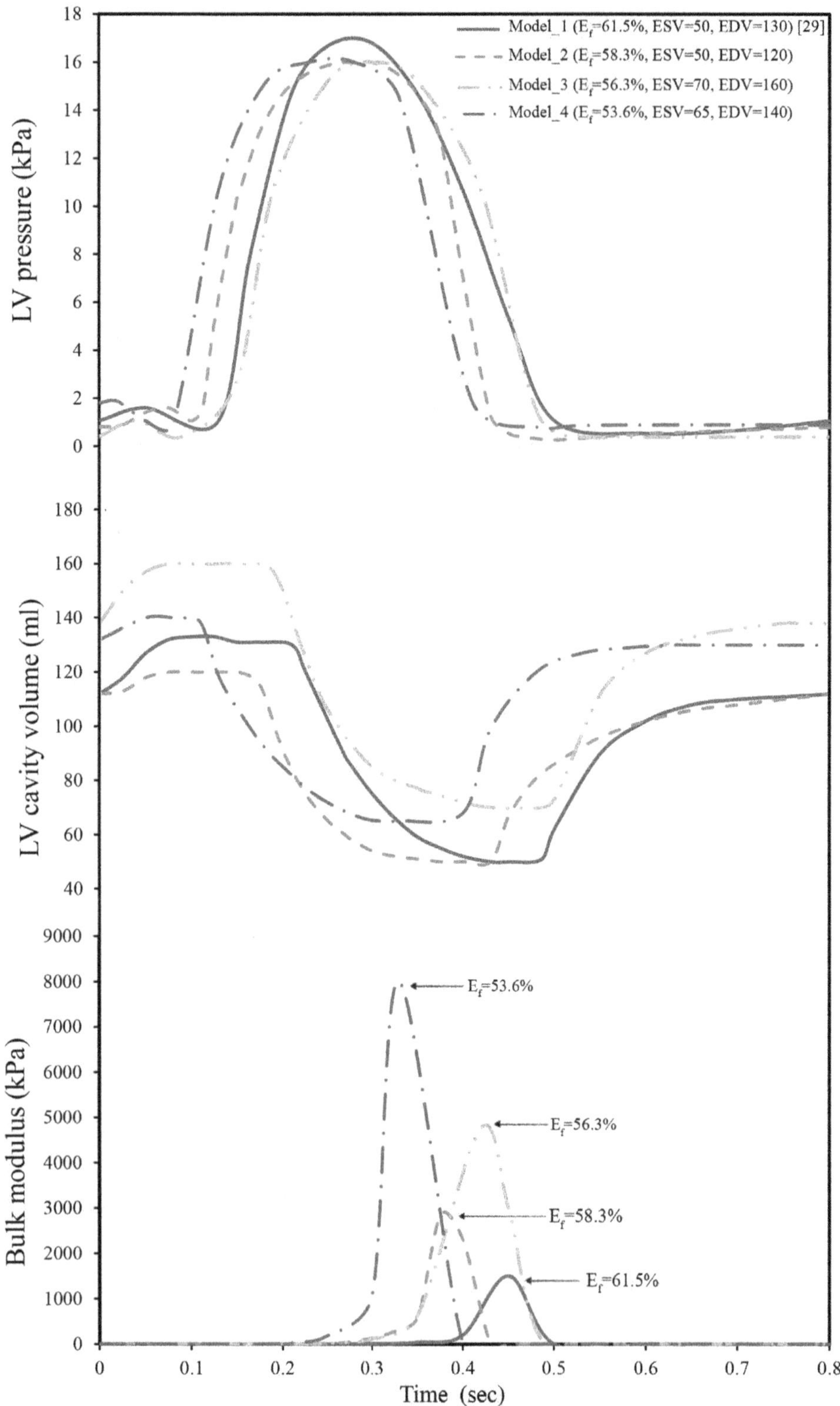

Figure 11. Variations of LV pressure, volume, and tissue bulk's modulus vs. time through one cardiac cycle. (A) Measured LV pressures for different cardiac cycles; (B) Measured LV cavity volumes; and (C) FE computed myocardium tissue bulk's modulus.

3. The calculations of active myofiber Young's modulus (myocardium active properties) based on the LV pressure proved their correctness.

With this research, the authors would like to recommend further investigations on the subject of compressibility of myocardium tissue, which is still debated and remains a challenging experimental topic.

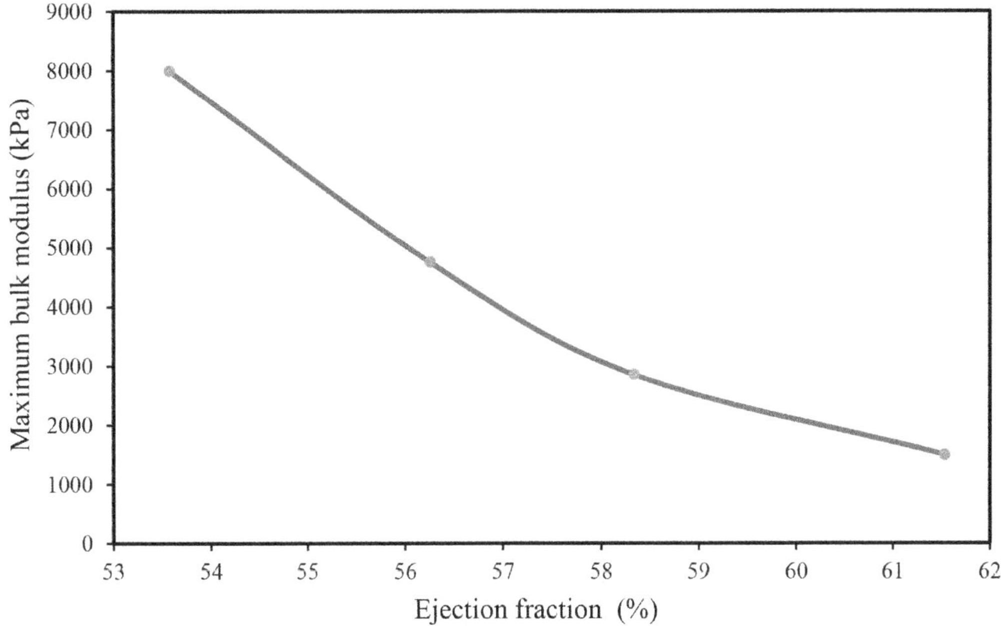

Figure 12. Comparison between the FE predicted maximum bulk modulus and ejection fraction.

Acknowledgments

Thanks to Prof. Ibrahim Mohamed Hassab-Allah (Assiut University) and to Prof. Asif Haleem (Jazan University) for their helpful discussions.

Author Contributions

Conceived and designed the experiments: AIH MAH. Performed the experiments: AIH ANM. Analyzed the data: AIH MH. Wrote the paper: AIH.

References

1. Kohl P, Sachs F, Franz MR (2011) Cardiac mechano-electric coupling and arrhythmias: OUP Oxford.
2. Fung Y, Cowin S (1994) Biomechanics: Mechanical properties of living tissues. Journal of Applied Mechanics 61: 1007–1007.
3. Yin F, Chan C, Judd RM (1996) Compressibility of perfused passive myocardium. American Journal of Physiology-Heart and Circulatory Physiology 271: H1864–H1870.
4. Bettendorff-Bakman DE, Schmid P, Lunkenheimer P, Niederer P (2006) A finite element study relating to the rapid filling phase of the human ventricles. J Theor Biol 238: 303–316.
5. Veress AI, Gullberg GT, Weiss JA (2005) Measurement of strain in the left ventricle during diastole with cine-MRI and deformable image registration.
6. Shim J, Grosberg A, Nawroth JC, Kit Parker K, Bertoldi K (2012) Modeling of cardiac muscle thin films: Pre-stretch, passive and active behavior. J Biomech 45: 832–841.
7. Dorri F, Niederer P, Lunkenheimer P (2006) A finite element model of the human left ventricular systole. Computer Methods in Biomechanics and Biomedical Engineering 9: 319–341.
8. Marchesseau S, Delingette H, Sermesant M, Sorine M, Rhode K, et al. (2012) Preliminary specificity study of the Bestel-Clément-Sorine electromechanical model of the heart using parameter calibration from medical images. Journal of the Mechanical Behavior of Biomedical Materials.
9. Yettram A, Beecham M (1998) An analytical method for the determination of along-fibre to cross-fibre elastic modulus ratio in ventricular myocardium–a feasibility study. Medical engineering & physics 20: 103–108.
10. Périé D, Dahdah N, Foudis A, Curnier D (2013) Multi-parametric MRI as an indirect evaluation tool of the mechanical properties of in-vitro cardiac tissues. BMC cardiovascular disorders 13: 1–9.
11. Augenstein KF, Cowan BR, LeGrice IJ, Young AA (2006) Estimation of cardiac hyperelastic material properties from MRI tissue tagging and diffusion tensor imaging. Medical Image Computing and Computer-Assisted Intervention–MICCAI 2006: Springer. 628–635.
12. Wang VY, Lam H, Ennis DB, Cowan BR, Young AA, et al. (2009) Modelling passive diastolic mechanics with quantitative MRI of cardiac structure and function. Med Image Anal 13: 773.
13. Dent CL, Scott MJ, Wickline SA, Hall CS (2000) High-frequency ultrasound for quantitative characterization of myocardial edema. Ultrasound in medicine & biology 26: 375–384.
14. Balaraman K, Mukherjee S, Chawla A, Malhotra R (2006) Inverse Finite Element Characterization of Soft Tissues Using Impact Experiments and Taguchi Methods. SAE Paper: 01–0252.
15. Zenker S, Rubin J, Clermont G (2007) From Inverse Problems in Mathematical Physiology to Quantitative Differential Diagnoses. PLoS Comput Biol 3: e204.
16. Xu Z-H, Yang Y, Huang P, Li X (2010) Determination of interfacial properties of thermal barrier coatings by shear test and inverse finite element method. Acta Materialia 58: 5972–5979.
17. Evans S, Avril S (2012) Editorial: Identification of material parameters through inverse finite element modelling. Computer Methods in Biomechanics and Biomedical Engineering 15: 1–2.
18. Hassaballah AIM, Hassan MA, Mardi NA, Hamdi MA (2013) Modeling the effects of myocardial fiber architecture and material properties on the left ventricle mechanics during rapid filling phase. Journal of applied mathematics and information sciences; in press.
19. LeGrice IJ, Smaill B, Chai L, Edgar S, Gavin J, et al. (1995) Laminar structure of the heart: ventricular myocyte arrangement and connective tissue architecture in the dog. American Journal of Physiology-Heart and Circulatory Physiology 269: H571–H582.
20. Stevens C, Remme E, LeGrice I, Hunter P (2003) Ventricular mechanics in diastole: material parameter sensitivity. J Biomech 36: 737–748.
21. Helm P, Beg MF, Miller MI, Winslow RL (2005) Measuring and mapping cardiac fiber and laminar architecture using diffusion tensor MR imaging. Ann Ny Acad Sci 1047: 296–307.
22. Sengupta PP, Korinek J, Belohlavek M, Narula J, Vannan MA, et al. (2006) Left ventricular structure and function: basic science for cardiac imaging. J Am Coll Cardiol 48: 1988–2001.
23. Arts T, Lumens J, Kroon W, Delhaas T (2012) Control of Whole Heart Geometry by Intramyocardial Mechano-Feedback: A Model Study. PLoS Comput Biol 8: e1002369.
24. Kerckhoffs R, Bovendeerd P, Kotte J, Prinzen F, Smits K, et al. (2003) Homogeneity of cardiac contraction despite physiological asynchrony of depolarization: a model study. Ann Biomed Eng 31: 536–547.
25. Chen J, Liu W, Zhang H, Lacy L, Yang X, et al. (2005) Regional ventricular wall thickening reflects changes in cardiac fiber and sheet structure during contraction: quantification with diffusion tensor MRI. American Journal of Physiology-Heart and Circulatory Physiology 289: H1898–H1907.
26. Lombaert H, Peyrat JM, Croisille P, Rapacchi S, Fanton L, et al. (2011) Statistical Analysis of the Human Cardiac Fiber Architecture from DT-MRI. Lect Notes Comput Sc 6666: 171–179.

27. Lombaert H, Peyrat JM, Croisille P, Rapacchi S, Fanton L, et al. (2012) Human Atlas of the Cardiac Fiber Architecture: Study on a Healthy Population. Ieee T Med Imaging 31: 1436–1447.
28. Rohmer D, Sitek A, Gullberg GT (2006) Reconstruction and visualization of fiber and laminar structure in the normal human heart from ex vivo DTMRI data. Tech. Rep., Lawrence Berkeley National Laboratory.
29. Hall JE (2011) Guyton and Hall Textbook of Medical Physiology: Enhanced E-book: Saunders.
30. Bettendorff-Bakman DE, Schmid P, Lunkenheimer P, Niederer P (2008) Diastolic ventricular aspiration: A mechanism supporting the rapid filling phase of the human ventricles. J Theor Biol 250: 581–592.
31. Zhong L, Ghista D, NG E, Chua T, Lee CN, et al. (2007) Left ventricular functional indices based on the left ventricular elastances and shape factor. Journal of Mechanics in Medicine and Biology 07: 107–116.
32. Watanabe S, Shite J, Takaoka H, Shinke T, Imuro Y, et al. (2006) Myocardial stiffness is an important determinant of the plasma brain natriuretic peptide concentration in patients with both diastolic and systolic heart failure. European heart journal 27: 832–838.
33. Venugopal JR, Prabhakaran MP, Mukherjee S, Ravichandran R, Dan K, et al. (2012) Biomaterial strategies for alleviation of myocardial infarction. J R Soc Interface 9: 1–19.
34. Hassan M, Hamdi M, Noma A (2012) The nonlinear elastic and viscoelastic passive properties of left ventricular papillary muscle of a Guinea pig heart. Journal of the Mechanical Behavior of Biomedical Materials 5: 99–109.
35. Bagnoli P, Malagutti N, Gastaldi D, Marcelli E, Lui E, et al. (2011) Computational finite element model of cardiac torsion. Int J Artif Organs 34: 44–53.
36. Le Rolle V, Hernández AI, Richard P-Y, Donal E, Carrault G (2008) Model-based analysis of myocardial strain data acquired by tissue Doppler imaging. Artificial Intelligence in Medicine 44: 201–219.
37. Niederer SA, Smith NP (2009) The role of the Frank–Starling law in the transduction of cellular work to whole organ pump function: A computational modeling analysis. PLoS computational biology 5: e1000371.
38. Evangelista A, Nardinocchi P, Puddu P, Teresi L, Torromeo C, et al. (2011) Torsion of the human left ventricle: Experimental analysis and computational modeling. Progress in biophysics and molecular biology 107: 112–121.
39. Kerckhoffs RC, Omens JH, McCulloch AD (2012) A single strain-based growth law predicts concentric and eccentric cardiac growth during pressure and volume overload. Mechanics research communications 42: 40–50.
40. Kroon W, Delhaas T, Arts T, Bovendeerd P (2007) Constitutive Modeling of Cardiac Tissue Growth. In: Sachse F, Seemann G, editors. Lect Notes Comput Sc: Springer Berlin Heidelberg. 340–349.
41. Eriksson T, Prassl A, Plank G, Holzapfel G (2013) Influence of myocardial fiber/sheet orientations on left ventricular mechanical contraction. Mathematics and Mechanics of Solids.
42. Lee LC, Wenk JF, Zhong L, Klepach D, Zhang Z, et al. (2013) Analysis of Patient-specific Surgical Ventricular Restoration-Importance of an Ellipsoidal Left Ventricular Geometry for Diastolic and Systolic Function. Journal of Applied Physiology.
43. Martina JR, Bovendeerd PH, de Jonge N, de Mol BA, Lahpor JR, et al. (2013) Simulation of Changes in Myocardial Tissue Properties During Left Ventricular Assistance With a Rotary Blood Pump. Artificial organs.
44. Teske AJ, De Boeck B, Melman PG, Sieswerda GT, Doevendans PA, et al. (2007) Echocardiographic quantification of myocardial function using tissue deformation imaging, a guide to image acquisition and analysis using tissue Doppler and speckle tracking. Cardiovasc Ultrasound 5: 27.
45. Masugata H, Mizushige K, Kinoshita A, Sakamoto S, Matsuo H, et al. (2000) Comparison of left ventricular diastolic filling with myocyte bulk modulus using doppler echocardiography and acoustic microscopy in pressure-overload left ventricular hypertrophy and cardiac amyloidosis. Clinical cardiology 23: 115–122.
46. Kolipaka A, Araoz PA, McGee KP, Manduca A, Ehman RL (2010) Magnetic resonance elastography as a method for the assessment of effective myocardial stiffness throughout the cardiac cycle. Magnetic Resonance in Medicine 64: 862–870.
47. Klabunde RE (2011) Cardiovascular physiology concepts: Wolters Kluwer Health.
48. Courneya CAM, Parker MJ (2010) Cardiovascular Physiology: A Clinical Approach [With Access Code]: Wolters Kluwer Health.
49. Stouffer G (2011) Cardiovascular hemodynamics for the clinician: Wiley. com.

A Neuro-Mechanical Model of a Single Leg Joint Highlighting the Basic Physiological Role of Fast and Slow Muscle Fibres of an Insect Muscle System

Tibor Istvan Toth[1], Joachim Schmidt[2], Ansgar Büschges[2], Silvia Daun-Gruhn[1]*

1 Emmy Noether Research Group of Computational Biology, Department of Animal Physiology, University of Cologne, Cologne, Germany, **2** Department of Animal Physiology, University of Cologne, Cologne, Germany

Abstract

In legged animals, the muscle system has a dual function: to produce forces and torques necessary to move the limbs in a systematic way, and to maintain the body in a static position. These two functions are performed by the contribution of specialized motor units, i.e. motoneurons driving sets of specialized muscle fibres. With reference to their overall contraction and metabolic properties they are called fast and slow muscle fibres and can be found ubiquitously in skeletal muscles. Both fibre types are active during stepping, but only the slow ones maintain the posture of the body. From these findings, the general hypothesis on a functional segregation between both fibre types and their neuronal control has arisen. Earlier muscle models did not fully take this aspect into account. They either focused on certain aspects of muscular function or were developed to describe specific behaviours only. By contrast, our neuro-mechanical model is more general as it allows functionally to differentiate between static and dynamic aspects of movement control. It does so by including both muscle fibre types and separate motoneuron drives. Our model helps to gain a deeper insight into how the nervous system might combine neuronal control of locomotion and posture. It predicts that (1) positioning the leg at a specific retraction angle in steady state is most likely due to the extent of recruitment of slow muscle fibres and not to the force developed in the individual fibres of the antagonistic muscles; (2) the fast muscle fibres of antagonistic muscles contract alternately during stepping, while co-contraction of the slow muscle fibres takes place during steady state; (3) there are several possible ways of transition between movement and steady state of the leg achieved by varying the time course of recruitment of the fibres in the participating muscles.

Editor: Vladimir Brezina, Mount Sinai School of Medicine, United States of America

Funding: Funding provided by Emmy Noether Programme DA 1182/1-1. The funders had no role in study design, data collection and analysis, decision to publish, or preparartion of the manuscript.

Competing Interests: The authors have declared that no competing interests exist.

* E-mail: sgruhn@uni-koeln.de

Introduction

In legged animals, the muscles of the limbs have two basic functions: i) to produce forces and torques in order to move the limbs of the body during fast and slow locomotion and other rhythmic or episodic behaviours, and ii) to hold the body or its parts in a static position (posture). In order to perform these tasks effectively, muscle fibres of differing contraction dynamics evolved in many species [1]. A muscle can be subdivided into motor units: a motoneuron (MN) and all of the muscle fibres it innervates. In mammals, the fibres of a motor unit show similar biochemical and histochemical properties (for review see [2].) By contrast, in arthropods, a single muscle fibre may be innervated by more than one MN, and the fibres innervated by one MN may exhibit different electrophysiological, histochemical and contractile properties (e.g. [3–7]). These properties may allow for fine tuned movements despite the low number of motoneurons that innervate an arthropod muscle. Motor units are usually recruited in the order of decreasing electrical input resistance (size principle, [8,9]), but this can be overruled (for reviews see [10,11]).

In the stick insect, for example, slow and fast muscle fibres were discovered in the extensor tibiae muscle. Moreover, they were found to be anatomically (spatially) separated [7,12]. It was also shown by [12] that the slow and fast fibres have different functional roles: both are active during stepping (locomotion) while only the former are active during maintaining the posture of the animal. The MNs innervating the fast fibres are normally not active during static positions of the stick insect. In addition, there exist common inhibitory MNs, which simultaneously inhibit the slow leg muscles during movement. In particular, the common inhibitory MN, denoted CI1, inhibits the slow muscle fibres of all main leg muscles, except for the m. flexor tibiae, which is inhibited by two different MNs CI2 and CI3. Up to recently, the presence of the differentiation between muscle fibres could only be confirmed with certainty in the extensor muscle. However, there is now experimental evidence that slow and fast muscle fibres are present in all three main muscle pairs (protractor-retractor, levator-depressor, and extensor-flexor) of the leg [13]. It therefore makes sense to use this property in models describing the neuronal control of muscle systems in insects.

In an earlier work [14], we constructed a neuro-mechanical model of the protractor-retractor muscle system, based on experimental data from the stick insect. This model included a central pattern generator (CPG), MNs that innervate the protractor and the retractor muscles, and interneurons (INs) connecting the CPGs to the MNs. It also comprised the models of the muscles just mentioned. The neurons of the CPG and the INs were non-spiking, and were described by the same, simple Hodgkin-Huxley-type model [15] but, of course, with different values of the model parameters. The MNs were also described by a Hodgkin-Huxley-type model but they could fire proper action potentials. We provide the model equations in Appendix S1. The model of the muscles was derived from Hill's model [16] with strong simplifications. It will be briefly described in the Methods below. This model is extended here to include slow muscle fibres beside the fast ones. The extension has been motivated by experimental results in which the leg, the femur in particular, showed only small-amplitude angular movements, or was held in a static horizontal position, for instance, during sideward stepping. Experimental findings (e.g. [7,12]) clearly proved that slow muscle fibres were necessary to carry out the tasks just mentioned. We also found that our original model, with only the fast muscle fibres, could not produce these types of behaviour. The inclusion of slow muscle fibres is to help remedy this shortcoming. For the same reason, gradual recruitment of the muscle fibres is also implemented in the present, extended version. This new property enables the model to produce arbitrary static angles at the thorax-coxa joint of the leg. Also, it increases the overall flexibility of the model. However, we do not take the variability of the electro-physiological properties of slow and fast MNs into account. Nor do we include, at this stage, the common inhibitor MNs in the model, and thus neglect the residual stiffness, which is discernible in the slow muscle fibres. The reason for this is to keep the model extension as simple as possible in order to be able to concentrate on the direct and specific effects produced by the slow and fast muscle fibre types. In the accompanying paper (Toth et al., unpublished results) in which we shall consider a model with both slow and fast muscle fibres in all main leg muscles and their recruitment implemented, we shall also investigate the effects of residual stiffness of the slow muscle fibres and of the common inhibitory MNs. We shall make use of them to elucidate the detailed mechanism of stop and start of the stepping movement (locomotion). In present paper, we report the results which relate to the basic functions of the slow and fast muscle fibres. Important points in the simulations are the presence or absence of co-contraction of antagonistic muscles, and the co-activation, or the lack of it, of the MNs driving them. The model makes predictions related to these points. We can, by means of the model, show how recruitment proves to be an effective mechanism to achieve and maintain (near) steady-state positions, and also during transition from steady state to angular movements.

Methods: The extended model of the protractor-retractor muscle system

Fig. 1 shows the network of the extended model. Its components are briefly described in the figure legend, but a more detailed description of them can be found in [14]. Its most important new property is that it now comprises slow muscle fibres together with their driving MNs, and inhibitory INs that connect the MNs to the CPG. As in the earlier version, the INs convey rhythmic inhibition from the CPG to the MNs (to both fast and slow.) The rhythmic inhibition can be modified or even abolished by increasing or decreasing the (central) inhibition to the INs (by changing the corresponding conductance g_d of the inhibitory current). The slow and fast muscle fibres differ by the dynamics of their response to neuronal excitation from the innervating MN. Thus the fast muscle fibres have fast response dynamics and the slow ones much slower response dynamics. The muscles are modelled as nonlinear springs [17] with variable spring constant (stiffness) and damping (viscosity) unit, as shown in Fig. 2. This is a gross simplification of Hill's muscle model [16]. In particular, our simplified model does not have explicit passive elements.

We also strongly simplified the force-velocity relationship of Hill's model by making it linear, assuming that the velocity range of the movements remains sufficiently narrow, as in the case of stick insects. The equation of mechanical motion of the femur under the influence of the (slow and fast) protractor and retractor muscles is given in Appendix S2. The elastic properties of the muscle fibres, as expressed by their spring constants, are identical. To be more specific, we recall the equations of the muscle model used in [14].

$$k(t)=k_{\infty}-[k_{\infty}-k(t_0)]\exp[-(a_0+b)(t-t_0)] \qquad (1)$$

$$k(t)=k(t_1)\exp[-b(t-t_1)] \qquad (2)$$

Here, $k(t)$ is the value of the spring constant at time t, k_{∞} is its stationary (end) value. Eqn. 1 is valid during a MN action potential, and eqn. 2 otherwise. Note that the spring constant will eventually vanish if the activity of the innervating MN ceases. However, at switching the direction of movement of the femur, vanishing angular velocity and acceleration are assumed. These conditions impose constraints on the stationary values (k_{∞}) of the spring constants. As a consequence, the spring constants can only vanish, if *neither* of the muscles of the antagonistic muscle pair receives neuronal drive from its MN (for a detailed explanation see [14]). Both fast and slow muscle fibres have been modelled this way. The only difference between the two muscle types therefore is their differing response dynamics.

The rate constants in eqn.s 1 and 2 are (a_0+b) and b, respectively, the former being much larger than the latter. These parameters characterize the kinetics of the muscle contraction. Slow muscle fibres have therefore small rate constants (a_0 values). Specifically, during retraction, the fast retractor muscle fibres have $a_0=5.0ms^{-1}$, and the protractor ones $a_0=2.0ms^{-1}$. During protraction, the rate constant of the fast retractor muscle fibres is $a_0=0.7ms^{-1}$, and that of the fast protractor muscle fibres $a_0=0.8ms^{-1}$. The values of the corresponding rate constants of the slow muscle fibres have been chosen to be 100 times smaller ($0.05ms^{-1}$ etc.). The relaxation rate constants (b values) have identical values in both muscle types ($b=0.01ms^{-1}$ for all muscle types). These choices ensure that the dynamics of the angular movement match that seen in the experiments. For further details, see [14].

Implementing muscle recruitment

So far, all muscles, fast or slow, have been regarded as "large", single muscle fibres that were either activated, i.e. recruited, or not. However, all muscles that are included in the model consist of several motor units, not all of which need to be activated during muscle activity in order to carry out a movement, or to maintain the spatial position, of an extremity. Moreover, partial recruitment of muscle fibres is an important tool for gradually increasing or decreasing the total muscle force. It is therefore important to take account of this fact in the model, too. The ability of gradual recruitment of the muscle fibres increases the flexibility of our muscle model. This flexibility will indeed be needed to simulate

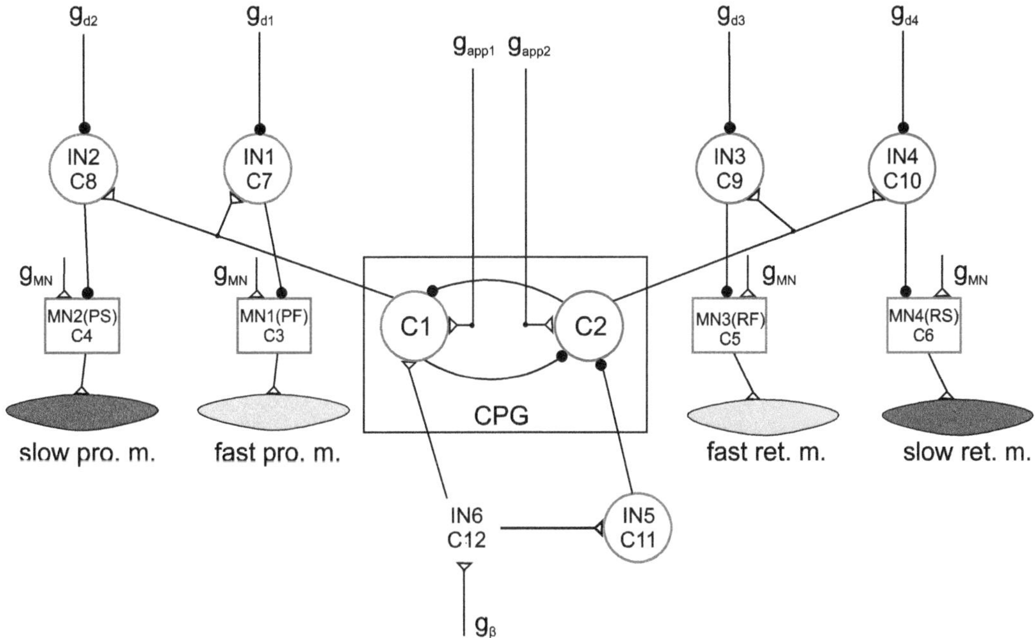

Figure 1. The extended model of the protractor-retractor muscle system. The model consists of a central pattern generator: CPG, slow and fast protractor and retractor muscles as indicated (slow pro. m. etc.), the corresponding motoneurons: MN(PS) etc., 4 inhibitory interneurons (IN1–IN4) connecting the CPG to the motoneurons, and two additional interneurons (IN5–IN6), which convey neuronal signals to the CPG from sense organs of other joints of the same leg, or possibly of other legs. g_{app1}, g_{app2} are conductances of the driving currents to C1 and C2, respectively. g_{MN} is the conductance of the common (central) input current to all motoneurons. g_{d1}–g_{d4} are conductances of the inhibitory currents to IN1–IN4, respectively. g_{β} is the conductance of the sensory input current from the levator-depressor muscle system. Empty triangles are excitatory synapses; filled black circles on neurons are inhibitory synapses. The tiny black circles on synaptic paths are branching points.

various static or dynamic conditions produced by the muscle activity.

The implementation of recruitment in the model is schematically illustrated in Fig. 3. The main idea is that a MN-muscle functional unit of a given type (slow or fast) in Fig. 1, now represents a number of motor units. The MNs of these units have identical properties and, if some of them are activated, it is done synchronously. That is the MN in Fig. 1 exhibits activity as long as at least one motor unit is active. The muscles in Fig. 1 are also thought to consist of several fibres belonging to different motor units of the same type. The mechanical and kinetic properties of

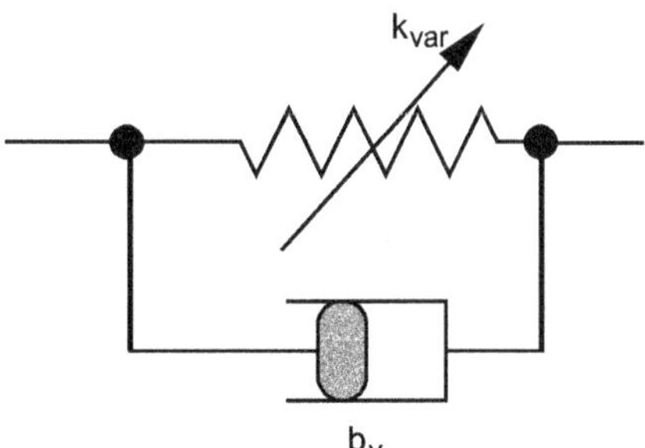

Figure 2. Schematic picture of the simplified muscle model. k_{var}: variable spring constant (elasticity modulus). The actual value of k_{var} is determined by the activity of the connecting motoneuron; k_{var} can be regarded as (actual) contractility of the muscle. b_v: coefficient of the damping produced by viscosity. The torque generated by the damping is assumed to be proportional to the contraction velocity of the muscle fibre with a constant value of b_v for a given muscle type.

the fibres are assumed to be identical. The only difference between them is that, at a given instant of time, some of them are activated, i.e. recruited, others are not. The quantitative formulation of the effect of recruitment is very simple: a linearly proportional relationship between muscle contractility and the proportion of recruited fibres in the whole muscle. That is,

$$k_{eff} = r_a \frac{k_c}{r_c} \quad (0 < r_a, r_c \leq 1) \tag{3}$$

where k_c is the total value of the spring constant of all recruited fibres of the muscle in "control conditions", which we take to be normal stepping. The quantities r_a and r_c are the proportions of the actually recruited muscle fibres and those in control conditions, respectively. Finally, k_{eff} is the effective (actual) total value of the spring constant of the muscle, which determines its actual contractility. Here, we additionally assume that not all muscle fibres are recruited in control conditions, thus $0 < r_c < 1$. We set $r_c = 0.7$ for all muscles. Unfortunately, there are no experimental data that would reveal the correct value of r_c. Hence, the value chosen for it remains somewhat arbitrary. In some muscles, there are a few motor units, only. The recruitment is, accordingly, rather coarse. In the muscle model, that means that r_c can assume a few discrete values, only, between 0 and 1. The number of the discrete values r_a can assume is equal to the number of motor units in the muscle. This means that the number of motor units determines the number of intermediate positions the femur (limb) can attain.

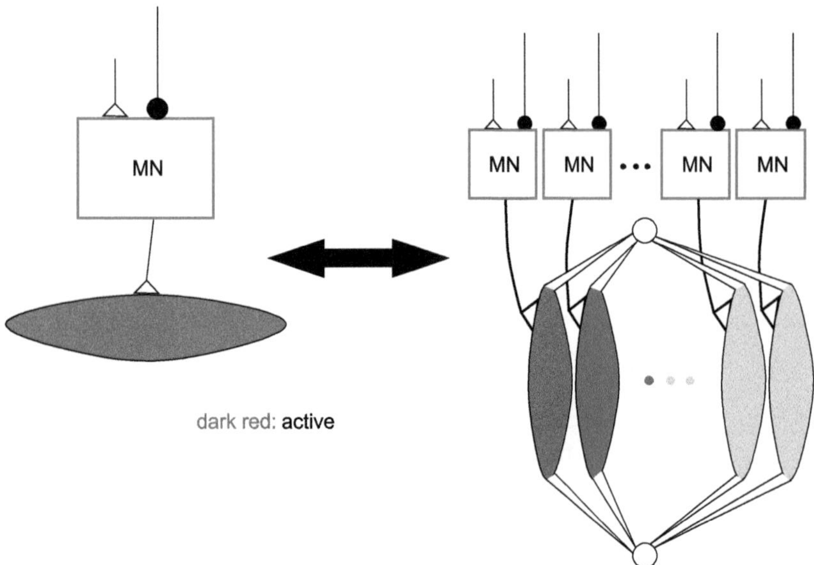

Figure 3. Modelling of recruitment. The single motor unit is symbolically replaced by a number of identical motor units in the model. The motoneurons are identical and the activated ones are synchronously driven. The mechanical and kinetic properties of the muscle fibres arranged in parallel are also identical for all fibres. Dark red fibres represent the recruited, i.e. active muscle fibres.

Results

Angular movement and network activity during forward stepping

First, the electrical activity of the CPG and the MNs during forward stepping, as well as the resulting angular movement of the femur were simulated. We tested the cases when both slow and fast MNs were simultaneously active (co-contraction of slow and fast muscle fibres) and when the activity of the slow MNs was blocked. The former case roughly corresponds to fast walking of the animal, whereas the latter one is admittedly rather artificial, since the slow MNs are normally recruited earlier during walking than the fast MNs [18]. The results are shown in Fig. 4. The rhythmic co-contraction of the slow and fast muscle fibres of the same muscle (protractor or retractor), as illustrated in panels 2,4 and 6,8 from the top of Fig. 4, respectively, moves the femur alternately forward or backward in the range between 30° and 128° (Fig. 4, top panel) in agreement with experimental data from the stick insect. Fig. 4 also displays the phase relations between CPG activity, MN discharge, muscle contraction, and angular movement during stepping. The activities of the slow and fast MNs innervating the same muscle type (protractor or rectractor) are, up to $t=6500ms$, in full synchrony (Fig. 4, panels 2–5, and 6–9 from the top, respectively). At $t=6500ms$, the activity of both the slow protractor and retractor MNs was blocked. The blockade completely abolished the forces in the slow muscles just after a short while (Fig. 4 panels 2 and 6 from the top). It had, however, a negligible effect, only on the angular movement, hardly discernible in Fig. 4. We can therefore conclude that, in the model, the large angular movements during forward stepping are determined by the contractions of the fast muscle fibres of the two muscle types (protractor and retractor). Consequently, if the fast muscle fibres are active, the omission of the slow muscle fibres when modelling angular movements during forward stepping will not lead to discernible simulation error.

Angular movement and network activity when the fast MNs are inhibited

Next we investigated the case when one or both fast MNs were inhibited, i.e. the conductances g_{d1} or g_{d3}, or both of the inhibitory inputs to IN1 and IN3 were strongly reduced. Fig. 5 shows the effect of the inhibition of both fast MNs. The amplitude of the angular movement strongly decreased after the onset of the inhibition (at $t=6500ms$). The new range of the angle α became 82°-100°, a peak-to-peak amplitude of 18°. (Compare it to the peak-to-peak amplitude of about 100° of the angular movement during stepping in Fig. 5A). This is a sign that the contraction kinetics of the slow muscle fibres cannot follow the relatively high frequency ($\approx 2Hz$) of the driving CPG. The decrease in the amplitude was even more striking if at the same time when the fast MNs were inhibited, the slow ones were activated by disinhibition, i.e. by strongly increasing the inhibition to the INs IN2 and IN4 (Fig. 5B). As a result, the peak-to-peak amplitude was reduced to about 3°. In both cases, the baseline of the small-amplitude oscillation lay at about 90°. In an earlier model with no slow muscle fibres [19], stationary states of the retraction position of the femur emerged when both (fast) protractor and (fast) retractor MNs were inhibited. This entailed that the forces in both the protractor and the retractor muscle vanished. In this way, a stationary position at $\alpha=102^o$ could be attained but the emerging stationary position was, in contrast to the present version of the model, prone to even small perturbations because of lack of stiffness in the muscles. Moreover, the stationary position in the earlier model heavily depended on the phase of the duty cycle in which the MN activity was stopped.

It is a quite important point to bear in mind that the diminution of the small amplitude to an almost negligible value was produced in the present model by the strong simultaneous activity of the slow MNs, hence by sustained co-contractions of the slow muscle fibres in agreement with the experimental results [12]. This mechanism turns out to be biologically more relevant and is in stark contrast to the behaviour of our previous model [19] in which the stationary position was due to the lack of muscle forces.

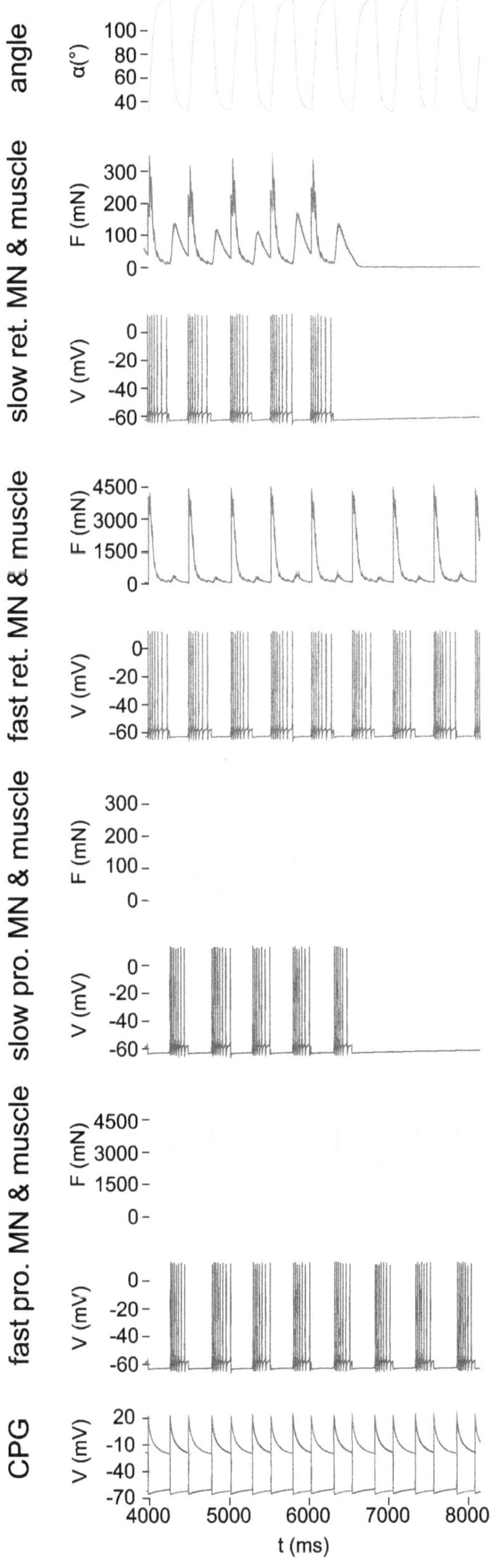

Figure 4. Angular movement and motoneuron and CPG activity in the protractor-retractor neuro-muscular system during forward stepping. The panels show the time evolution of the quantities indicated at the panels. Slow and fast relate to motoneurons and corresponding muscles they innervate. The small and wide peaks between the larger and narrower ones in the activity of the slow muscles are generated by the contraction of the antagonistic muscles (passive stretching). The colour code of the activity of the CPG neurons signalizes the association with the motoneuron type. Note that at $t = 6500ms$, the activity of the slow motoneurons was blocked.

When only one of the fast MNs was inhibited and the other kept on firing, the small-amplitude oscillation appeared near one of the extremal values of the angular movements after the onset of the MN inhibition. This is shown in Fig. 6, the inhibition starting at $t = 6500ms$ in the simulations. As indicated in Fig. 6, the column on the left comprises the cases when the fast protractor MN was inhibited, the other column those when the fast retractor MN underwent inhibition. Accordingly, the small-amplitude oscillation took place near to the extremal retraction and protraction angle, respectively. The peak-to-peak amplitude of the small-amplitude oscillation varied between 9° and 20° in the former case, and between 11° and 25° in the latter (Fig. 6). We see thus a certain asymmetry between the two cases. The minimum of the peak-to-peak amplitude of the small-amplitude oscillation was attained in both groups of cases when both slow MNs were strongly disinhibited ($g_d = 16nS$), (i.e. activated). When only one of the slow MNs were inhibited, the size of the amplitude of the small-amplitude oscillation depended on which of the slow MNs was inhibited. For example, in the left column of Fig. 6 (inhibition of the fast protractor MN), the peak-to-peak amplitude stayed close to its minimum (9°) when the slow protractor MN was strongly disinhibited, i.e. activated, (row 3 and 4 in the left column of Fig. 6). Otherwise, the peak-to-peak amplitude was close to that in the case when both slow MNs received normal activation (disinhibition) ($g_d = 1.6nS$). Analogously, the peak-to-peak amplitude of the small-amplitude oscillation was near to its minimum (11°) when the slow retractor MN was strongly activated (disinhibited) (row 2 and 3 in the right column of Fig. 6). It is an interesting property of our model that in both cases, the inhibition of the fast MN of a specific type and strong activation (disinhibition) of the *same* type of slow MN produced smaller amplitudes than when the slow MN of the antagonistic type was activated (disinhibited).

In summary, we found that the small-amplitude oscillation of the angle α driven by the slow MNs can be positioned near to one of the extremal angles if only one of the fast MNs is inhibited. Again, the peak-to-peak amplitude of this oscillation depends on the degree of activation (disinhibition) of the slow MNs.

Producing static protraction-retraction positions in the model by using recruitment of the muscle fibres

In the protractor-retractor muscle system, the pool of the protractor MNs consists of about 17, that of the retractor ones of about 25 MNs [20]. Hence our model assumptions concerning the recruitment of muscle fibres appear to be acceptable in this case. There are, however, no data on the proportion of MNs supplying fast or slow muscle fibres. We assumed that, in the model, there were equally many (10) fast and slow MNs in each MN pool. This allows a resolution of 0.1 of the recruitment levels (r_a and r_c in eqn. 3). Moreover, we chose $r_c = 0.7$ for both the protractor and retractor muscles (cf. Methods). That is, during stepping, 7, out of the 10 motor units, are assumed to be recruited, hence involved in producing muscle force in both of the antagonistic muscle pairs during stepping. We have made this assumption because it seems physiologically unreasonable that during normal locomotion, i.e. when the animal is not exposed to any additional load, only to its own weight, all muscle fibres would be recruited. On the other hand, during locomotion, the muscles of the legs move the mass of the whole body. One could therefore reckon with a substantial

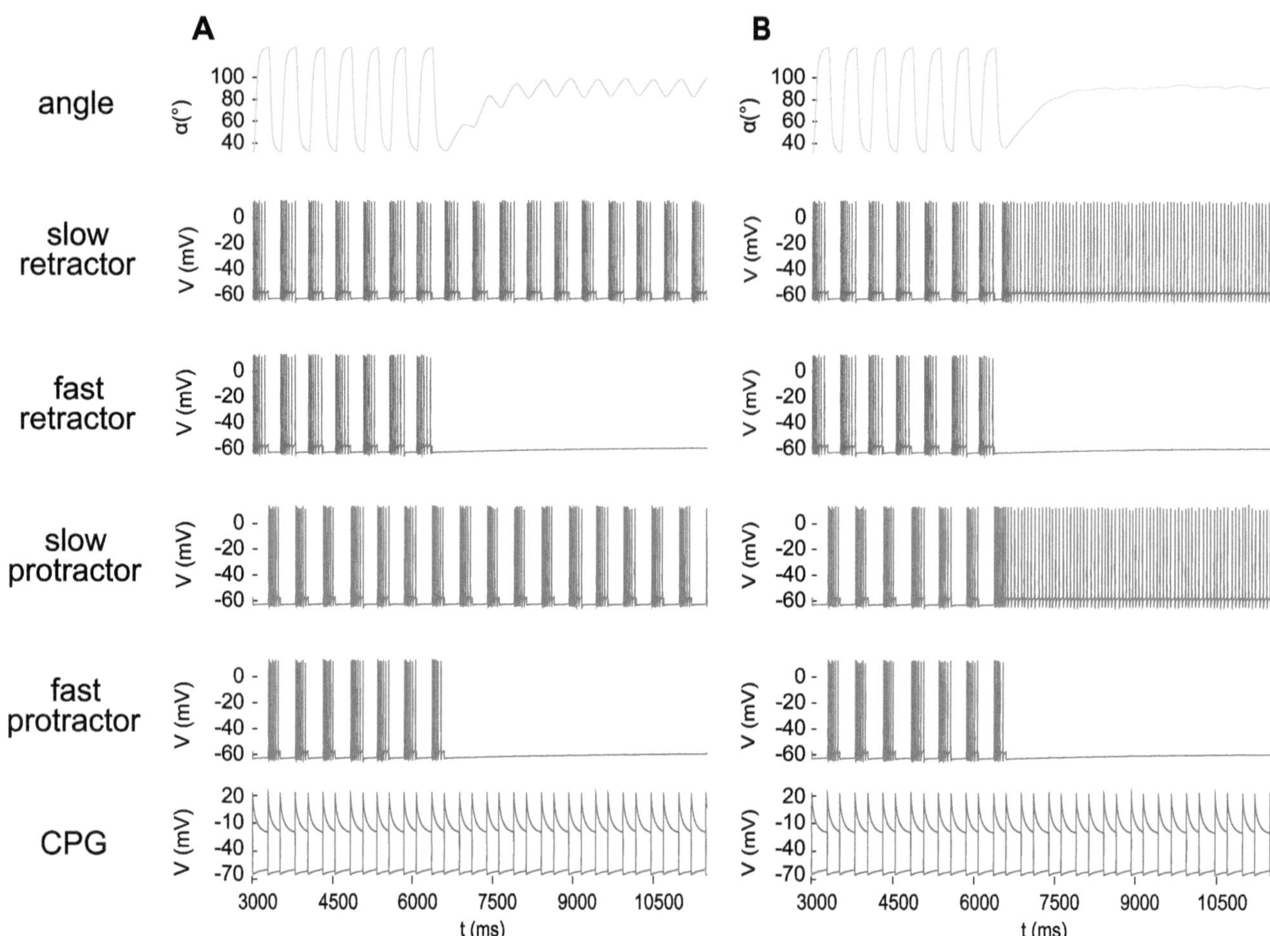

Figure 5. The effect of inhibition of the fast motoneurons. The angular movement and the neuronal activities displayed in the panels are the same as in Fig. 4. Inhibition was brought about in the model by reducing the value of both conductances g_{d1} and g_{d3} of the inhibitory currents to the interneurons IN1 and IN3, respectively (cf. Fig. 1), from $g_{d1}=g_{d3}=1.6nS$ to $1.0nS$ A: leaving the values of the conductances g_{d2} and g_{d4} at IN2 and IN4, respectively, unchanged at $g_{d2}=g_{d4}=1.6nS$ (no change to the input of the slow MNs); B: increasing the values of these conductances to $g_{d2}=g_{d4}=16.0nS$ (disinhibition of the slow MNs). Note the large difference in the amplitude of the oscillation after the onset (at $t=6500ms$) of the inhibition to the fast MNs.

degree of recruitment of muscle fibres in this condition. Investigations in the locust [21] showed that the locust does have "recruitment reserve" when horizontally walking, since at vertical climbing, additional protractor-retractor muscles are recruited. Hence, the control recruitment level of $r_c=0.7$ does not appear unrealistic.

Next we carried out simulations using various recruitment levels of the slow and fast muscle fibres in order to study the role muscle recruitment plays in shaping the mechanical movement of a limb. To be more precise, the fast MNs of both muscle types were first inhibited. Thus only the slow muscle fibres showed activity at a number of recruitment levels. We found that the relation between the recruitment levels in the antagonistic muscles determined the stationary retraction position of the femur. Fig. 7 illustrates this for a number of positions. Fig. 7A shows the results when only the recruitment level of muscle fibres in the slow protractor muscle was varied, but the recruitment level in the retractor muscle was kept at its control value ($r_a=r_c=0.7$). In Fig. 7B, the situation is analogous to that in Fig. 7A, only the roles of the muscles are exchanged. It can be seen that by suitable choices of the recruitment levels (r_a values) in the protractor and retractor muscles, a steady state at any angle α within the range $[30^o,128^o]$ can be attained within the error limits due to the finite (0.1) resolution of the muscle fibre recruitment. One can thus conclude that the slow antagonistic muscle fibres can be driven by the associated neuronal network so as to keep the femur in any desired steady-state position.

In another series of simulations, we aimed at emulating the transition from steady state to rhythmic stepping (locomotion) by using increasing recruitment in time of the fast muscle fibres, while the slow ones remained at their normal (control) recruitment level. Fig. 8 shows the results of these simulations. We considered three cases: very fast (instantaneous) (Fig. 8A), gradual (Fig. 8B), and partial restoration of the stepping movement (Fig. 8C). In the first case, the recruitment of both the fast protractor and retractor muscle fibres occurred very fast, implemented by a pulse (jump) time function (Fig. 8A), whereas in the second case, ramp time functions were used to control the actual level of recruitment of the fast muscle fibres (Fig. 8B). Note that although the fast, both protractor and retractor, muscle fibres had linearly increasing recruitment in time, the amplitude of the angular movement α of the femur was increasing nonlinearly (Fig. 8B). Finally, Fig. 8C shows a case of partial restoration of the protraction-retraction angular movement during stepping. Here, no recruitment of the

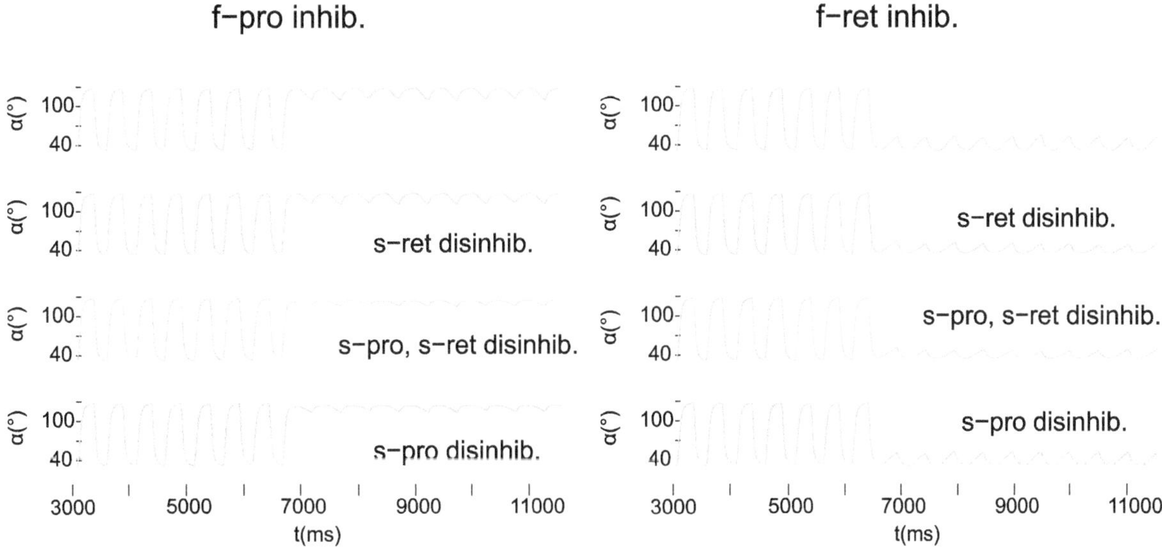

Figure 6. Selective inhibition of the fast motoneurons. Left column: only the fast protractor motoneuron is inhibited. Right column: only the fast retractor motoneuron is inhibited. In both columns: top panel: normal disinhibition of both slow motoneurons ($g_{d2} = g_{d4} = 1.6nS$); 2nd panel: strong disinhibition of the slow retractor motoneuron, only ($g_{d2} = 1.6nS$, $g_{d4} = 16.0nS$); 3rd panel: strong disinhibition of both slow motoneurons ($g_{d2} = g_{d4} = 16.0nS$); bottom panel: strong disinhibition of the slow protractor motoneuron, only ($g_{d2} = 16.0nS$, $g_{d4} = 1.6nS$). Note that the small-amplitude oscillation due to the activity of the slow motoneurons is positioned close to the extremal angle corresponding to the *uninhibited* fast motoneuron, e.g. to the maximal retraction position if only the fast retractor motoneuron remains active (left column).

fast retractor muscles took place, while the fast protractor ones were gradually recruited. As a result, the full range of the angular movement was not restored, and the angular oscillation remained near the extremal protraction position, and had a reduced peak-to-peak amplitude. A later recruitment of the fast retractor muscle fibres would have restored the full range of the angular movement during stepping (not illustrated).

Muscle forces during inhibition of the fast MNs

It is of considerable interest to find out what the acting muscle forces are during the small-amplitude oscillation, or in a nearly static state, when one or both fast MNs are inhibited. The muscle forces produced by the model in these conditions are shown in Fig. 9 together with the control case, i.e. when both slow and fast muscles are active.

In control conditions (i.e. during stepping), the antagonistic fast muscles contract alternately, with negligible co-contraction (Fig. 9A, top panel). In the slow muscles, co-contraction is discernible but the alternate contractions are still dominant (Fig. 9B, top panel). This situation is also depicted in Fig. 4, although in a different context. When both fast muscles are inhibited, the contraction forces of both fast muscles vanish in the model (Fig. 9A, second panel). The reason for this is that there is no explicit passive elastic component in our muscle model, hence

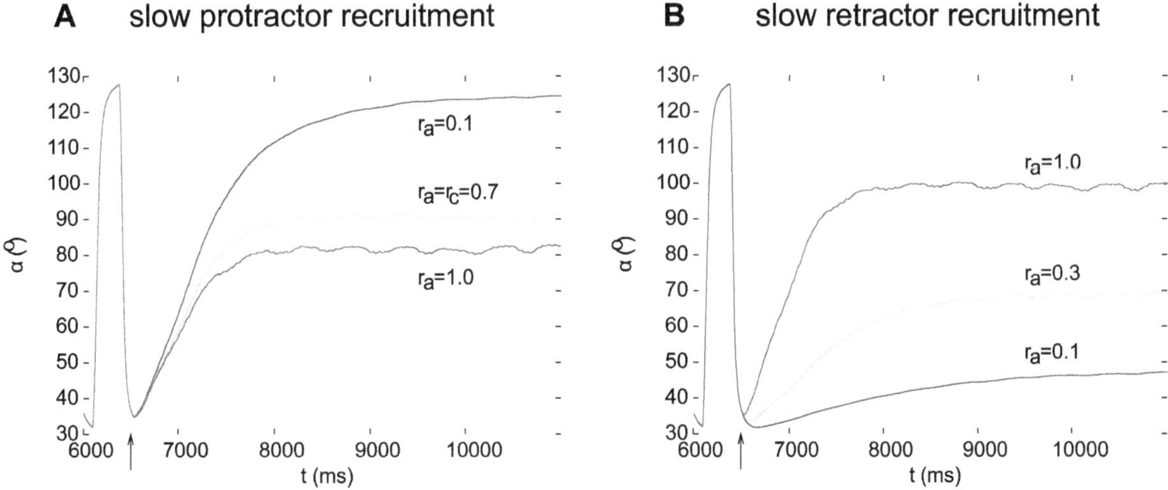

Figure 7. Steady states and recruitment levels. Different steady states are brought about by different recruitment levels of the slow muscle fibres in the protractor (A) or retractor (B) muscle. The actual recruitment levels are indicated in the panels next to the individual curves. All fast motoneurons were inhibited in these simulations. The arrows mark the start of the inhibition of the fast motoneurons ($t = 6500ms$).

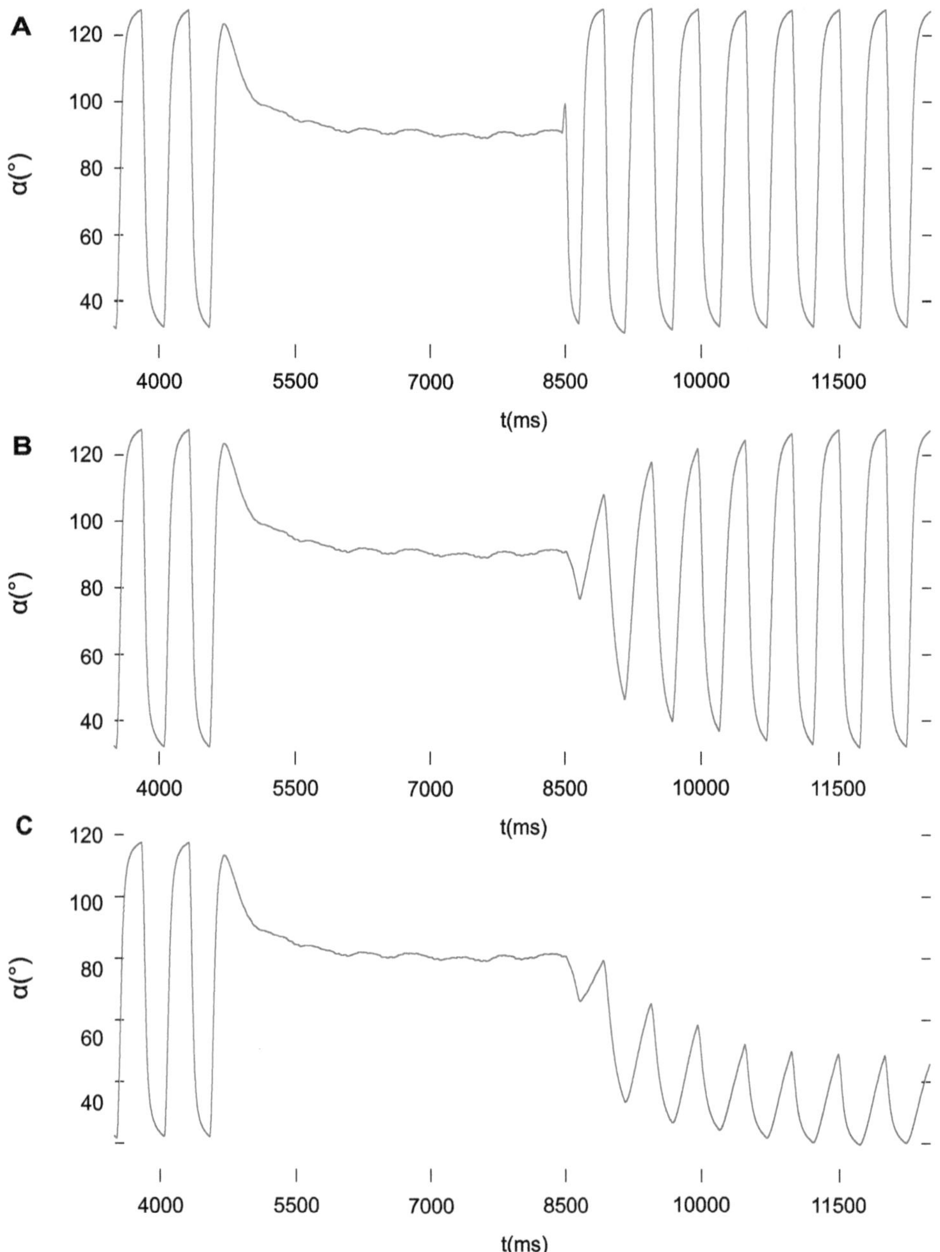

Figure 8. Restoring normal stepping from steady state (standing still). A: instantaneously, B: gradually, C: partially. At $t=4700ms$, the fast motoneurons are inhibited, and the slow ones disinhibited, hence the steady state. At the same time, the recruitment of the fast fibres decreases to virtually zero, whereas that of the slow ones remains unchanged. At $t=8460ms$, the inhibition of the fast motoneurons and the disinhibition of the slow motoneurons are stopped, and, in A and B, the recruitment of the fast protractor and retractor muscle fibres starts, while in C, only the fast protractor muscle fibres are recruited. The recruitment plays a crucial part in the restoration process. In case A, the recruitment of the fast fibres occurs very fast (instantaneously), while in the cases B and C, it does so linearly over a time interval of 3 s. Note, however, that in B, the increase of the amplitude of the angular movement α is nonlinear. In C, the full amplitude of the angular movement α is not restored, because the fast retractor muscle fibres are not recruited.

the variable elasticity modulus k eventually decays to zero if there is no drive from the MNs of an antagonistic muscle pair (see eqn.s 1 and 2). However, there are still antagonistic forces of the slow muscle fibres present (Fig. 9B, second panel). They are, in the present case, almost exactly equal, since the steady state is around $\alpha=90^o$, i.e. both types of slow muscle fibres are at their control level of recruitment ($r_c=0.7$). If only one of the fast muscles is inhibited, the other, the active one evokes co-contraction of the antagonistic fast muscle, even with no MN drive to the inhibited one (Fig. 9A, the two bottom panels). This apparent passive force arises because at the switch of direction of movement of the femur stationary conditions (vanishing angular velocity and acceleration) have to be fulfilled. These conditions impose constraints on the stationary values of the spring constants (k_∞ values in eqn. 1) of an antagonistic muscle pair (see Methods and, for a detailed

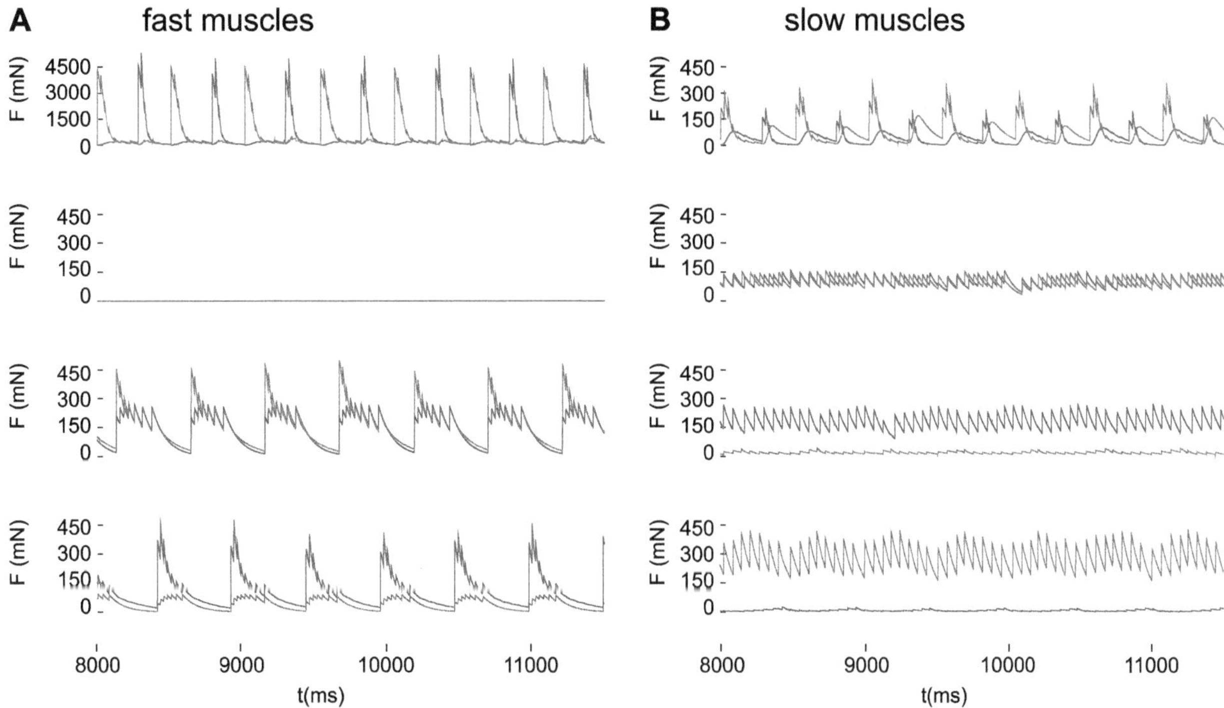

Figure 9. Muscle forces in control conditions and during inhibition of one or both fast motoneurons. A: forces in the fast protractor (red) and retractor (blue) muscles. B: forces in the slow protractor (red) and retractor (blue) muscles. Top row of panels: control condition when both the fast and the slow muscles are active; 2nd row of panels: both fast motoneurons are inhibited ($g_{d1} = g_{d3} = 1.0nS$); 3rd row of panels: only the fast protractor motoneuron is inhibited ($g_{d1} = 1.0nS$, $g_{d3} = 1.6nS$); bottom row of panels: only the fast retractor motoneuron is inhibited ($g_{d1} = 1.6nS$, $g_{d3} = 1.0nS$).

explanation, [14]). Hence, neither of the spring constants will be zero.

As for the slow muscles, the force in the slow muscle whose fast counterpart is inhibited is much larger than the force in its antagonistic counterpart, compensating for the lack of force in the corresponding fast muscle (Fig. 9B, the two bottom panels). For example, the bottom panels of Fig. 9 show the case when the fast retractor muscle is inhibited. Accordingly, the fast muscles show co-contraction, with the force of the retractor muscle (blue) being much smaller than that of the fast protractor muscle (red) (Fig. 9A, bottom panel). At the same time, the force of the slow retractor muscle (blue) is much larger than that of the slow protractor muscle (red) (Fig. 9B, bottom panel).

Discussion

In this study, we investigated, by means of a neuro-mechanical model, possible mechanisms that can produce and maintain steady-state positions of limb joints, as well as the transition between angular movements during stepping and the above positions. The mechanisms suggested can serve as elements of more complex neuro-muscular coordination which produces stable postures or aimed movements in animals, in our specific case, in the stick insect. The model we used is an extension of the one by [14] and includes separate slow and fast muscle fibres and their dedicated neuronal control network. One should, however, bear in mind that this is a strong simplification of the real situation. The separation between slow and fast muscle fibres is not as sharp in the animals as we implemented it in our model. Rather, experimental data indicate a gradual transition between fast and slow muscle fibres, i.e. a continuum of muscle properties [4,7]. We, for the sake of simplicity, 'discretized' this continuum by dividing the muscle fibres into just two groups of contrasting properties. In addition, we implemented the differential recruitment of muscle fibres. As far as we are aware of, this is the first model for insects that possesses such properties. Previous muscle models were more specialized. They either did not take the differing properties of the slow and fast muscle fibres into account, e.g. [22–25], or did not include the dedicated neuronal control network of the muscles [26,27]. They concentrated on producing specific muscle behaviour using certain aspects of the muscle function. In contrast, our integrated model enables us to study a more complex phenomenon: the functional differentiation between static and dynamic aspects of movement control.

We constructed this extended model only for the protractor-retractor neuro-muscular system as it plays an important part in maintaining posture, i.e. when an insect is standing still, or when the joint is fixed during sideward stepping. However, the same type of extension can be done, with some constraints due to the much fewer motor units, for the other neuro-muscular systems (joints), too. Indeed, a model that has fast and slow muscle fibres in each of the three pairs of main leg muscles complete with their neuronal control (MNs) will be introduced in the accompanying paper (Toth et al., unpublished results). Simulations with the extended model, presented in this paper, highlighted some model properties that might be of physiological relevance in insects, or, possibly in other animals, too. First of all, we found in the simulations that during (fast) stepping (also regarded as control conditions in this study), the fast muscles determine the stepping, more precisely, the protraction and retraction movement. The effect of the slow muscle fibres in this case is minute. Although there exists no direct experimental evidence for this simulation

Table 1. Locomotion status and motoneuron (MN) activity that produces it.

Locomotion status	MN type	
	fast	slow
normal stepping	+	(+)
small-amplitude oscillation	−	+
(near) steady state	−	++

"+": excited, "++": strongly excited (disinhibited), "(+)": activated but not effective, "−": inhibited.

Table 2. The physiological functions responsible for changing the attributes of the angular movement.

Angular movement	MN activity	Muscle recruitment
amplitude	fast	fast
average position	slow (+fast)	slow (+fast)
frequency	CPG	

Fast and slow relate to fast and slow muscle fibres or motoneurons (MNs), respectively. (+fast) means that additional activity of the fast muscle fibres (or MNs) substantially contributes to producing the average position of the protractor-retractor angle α during oscillation.

result, indirect evidence can be derived from [18], [12], and [17]. In [18], higher treadwheel velocities led to recruitment of fast MNs resulting in large depolarizations in the fast fibres of the stick insect's flexor tibiae muscle. Similarly, [12] showed that the fast MN of the extensor tibiae muscle of the stick insect produced much larger depolarizations in the muscle fibres it innervated than the slow MN driving the slow muscle fibres. In the experiments in [17], additional stimulation of the slow extensor MN (SETi) did not result in a discernible increase of the muscle force due to the activity of the fast extensor MN (FETi). The simulations further showed that when the MNs that innervate the fast muscle fibres (fast MNs) are inhibited but the slow MNs are not, the angular movement becomes a small-amplitude oscillation about the angle 90°. By further disinhibition (activation) of the slow MNs, the amplitude of this oscillation can be reduced to become negligible. However, the nearly steady state, too, represented by the small-amplitude oscillation in the model, has its experimental analogue: the extremities of a standing stick insect do not remain in a strictly static position but show slight rocking (oscillatory) movements [28]. This small-amplitude oscillation most likely occurs because the slow inherent contraction kinetics of the slow muscle fibres cannot cope with the relatively high frequency ($\approx 2Hz$) of the CPG that ultimately drives these fibres. Most importantly, [28] found that rocking was produced by the slow muscle fibres, only, and that the frequency of rocking was about $2Hz$. This is in excellent agreement with the properties of our model and the simulation results.

Taking, in addition, the gradual recruitment of the muscle fibres into account in the model, the steady state of the protractor-rectractor angle α can be set at any position within the angular range of $[30^o, 128^o]$. The simulation results produced by the model are in agreement with the important experimental finding that steady states are maintained by co-contraction of antagonistic (slow) muscle pairs, and not because of the lack of muscle forces [12,25]. Co-activation of the MNs driving the antagonistic slow muscles can improve the steady state, i.e. reduce the amplitude of the remaining small-amplitude oscillation to a negligible size. In Table 1, the locomotion status of a leg and the functional modes of the MNs that produce this status are summarized. Table 2, in turn, lists the physiological functions that shape the properties of the angular movement. Clearly, the frequency of the rhythmic angular movement (α) is determined by that of the CPG. The amplitude of the oscillation depends on whether the fast MNs are active at all, and if so, how many fast motor units are actually recruited (recruitment). The average position of the oscillation, or the static position is mainly determined by the activity of the slow MNs and the recruitment of the slow motor units but partial recruitment of the fast muscle fibres can also make a substantial contribution (cf. Fig. 6). Our model suggests that the steady-state position is more likely maintained by the recruitment ratio of the slow fibres in the antagonistic (protractor-retractor) muscle pair, than by the forces in the individual muscle fibres.

The transition between the angular movement during stepping and steady-state position could also be simulated by the model. Here, the time-dependent recruitment levels of the *fast* muscle fibres play a crucial part in the transition process. Depending on the dynamics of the recruitment changes, the transition can take different shapes. The movements simulated here can be regarded as elements of more complex movements of the limbs in which, of course, several joints will be involved [29–31]. In the accompanying paper (Toth et al., unpublished results), we shall present simulation results on the intra-leg coordination of the activities of the three main leg muscle pairs.

Our model provides information on the muscle forces that arise in different conditions (Fig. 9). While in the majority of conditions, the size of the forces in the slow and fast muscle fibres seem to be reasonable, the forces generated by the fast muscle fibres of the model in control conditions (normal stepping) appear to be somewhat too large. Since there do not exist direct force measurements in the protractor or retractor muscles, it is hard to judge the possible error occurring in the model in this condition. However, when we applied the same muscle model, with suitable numerical values of the parameters to the extensor and flexor muscles, in which force measurement were made [17], we found comparable muscle forces in experiment and simulation (data not shown).

Irrespective of this problem, our model makes interesting predictions with regard to the muscle forces arising in various conditions, e.g. during stepping, or in (near) steady state. The model predicts that during stepping, the alternate contraction of the antagonistic muscles, protractor and retractor, is dominant in both the fast and the slow muscle fibres. These forces are generated by the excitatory drive by the corresponding MNs. In (near) steady state, however, when the fast MNs are inhibited, only the slow muscle fibres stay active, the fast ones do not contribute to the total muscle force. The forces in the slow muscle fibres are generated actively by the excitatory drive, occasional co-activation, of the slow MNs. There is some experimental evidence, although in the extensor tibiae muscle of the stick insect [7,12], that fast muscle fibres do not develop substantial force during steady state and it is the slow muscle fibres that maintain this state. It is also predicted by the model that when only either the fast protractor or fast retractor muscle fibres are inhibited, co-contraction becomes dominant in the fast muscle fibres. The contraction in the fast muscle fibres that do not receive MN activity is due to the nonlinear elasticity of the muscle represented by the, in this case, non-vanishing spring constant that produces an apparently passive component of the muscle function. The slow muscle fibres will perform co-contractions, only if their respective MNs are co-activated. The force in those slow muscle fibres whose fast counterparts are inhibited (e.g. retractor in the bottom panel of Fig. 9B) is now much larger than in the antagonistic slow fibres. Thus the force produced by the slow fibres, to some extent, compensates for the lack of force in the corresponding fast fibres.

Some of these properties can be deduced from the way our muscle model has been constructed. Contrary to some other muscle models (e.g. [22–25]), it does not have passive elastic elements. The variable spring constants will therefore tend to zero, if *neither* of the antagonistic muscles receives any excitatory signals from their corresponding MN. However, if one of the muscles receives electrical excitation from its MN, *neither* of the spring constants will vanish. This seems reasonable, since the active muscle, with MN driving, stretches its antagonist evoking elastic contraction force in it. Thus our muscle model is capable of producing apparently passive (elastic) contraction force in the muscle with no MN drive. The underlying property of the model which results in this behaviour is that the spring constants of the antagonistic muscles are not independent of each other. They are subject to a constraint that arises from the switch conditions from protraction to retraction and *vice versa* (cf. Methods and Results and [14]). But note that the muscle fibres in our model do not possess residual stiffness.

Closely related to this fact is that our neuro-muscular model does not include the common inhibitor MNs, either. Slow muscle fibres, but no fast ones, are innervated by them in the stick insect and locust [7,12] and also in the cockroach [32]. Their physiological role is to remove the residual stiffness of the slow muscle fibres during locomotion (stepping) in order to improve the dynamics of the movement [12,33–35]. The common inhibitory MN CI1 acts on all main leg muscles, except for the m. flexor tibiae, which receives input from the inhibitory MNs CI2 and CI3. We omitted the common inhibitory MNs from the present model, comprising one single antagonistic muscle pair, for the sake of simplicity. CI1 (and CI2–CI3), and the residual stiffness of the slow muscle fibres will become quite important when we deal with intra-leg coordination of the activities of the three pairs of antagonistic leg muscles (cf. accompanying paper, Toth et al., unpublished results).

Our simulation results highlight the differing roles of the fast and slow muscles during locomotion and maintaining body posture. They receive support from experimental findings. [7] showed the spatial separation of slow and fast muscle fibres in the extensor muscle. Here, however, it should again be remembered that the strict classification into slow and fast muscle fibres is a simplification in the model. Even though there are no direct data from the protractor-retractor muscles, we would assume to find a similar situation there, as well. Furthermore, [12] found differing functions of the slow and fast muscle fibres in the stick insect's extensor muscle similar to those observed in the simulations. Again, these experimental findings relate to the extensor muscle but there is recent evidence [13] that slow and fast muscle fibres do exist in both the protractor and the retractor muscle of the stick insect. We suggest that they share functional roles similar to those in the extensor muscle as observed in the experiments [12], and to those produced by the simulations with the extended neuro-muscular model. As a general tool, selective blockade or (partial) elimination of the fast or slow muscle fibres from the protractor or rectractor muscle in experiments could help test the predictions of our model.

Author Contributions

Conceived and designed the experiments: TT SD-G. Performed the experiments: TT SD-G. Analyzed the data: TT JS SD-G. Contributed reagents/materials/analysis tools: AB SD-G. Wrote the paper: TT JS AB SD-G.

References

1. Schmidt-Nielsen K (1997) Animal Physiology. Cambridge (UK): Cambridge University Press. 607 p.
2. Monti RJ, Roy RR, Edgerton VR (2001) Role of motor unit structure in defining function. Muscle Nerve 24: 848–866.
3. Hoyle G (1978) Distribution of nerve and muscle fibre types in locust jumping muscle. J Exp Biol 78: 205–233.
4. Rathmayer W, Maier L (1987) Muscle fiber types in crabs: Studies on single identified muscle fibers. Am Zool 27: 1067–1077.
5. Rathmayer W, Hammelbeck M (1985) Identified muscle fibres in a crab. Differences in facilitation properties. J Exp Biol 116: 291–300.
6. Müller AR, Wolf H, Galler S, Rathmayer W (1992) Correlation of electrophysiological, histochemical, and mechanical properties in fibres of the coxa rotator muscle of the locust, Locusta migratoria. J Comp Physiol B 162: 5–15.
7. Bässler D, Büschges A, Meditz S, Bässler U (1996) Correlation between muscle structure and filter characteristics of the muscle-joint system in three orthopteran insect species. J Exp Biol 199: 2169–2183.
8. Henneman E, Somjen G, Carpenter DO (1965) Functional significance of cell size in spinal motoneurons. J Neurophysiol 28: 560–580.
9. Henneman E, Somjen G, Carpenter DO (1965) Excitability and inhibitability of motoneurons of different sizes. J Neurophysiol 28: 599–620.
10. Powers RK, Binder MD (2001) Input-output functions of mammalian motoneurons. Rev Physiol Biochem Pharmacol 143: 137–263.
11. Kernell D (2003) Principles of force generation in skeletal muscles. Neural Plasticity 10: 69–76.
12. Bässler U, Stein W (1996) Contributions of structure and innervation pattern of the stick insect extensor tibiae muscle to the filter characteristics of the muscle-joint system. J Exp Biol 199: 2185–2198.
13. Godlewska E (2012) The histochemical characterization of muscle fiber types in an insect leg. Master Thesis, University of Cologne, Germany.
14. Tóth TI, Knops S, Gruhn S (2012) A neuro-mechanical model explaining forward and backward stepping in the stick insect. J Neurophysiol 107: 3267–3280.
15. Hodgkin AL, Huxley AF (1952) A quantitative description of membrane current and its application to conduction and excitation in nerve. J Physiol 117: 500–544.
16. Hill AV (1953) The mechanics of active muscle. Proc Roy Soc Lond (Biol), 141: 104–117.
17. Guschlbauer Ch, Scharstein H, Büschges A (2007) The extensor tibiae muscle of the stick insect: biomechanical properties of an insect walking leg muscle. J Exp Biol 210: 1092–1108.
18. Gabriel JP, Scharstein H, Schmidt J, Büschges A (2003) Control of flexor motoneuron activity during single leg walking of the stick insect on an electronically controlled treadwheel. J Neurobiol 56: 237–251.
19. Knops S, Tóth TI, Guschlbauer C, Gruhn M, Daun-Gruhn S (2013) A neuro-mechanical model for the neuronal basis of curve walking in the stick insect. J Neurophysiol 109: 679–691.
20. Goldammer J, Büschges A, Schmidt J (2012) Motoneurons, DUM cells, and sensory neurons in an insect thoracic ganglion: a tracing study in the stick insect carausius morosus. J Comp Neurology 520: 230–257.
21. Duch J, Pflüger H-J (1995) Motor patterns for horizontal and upside-down walking and vertical climbing in the locust. J Exp Biol 198: 1963–1978.
22. Blümel M, Hooper SL, Guschlbauer C, White WE, Büschges A (2012a) Determining all parameters necessary to build Hill-type muscle models from experiments on single muscles. Biol Cybern 106: 543–558.

23. Blümel M, Guschlbauer C, Gruhn S, Hooper SL, Büschges A (2012b) Hill-type muscle model parameters determined from experiments on single muscle show large animal-to-animal variation. Biol Cybern 106: 559–571.
24. Blümel M, Guschlbauer C, Hooper SL, Büschges A (2012c) Using individual-muscle specific instead of across-muscle mean data halves muscle simulation error. Biol Cybern 106: 573–585.
25. Zakotnik J, Matheson T, Dürr V (2006) Co-contraction and passive forces facilitate load compensation of aimed limb movements. J Neurosci 26: 4995–5007.
26. Wilson E, Rustighi E, Mace BR, Newland PR (2011) Modelling the isometric force response to multiple pulse stimuli in locust skeletal muscle. Biol Cybern 104: 121–136.
27. Wilson E, Rustighi E, Newland PR, Mace BR (2011) Slow motor neuron stimulation of locust skeletal muscle: model and measurement. Biomech Model Mechanobiol DOI 10.1007/s10237- 012-0427-2
28. Pflüger H-J (1977) The control of rocking movements of the phasmid Carausius morosus Br. J Comp Physiol A 120: 181–202.
29. Bässler U, Rohrbacher J, Karg G, Breutel G (1991) Interruption of searching movements of partly restrained front legs of stick insects, a model situation for the start of a stance phase? Biol Cybern 65: 507–514.
30. Berg E, Büschges A, Schmidt J (2013) Single perturbations cause sustained changes in searching behavior in stick insects. J Exp Biol 216: 1064–1074.
31. Karg G, Breutel G, Bässler U (1991) Sensory influences on the coordination of two leg joints during searching movements of stick insects. Biol Cybern 64: 329–335.
32. Pearson KG, Iles JF (1971) Innervation of coxal depressor muscles in the cockroach, *periplaneta americana*. J Exp Biol 54: 215–232.
33. Ballantyne D, RathmayerW(1981) On the function of the common inhibitory neuron in walking legs of the crab, *eriphia spinifrons*. J Comp Physiol A 143: 111–122.
34. Wolf H (1990) Activity patterns of inhibitory motoneurones and their impact on leg movement in tethered walking locusts. J Exp Biol 152: 281–304.
35. Iles JF, Pearson KG (1971) Coxal depressor muscles of the cockroach and the role of peripheral inhibition. J Exp Biol 55: 151–164.

11

Impaired Adaptive Response to Mechanical Overloading in Dystrophic Skeletal Muscle

Pierre Joanne[1], Christophe Hourdé[2], Julien Ochala[3], Yvain Caudéran[2], Fadia Medja[2], Alban Vignaud[2], Etienne Mouisel[2], Wahiba Hadj-Said[2], Ludovic Arandel[2], Luis Garcia[2], Aurélie Goyenvalle[2], Rémi Mounier[4], Daria Zibroba[5], Kei Sakamato[5], Gillian Butler-Browne[2], Onnik Agbulut[1], Arnaud Ferry[2,6]*

1 Université Paris Diderot, Sorbonne Paris Cité, CNRS EAC4413, Unit of Functional and Adaptive Biology, Laboratory of Stress and Pathologies of the Cytoskeleton, Paris, France, **2** Université Pierre et Marie Curie-Paris6, Sorbonne Universités, UMR S794, INSERM U974, CNRS UMR7215, Institut de Myologie, Paris, France, **3** Department of Neuroscience, Uppsala University, Uppsala, Sweden, **4** Université Paris Descartes, Sorbonne Paris Cité, INSERM U1016, CNRS UMR8104, Institut Cochin, Paris, France, **5** MRC Protein Phosphorylation Unit, College of Life Sciences, University of Dundee, Dundee, United Kingdom, **6** Université Paris Descartes, Sorbonne Paris Cité, Paris, France

Abstract

Dystrophin contributes to force transmission and has a protein-scaffolding role for a variety of signaling complexes in skeletal muscle. In the present study, we tested the hypothesis that the muscle adaptive response following mechanical overloading (ML) would be decreased in MDX dystrophic muscle lacking dystrophin. We found that the gains in muscle maximal force production and fatigue resistance in response to ML were both reduced in MDX mice as compared to healthy mice. MDX muscle also exhibited decreased cellular and molecular muscle remodeling (hypertrophy and promotion of slower/oxidative fiber type) in response to ML, and altered intracellular signalings involved in muscle growth and maintenance (mTOR, myostatin, follistatin, AMPKα1, REDD1, atrogin-1, Bnip3). Moreover, dystrophin rescue via exon skipping restored the adaptive response to ML. Therefore our results demonstrate that the adaptive response in response to ML is impaired in dystrophic MDX muscle, most likely because of the dystrophin crucial role.

Editor: Daniel Tomé, Paris Institute of Technology for Life, Food and Environmental Sciences, France

Funding: Financial support has been provided by Université Pierre et Marie Curie (UPMC), CNRS, INSERM, Université Paris Descartes, ANR-Genopath In-A-Fib, ANR-Blanc Androgluco, the Association Française contre les Myopathies (AFM), MyoAge (EC 7th FP, contract 223576), and Agence Française de Lutte contre le Dopage. The funders had no role in study design, data collection and analysis, decision to publish, or preparation of the manuscript.

Competing Interests: The authors have declared that no competing interests exist.

* E-mail: arnaud.ferry@upmc.fr

Introduction

Skeletal muscle exhibits a crucial capacity to adapt to changing use. In response to repeated high-force contractions, i.e., mechanical overloading (ML), both absolute maximal force production and fatigue resistance of the muscle markedly increase. Tension, stretch and deformation generated during ML, together with other activity-related signals (*e.g.* muscle action potential, metabolites…), are sensed and in turn activate different intracellular signaling pathways that converge to induce muscle cellular and molecular adaptations, such as hypertrophy and fiber-type conversion, resulting in muscle performance improvement [1,2,3,4,5].

The gain in absolute maximal force induced by ML is, at least partly, attributed to muscle hypertrophy, since absolute maximal force is roughly proportional to muscle cross-sectional area. Muscle hypertrophy in response to ML results from increased protein synthesis via activation of the mammalian target of rapamycin (mTOR) signaling pathway [6,7]. More precisely, it is the mTOR complex-1 (mTORC1) that contains mTOR and the rapamycin-sensitive raptor subunit that promotes protein synthesis via the phosphorylation of the initiation factor-4E binding protein-1 and the S6 kinase (S6K) that in turn phosphorylates at the S240/244 site the ribosomal S6 protein (rS6)[1,2]. Akt is also activated by ML [6] and it is known that genetic activation of Akt promotes muscle hypertrophy [8,9]. Recently, we demonstrated that the alpha-1 isoform of the AMP-activated protein kinase (AMPK-α 1) plays an important role in limiting muscle growth during ML, via the reduced activation of mTOR signaling [10]. In addition, it has been shown that myostatin is down-regulated in response to ML [11]. Since myostatin deactivates mTOR [12,13,14], these results suggest that together with AMPK, myostatin also limits muscle hypertrophy induced by ML. In addition, the myostatin inhibitor follistatin [15] and the stress response genes REDD1 and REDD2 (regulated in development and DNA damage response)[1,16] are possibly involved in the control of mTOR signaling in response to ML. Of note, the activation of the mitogen-activated protein kinase pathway (MAPK) may be not sufficient to induce muscle growth [17,18] and a recent study reported that satellite cells are not necessary for a robust ML-induced hypertrophy [19].

The fast/glycolytic -to slow/oxidative fiber conversion is likely the cellular and molecular adaptation responsible for the increase in fatigue resistance induced by ML. Indeed, it is well established that slow/oxidative fibers expressing type-1 and -2a myosin heavy chain (MHC-1 and MHC-2a) are more fatigue-resistant than fast/glycolytic fibers expressing MHC-2x and MHC-2b [20]. Calcineurin/NFAT signaling is a key player in the promotion of the slow/oxidative fiber phenotype [3,21]. Pharmacological inhibition or genetic loss of calcineurin blocks the fast/glycolytic -to slow/oxidative fiber-type conversion induced by ML [22,23,24]. The peroxisome proliferator-activated receptor γ coactivator-1 (PGC-

1), peroxisome proliferator-activated receptor (PPAR) and AMPK signaling pathways have also been proposed to promote the formation of slow/oxidative fibers [3,5,21,25].

Dystrophin, a costameric protein, is known to operate as a physical link between the actin cytoskeleton and laminin in the extracellular matrix, allowing likely the force to be transmitted outside of the cell and vice-versa [26]. This is supported by the findings that in the MDX mice that lacks dystrophin, muscle specific maximal force (force adjusted to muscle size) production is reduced [27] whereas exon skipping-mediated dystrophin rescue improves it [28]. Thus, force transmission with the participation of dystrophin possibly contributes to the sensing of the tension/deformation. Dystrophin may be also required for the membrane localization and function of certain components of signaling pathways (e.g. mechanoreceptor, dihydropyridine receptor, nNOS) acting in muscle growth and maintenance [29,30,31,32,33]. Several studies support this hypothesis by showing aberrant activation of Akt and mTOR, calcineurin, and MAPK pathways in the MDX mice [34,35,36,37,38]. Together these results suggest that dystrophin may contribute to the mechanotransduction and other activity-signaling pathways mediating muscle adaptations in response to ML.

The general aim of this study was to determine the adaptive response to ML of skeletal muscle from MDX mice, a murine model of Duchenne muscular dystrophy (DMD) causing severe muscle weakness for yet not fully understood reasons. We studied the effect of ML on MDX dystrophic muscle performance (maximal force production, fatigue resistance) and cellular and molecular remodeling (hypertrophy, fiber-type conversion…). ML was induced by surgical removal of the synergic muscles of the plantaris hindlimb muscle, a well-established rodent model [6,7,10,19,22,23,24,39,40,41,42,43]. More specifically, we tested the hypothesis that the muscle adaptive response following ML would be decreased in MDX mice as compared to healthy mice. We also determined whether dystrophin rescue via exon skipping would restore dystrophic muscle adaptations to ML. To our knowledge, this has not yet been studied.

Results

Reduced gain in muscle performance: maximal force

In situ plantaris muscle force production in response to nerve stimulation showed important changes 2 months after ML. The muscle absolute maximal force in MDX mice with mechanical loading (MDX+ML) and C57+ML mice were markedly increased as compared to MDX mice and C57 mice (Figure 1a). However, muscle absolute maximal force in MDX+ML mice was lower as compared to C57+ML mice, indicating that the increase in muscle absolute maximal force is lower in MDX+ML mice (+40%) as compared to C57+ML mice (+204%) mice. This difference between the 2 strains of mice was first explained by the reduced increase in muscle weight in response to 2-month ML in MDX+ML mice (+24%) as compared to C57+ML mice (+80%) mice (Figure 1b). The fact that in contrast to C57+ML mice, muscle specific maximal force was not increased in MDX+ML mice in response to 2 months of ML (Figure 1c) was also responsible for the smaller increase in muscle absolute maximal force in MDX+ML mice.

To test the possibility that a defect in the contractile machinery (myofilaments) could be directly responsible for the maintained muscle specific maximal force observed in the MDX+ML mice, we also determined the force generation of plantaris skinned muscle fibers in response to maximal activation by calcium 2 months after ML. Data obtained from skinned fibers expressing MHC-2b and MHC-2x were pooled since no difference was observed between these 2 types of fibers. We found that fiber specific maximal force of MDX+ML mice was reduced when compared to MDX mice (−18%) whereas that of C57+ML mice did not change following ML (Figure 1d).

We also observed an increased fibrosis (decreased concentration of contractile material) in the MDX mice in response to 2 month-ML as shown with Sirius red staining (Figures 2a and 2b), which may partly explain the deficit in muscle specific maximal force observed in MDX+ML. Regenerating fibers were recently reported following ML [19,54] and are thought to produce less specific maximal force than mature fibers. Therefore, we checked the possibility that ML induced a greater increase in the number of regenerating fibers in MDX+ML mice as compared to C57+ML mice. These regenerating fibers would consequently have a greater contribution to force production in the MDX+ML mice. Nuclei and laminin were stained to count the number of regenerating/regenerated fibers that contain one or more centronuclei 2 months after ML. However, in contrast to C57+ML mice, we observed that there was no increase in the percentage of centronucleated fibers in response to ML in MDX+ML (Figure 2c). No notable expression of neonatal or embryonic MHC was found in both strains 2 months after ML (data not shown), indicating that these centronucleated fibers were regenerated. Since the fast muscle fibers expressing MHC-2b could produce a higher specific maximal force, we tested the possibility that ML reduced more efficiently the percentage of fast fibers in MDX+ML mice as compared to C57+ML mice. However, in contrast to C57+ML mice, immunostaining for MHC isoform revealed that the percentage of fibers expressing MHC-2b did not decrease in MDX+ML mice in response to 2 months ML (Figure 2d). It should ne noted that a substantial number of these fibers co-expressed MHC-2x. Unfortunately, it was not possible to distinguish pure and hybrid fibers expressing MHC-2b.

Reduced gain in muscle performance: fatigue resistance

Together with the increase in absolute maximal force production, muscles from both MDX+ML mice and C57+ML mice improved their fatigue resistance in response to 2-month ML (Figure 1e). However, the improvement in muscle fatigue resistance was less marked in MDX+ML mice (+36%) as compared to C57+ML mice (+85%). The fact that in contrast to C57+ML mice the percentage of fibers expressing MHC-2b (less fatigue resistant fibers) did not decrease in MDX+ML mice (Figure 2d) might be responsible for this difference. Since the calcineurin/NFAT, PGC-1, and PPAR signaling pathways promote the formation of slow/oxidative/fatigue-resistant fibers [3], we further analysed these pathways 7 days after ML [41] to test the possibility that they are less activated in MDX+ML mice. We found that the transcript levels of NFATc1a, PGC1α1a and PPARß were globally reduced by ML in both mice strains (Figure S1a–c).

Fiber atrophy and altered catabolic processes

To further analyze the reduced muscle hypertrophy in MDX+ML mice in response to ML, we counted the fiber number observed in a muscle cross-section, using laminin labeling 2 months after ML. We found that in response to ML, the fiber number increased in both MDX+ML mice and C57 +ML mice, with no notable difference between the two mice strains (+71% versus + 84%)(Figure 3a). In contrast to C57+ML mice, MDX+ML mice increased the number of fibers expressing MHC-2b and did not change those expressing MHC-2x (Figure 3b). In both strains however, the number of fibers expressing MHC-2a or MHC-1 increased (Figure 3b).

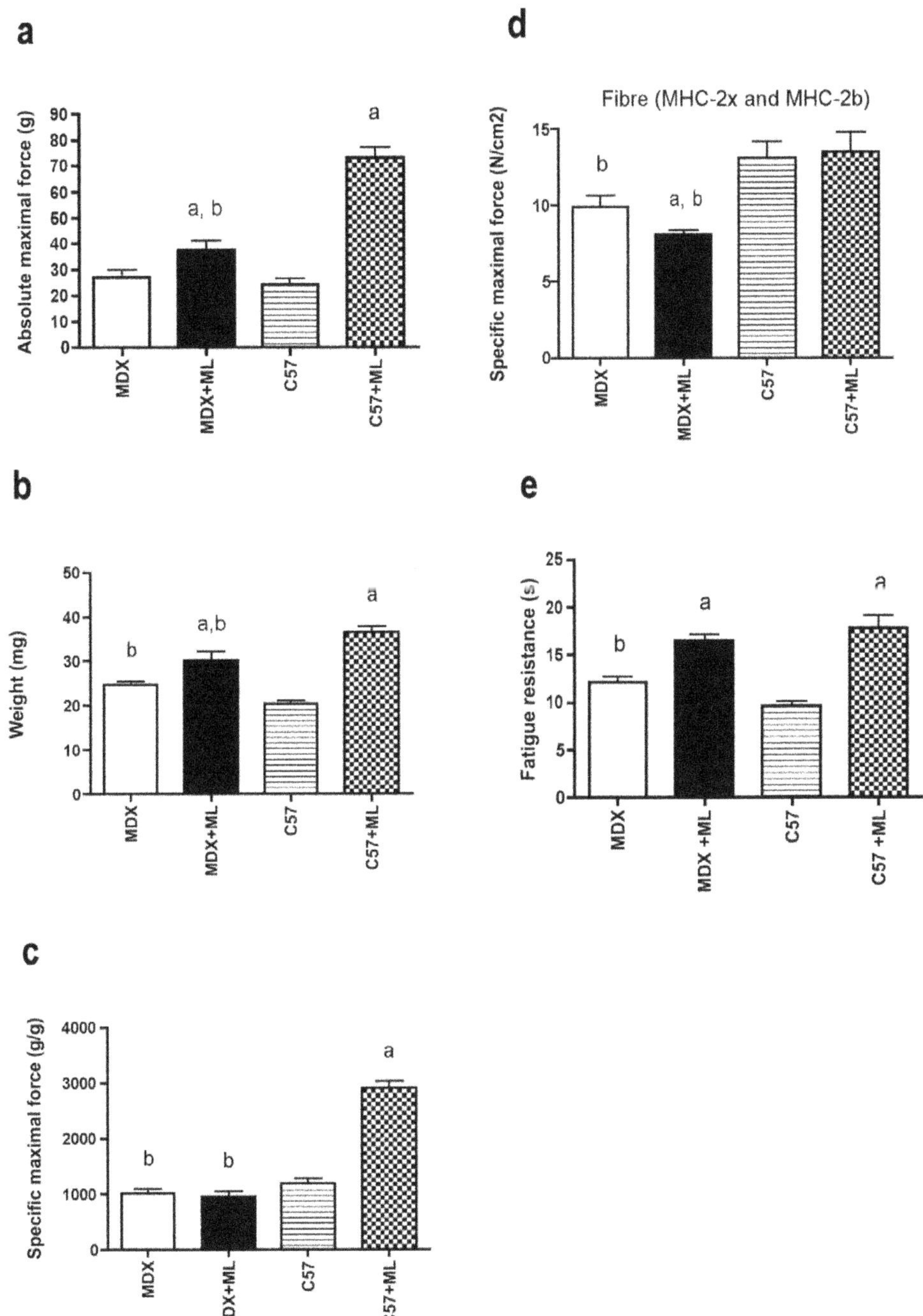

Figure 1. Reduced muscle performance gain and hypertrophy and decrease in contractile machinery function following 2 month-ML in MDX mice. Absolute muscle maximal force (a), muscle weight (b), muscle specific maximal force (c), specific maximal force of skinned muscle fibers (d), and muscle fatigue resistance (e) after 2 months of ML. a: significantly different from unoverloaded muscle ($p<0.05$). b: significantly different from corresponding C57 mice ($p<0.05$). n = 14–26/group for absolute and specific muscle maximal forces and n = 30/group (at least 7 per animal) for specific maximal force skinned fibers.

Moreover, we examined the size (diameter) of the fibers 2 months after ML to confirm that the reduced muscle hypertrophy in MDX+ML mice resulted from a smaller fiber diameter in MDX+ML mice. This was in fact the case since the mean diameter of fibers in MDX+ML mice was reduced by ML (Figure 3c). However, this was not explained by a smaller percentage of large diameter fibers expressing MHC-2b (Figure 3d), but by the diameter of the fibers expressing MHC-2b or MHC-2a that was reduced by ML in MDX+ML mice (Figures 3d–e).

Together with the anabolic processes (regulated by the mTOR pathway, see below), the catabolic processes control muscle size. Thus, we addressed the role of catabolic processes in the reduced muscle hypertrophy (reduced diameter of the fibers) induced by ML in MDX mice. We studied the ubiquitin-proteasomal pathway responsible for the myofibrillar muscle protein degradation, possibly

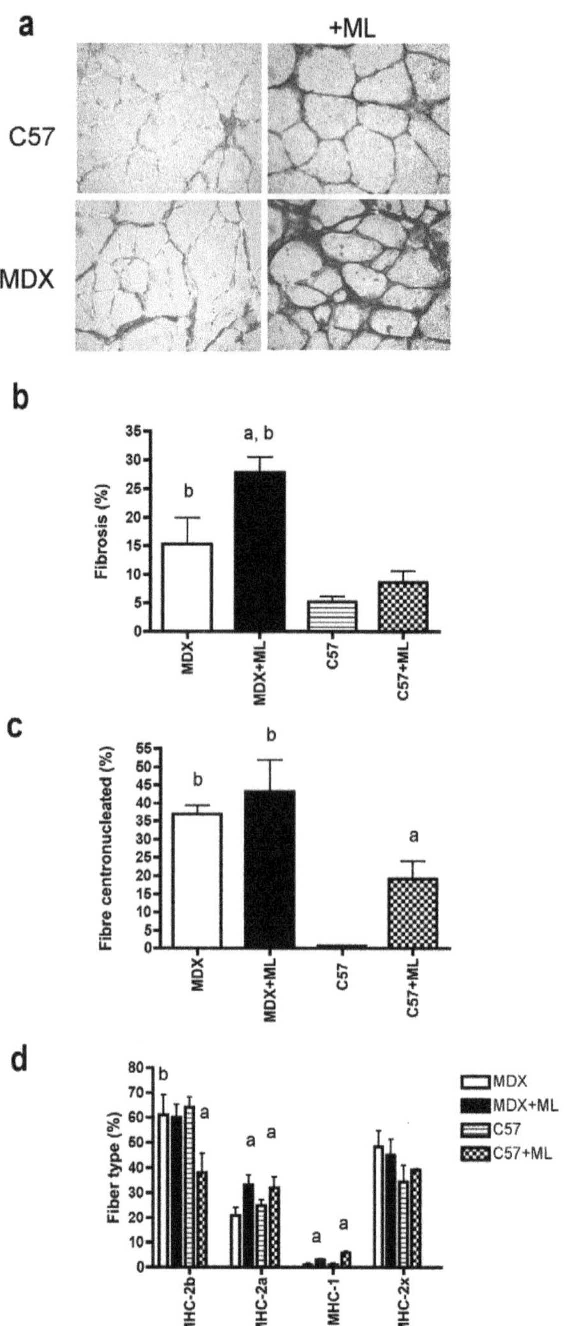

Figure 2. Muscle histology following 2 month-ML in MDX mice. Fibrosis (a and b), percentage of centronucleated muscle fibers (c) and percentage of the different types of muscle fibers (d) after 2 months of ML. Representative images of fibrosis (red) on Sirius red staining cross-section (a) shown increased fibrosis in MDX and MDX+ML mice. Of note, since muscle fiber can express more than one MHC, the total percentage of the different muscle fiber types added up to well over 100%. n = 3–4/group for fibrosis and n = 5–8 for percentage of fibers. a: significantly different from unoverloaded muscle ($p<0.05$). b: significantly different from corresponding C57 mice ($p<0.05$).

more activated in MDX+ML as compared to C57+ML. This pathway is negatively controlled via a set of E3 ligase-encoding genes, such as atrogin-1 [55]. Atrogin-1 mRNA decreased globally less in response to ML in MDX+ML than in C57+ML mice (Figure S2a). Autophagy, involving a battery of genes such as LC3 and Bnip3, also plays an important role in the degradation of muscle proteins [55]. We found that LC3 mRNA similarly decreased in MDX+ML and C57+ML mice (at day 7 respectively –31% versus -33%)(Figure S2b). However Bnip3 mRNA decreased to a somewhat lesser extent in MDX+ML as compared to C57+ML (−63% versus −82% at day 7)(Figure S2c).

Altered anabolic signaling pathways

To determine whether the reduced hypertrophy in response to ML in MDX+ML mice is also caused by a lower activation of mTOR signaling, we measured the phosphorylation level of the key downstream effector of mTOR, rS6, after 7 days of ML [10,41,56]. We found a smaller increase in rS6 phosphorylation in MDX+ML mice (+360%) as compared to C57+ML mice (+796%)(Figures 4a–b). Of note the level of rS6 phosphorylation was lower in MDX+ML mice than in C57+ML mice. In line with this finding, we also observed that ML caused Akt phosphorylation to a reduced extent in MDX+ML mice (+88%) than in C57+ML mice (+198%)(Figure 4c).

We measured the AMPKα1 activity at day 7 [10,41] to test the hypothesis that the reduced mTOR activation was due to hyper-activation of AMPKα1 activity. We found that AMPKα1 activity was increased in a similar way in MDX+ML mice (+1,141%) and C57+ML mice (+1,006%) 7 days after ML; however AMPKα1 activity was higher in MDX+ML mice as compared to C57+ML mice (Figure 4d).

We also determined whether there was a smaller reduction in myostatin expression, a mTOR deactivator, in MDX+ML mice in response to ML as compared to C57+ML mice at day 7. We observed that the level of myostatin mRNA decreased less in the MDX+ML mice in response to ML (−74%) than in the C57+ML mice (−93%)(Figure 4e). Follistatin is known to antagonize myostatin, to be regulated by mTOR and to play an important role as a myoblast fusion/growth promoting factor [15]. We found that the increase in follistatin mRNA induced by 7-day ML was reduced in MDX+ML (+119%) as compared to C57+ML (+331%)(Figure 4f).

Both REDD1 and REDD2 genes (regulated in development and DNA damage responses 1 and 2) are negative regulators of mTOR signaling, REDD2 overexpression diminishing the activation of mTOR in response to mechanical signal [16]. Therefore, we also measured the expression of both genes at day 7. In contrast to C57+ML mice, there was no ML-induced decrease in REDD1 mRNA in MDX+ML mice (Figure 4g). Concerning REDD2 mRNA, it was reduced in a similar way in MDX+ML mice (−73%) and C57+ML mice (–82%) 7 days after ML (Figure 4h).

Dystrophin rescue restored the adaptive response

Together, our results suggest that dystrophin is essential for a normal response to ML. To further substantiate the role of dystrophin in the adaptive response to ML, we performed a dystrophin rescue experiment. We evaluated the effect of U7-mediated dystrophin (U7-DYS) rescue in plantaris muscle [44]. We injected U7-DYS contruct to MDX mice 1 month before ML (MDX+ML+DYS) and we studied the muscle following 1-month ML.

In contrast to C57+ML mice, MDX+ML mice did not increase absolute maximal force and fatigue resistance and reduce specific maximal force in response to 1-month ML (Figures 5a–c), confirming that the adaptative response was blunted in MDX+ML mice as compared to C57+ML mice. MDX+ML+DYS muscles immunostained for dystrophin expression revealed high levels of dystrophin expression properly localized to the fiber sarcolemma

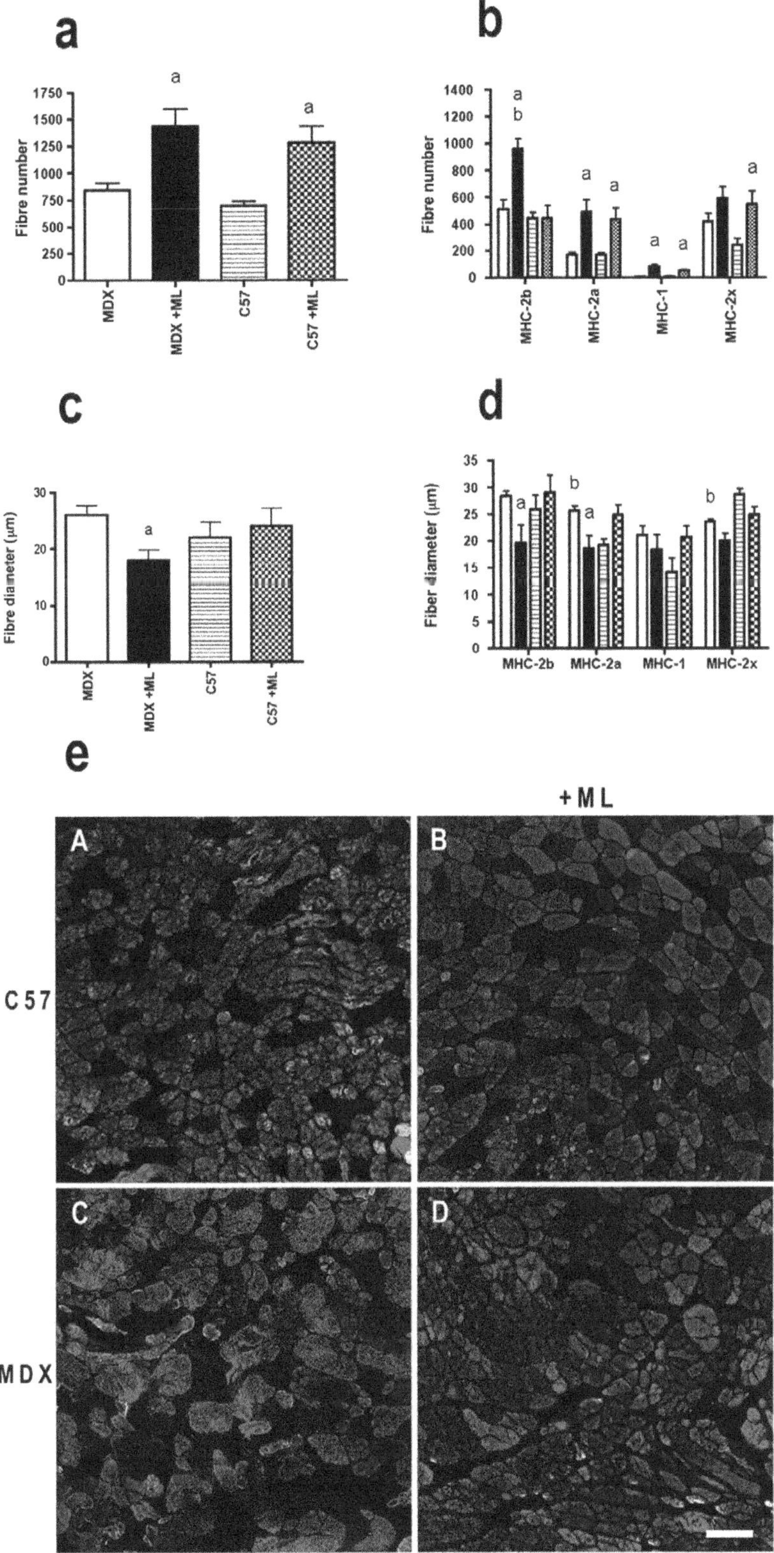

Figure 3. Cellular aspects of the attenuation of muscle hypertrophy following 2 month-ML in MDX mice. Number (a and b) and diameter (c,d and e) of the muscle fibers after 2 months of ML. Of note, since muscle fiber can express more than one MHC, the sum of the number of the different types of muscle fibers exceeded the total number of fibers. The representative images (e) show reduced size of fibers expressing MHC-2b following ML. Cross-sections were revealed for MHC-2b (red), MHC-2a (green) and MHC-1 (blue) reactivity. Scale bar = 20 µm. a: significantly different from unoverloaded muscle ($p<0.05$). b: significantly different from corresponding C57 mice ($p<0.05$). n = 5–8/group.

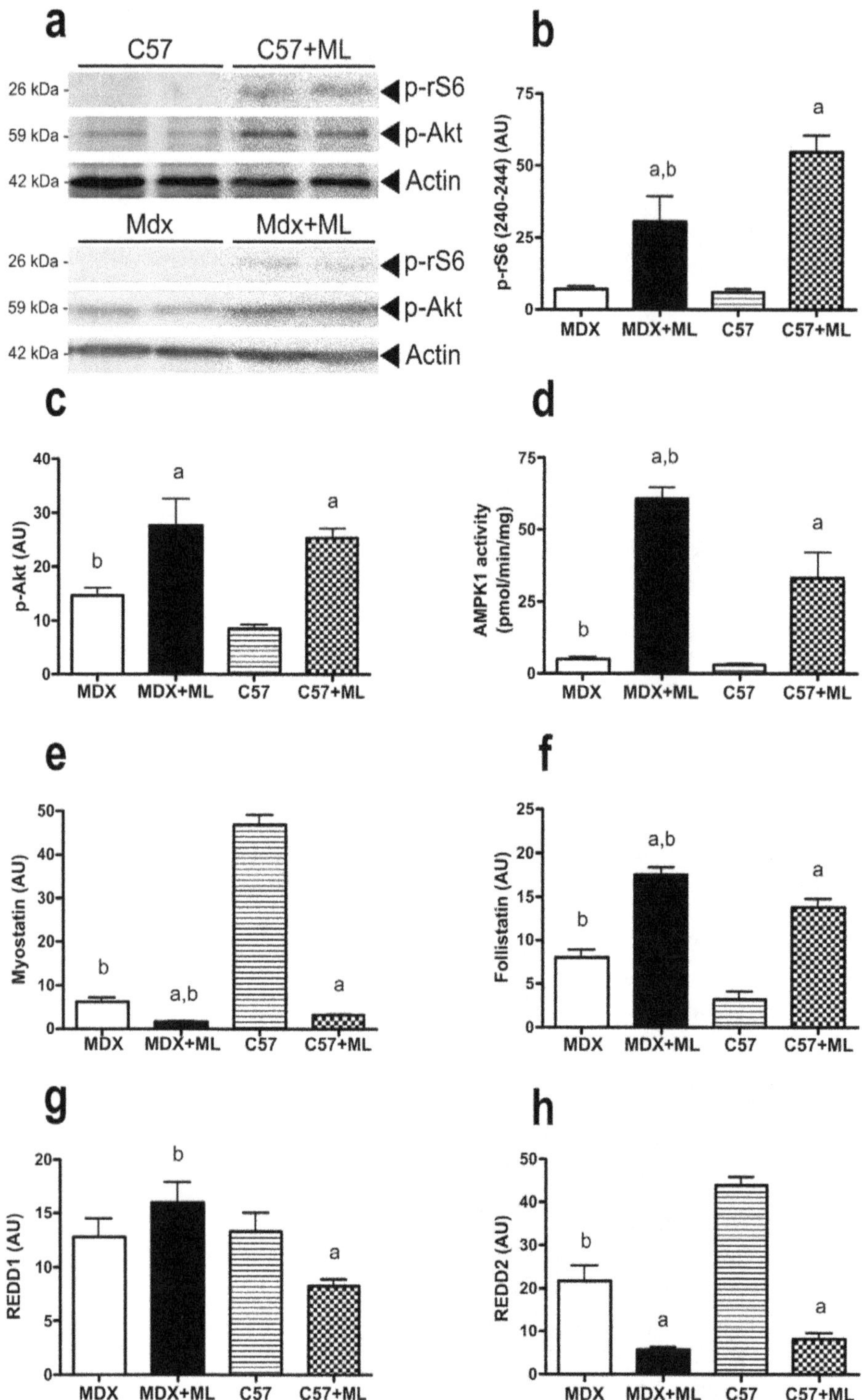

Figure 4. Altered activation (p-rS6 and p-Akt) and regulation (AMPKα1, myostatin, follistatin, REDD1 and REDD2) of mTOR signaling pathway at 7 days following ML in MDX mice. p-rS6 (a, b), p-Akt (a, c), AMPKα1 activity (d), myostatin (e), follistatin (f), REDD1 (g) and REDD2 (h) mRNA after 7 days of ML. The image (a) show representative blots of p-rS6 and p-Akt. a: significantly different from unoverloaded muscle ($p<0.05$). b: significantly different from corresponding C57 mice ($p<0.05$). n = 5–12/group.

(Figure S3a), confirming that dystrophin rescue was effective. Interestingly, the delivery of U7-DYS construct in MDX mice was able to fully restore the gain of absolute maximal force induced by 1 month ML. Indeed, ML combined with U7-DYS in MDX induced similar increase in absolute maximal force (+90%) as ML alone in C57 mice (+77%). This was explained by the fact that U7-DYS prevented the drop in specific maximal force in MDX+ML+DYS (Figure 5c), without affecting fibrosis (Figure S3b–c). Moreover, U7-DYS partially restored the increase in muscle fatigue resistance induced by ML in MDX+ML+DYS

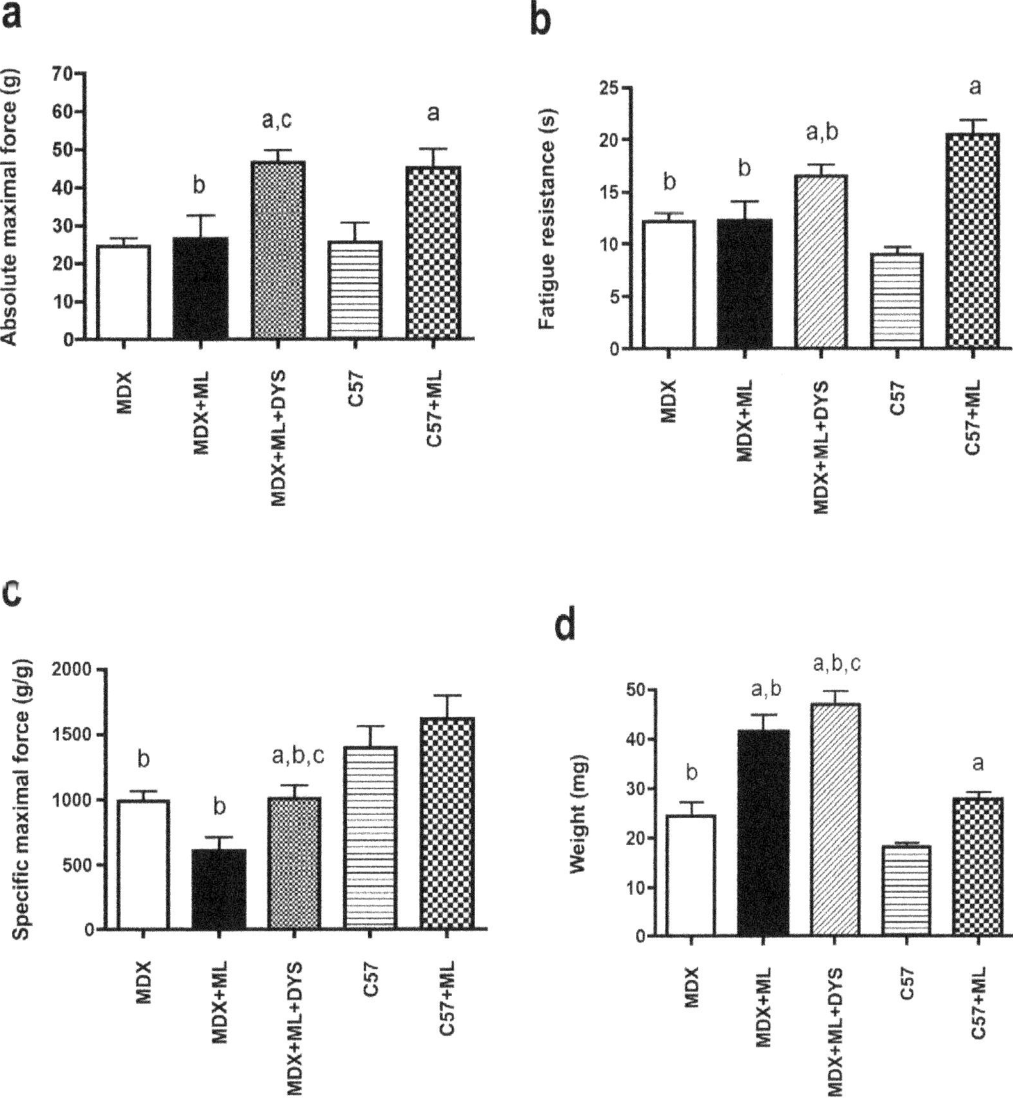

Figure 5. Restoration of the adaptive response to 1 month ML by dystrophin rescue. Absolute (a) and specific (b) muscle maximal forces, weight (c) and fatigue resistance (d) and after 1-month of ML combined with U7-mediated dystrophin rescue. a: significantly different from unoverloaded muscle ($p<0.05$). b: significantly different from corresponding C57 mice ($p<0.05$). c: significantly different from MDX+ML ($p<0.05$). n = 6/group.

mice (Figure 5b). Finally, it induced a modest increase in muscle weight in MDX+ML+DYS (Figure 5d) that was associated with a greater diameter for the fibers expressing dystrophin as compared to the fibers not expressing dystrophin (Figure S3d).

Discussion

In the present study, we reported for the first time that the muscle adaptive response following ML was impaired in MDX mice and dystrophin rescue restored it. Our study strongly suggests that dystrophin plays an important role in the muscle performance gain and remodeling following ML.

Reduced performance gain

Muscle performance was improved to a lesser extent in MDX+ML mice as compared to C57+ML mice. The markedly reduced increase in muscle absolute maximal force (both 1 and 2 months after ML; at month 2:+40% versus+204%) resulted from the fact that muscle specific maximal force was reduced (1 month-ML) or did not increase (2 month-ML) in MDX mice. The reduced specific maximal force of the fast fibers in MDX+ML mice explains this difference between the two mice strains. We would suggest that the reduced specific maximal force of the muscle fibers was caused by a lower concentration of contractile proteins since we found that fibers were atrophied in the MDX+ML mice and dystrophin rescue increased their diameter (see below). In addition, we cannot exclude the possibility that ML increased the alterations in subcellular sarcomere microarchitecture in MDX mice [57]. The smaller increase in muscle absolute maximal force induced by 2 month-ML in MDX+ML mice was also caused by a reduced muscle hypertrophy (see below).

Together with the reduced gain in muscle absolute maximal force, we also reported an attenuated increase in muscle fatigue resistance in response to ML in MDX mice (both at 1 and

2 months; at 2 months:+36 versus +85%). This was associated with a reduction in the fast/glycolytic to slow/oxidative fiber-type conversion in response to ML (higher percentage of fibers expressing MHC-2b) in MDX mice. It is well established that slow/oxidative fiber are more fatigue resistant than fast/glycolytic fibers [20]. Since the calcineurin, PGC-1α, and PPAR signaling pathways promote the formation of slow/oxidative/fatigue resistant fiber [3], these pathways could be less activated in response to ML in MDX mice. The data concerning the expression of NFATc, PGC-1α and PPAR-ß mRNAs in response to ML in both strains did not support this hypothesis. However, activation of these signaling pathways, in addition to modulation of gene transcripts as analyzed in the present study, involves also post-transcriptional modifications.

Interestingly, dystrophin rescue restored these aspects of the adaptive response to ML, substantiating the idea that the absence of dystrophin is responsible of the defect. It should be noted that partial dystrophin replacement appears to be enough, confirming previous studies [58]. Apparently, the dystrophic state does not play a role in the reduced adaptive response since dystrophin rescue restores it, whithout affecting the level of fibrosis. Therefore, a key finding of the present study is that dystrophin is very likely a new player in the adaptive response to ML.

Potential mechanisms of the fiber atrophy

In the present study, the reduced muscle hypertrophy (increase in muscle weight) in response to 2 month-ML in MDX mice is not caused by a smaller increase in fiber number per muscle cross-sectional area (similar increase). Fiber number increase following ML have been previously reported [7,19,24,40], and most probably results from both de novo fiber formation from satellite cells and fiber splitting/branching since the increased fiber number is only partially attenuated with satellite cell ablation [19]. This is the atrophy of the fibers expressing MHC-2b and MHC-2a that is responsible for the reduced muscle hypertrophy in MDX+ML mice. This may result from the lower reduction in catabolic processes (ubiquitin-proteasomal pathway and autophagy) in MDX+ML, in agreement with the lower increase in Akt phosphorylation. It is also likely that split/branched and newly formed fibers did not grow enough in the MDX+ML mice. A possible lower contribution of satellite cells to muscle hypertrophy resulting from dystrophic environment is not supported by our results concerning the increase in fiber number (similar between the 2 strains) and the effect of dystrophin rescue (restoration of the adaptive response without notable change in the dystrophic environment), and the recent finding that satellite cells are not necessary for robust ML-induced hypertrophy [19].

The increase in fiber number following ML is independent of mTOR signaling whereas fiber growth is not [6]. Therefore, we propose that the splitted/branched and newly formed fibers did not grow enough in the MDX+ML mice due to reduced mTOR signaling in response to ML. In support of this hypothesis, we found a lower increase in phosphorylation of rS6 in MDX+ML mice. Moreover, phosphorylation of Akt is also increased to a lesser extent; activation of Akt also promoting muscle hypertrophy [8,9]. The reduced augmentation of follistatin and the reduced attenuation of myostatin and REDD1 in response to ML in MDX mice were consistent with the inhibition of mTOR activation [12,13,15,16]. We have recently reported that AMPKα1 plays a key role in suppressing mTOR activation and limits hypertrophy in response to ML [10]. In the present study, we found that AMPKα1 activity increased to a similar extent in response to ML in MDX mice as compared to C57+ML; however AMPKα1 actvity was higher in MDX+ML mice.

Together with an inhibition of the mTOR pathway, it is also possible that reduced mTOR signaling in MDX+ML mice resulted from a lower input from mTOR activation during ML. Recent studies have ruled out the theory that local production of insulin-like growth factor (IGF-1) and IGF-1 signaling is responsible for mTOR activation in response to ML [17,43,59]. This is consistent with the fact that IGF-1 does not either cause hypertrophy nor activate Akt/mTOR signaling in (adult) muscle [60]. How mTOR signaling is activated by mechanical signals is not well understood [2,61]. However, mTOR activation in response to ML is reduced by inhibition of mechanoreceptors such as stretch-activated channels [62]. Therefore, the lower activation of mTOR in MDX+ML mice may result from a dysfunction in the mechanoreceptors due to colocalization of dystrophin and mechanoreceptors [30,31].

Since dystrophin rescue increased the fiber diameter in MDX+ML+DYS mice, this result substantiates the idea that dystrophin plays an important role both in anabolic and catabolic pathways, possibly due to the fact that dystrophin contributes to force transmission [26] and serves as a scaffold for signaling complexes [29,30,31]. Consistent with our results, it was reported that dystrophin may be critical for muscle growth/maintenance [63,64].

Conclusion

The extent of the improvement in muscle performance (gains in absolute maximal force and fatigue resistance) in response to ML was lower in dystrophic MDX mice. Decreased cellular and molecular adaptations (hypertrophy, promotion of slower/oxidative fibers) in response to ML and altered intracellular signaling pathways involved in muscle growth and maintenance were also found in MDX mice. The fact that dystrophin rescue restored the muscle response to ML further substantiates the idea that dystrophin plays an important role. Future studies are required to dissect the detailed link between dystrophin and muscle growth and maintenance. Additional studies are also needed to test the possibility that long-term physical rehabilitation using high-force contractions could be a safe therapeutic strategy to ameliorate dystrophic muscle weakness.

Methods

Animals and mechanical overloading

All procedures were performed in accordance with national and European legislations. Male MDX mice (MDX, C57BL/10ScSc-DMD^{mdx}/J) and their control (C57, C57BL/10) were used at 4–6 months of age. The *MDX* mice were kindly provided by D. Sassoon and A. Pannerec (INSERM U787 Paris). All animals were housed in conventional conditions. The animals were anaesthetized with pentobarbital (ip, 50 mg/kg body weight). The plantaris muscles of both legs from each mouse were mechanically overloaded (ML) by the surgical removal of soleus muscles and a major portion of the gastrocnemius muscles as described [39]. Body weight was not changed by 2 month ML in both MDX and C57 mice. The plantaris muscles were recovered 3 and 7 days, and 1 and 2 months following ML. The animals were euthanized with an overdose of pentobarbital.

Dystrophin rescue strategy

The restoration of a quasi-dystrophin was mediated by the vectorized U7 exon-skipping technique (U7-DYS)[44]. Vectors were prepared according to published protocols [45]. Adeno-associated vectors (AAV2/1) carrying the U7-DYS construct were injected in 6 MDX animals through intra-arterial perfusion of the right hind limb. Titer for AAV2/1-U7 was 1.10^{12} vector genomes (vg).ml^{-1}. Detailed procedure for intra-arterial injection was previously described [46]. Briefly, anesthetized mice (2–4% isoflurane) underwent femoral artery and vein isolation of the right hindlimb. After clamping the femoral vein and two collaterals, a catheter was introduced in the femoral artery and we injected 1 ml per 20 g of body weight at a rate of 100 µl.s^{-1}. Control muscle was obtained from left hind limb in which femoral artery was injected with saline solution only. Muscles were collected 1 month after ML.

Whole muscle force measurement

Skeletal muscle function was evaluated by measuring *in situ* muscle contraction, as described previously [47,48]. At different times after ML (1 and 2 months after ML), animals were anesthetized (ip, pentobarbital sodium, 50 mg/kg). During physiological experiments, supplemental doses were given as required to maintain deep anesthesia. The knee and foot were fixed with clamps and stainless steel pins. The plantaris muscle was exposed and the distal tendon of the gastronecmius and soleus muscle complex was cut. The distal tendon of the plantaris muscle was attached to an isometric transducer (Harvard Bioscience) using a silk ligature. The sciatic nerves were proximally crushed and distally stimulated by a bipolar silver electrode using supramaximal square wave pulses of 0.1 ms duration. Responses to tetanic stimulation (pulse frequency 50–143 Hz) were successively recorded. At least 1 min was allowed between contractions. Absolute maximal forces were determined at optimal length (length at which maximal tension was obtained during the tetanus). Force was normalized to the muscle mass (m) as an estimate of specific maximal force. Fatigue resistance was then determined after a 5-min rest period. The muscle was continuously stimulated at 50 Hz for 2 min (sub maximal continuous tetanus). The duration corresponding to a 20% decrease in force was noted. Body temperature was maintained at 37°C using radiant heat.

Single muscle fiber force measurement

Plantaris muscles were collected 2 months after ML and immediately placed in an ice-cold relax solution (in mmol/l: 100 KCl, 20 Imidazole, 7 $MgCl_2$, 2 EGTA, 4 ATP, pH 7.0; 4°C). Small bundles of ~25–50 fibers were dissected free from the muscle and tied to a glass micro capillary tube at ~110% resting length. The bundles were then placed in a skinning solution (relax solution containing glycerol; 50:50 v/v) at 4°C for 24 h and subsequently treated with a cryoprotectant (sucrose solution) for long-term storage at −80°C as described earlier [49]. On the day of experiment, a bundle was desucrosed and single fibers isolated. A fiber segment length of 1 to 2 mm was then left exposed to the relax solution between connectors leading to a force transducer (model 400A, Aurora Scientific) and a lever arm system (model 308B, Aurora Scientific). The apparatus was mounted on the stage of an inverted microscope (model IX70; Olympus). While the fiber segment was in relax solution, sarcomere length was set to 2.50±0.05 µm by adjusting the overall segment length. The sarcomere length was controlled during the experiments using a high-speed video analysis system (model 901A HVSL, Aurora Scientific). The fiber segment width, depth and length between the connectors were measured. Fiber cross-sectional area (CSA) was calculated from the diameter and depth, assuming an elliptical circumference, and was corrected for the 20% swelling that is known to occur during skinning. At 15°C, immediately preceding each activation, the fiber segment was immersed for 10–20 s in a solution with a reduced Ca^{2+}-EGTA buffering capacity. This solution is identical to the relax solution except that the EGTA concentration is reduced to 0.5 mM, which results in more rapid attainment of steady force during subsequent activation. Maximal isometric force was calculated as the difference between the total force in activating solution (pCa 4.5) and the resting force measured in the same segment while in the relax solution. Maximal force was adjusted for fiber CSA (specific maximal force). After mechanical measurements, each fiber was placed in urea buffer in a plastic microcentrifuge tube and stored at −80°C until analyzed by gel electrophoresis. The myosin heavy chain (MHC) isoform composition of fibers was determined by 6% SDS-PAGE. The acrylamide concentration was 4% (wt/vol) in the stacking gel and 6% in the running gel, and the gel matrix included 30% glycerol. Sample loads were kept small (equivalent to ~0.05 mm of fiber segment) to improve the resolution of the MHC bands (slow and fast MyHC: type I, IIa, IIx and IIb). Electrophoresis was performed at 120 V for 24 h with a Tris–glycine electrode buffer (pH 8.3) at 15°C (SE 600 vertical slab gel unit, Hoefer Scientific Instruments). The gels were silver-stained and subsequently scanned in a soft laser densitometer (Molecular Dynamics) with a high spatial resolution (50 µm pixel spacing) and 4096 optical density levels.

Histology

Transverse serial sections (8 µm) of muscles (collected 1 and 2 months after ML) were obtained using a cryostat, in the mid-belly region. The muscles were sectioned at different intervals to determine the maximal muscle CSA and the corresponding sections were studied. Some of the sections were processed for histological analysis according to standard protocols (stained for H&E, Sirius red, dapi). Others were used for immunohistochemistry as described previously [50,51]. For determination of muscle fiber diameter and myosin heavy chain (MHC) analysis, frozen unfixed sections were blocked 1 h in PBS plus 2% BSA, 2% sheep serum and incubated 30 min with mouse Fab 1/100 in PBS. Sections were then incubated overnight with primary antibodies against laminin (Z0097, Dako), dystrophin (anti-Dys1, Novocastra) and MHC isoforms (BAD5/MHC-1, BF3/MHC-2b, SC71/MHC-2a, 6H1/MHC-2x, F1652/MHC-dev, Hybridoma bank). After washes in PBS, sections were incubated 1 h with secondary antibodies (alexa fluor). After washes in PBS, slides were finally mounted in Fluoromont (Southern Biotech). Morphometric analyses were made on two serial sections of muscles. Images were captured using a digital camera (Hamamatsu ORCA-AG) attached to a motorized fluorescence microscope (Zeiss AxioImager.Z1), and morphometric analyses were made using the software MetaMorph 7.5 (Molecular Devices). The smallest diameter of the fibers was measured. For muscle fiber diameter and fiber typing analyses all of the muscle fibers of the muscle section were measured. Unfortunately, it was not possible to distinguish pure and hybrid fibers expressing MHC-2b and MHC-2x since the isotype and species of the 2 primary antibodies were similar. To evaluate the amount of fibrosis, we measured the cross-sectional area occupied by Sirius red stained interstitial tissue.

AMPK activity assay

Muscles were recovered 7 days after ML (they were not previously electrically stimulated) in order to assay AMK activity. AMPK was immunoprecipitated from 30 µg lysate with antibodies against the α1 catalytic subunit and assayed for phosphotransferase activity towards *AMARA* peptide (AMARAASAAALARRR) using [γ-^{32}P]-ATP as previously described [52]. AMPKα1 antibodies used for immunoprecipitation was generated and donated by Professor D. Grahame Hardie (University of Dundee)

Western blot analysis

Immunoblotting was carried out as described previously [47,53] using muscles 7 days after ML (muscles were not previously electrically stimulated) from overnight fasted mice. Muscle tissues were snap frozen in liquid nitrogen immediately after dissection. Frozen muscles were placed into an ice-cold homogenization buffer containing: 50 mM Tris (pH 7.6), 250 mM NaCl, 3 mM EDTA, 3 mM EGTA, 0.5% NP40, 2 mM dithiothreitol, 10 mM sodium orthovanadate, 10 mM NaF, 10 mM glycerophosphate and 2% of protease inhibitor cocktail (Sigma, P8340). Samples were finely minced with scissors and then homogenized using plastic pestles, incubated 30 minutes on ice, sonicated 3 times for 5 s with 30 s intervals on ice and then centrifuged at 12,000 *g* for 30 min at 4°C. Protein concentration was measured using the Bradford method with BSA as a standard. Equal amounts of protein extracts, ie. 10 µg (phosphorylated-Ak, p-Akt), or 20 µg (phosphorylated-ribosomal S6 protein, p-rS6) were separated by SDS-PAGE before electrophoretic transfer onto a nitrocellulose membrane (Amersham Hybond-ECL, GE Healthcare). Western-blot analysis was carried out using p-rS6 (Ser240/244) antibody (1:2000, Cell Signaling #2215S); p-Akt (Ser473) antibody (1:2000, Cell Signaling #9271S), and a pan-actin Antibody (Clone C4, 1:20000, Millipore). Antibody reacting bands were visualized with peroxidase-conjugated secondary antibodies (Pierce Biotechnology) and a chemiluminescent detection system (ECL-Plus; GE Healthcare). Bands of actin were used to check that the protein load was correct. Bands were quantified by densitometric software (Multi Gauge, Fujifilm).

Relative quantification of gene expression by qPCR

Unstimulated muscles were collected 3 and 7 days after ML. Total RNA was extracted from plantaris muscle using miRNeasy Mini Kit (Qiagen SA) following the manufacturer's instructions. RNA quality for each sample was checked with Experion RNA StdSens Analysis Kit and the Experion automated electrophoresis station according to the manufacturer's instructions. Only samples with a RQI (RNA quality indicator) superior to 7 were used for further studies. The first-strand cDNA was then synthesized using Transcriptor First Strand cDNA Synthesis Kit (Roche Diagnostics) with Anchored-oligo(dT)$_{18}$ primer and according to the manufacturer's instructions. PCR analysis was then carried out with SYBR green PCR technology using Light Cycler 480 system (Roche Diagnostics). The reaction was carried out in duplicate for each sample in a 8 µl reaction volume containing 4 µl of SYBR Green Master Mix and 500 nM each the forward and reverse primer, and 4 µl of diluted (1:25) cDNA. The thermal profile for SYBR Green qPCR was 95°C for 8 min, followed by 40 cycles at 95°C for 15 s, 60°C for 15 s, 72°C 30 s. Primers sequences used in this study are available on request. The gene expression stability of GAPDH, HPRT and P0 were calculated using geNorm software and after analysis only HPRT and P0 were used as the references transcripts.

Statistical analysis

Groups were statistically compared using analysis of variance. If necessary, subsequent contrast analysis was also performed. For groups that did not pass tests of normality and equal variance, non-parametric tests were used (Kruskal Wallis and Wilcoxon). Values are means ± SEM.

Supporting Information

Figure S1 Factors promoting fast/glycolytic to slow/oxidative fiber-type conversion after 7 days of ML. PPARß (a), PGC1α (b) and NFATc1a (c) mRNA after 7 days of ML. a: significantly different from unoverloaded muscle ($p<0.05$). b: significantly different from corresponding C57 mice ($p<0.05$). n = 6/group.

Figure S2 Changes in catabolic processes following ML in MDX mice after 3 and 7 days of ML. Atrogin-1 (ubiquitin-proteasomal pathway)(a), LC3 (b) and Bnip3 (autophagy)(c) mRNA at 3 and 7 days. a: significantly different from unoverloaded muscle ($p<0.05$). b: significantly different from corresponding C57 mice ($p<0.05$). n = 5–10/group.

Figure S3 Cellular effects of dystrophin rescue at 1 month following ML in MDX mice. (a) representative image of fibers expressing dystrophin in MDX+ML+DYS mice, (b, c) fibrosis using red Sirius staining and (d) diameter of fibers expressing (DYS positive) or not dystrophin (DYS negative) in MDX+ML mice. c: significantly different from fiber expressing not dystrophin ($p<0.05$). n = 4–6/group.

Acknowledgments

We thank Athanassia Sotiropoulos (INSERM U1016) for helpful critical reading of the manuscript. We are grateful to Cyriaque Beley, Isabelle Lachaize, and Guillaume Précigout (INSERM U974) for technical assistance during the experiments.

Author Contributions

Conceived and designed the experiments: AF GBB OA. Performed the experiments: PJ CH JO YC FM AV WH LA DZ AF. Analyzed the data: PJ CH YC FM JO RM KS AF. Contributed reagents/materials/analysis tools: EM AG LG. Wrote the paper: AF OA GBB.

References

1. Miyazaki M, Esser KA (2009) Cellular mechanisms regulating protein synthesis and skeletal muscle hypertrophy in animals. J Appl Physiol 106: 1367–1373.
2. Spangenburg EE (2009) Changes in muscle mass with mechanical load: possible cellular mechanisms. Appl Physiol Nutr Metab 34: 328–335.
3. Schiaffino S, Sandri M, Murgia M (2007) Activity-dependent signaling pathways controlling muscle diversity and plasticity. Physiology (Bethesda) 22: 269–278.
4. Fluck M, Hoppeler H (2003) Molecular basis of skeletal muscle plasticity–from gene to form and function. Rev Physiol Biochem Pharmacol 146: 159–216.
5. Gundersen K (2010) Excitation-transcription coupling in skeletal muscle: the molecular pathways of exercise. Biol Rev Camb Philos Soc 86: 564–600.
6. Bodine SC, Stitt TN, Gonzalez M, Kline WO, Stover GL, et al. (2001) Akt/mTOR pathway is a crucial regulator of skeletal muscle hypertrophy and can prevent muscle atrophy in vivo. Nat Cell Biol 3: 1014–1019.
7. Goodman CA, Frey JW, Mabrey DM, Jacobs BL, Lincoln HC, et al. (2011) The role of skeletal muscle mTOR in the regulation of mechanical load-induced growth. J Physiol 589: 5485–5501.
8. Lai KM, Gonzalez M, Poueymirou WT, Kline WO, Na E, et al. (2004) Conditional activation of akt in adult skeletal muscle induces rapid hypertrophy. Mol Cell Biol 24: 9295–9304.
9. Blaauw B, Canato M, Agatea L, Toniolo L, Mammucari C, et al. (2009) Inducible activation of Akt increases skeletal muscle mass and force without satellite cell activation. Faseb J 23: 3896–3905.
10. Mounier R, Lantier L, Leclerc J, Sotiropoulos A, Pende M, et al. (2009) Important role for AMPKalpha1 in limiting skeletal muscle cell hypertrophy. Faseb J 23: 2264–2273.
11. Xu Z, Ichikawa N, Kosaki K, Yamada Y, Sasaki T, et al. (2010) Perlecan deficiency causes muscle hypertrophy, a decrease in myostatin expression, and changes in muscle fiber composition. Matrix Biol 29: 461–470.
12. Trendelenburg AU, Meyer A, Rohner D, Boyle J, Hatakeyama S, et al. (2009) Myostatin reduces Akt/TORC1/p70S6K signaling, inhibiting myoblast differentiation and myotube size. Am J Physiol Cell Physiol 296: C1258–1270.
13. Sartori R, Milan G, Patron M, Mammucari C, Blaauw B, et al. (2009) Smad2 and 3 transcription factors control muscle mass in adulthood. Am J Physiol Cell Physiol 296: C1248–1257.
14. Amirouche A, Durieux AC, Banzet S, Koulmann N, Bonnefoy R, et al. (2009) Down-regulation of Akt/mammalian target of rapamycin signaling pathway in response to myostatin overexpression in skeletal muscle. Endocrinology 150: 286–294.

15. Sun Y, Ge Y, Drnevich J, Zhao Y, Band M, et al. (2010) Mammalian target of rapamycin regulates miRNA-1 and follistatin in skeletal myogenesis. J Cell Biol 189: 1157–1169.
16. Miyazaki M, Esser KA (2009) REDD2 is enriched in skeletal muscle and inhibits mTOR signaling in response to leucine and stretch. Am J Physiol Cell Physiol 296: C583–592.
17. Miyazaki M, McCarthy JJ, Fedele MJ, Esser KA (2011) Early activation of mTORC1 signalling in response to mechanical overload is independent of phosphoinositide 3-kinase/Akt signalling. J Physiol 589: 1831–1846.
18. Dupont E, Cieniewski-Bernard C, Bastide B, Stevens L (2011) Electrostimulation during hindlimb unloading modulates PI3K-AKT downstream targets without preventing soleus atrophy and restores slow phenotype through ERK. Am J Physiol Regul Integr Comp Physiol 300: R408–417.
19. McCarthy JJ, Mula J, Miyazaki M, Erfani R, Garrison K, et al. (2011) Effective fiber hypertrophy in satellite cell-depleted skeletal muscle. Development 138: 3657–3666.
20. Burke RE, Levine DN, Tsairis P, Zajac FE 3rd (1973) Physiological types and histochemical profiles in motor units of the cat gastrocnemius. J Physiol 234: 723–748.
21. Bassel-Duby R, Olson EN (2006) Signaling pathways in skeletal muscle remodeling. Annu Rev Biochem 75: 19–37.
22. Dunn SE, Burns JL, Michel RN (1999) Calcineurin is required for skeletal muscle hypertrophy. J Biol Chem 274: 21908–21912.
23. Dunn SE, Chin ER, Michel RN (2000) Matching of calcineurin activity to upstream effectors is critical for skeletal muscle fiber growth. J Cell Biol 151: 663–672.
24. Parsons SA, Millay DP, Wilkins BJ, Bueno OF, Tsika GL, et al. (2004) Genetic loss of calcineurin blocks mechanical overload-induced skeletal muscle fiber type switching but not hypertrophy. J Biol Chem 279: 20192–20200.
25. Lira VA, Benton CR, Yan Z, Bonen A (2010) PGC-1alpha regulation by exercise training and its influences on muscle function and insulin sensitivity. Am J Physiol Endocrinol Metab 299: E145–161.
26. Ramaswamy KS, Palmer ML, van der Meulen JH, Renoux A, Kostrominova TY, et al. (2011) Lateral transmission of force is impaired in skeletal muscles of dystrophic mice and very old rats. J Physiol.
27. Lynch GS, Hinkle RT, Chamberlain JS, Brooks SV, Faulkner JA (2001) Force and power output of fast and slow skeletal muscles from mdx mice 6–28 months old. J Physiol 535: 591–600.
28. Dumonceaux J, Marie S, Beley C, Trollet C, Vignaud A, et al. (2010) Combination of myostatin pathway interference and dystrophin rescue enhances tetanic and specific force in dystrophic mdx mice. Mol Ther 18: 881–887.
29. Friedrich O, von Wegner F, Chamberlain JS, Fink RH, Rohrbach P (2008) L-type Ca2+ channel function is linked to dystrophin expression in mammalian muscle. PLoS One 3: e1762.
30. Allen DG, Zhang BT, Whitehead NP (2010) Stretch-Induced Membrane Damage in Muscle: Comparison of Wild-Type and mdx Mice. Adv Exp Med Biol 682: 297–313.
31. Rolland JF, De Luca A, Burdi R, Andreetta F, Confalonieri P, et al. (2006) Overactivity of exercise-sensitive cation channels and their impaired modulation by IGF-1 in mdx native muscle fibers: beneficial effect of pentoxifylline. Neurobiol Dis 24: 466–474.
32. Sellman JE, DeRuisseau KC, Betters JL, Lira VA, Soltow QA, et al. (2006) In vivo inhibition of nitric oxide synthase impairs upregulation of contractile protein mRNA in overloaded plantaris muscle. J Appl Physiol 100: 258–265.
33. Pietri-Rouxel F, Gentil C, Vassilopoulos S, Baas D, Mouisel E, et al. (2010) DHPR alpha1S subunit controls skeletal muscle mass and morphogenesis. Embo J 29: 643–654.
34. Kumar A, Khandelwal N, Malya R, Reid MB, Boriek AM (2004) Loss of dystrophin causes aberrant mechanotransduction in skeletal muscle fibers. Faseb J 18: 102–113.
35. Barton ER (2006) Impact of sarcoglycan complex on mechanical signal transduction in murine skeletal muscle. Am J Physiol Cell Physiol 290: C411–419.
36. Stupka N, Michell BJ, Kemp BE, Lynch GS (2006) Differential calcineurin signalling activity and regeneration efficacy in diaphragm and limb muscles of dystrophic mdx mice. Neuromuscul Disord 16: 337–346.
37. Nakamura A, Yoshida K, Ueda H, Takeda S, Ikeda S (2005) Up-regulation of mitogen activated protein kinases in mdx skeletal muscle following chronic treadmill exercise. Biochim Biophys Acta 1740: 326–331.
38. Lang JM, Esser KA, Dupont-Versteegden EE (2004) Altered activity of signaling pathways in diaphragm and tibialis anterior muscle of dystrophic mice. Exp Biol Med (Maywood) 229: 503–511.
39. Baldwin KM, Valdez V, Herrick RE, MacIntosh AM, Roy RR (1982) Biochemical properties of overloaded fast-twitch skeletal muscle. J Appl Physiol 52: 467–472.
40. Ianuzzo CD, Gollnick PD, Armstrong RB (1976) Compensatory adaptations of skeletal muscle fiber types to a long-term functional overload. Life Sci 19: 1517–1523.
41. McGee SL, Mustard KJ, Hardie DG, Baar K (2008) Normal hypertrophy accompanied by phosphoryation and activation of AMP-activated protein kinase alpha1 following overload in LKB1 knockout mice. J Physiol 586: 1731–1741.
42. Roy RR, Edgerton VR (1995) Response of mouse plantaris muscle to functional overload: comparison with rat and cat. Comp Biochem Physiol A Physiol 111: 569–575.
43. Spangenburg EE, Le Roith D, Ward CW, Bodine SC (2008) A functional insulin-like growth factor receptor is not necessary for load-induced skeletal muscle hypertrophy. J Physiol 586: 283–291.
44. Goyenvalle A, Vulin A, Fougerousse F, Leturcq F, Kaplan JC, et al. (2004) Rescue of dystrophic muscle through U7 snRNA-mediated exon skipping. Science 306: 1796–1799.
45. Riviere C, Danos O, Douar AM (2006) Long-term expression and repeated administration of AAV type 1, 2 and 5 vectors in skeletal muscle of immunocompetent adult mice. Gene Ther 13: 1300–1308.
46. Gonin P, Arandel L, Van Wittenberghe L, Marais T, Perez N, et al. (2005) Femoral intra-arterial injection: a tool to deliver and assess recombinant AAV constructs in rodents whole hind limb. J Gene Med 7: 782–791.
47. Mouisel E, Vignaud A, Hourde C, Butler-Browne G, Ferry A (2010) Muscle weakness and atrophy are associated with decreased regenerative capacity and changes in mTOR signaling in skeletal muscles of venerable (18–24-month-old) dystrophic mdx mice. Muscle Nerve 41: 809–818.
48. Risson V, Mazelin L, Roceri M, Sanchez H, Moncollin V, et al. (2009) Muscle inactivation of mTOR causes metabolic and dystrophin defects leading to severe myopathy. J Cell Biol 187: 859–874.
49. Frontera WR, Larsson L (1997) Contractile studies of single human skeletal muscle fibers: a comparison of different muscles, permeabilization procedures, and storage techniques. Muscle Nerve 20: 948–952.
50. Trollet C, Anvar SY, Venema A, Hargreaves IP, Foster K, et al. (2010) Molecular and phenotypic characterization of a mouse model of oculopharyngeal muscular dystrophy reveals severe muscular atrophy restricted to fast glycolytic fibres. Hum Mol Genet 19: 2191–2207.
51. Agbulut O, Vignaud A, Hourde C, Mouisel E, Fougerousse F, et al. (2009) Slow myosin heavy chain expression in the absence of muscle activity. Am J Physiol Cell Physiol 296: C205–214.
52. Sakamoto K, Goransson O, Hardie DG, Alessi DR (2004) Activity of LKB1 and AMPK-related kinases in skeletal muscle: effects of contraction, phenformin, and AICAR. Am J Physiol Endocrinol Metab 287: E310–317.
53. Hourde C, Jagerschmidt C, Clement-Lacroix P, Vignaud A, Ammann P, et al. (2009) Androgen replacement therapy improves function in male rat muscles independently of hypertrophy and activation of the Akt/mTOR pathway. Acta Physiol (Oxf) 195: 471–482.
54. Marino JS, Tausch BJ, Dearth CL, Manacci MV, McLoughlin TJ, et al. (2008) Beta2-integrins contribute to skeletal muscle hypertrophy in mice. Am J Physiol Cell Physiol 295: C1026–1036.
55. Sandri M (2008) Signaling in muscle atrophy and hypertrophy. Physiology (Bethesda) 23: 160–170.
56. Borst SE (2004) Interventions for sarcopenia and muscle weakness in older people. Age Ageing 33: 548–555.
57. Friedrich O, Both M, Weber C, Schurmann S, Teichmann MD, et al. (2010) Microarchitecture is severely compromised but motor protein function is preserved in dystrophic mdx skeletal muscle. Biophys J 98: 606–616.
58. Koo T, Malerba A, Athanasopoulos T, Trollet C, Boldrin L, et al. (2011) Delivery of AAV2/9-Microdystrophin Genes Incorporating Helix 1 of the Coiled-Coil Motif in the C-Terminal Domain of Dystrophin Improves Muscle Pathology and Restores the Level of alpha1-Syntrophin and alpha-Dystrobrevin in Skeletal Muscles of mdx Mice. Hum Gene Ther 22: 1379–1388.
59. Hamilton DL, Philp A, MacKenzie MG, Baar K (2010) A limited role for PI(3,4,5)P3 regulation in controlling skeletal muscle mass in response to resistance exercise. PLoS One 5: e11624.
60. Shavlakadze T, Chai J, Maley K, Cozens G, Grounds G, et al. (2010) A growth stimulus is needed for IGF-1 to induce skeletal muscle hypertrophy in vivo. J Cell Sci 123: 960–971.
61. Hornberger TA (2011) Mechanotransduction and the regulation of mTORC1 signaling in skeletal muscle. Int J Biochem Cell Biol 43: 1267–1276.
62. Spangenburg EE, McBride TA (2006) Inhibition of stretch-activated channels during eccentric muscle contraction attenuates p70S6K activation. J Appl Physiol 100: 129–135.
63. Acharyya S, Butchbach ME, Sahenk Z, Wang H, Saji M, et al. (2005) Dystrophin glycoprotein complex dysfunction: a regulatory link between muscular dystrophy and cancer cachexia. Cancer Cell 8: 421–432.
64. Judge LM, Arnett AL, Banks GB, Chamberlain JS (2011) Expression of the dystrophin isoform Dp116 preserves functional muscle mass and extends lifespan without preventing dystrophy in severely dystrophic mice. Hum Mol Genet 20: 4978–4990.

12

Biomechanical Analysis of the Human Finger Extensor Mechanism during Isometric Pressing

Dan Hu[1,3], David Howard[2], Lei Ren[1]*

1 School of Mechanical, Aerospace and Civil Engineering, University of Manchester, Manchester, United Kingdom, **2** School of Computing, Science and Engineering, University of Salford, Manchester, United Kingdom, **3** State Key Laboratory of Automotive Simulation and Control, Jilin University, Changchun, P.R. China

Abstract

This study investigated the effects of the finger extensor mechanism on the bone-to-bone contact forces at the interphalangeal and metacarpal joints and also on the forces in the intrinsic and extrinsic muscles during finger pressing. This was done with finger postures ranging from very flexed to fully extended. The role of the finger extensor mechanism was investigated by using two alternative finger models, one which omitted the extensor mechanism and another which included it. A six-camera three-dimensional motion analysis system was used to capture the finger posture during maximum voluntary isometric pressing. The fingertip loads were recorded simultaneously using a force plate system. Two three-dimensional biomechanical finger models, a minimal model without extensor mechanism and a full model with extensor mechanism (tendon network), were used to calculate the joint bone-to-bone contact forces and the extrinsic and intrinsic muscle forces. If the full model is assumed to be realistic, then the results suggest some useful biomechanical advantages provided by the tendon network of the extensor mechanism. It was found that the forces in the intrinsic muscles (interosseus group and lumbrical) are significantly reduced by 22% to 61% due to the action of the extensor mechanism, with the greatest reductions in more flexed postures. The bone-to-bone contact force at the MCP joint is reduced by 10% to 41%. This suggests that the extensor mechanism may help to reduce the risk of injury at the finger joints and also to moderate the forces in intrinsic muscles. These apparent biomechanical advantages may be a result of the extensor mechanism's distinctive interconnected fibrous structure, through which the contraction of the intrinsic muscles as flexors of the MCP joint can generate extensions at the DIP and PIP joints.

Editor: Steve Milanese, University of South Australia, Australia

Funding: The China Scholarship Council (CSC) had partly supported the study design, data collection and analysis. The additional part of the funding of the study has been supported by the UK EPSRC from grant number EP/I033602/1. The funders had no role in study design, data collection and analysis, decision to publish, or preparation of the manuscript.

Competing Interests: The authors have declared that no competing interests exist.

* E-mail: lei.ren@manchester.ac.uk

Introduction

The structural and functional complexities of the human finger have long been recognised [1–5]. Effective function of the finger requires precise coordination of multiple muscles and the resulting finger motion is constrained by the forces exerted by the joint capsules, ligaments and joint articular surfaces. In manual activities, the highly complex musculoskeletal system of the hand and forearm is well coordinated to generate appropriate fingertip forces and finger postures. A good understanding of the biomechanical mechanisms of the finger would not only improve our knowledge of normal finger function and the etiology of hand diseases, but may also significantly improve prosthetic and biomimetic hand design.

However, finger mechanics is complicated by the finger extensor mechanism (also referred to as the extensor apparatus, extensor assembly or extensor expansion), which is a complex tendon network that brings together the forces of the lumbrical, interossei, and long extensor to produce precise functional movements of the phalanxes (see Figure 1). In recent decades, a number of studies have been conducted to investigate its anatomical structure [6–16] and the spatial relationships between its different components, to quantify its geometric configuration [17] and material properties [18]. In addition, recently there has been increasing use of extensor mechanism models for the biomechanical analysis of finger function [19–27]. However, despite this, little is known about how the extensor mechanism affects the mechanical loadings at finger joints and muscles.

Therefore, in this study, we aim to investigate the biomechanical effect of the extensor mechanism (tendon network) during isometric pressing using a combined experimental and modelling approach. Fingertip force and finger posture were recorded using a force plate and a three-dimensional (3D) motion analysis system. Force analysis was conducted using two different finger models, a minimal model excluding the extensor mechanism and a full model including the extensor mechanism. In this way, the effects of this complex tendon network on finger joint contact forces and extrinsic and intrinsic muscle forces were analysed. However, it should be noted that the conclusions drawn are based on interpreting the differences between the results generated by the two models and, as such, cannot be quoted with the confidence one would associate with wholly experimental results.

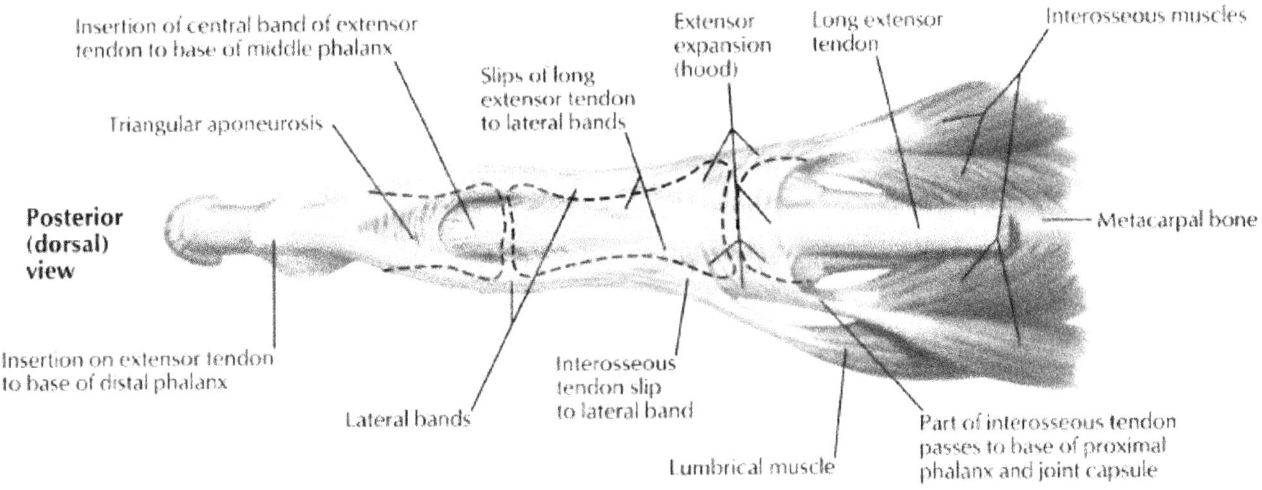

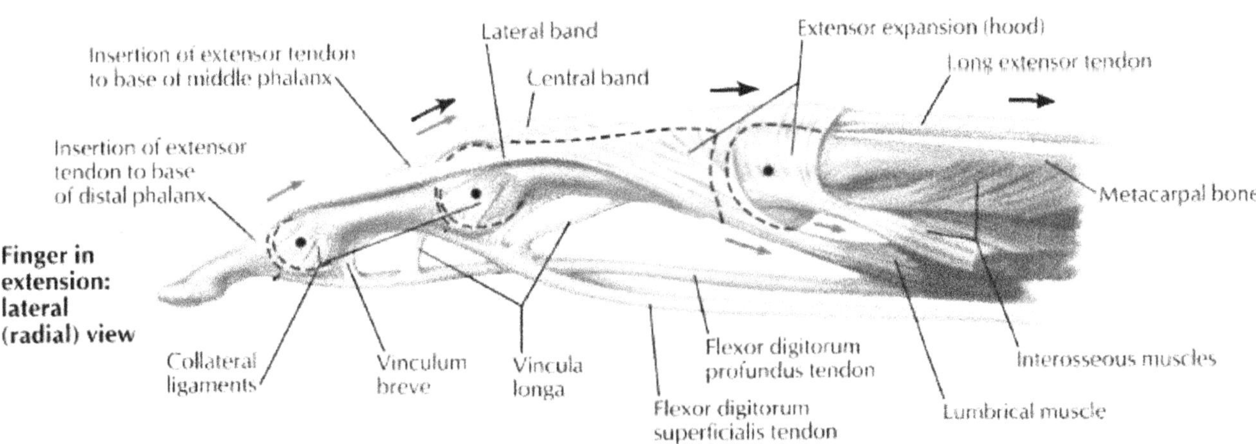

Figure 1. Musculotendonal structure of the human finger. The musculotendonal structure of the human finger from posterior (dorsal) and lateral (radial) views (from Netter, 2002)

Methods

Notation

PF: primary flexor

PE: primary extensor

FDP: flexor digitorum profundus

FDS: flexor digitorum superficials

TE: terminal extensor

ES: extensor slip

LE: long extensor

RI: radial interosseous

UI: ulnar interosseous

LU: lumbrical

RB: radial band

UB: ulnar band

DIP: distal interphalangeal

PIP: proximal interphalangeal

MCP: metacarpophalangeal

$a_{PF\_DIP\_FL}$, $a_{PF\_PIP\_FL}$, $a_{PF\_MCP\_FL}$: flexion/extension moment arm of *PF* around DIP, PIP and MCP joint

$a_{PE\_DIP\_FL}$, $a_{PE\_PIP\_FL}$, $a_{PE\_MCP\_FL}$: flexion/extension moment arm of *PE* around DIP, PIP and MCP joint

$a_{RI\_MCP\_FL}$, $a_{UI\_MCP\_FL}$: flexion/extension moment arm of *RI* and *UI* around MCP joint

$a_{RI\_MCP\_AD}$, $a_{UI\_MCP\_AD}$: adduction/abduction moment arm of *RI* and *UI* around MCP joint

$a_{TE\_DIP\_FL}$: flexion/extension moment arm of *TE* around DIP joint

$a_{FDP\_DIP\_FL}$, $a_{FDP\_PIP\_FL}$, $a_{FDP\_MCP\_FL}$: flexion/extension moment arm of *FDP* around DIP, PIP and MCP joint

$a_{ES\_PIP\_FL}$, $a_{UB\_PIP\_FL}$, $a_{RB\_PIP\_FL}$: flexion/extension moment arm of *ES*, *UB* and *RB* around PIP joint

$a_{LE\_MCP\_FL}$, $a_{RI\_MCP\_FL}$, $a_{UI\_MCP\_FL}$, $a_{LU\_MCP\_FL}$: flexion/extension moment arm of *LE*, *RI*, *UI* and *LU* around MCP joint

$a_{RI\_MCP\_AD}$, $a_{UI\_MCP\_AD}$, $a_{LU\_MCP\_AD}$: adduction/abduction moment arm of *RI*, *UI* and *LU* around MCP joint

$\theta_1,\theta_2,\theta_3,\theta_4$: angles between phalange segments and X axis of global coordinate system (which is horizontal)

θ_{PF_DIP}, θ_{PF_PIP}, θ_{PF_MCP}: angle between *PF* and X axis of global coordinate system at DIP,PIP and MCP joint

θ_{PE_DIP}, θ_{PE_PIP}, θ_{PE_MCP}: angle between *PE* and X axis of global coordinate system at DIP, PIP and MCP joint

$\theta_{x\_RI\_MCP}$, $\theta_{y\_RI\_MCP}$, $\theta_{z\_RI\_MCP}$: angles between *RI* and the X,Y,Z axes of the global coordinate system at MCP joint

$\theta_{x\_UI\_MCP}$, $\theta_{y\_UI\_MCP}$, $\theta_{z\_UI\_MCP}$: angles between *UI* and the X,Y,Z axes of the global coordinate system at MCP joint

θ_{FDP_DIP}, θ_{FDP_PIP}, θ_{FDP_MCP}: angle between *FDP* and X axis of global coordinate system at DIP, PIP and MCP joint

θ_{TE_DIP}: angle between TE and X axis of global coordinate system at DIP joint

θ_{ES_PIP}: angle between ES and X axis of global coordinate system at PIP joint

θ_{LE_MCP}: angle between LE and X axis of global coordinate system at MCP joint

$\theta_{x\_UB\_PIP}$, $\theta_{y\_UB\_PIP}$, $\theta_{z\_UB\_PIP}$: angles between UB and the X,Y,Z axes of the global coordinate system at PIP joint

$\theta_{x\_RB\_PIP}$, $\theta_{y\_RB\_PIP}$, $\theta_{z\_RB\_PIP}$: angles between RB and the X,Y,Z axes of the global coordinate system at PIP joint

$\theta_{x\_LU\_MCP}$, $\theta_{y\_LU\_MCP}$, $\theta_{z\_LU\_MCP}$: angles between LU and the X,Y,Z axes of the global coordinate system at MCP joint

l_1, l_2, l_3: phalangeal lengths

P_x, P_y, P_z: measured fingertip forces

Ethics Statement

This study was approved by Manchester University's Institutional Review Board, and the subjects provided written informed consent to participate in the experimental work.

Static pressing measurements

The experimental work involved six male subjects (age: 26±1years, weight: 75.8±8.1 kg, height: 174±4 cm) recruited from the University's population of postgraduate students. The subjects were instructed to press the force plate surface using their index finger for approximately 3 seconds using maximum voluntary isometric force (see Figure 2), while other parts of the body were not allowed to touch the force plate. Four different finger postures were adopted during static pressing, ranging from very flexed to fully extended (see Figure 3). Each experimental condition was measured ten times. Motion data were recorded at 200 Hz using a six-camera motion analysis system (Vicon, Oxford, UK) and the 3D external force acting on the fingertip was recorded at 1000 Hz using a force plate (Kistler, Switzerland). Referring to Figure 3, to capture finger motion, five semi-reflective markers of 8 mm diameter were attached to the distal phalange dorsal head (Marker01), middle phalange dorsal head (Marker02), proximal phalange dorsal head (Marker03), metacarpal bone dorsal head (Marker04), and metacarpal bone dorsal base (Marker05).

The raw marker data were processed using bespoke programs written in Matlab (Mathworks, MA, USA). All trials with more than 10 consecutive missing frames were discarded. After fill-gap processing, the data were filtered using a low-pass zero-lag fourth-order Butterworth digital filter with a cut-off frequency of 6.0 Hz. For both marker and force plate records, only the data in the middle of the trials was used when the subject had reached a steady isometric pressing condition. After data processing, the measured 3D external fingertip load P (P_x, P_y, P_z) and phalange angles ($\theta_1,\theta_2,\theta_3,\theta_4$) at a representative instant in time were used for the following biomechanical force analyses.

Minimal model without extensor mechanism

To represent the index finger musculoskeletal structure without the extensor mechanism, a simple 3D multi-segment model was constructed by scaling a standard finger model provided in the OpenSim biomechanical simulation environment [28]. The geometry of the digital bones was extracted from the OpenSim software and all other geometry (e.g. muscle insertion, origin positions etc.) was defined by referring to the Primal Pictures 3D anatomical software (Primal Picture Ltd., London, UK) and the literature [12]. The model consists of four segments, namely the distal, middle and proximal phalanxes, and the metacarpal bone, and three joints, namely the DIP, PIP and MCP. Both the DIP and PIP were modelled as hinge joints, each with 1 degree of freedom (DoF), and the MCP was modelled as a saddle joint with 2 DoF (see Figure 4). For this 4-DoF multi-segment system, a minimum of four muscles are needed to balance the external load during static pressing. Referring to Figure 4, a primary extensor (PE) was included to represent the combined action of the extensor muscles (mainly the long extensor) spanning the three joints. A primary flexor (PF) was used to represent the action of the flexor muscles (mainly the FDP and FDS). Two lateral muscles (UI and RI) are included on each side of the finger. This is analysed as a statically determinate system at equilibrium with the required minimum number of muscles. The force and moment equilibrium equations were derived as follows for each of the three joints (DIP, PIP and MCP respectively)

$$\begin{cases} F_{PE}\cos\theta_{PE\_DIP}+F_{PF}\cos\theta_{PF\_DIP}-F_{x\_DIP}+P_x=0 \\ F_{PE}\sin\theta_{PE\_DIP}+F_{PF}\sin\theta_{PF\_DIP}-F_{y\_DIP}+P_y=0 \\ -F_{z\_DIP}+P_z=0 \\ -F_{PE}a_{PE\_DIP\_FL}-P_y l_1\cos\theta_1+F_{PF}a_{PF\_DIP\_FL}+P_x l_1\sin\theta_1=0 \end{cases} \quad (1)$$

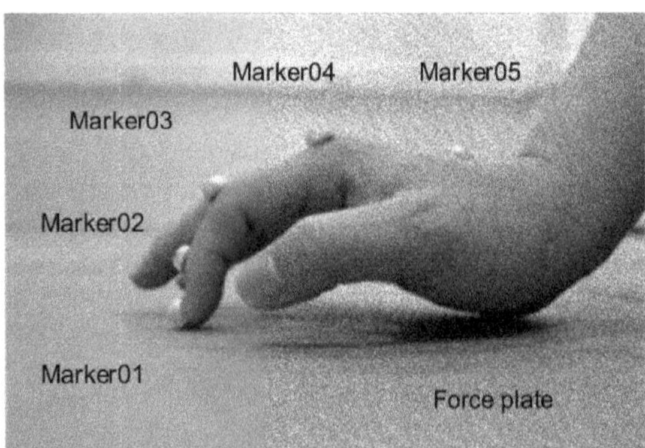

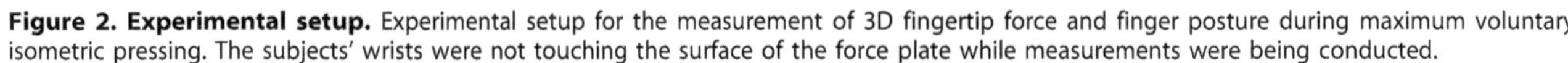

Figure 2. Experimental setup. Experimental setup for the measurement of 3D fingertip force and finger posture during maximum voluntary isometric pressing. The subjects' wrists were not touching the surface of the force plate while measurements were being conducted.

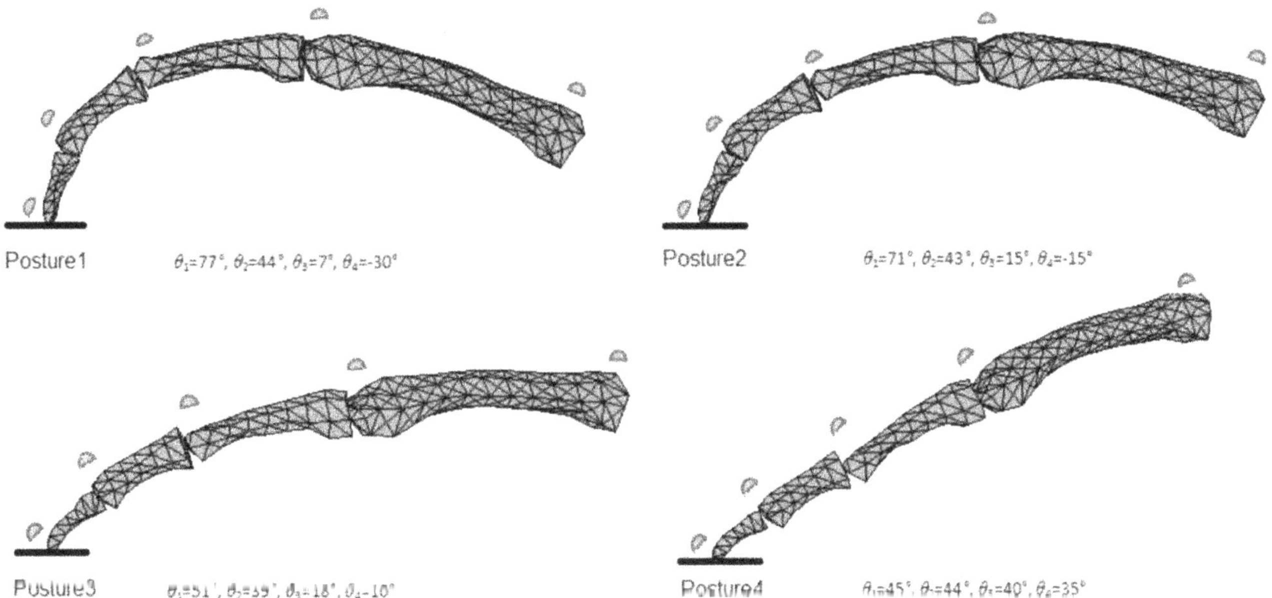

Figure 3. The four finger pressing postures. The four pressing postures, varying from flexed to fully extended, used in the experimental work. The segmental angles (θ_1, θ_2, θ_3, θ_4) are defined in Figure 4.

$$\begin{cases} F_{PE}\cos\theta_{PE\_PIP}+F_{PF}\cos\theta_{PF\_PIP}-F_{x\_PIP}+P_x=0 \\ F_{PE}\sin\theta_{PE\_PIP}+F_{PF}\sin\theta_{PF\_PIP}-F_{y\_PIP}+P_y=0 \\ -F_{z\_PIP}+P_z=0 \\ -F_{PE}a_{PE\_PIP\_FL}-P_y(l_1\cos\theta_1+l_2\cos\theta_2)+F_{PF}a_{PF\_PIP\_FL} \\ +P_x(l_1\sin\theta_1+l_2\sin\theta_2)=0 \end{cases} \tag{2}$$

$$\begin{cases} F_{PE}\cos\theta_{PE\_MCP}+F_{PF}\cos\theta_{PF\_MCP}+F_{RI}\cos\theta_{x\_RI\_MCP}+ \\ F_{UI}\cos\theta_{x\_UI\_MCP}-F_{x\_MCP}+P_x=0 \\ F_{PE}\sin\theta_{PE\_MCP}+F_{PF}\sin\theta_{PF\_MCP}+F_{RI}\cos\theta_{y\_RI\_MCP}+ \\ F_{UI}\cos\theta_{y\_UI\_MCP}-F_{y\_MCP}+P_y=0 \\ F_{RI}\cos\theta_{z\_RI\_MCP}+F_{UI}\cos\theta_{z\_UI\_MCP}-F_{z\_MCP}+P_z=0 \\ -F_{PE}a_{PE\_MCP\_FL}-P_y(l_1\cos\theta_1+l_2\cos\theta_2+l_3\cos\theta_3)+F_{PF}a_{PF\_MCP\_FL} \\ +F_{RI}a_{RI\_MCP\_FL}+F_{UI}a_{UI\_MCP\_FL}+ \\ P_x(l_1\sin\theta_1+l_2\sin\theta_2+l_3\sin\theta_3)=0 \\ F_{RI}a_{RI\_MCP\_AD}-F_{UI}a_{UI\_MCP\_AD}+P_z(l_1\cos\theta_1+l_2\cos\theta_2+l_3\cos\theta_3)=0 \end{cases} \tag{3}$$

Where the various muscle and tendon forces ($F_{\text{identifier}}$), moment arms ($a_{\text{identifier}}$), angles ($\theta_{\text{identifier}}$), and segment lengths ($l_{\text{identifier}}$) are defined in the notation list.

Equations 1 to 3 result in a total of 13 equilibrium equations with 13 unknowns (4 muscle forces and 9 bone-to-bone contact forces at the 3 joints). Therefore, the system is statically determinate and all of the unknowns can be determined from the measured finger posture and fingertip load during static pressing.

Full model with extensor mechanism

To investigate the effect of the extensor mechanism, a second multi-segment finger model was developed that represents the extensor apparatus as an interconnected tendon network (see Figure 5). The model shares the same segments, joint configurations, and bone geometry as the minimal model but with additional muscles and tendons. Referring to Figure 5, the five muscles included are the *LE*, *FDP*, *RI*, *UI* and *LU*. As the major extensor, *LE* has a similar function to that of the *PE* muscle in the minimal model. As the major flexor, *FDP* has a similar function to that of the *PF* muscle in the minimal model. In order to represent the key structural features of the extensor mechanism, another muscle (*LU*) is added to the full model on the radial side in addition to the *RI* and *UI* muscles. The force and moment equilibrium equations were derived as follows for each of the three joints (DIP, PIP and MCP respectively).

$$\begin{cases} F_{TE}\cos(\theta_{TE\_DIP})+F_{FDP}\cos(\theta_{FDP\_DIP})-F_{x\_DIP}+P_x=0 \\ F_{TE}\sin(\theta_{TE\_DIP})+F_{FDP}\sin(\theta_{FDP\_DIP})-F_{y\_DIP}+P_y=0 \\ -F_{z\_DIP}+P_z=0 \\ -F_{TE}a_{TE\_DIP}+F_{FDP}a_{FDP\_DIP}+P_xl_1\sin\theta_1-P_yl_1\cos\theta_1=0 \end{cases} \tag{4}$$

$$\begin{cases} F_{ES}\cos(\theta_{ES\_PIP})+F_{FDP}\cos(\theta_{FDP\_PIP})+F_{UB}\cos(\theta_{x\_UB\_PIP}) \\ +F_{RB}\cos(\theta_{x\_UB\_PIP})-F_{x\_PIP}+P_x=0 \\ F_{ES}\sin(\theta_{ES\_PIP})+F_{FDP}\sin(\theta_{FDP\_PIP})+F_{UB}\cos(\theta_{y\_UB\_PIP}) \\ +F_{RB}\cos(\theta_{y\_UB\_PIP})-F_{y\_PIP}+P_y=0 \\ F_{UB}\cos(\theta_{z\_UB\_PIP})+F_{RB}\cos(\theta_{z\_RB\_PIP})-F_{z\_PIP}+P_z=0 \\ F_{FDP}a_{FDP\_PIP\_FL}-F_{ES}a_{ES\_PIP\_FL}-F_{UB}a_{UB\_PIP\_FL}-F_{RB}a_{RB\_PIP\_FL} \\ +P_x(l_1\sin\theta_1+l_2\sin\theta_2)-P_y(l_1\cos\theta_1+l_2\cos\theta_2)=0 \end{cases} \tag{5}$$

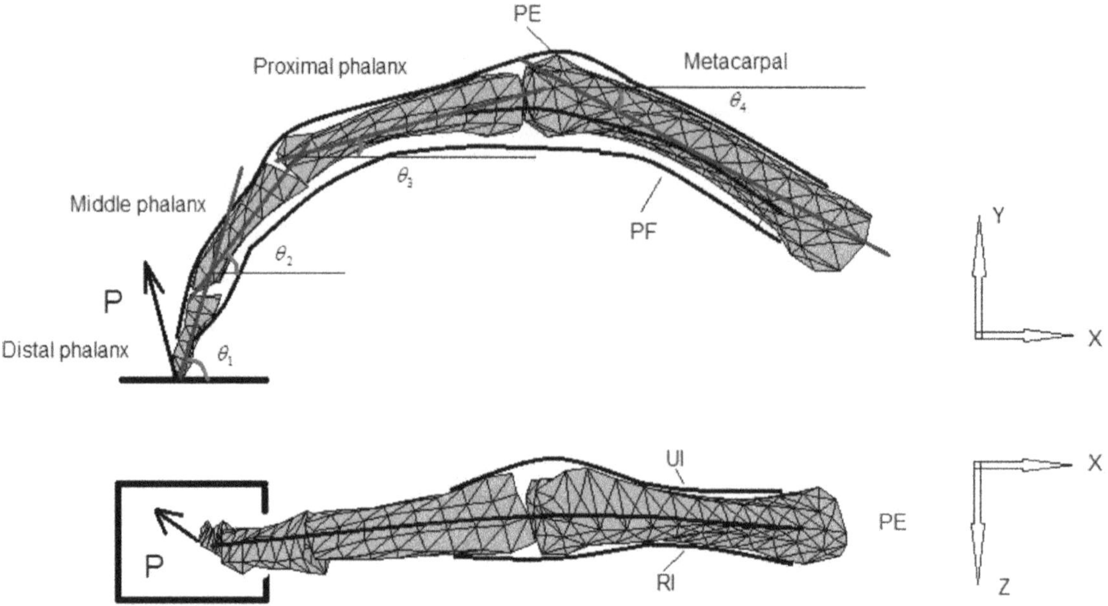

Figure 4. Minimal Model of the finger without extensor mechanism. Posterior (dorsal) and lateral (radial) views of the Minimal Model of the index finger without extensor mechanism. Four equivalent muscles (*PF, PE, UI, RI*) are considered to represent the actions of the finger flexor, extensor, lateral ulnar and lateral radial muscle groups respectively.

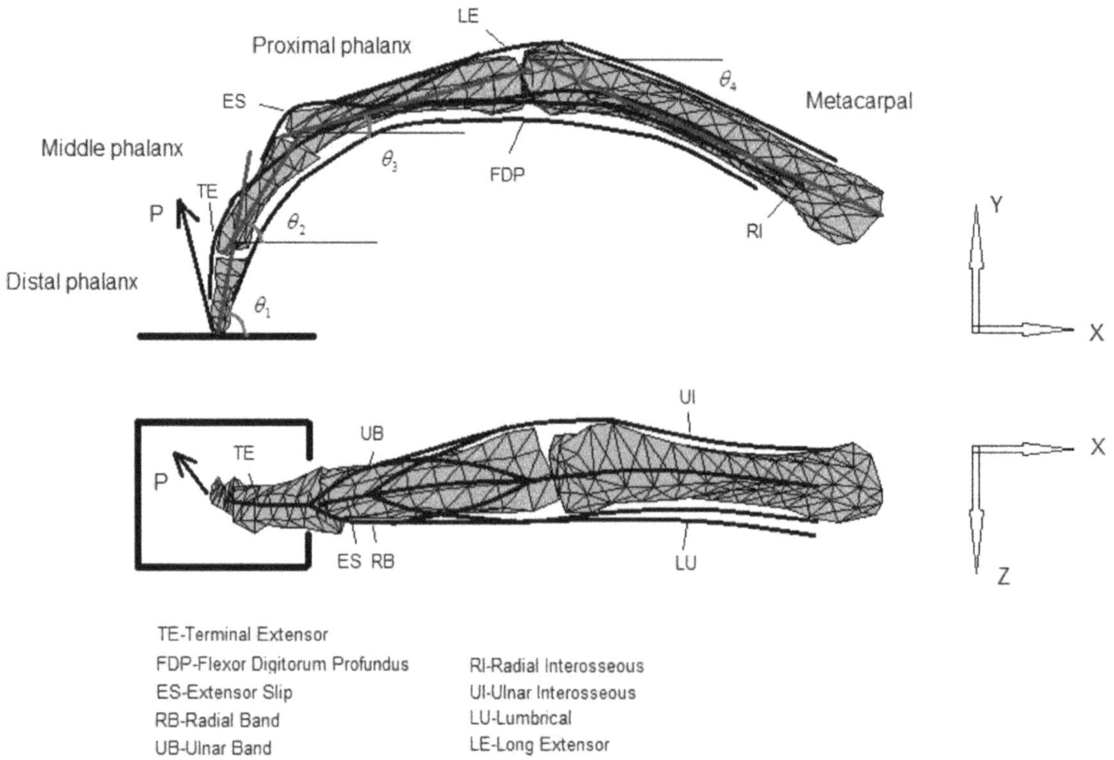

Figure 5. Full Model of the finger with extensor mechanism. Posterior (dorsal) and lateral (radial) views of the Full Model of the index finger with extensor mechanism (tendon network). In addition to the finger extensor muscle LE and flexor muscle FDP, the three major intrinsic muscles (*UI, RI* and *LU*) are included.

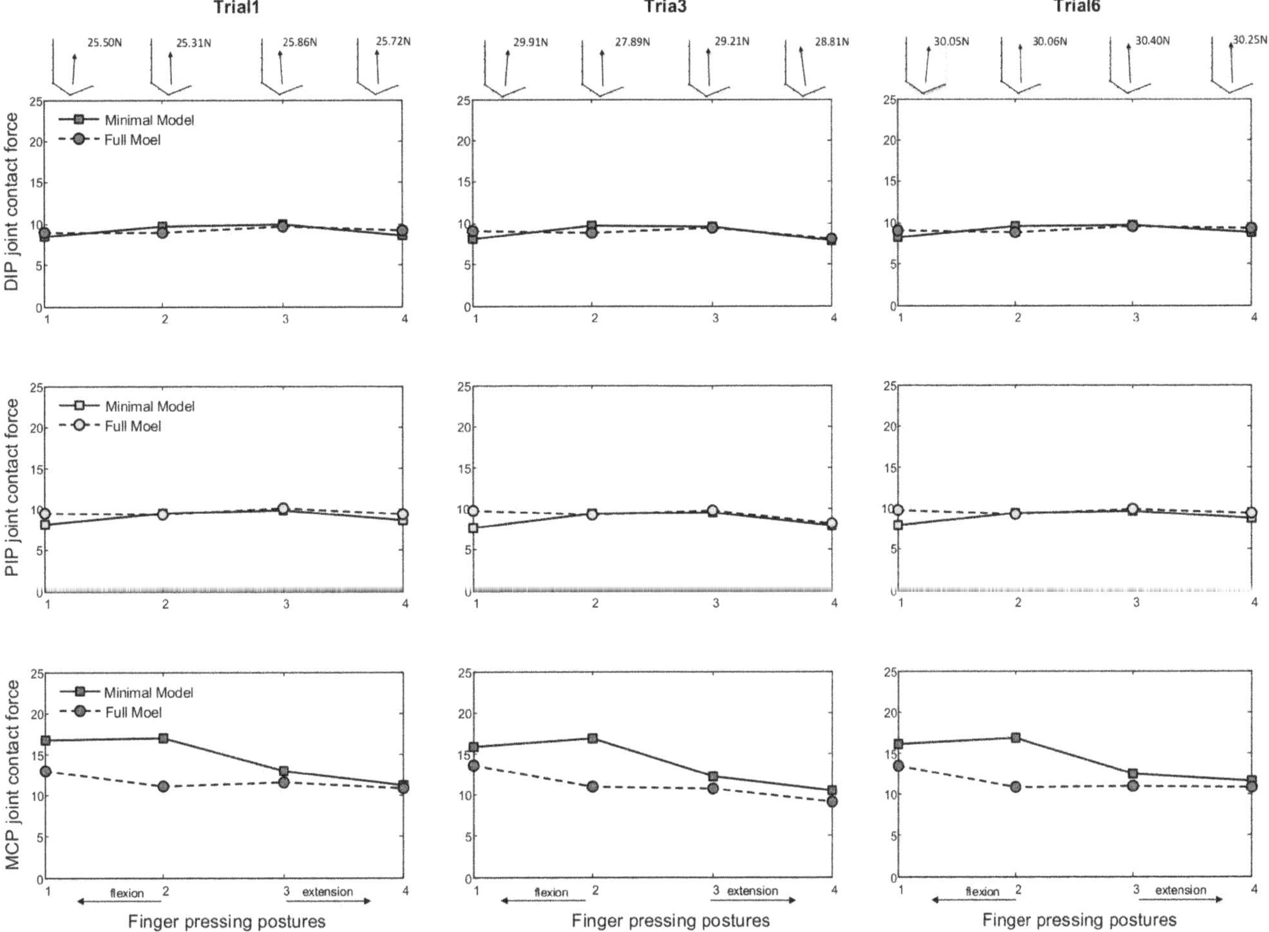

Figure 6. Bone-to-bone contact force calculation results. Calculated bone-to-bone contact forces (normalized by applied load) at the DIP, PIP and MCP joints obtained from both models for all finger postures. Based on measurement data from three typical trials (Trial 1, 3 and 6) for a representative subject (age: 25, weight: 75 kg, height: 1.72 m). The insets at the top show the measured 3D fingertip force vector for each posture.

$$
\begin{cases}
F_{LE}\cos(\theta_{LE\_MCP})+F_{FDP}\cos(\theta_{FDP\_MCP})+ \\
F_{RI}\cos(\theta_{x\_RI\_MCP})+F_{UI}\cos(\theta_{x\_UI\_MCP})+F_{LU}\cos(\theta_{x\_LU\_MCP})-F_{x\_MCP}+P_x=0 \\
F_{LE}\sin(\theta_{LE\_MCP})+F_{FDP}\sin(\theta_{FDP\_MCP})+ \\
F_{RI}\cos(\theta_{y\_RI\_MCP})+F_{UI}\cos(\theta_{y\_UI\_MCP})+F_{LU}\sin(\theta_{y\_LU\_MCP})-F_{y\_MCP}+P_y=0 \\
F_{RI}\cos(\theta_{z\_RI\_MCP})+F_{UI}\cos(\theta_{z\_UI\_MCP})+F_{LU}\cos(\theta_{z\_LU\_MCP})-F_{z\_MCP}+P_z=0 \\
F_{FDP}a_{FDP\_MCP\_FL}- \\
F_{LE}a_{LE\_MCP\_FL}+F_{RI}a_{RI\_MCP\_FL}+F_{UI}a_{UI\_MCP\_FL}+F_{LU}a_{LU\_MCP\_FL}+ \\
P_x(l_1\sin\theta_1+l_2\sin\theta_2+l_3\sin\theta_3)-P_y(l_1\cos\theta_1+l_2\cos\theta_2+l_3\cos\theta_3)=0 \\
F_{RI}a_{RI\_MCP\_AD}- \\
F_{UI}a_{UI\_MCP\_AD}+F_{LU}a_{LU\_MCP\_AD}+P_z(l_1\cos\theta_1+l_2\cos\theta_2+l_3\cos\theta_3)=0
\end{cases} \quad (6)
$$

Where the various muscle and tendon forces ($F_{\text{identifier}}$), moment arms ($a_{\text{identifier}}$), angles ($\theta_{\text{identifier}}$), and segment lengths ($l_{\text{identifier}}$) are defined in the notation list.

Equations 4-6 define a statically indeterminate system at equilibrium with 13 equations and 18 unknowns. To resolve the static indeterminacy problem, the equations below are included, which are based on previous anatomical studies and cadaveric testing [29]. These equations describe the empirical distribution of forces between the muscles (F_{RI}, F_{UI}, F_{LU}, F_{LE}) and the tendon components (F_{RB}, F_{UB}, F_{TE}, F_{ES}) of the extensor mechanism [30,31].

$$F_{RB}=2/3F_{LU}+1/6F_{LE} \quad (7)$$

$$F_{UB}=1/3F_{UI}+1/6F_{LE} \quad (8)$$

$$F_{TE}=F_{RB}+F_{UB} \quad (9)$$

$$F_{ES}=1/3F_{RI}+1/3F_{UI}+1/3F_{LU}+1/6F_{LE} \quad (10)$$

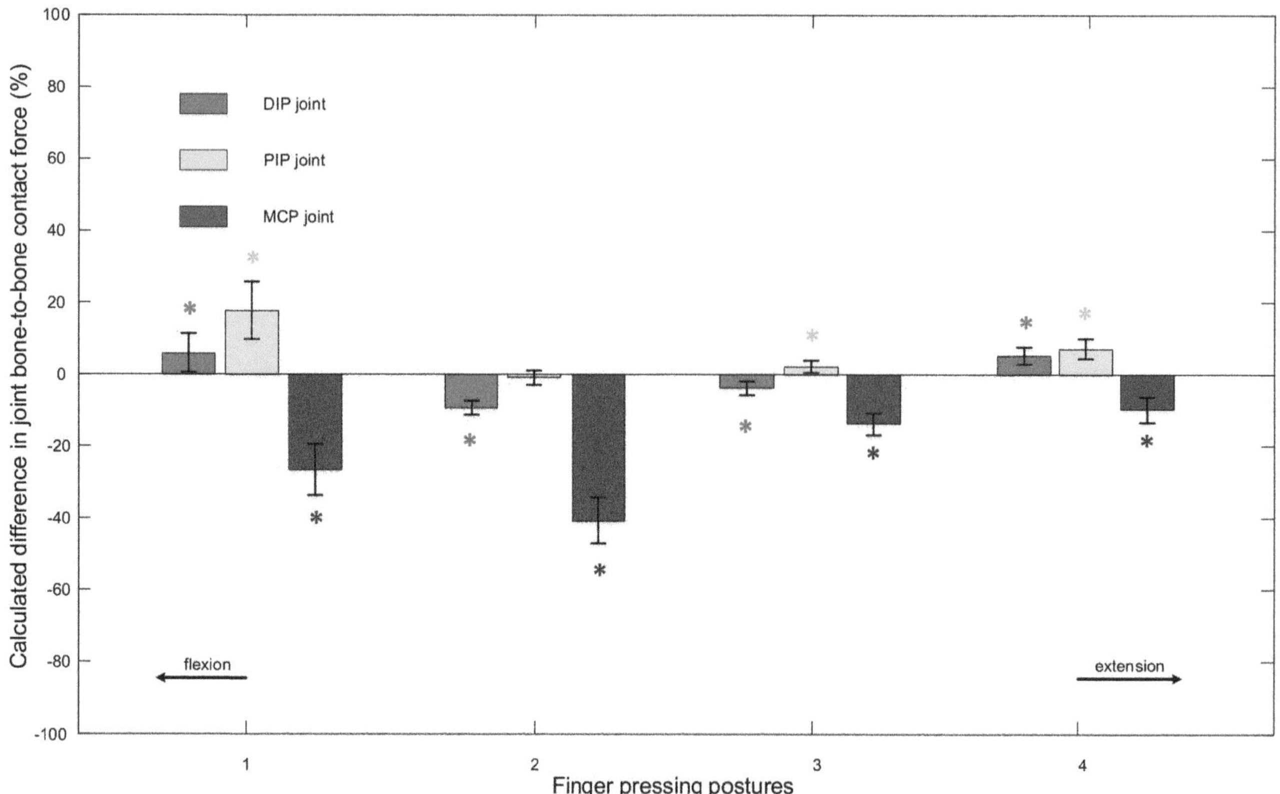

Figure 7. Percentage difference in bone-to-bone contact forces. The differences between the calculated bone-to-bone contact forces at the DIP, PIP and MCP joints obtained from the two models for all finger postures. The means and standard deviations were calculated across all trials and all subjects. A '*' indicates a significant difference between the results of the two models.

$$F_{LE} = F_{ES} \tag{11}$$

A more sophisticated optimisation based method could be employed to improve the solution of this statically indeterminate system [35–38]. However, finding an appropriate optimisation criterion may be challenging. Equations 4–11 can be used to solve for the bone-to-bone contact forces at all three joints and also the forces within the musculotendon network of the extensor mechanism for each measured finger posture and fingertip force.

Statistical analysis

All statistical analyses were conducted using SPSS 20.0 software (IBM, Armonk, NewYork, USA). The effects of finger model and posture on joint bone-to-bone contact forces and muscle forces were analysed using analysis of variance (ANOVA) with repeated measurements using a linear mixed model approach taking into account intra- and inter-subject variability. The different finger models and postures were the fixed effects, and subjects and trials were random effects. Differences between the two models and between each pair of postures were tested using Fisher's least significant difference (LSD) multiple comparison based on the least-squared means.

Table 1. Statistical analysis of results from the Minimal Model.

	Muscle forces				**Bone-to-bone contact forces**		
	F_{PE}	F_{PF}	F_{RI}	F_{UI}	F_{DIP}	F_{PIP}	F_{MCP}
Posture1	2.863 ± 0.571^a	5.150 ± 0.802^a	4.218 ± 0.892^a	4.121 ± 0.832^a	8.946 ± 0.998^a	8.641 ± 0.917^a	15.719 ± 1.921^a
Posture2	4.033 ± 1.110^b	8.293 ± 1.987^b	4.800 ± 1.378^b	7.437 ± 3.502^b	13.159 ± 2.562^b	12.879 ± 2.557^b	23.731 ± 6.568^b
Posture3	3.657 ± 1.024^c	8.817 ± 1.442^c	3.847 ± 1.156^c	7.059 ± 2.562^b	13.268 ± 1.777^b	13.032 ± 1.731^b	22.586 ± 4.840^b
Posture4	1.772 ± 0.613^d	7.565 ± 1.793^d	1.132 ± 0.259^d	2.375 ± 0.649^c	10.098 ± 2.164^c	10.092 ± 2.166^c	13.464 ± 2.797^c

Statistical analysis of the effect of finger posture on normalised muscle forces and joint bone-to-bone contact forces based on results from the Minimal Model. Values are means ± s.e.m. for all trials and all subjects. Identical letters indicate posture groups within a column do not differ significantly from each other ($p > 0.05$).

Table 2. Statistical analysis of results from the Full Model.

	Muscle forces				Bone-to-bone contact forces		
	F_{LE}	F_{FDP}	F_{RI}+F_{LU}	F_{UI}	F_{DIP}	F_{PIP}	F_{MCP}
Posture1	2.293±0.497[a]	4.992±0.932[a]	2.503±0.712[a]	2.287±0.788[a]	8.630±1.031[a]	9.028±1.348[a]	11.755±2.101[a]
Posture2	3.066±0.905[b]	7.999±2.308[b]	3.017±0.754[b]	3.066±1.598[b]	12.575±2.913[b]	13.693±3.502[b]	16.742±4.488[b]
Posture3	3.080±1.292[b]	8.671±1.498[c]	2.448±0.643[a]	3.075±1.287[b]	12.977±1.798[b]	14.025±2.173[b]	16.921±3.030[b]
Posture4	1.760±0.618[c]	7.446±1.728[d]	0.953±0.232[c]	1.294±0.446[c]	9.860±1.979[c]	10.064±2.041[c]	12.093±2.583[a]

Statistical analysis of the effect of finger posture on normalised muscle forces and joint bone-to-bone contact forces based on results from the Full Model. Values are means ± s.e.m. for all trials and all subjects. Identical letters indicate posture groups within a column do not differ significantly from each other (p>0.05).

Results

For all subjects, the measured finger joint angles (θ_1,θ_2,θ_3,θ_4) and fingertip forces (P_x, P_y, P_z) for each static pressing trial were used as inputs to both the minimal model and the full model. These models were implemented using bespoke programs written in Matlab (Mathworks, MA, USA). In this way, biomechanical analyses were conducted to assess the bone-to-bone contact forces at each joint and also the forces in the muscles and tendon components.

Figure 6 compares the calculated bone-to-bone contact forces at the DIP, PIP and MCP joints obtained from the two finger models, for all four pressing postures, using measurement data from three typical trials (Trial 1, 3, 6) for a representative subject (age: 25, weight: 75 kg, height: 1.72 m). The corresponding numerical data are presented in Tables S1 and S2. The DIP and

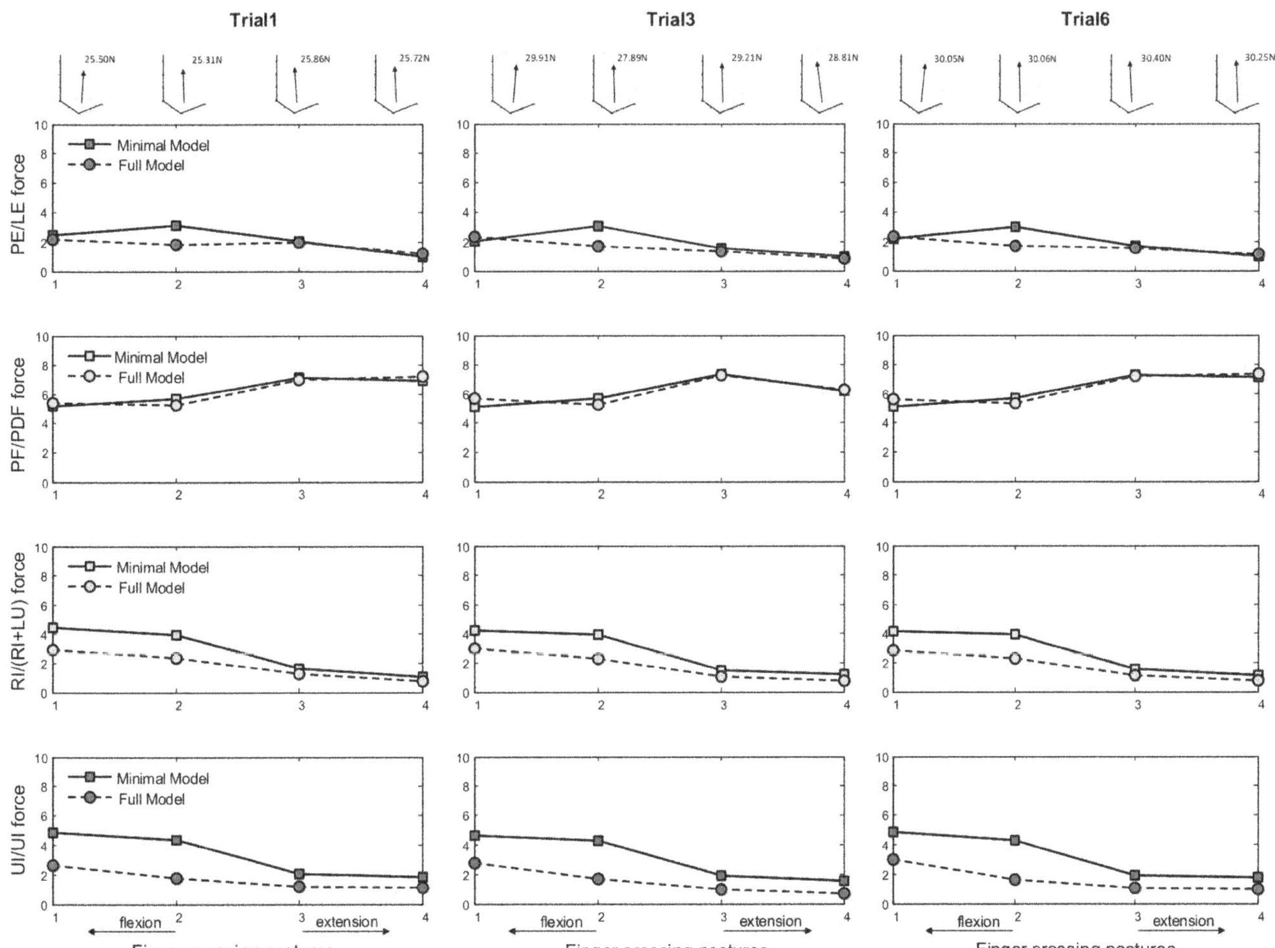

Figure 8. Muscle force calculation results. Calculated muscles forces (normalized by applied load) for the *PE* (*LE*), *PF* (*PDF*), *RI* (*RI+LU*) and *UI* muscles obtained from both models for all finger postures. Based on measurement data from three typical trials (Trial 1, 3 and 6) for a representative subject (age: 25, weight: 75 kg, height: 1.72 m). The insets at the top show the measured 3D fingertip force vector for each posture.

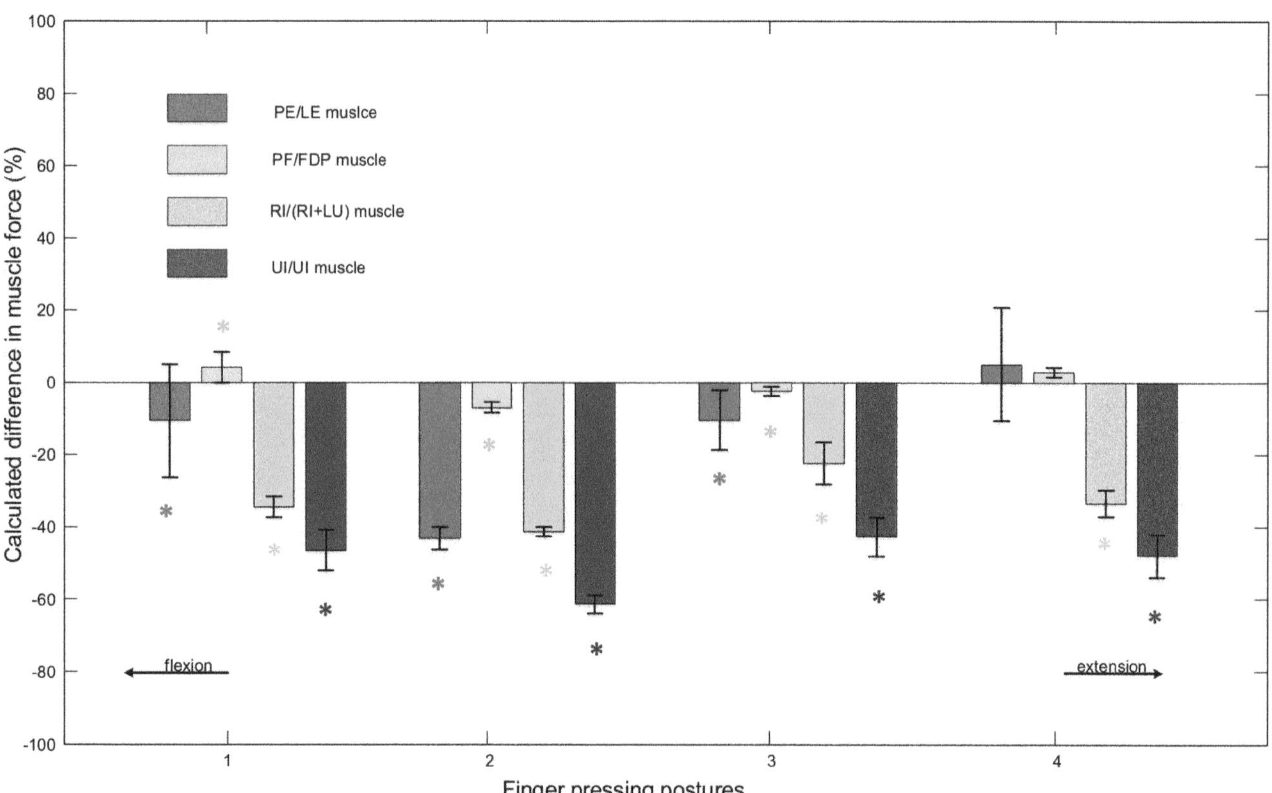

Figure 9. Percentage difference in muscle forces. The differences between the calculated muscle forces for the *PE* (*LE*), *PF* (*PDF*), *RI* (*RI+LU*) and UI muscles obtained from the two models for all finger postures. The means and standard deviations were calculated across all trials and all subjects. A '*' indicates a significant difference between the results of the two models.

PIP joint contact forces calculated by both models, normalized by the applied fingertip load, are in the range 7.7–9.8 for all finger postures. The MCP joint contact forces calculated by both models are in the range 10.5–17.0 times the applied fingertip load. This agrees well with the estimated contact force ranges for the index finger interphalangeal and metacarpal joints from previous studies for isometric key pinching [32]. However, it should be noted that, in this study, maximum voluntary isometric pressing was conducted on a large force plate surface, which differs slightly from key pinching. It can be seen from Figure 6 that both models show the MCP joint contact force increasing with more flexed postures. This is in general agreement with the posture-dependent pattern of MCP joint contact force reported by Harding et al. [21]. Comparing the joint contact forces generated by the minimal model and the full model in Figure 6, it appears that including the extensor mechanism does not have a significant effect on the calculated DIP and PIP joint contact forces. However, an appreciable effect can be observed on the calculated MCP joint contact force, where the full model predicts much lower values, especially in more flexed finger postures.

Figure 7 shows the percentage differences between the contact forces calculated by the full model and those calculated by the minimal model for each pressing posture (means and standard deviations across all trials and all subjects). This further supports the observation that including the extensor mechanism has a limited effect on the calculated DIP and PIP joint contact forces. With the exception of the PIP joint in the most flexed posture, the mean differences for the DIP and PIP joints are within ±9% and there is no consistent trend as the finger becomes more flexed or more extended. However, there is a consistent negative difference for the calculated MCP joint contact force across all finger postures (i.e. the full model produces lower force estimates). This difference becomes more pronounced when the finger becomes more flexed. For the two most flexed postures, mean decreases of 27% and 41% in estimated MCP contact force are obtained when the extensor mechanism is included. If the full model is assumed to be realistic, this suggests that the tendon network of the extensor mechanism might help to moderate the joint contact loads at the MCP during isometric pressing and hence may reduce the risk of injury or osteoarthritis [33,34].

In Figure 7, statistically significant differences ($p<0.05$) between models are labelled with a '*', which indicates that the mean bone-to-bone contact forces calculated by the two models differ significantly. With the exception of the PIP joint in posture 2, the differences between the results from the two models are all statistically significant (i.e. the calculated joint contact forces are significantly different when the extensor mechanism is included). Statistically significant differences between postures for both models are presented in Tables 1 and 2.

Figure 8 compares the calculated muscle forces obtained from the two finger models, for all four pressing postures, using measurement data from three typical trials (Trial 1, 3, 6) for a representative subject (age: 25, weight: 75 kg, height: 1.72 m). The corresponding numerical data are presented in Tables S1 and S2. The muscles from the two models are compared based on their anatomical functions, i.e. *PE* versus *LE* as extensors, *PF* versus *FDP* as flexors, *RI* versus *RI+LU* as lateral radial muscles and *UI* versus *UI* as lateral ulnar muscle. The range of muscle forces is approximately 1.2 to 7.0 times the applied fingertip load, which is in general agreement with the muscle force data reported in previous research on isometric pinching [30,32], which is similar to pressing on a flat surface. It can be seen from Figure 8 that posture-dependent trends are present for the *PF* or *FDP*, *RI* or *RI+LU* and *UI* muscles. The intrinsic muscle forces (*RI* or *RI+LU* and *UI*) increase with more flexed postures. However, the extrinsic flexor muscle (*PF* or *FDP*) shows decreasing force when the finger becomes more flexed. This is in a good agreement with the posture-dependent trends of the *FDP* muscle reported in the study by Weightman and Amis [20]. If the full model is assumed to be realistic, then the results from the two models suggest that the extensor mechanism may have a significant effect on the *RI+LU* and *UI* muscles for all finger postures. The full model, including the extensor mechanism, predicts much lower *RI+LU* and *UI* muscle forces than those predicted by the minimal model without the extensor mechanism.

Figure 9 shows the percentage differences between the muscle forces calculated by the full model and those calculated by the minimal model for each pressing posture (means and standard deviations across all trials and all subjects). It can be seen that the *RI+LU* and *UI* muscle forces are notably reduced when the extensor mechanism is included. The differences increase in magnitude with more flexed pressing postures, reaching 34% to 61% at the two most flexed postures. The differences are very small for the *PF* or *FDP* muscle forces. This agrees with the results obtained by Li et al. [23] who used simple 2D models without extensor forces to investigate the effect of fingertip load on flexor forces during isometric pressing with a fully extended finger. It can be seen from Figure 9 that mixed results are obtained for the *PE* or *LE* muscles. At postures 1, 3 and 4 the differences are small but at posture 2 there is a large negative difference (43%). In conclusion, if the full model is assumed to be realistic, the muscle force results suggest that the extensor mechanism helps to reduce the intrinsic muscle forces (*RI*, *LU* and *UI*), and this may also be the case for the extrinsic extensor muscles at moderately flexed postures.

In Figure 9, statistically significant differences ($p<0.05$) between models are labelled with a '*', which indicates that the mean muscle forces calculated by the two models differ significantly. With the exception of the *PE* (*LE*) and *PF* (*FDP*) in posture 4, the differences between the results from the two models are all statistically significant (i.e. the calculated muscle forces are significantly different when the extensor mechanism is included). Statistically significant differences between postures for both models are presented in Tables 1 and 2.

Discussion and Conclusion

By combining experimental measurement with biomechanical modelling, this study has investigated the calculated effects of the finger extensor mechanism on the contact forces at the interphalangeal and metacarpal joints and also on the forces exerted by the intrinsic and extrinsic muscles. If the full model is assumed to be realistic, then the results from the two models suggest some biomechanical advantages that may be provided by the tendon network of the extensor mechanism. The estimated forces in the intrinsic muscles (interosseus group and lumbrical) are significantly reduced by 22% to 61% when the extensor mechanism is included, especially in more flexed postures. The estimated contact force at the MCP joint is decreased by 10% to 41%, with larger reductions in more flexed postures, when the extensor mechanism is included. These effects may help to reduce the risk of injury at the finger joints and may also help to moderate the muscular effort required of the finger's intrinsic muscles.

The apparent biomechanical advantages provided by the finger extensor mechanism may be a result of its distinctive anatomical arrangement. The extensor apparatus surrounding the MCP joint receives muscle forces from the lumbricals (*LU*) and interossei (*RI* and *UI*). The contraction of these intrinsic muscles produces PIP and DIP extension by transmitting tension through the tendon network of the extensor mechanism (see Figures 1 and 5). The extensor slip (*ES*) attaches to the intermediate phalanx, where tension transmitted through the tendon network due to the intrinsic muscles extends the PIP joint. The lateral bands (radial band *RB* and ulnar band *UB*) on the dorsal side of the PIP joint merge over the dorsum of the intermediate phalanx, forming the terminal extensor (*TE*) slip, and insert into the distal phalanx, where the intrinsic muscle contraction leads to extension of the DIP joint. The tension generated by the contraction of the intrinsic muscles at the DIP and PIP joints tends to increase the force at the *FDP* muscle which further contributes to the flexion moment at the MCP joint, and thereby reduces the force demand imposed on the intrinsic muscles and hence moderates the bone-to-bone contact force at the MCP joint.

The biomechanical models used in this study have some limitations. The extensor apparatus is modelled as a tendon network with the individual tendon components represented by lines. However, in reality the finger extensor mechanism is a complex assembly of multi-directional fibres of varying viscoelastic properties. Three-dimensional solid mechanics models (e.g. based on the finite-element method) would be needed to better represent this interconnected fibrous structure in the future. To calculate the muscle and tendon forces in the full model, a set of empirical equations obtained from previous studies (Equations 7–11) was used to resolve the static indeterminacy problem. A more sophisticated optimisation based method could be employed to improve the solution of this statically indeterminate system of muscles and tendons [35–38]. However, finding an appropriate optimisation criterion may be challenging.

Supporting Information

Table S1 Calculation results from the Minimal Model. Force plate data and normalized calculation results from the Minimal Model for three typical trials (Trial 1, 3 and 6) with a representative subject (age: 25, weight: 75 kg, height: 1.72 m)

Table S2 Calculation results from the Full Model. Force plate data and normalized calculation results from the Full Model for three typical trials (Trial 1, 3 and 6) with a representative subject (age: 25, weight: 75 kg, height: 1.72 m)

Acknowledgments

Manxu Zheng's assistance with measurement data collection has been invaluable.

Author Contributions

Conceived and designed the experiments: LR D. Hu D. Howard. Performed the experiments: D. Hu LR. Analyzed the data: D. Hu. Contributed reagents/materials/analysis tools: D. Hu. Wrote the paper: D. Hu LR D. Howard.

References

1. Landsmeer JMF (1955) Anatomical and functional investigations on the articulation of the human fingers. Acta Anat Suppl 25: 1–69
2. Smith EM, Juvinall RC, Bender LF, Pearson JR (1964) Role of the finger flexors in Rheumatoid deformities of the metacarpophalangeal joints. Arthritis Rheum 7: 467–480
3. Cooney WP, Chao EY (1977) Biomechanical analysis of static forces in the thumb during hand function. J Bone Joint Surg 59: 27–36
4. Berme PW, Paul JP, Purves WK (1977) A biomechanical analysis of the metacarpophalangeal joint. J Biomech 10: 409–412
5. Fowler NK, Nicol AC (2000) Interphalangeal joint and tendon forces: normal model and biomechanical consequences of surgical reconstruction. J Biomech 33: 1055–1062
6. Eyler DL, Markee JE (1954) The anatomy and function of the intrinsic musculature of the fingers. J Bone Joint Surg (A) 36: 1–9
7. Landsmeer JMF (1961) Studies in the anatomy of articulation. 1. The equilibrium of the 'intercalated' bone. Acta Morph Neerl Scand 3: 287–303
8. Landsmeer JMF (1963) The coordination of finger-joint motions. J Bone Joint Surg 45: 1654–1662
9. Long C (1968) Intrinsic-extrinsic muscle control of the fingers. J Bone Joint Surg(A) 50: 973–984
10. Smith RJ (1974) Balance and kinetics of the finger under normal and pathological conditions. Clin Orthop Rel Res 104: 92–11
11. Ketchum LD, Thompson D, Pocock G, Wallingford D (1978) A clinical study of forces generated by the intrinsic muscles of the index finger and the extrinsic flexor and extensor muscles of the hand. J Hand Surg 3: 571–578
12. An KN, Chao EYS, Cooney WP, Linscheid RL (1979) Normative model of human hand for biomechanical analysis. J Biomech 12: 775–788
13. Darling WG, Cole KJ, Miller GF (1994) Coordination of index finger movements. J Biomech 12: 479–491
14. Dennerlein JT, Diao E, Mote CD, Rempel DM (1998) Tensions of the flexor digitorum superficialis are higher than a current model predicts. J Biomech 31: 295–301
15. Valero-Cuevas FJ, Zajac FE, Burgar CG (1998) Large index fingertip forces are produced by subject-independent patterns of muscle excitation. J Biomech 31: 693–703
16. Kursa K, Diao E, Lattanza L, Rempel D (2005) In vivo forces generated by finger flexor muscles do not depend on the rate of fingertip loading during an isometric task. J Biomech 38: 2288–2293
17. Garcia-Elias M, An KN, Berglund L, Linscheid RL, et al. (1991) Extensor mechanism of the fingers. I. A quantitative geometric study. J Hand Surg (A) 16: 1130–1136
18. Garcia-Elias M, An KN, Berglund L, Linscheid RL, et al. (1991) Extensor mechanism of the fingers. II. Tensile properties of components. J Hand Surg (A) 16: 1136–1140
19. Harris C, Rutledge AL (1972) The functional anatomy of the extensor mechanism of finger. J Bone Joint Surg (A) 54: 713–726
20. Weightman B, Amis AA (1982) Finger joint force predictions related to design of joint replacements. J Biomed Eng 4: 197–205
21. Harding DC, Brand KD, Hillberry BM (1993) Finger joint force minimization in pianists using optimization techniques. J Biomech 26: 1403–1412
22. Li ZM, Zatsiorsky VM, Latash ML (2000) Contribution of the extrinsic and intrinsic hand muscles to the moments in finger joints. Clin Biomech 15: 203–211
23. Li ZM, Zatsiorsky VM, Latash ML (2001) The effect of finger extensor mechanism on the flexor force during isometric tasks. J Biomech 34: 1097–1102
24. Lee SW, Chen H, Towles JD, Kamper DG (2008) Effect of finger posture on the tendon force distribution within the finger extensor mechanism. J Biomech Eng 130: 1–9
25. Vigouroux L, Quaine F, Labarre-Vila A, Amarantini D, Moutet F (2006) Estimation of finger muscle tendon tensions and pulley forces during specific sport-climbing grip techniques. J Biomech 39: 2583–2592
26. Valero-Cuevas FJ, Lipson H (2004) A computational Environment to simulate complex tendinous topologies. Proceedings of the 26th Annual International Conference of the IEEE EMBS, San Francisco, US
27. Valero-Cuevas FJ, Jae-Woong Y, Brown D, McNamara RV, Paul C (2007) The tendon network of the fingers performs anatomical computation at a macroscopic scale. IEEE Trans on Biomed Eng 54: 1161–1166
28. Scott LD, Frank CA, Allison SA, Peter L, Ayman H (2007) OpenSim: Open-source software to create and analyze dynamic simulations of movement. IEEE Trans Biomed Eng 54: 1940–1950
29. Chao EY, An KN (1978) Graphical interpretation of the solution to the redundant problem in biomechanics. J Biomech Eng 100: 159–167
30. Chao EY, Opgrance JD, Axmear FE (1976) Three-dimensional force analysis of finger joints in selected isometric hand functions. J Biomech 9: 387–396
31. Brook N, Mizrahi J, Shoham M, Dayan J (1995) A biomechanical model of index finger dynamics. Med Eng Phys 15: 54–63
32. An KN, Chao EYS, Cooney WP, Linscheid RL (1985) Forces in the normal and abnormal hand. J Orthop Res 3: 202–211
33. Kaab MJ, Ito K, Clark JM, Notzli HP (1998) Deformation of articular cartilage collagen structure under static and cyclic loading. J Orthop Res 16: 743–751
34. Arokoski JPA, Jurvelin JS, Vaatainen U, Helminen HJ (2000) Normal and pathological adaptions of articular cartilage to joint loading. Scand J Med Sci Sports 10: 186–198
35. Crowninshield RD, Brand RA (1981) A physiologically based criterion of muscle force prediction in locomotion. J Biomech 14:793–801
36. Sancho-Bru JL, Perez-Gonzalez A, Vergara-Monedero M, Giurintano D (2001) A 3-D dynamic model of human finger for studying free movements. J Biomech 34:1491–1500
37. Vigouroux L, Quaine F, Labarre-Vila A, Amarantini D, Moutet F (2007) Using EMG data to constrain optimization procedure improves finger tendon tension estimations during static fingertip force production. J Biomech 40:2846–2856
38. Fok KS, Chou SM (2010) Development of a finger biomechanical model and its considerations. J Biomech 43:701–713

13

Cross-Talk in Mechanomyographic Signals from the Forearm Muscles during Sub-Maximal to Maximal Isometric Grip Force

Md. Anamul Islam[1]*, Kenneth Sundaraj[1], R. Badlishah Ahmad[1], Sebastian Sundaraj[2], Nizam Uddin Ahamed[1], Md. Asraf Ali[1]

1 Al-Rehab Research Group, Universiti Malaysia Perlis (UniMAP), Arau, Perlis, Malaysia, **2** Medical Officer, Malaysian Ministry of Health, Klang, Selangor, Malaysia

Abstract

Purpose: This study aimed: i) to examine the relationship between the magnitude of cross-talk in mechanomyographic (MMG) signals generated by the extensor digitorum (ED), extensor carpi ulnaris (ECU), and flexor carpi ulnaris (FCU) muscles with the sub-maximal to maximal isometric grip force, and with the anthropometric parameters of the forearm, and ii) to quantify the distribution of the cross-talk in the MMG signal to determine if it appears due to the signal component of intramuscular pressure waves produced by the muscle fibers geometrical changes or due to the limb tremor.

Methods: Twenty, right-handed healthy men (mean ± SD: age = 26.7±3.83 y; height = 174.47±6.3 cm; mass = 72.79±14.36 kg) performed isometric muscle actions in 20% increment from 20% to 100% of the maximum voluntary isometric contraction (MVIC). During each muscle action, MMG signals generated by each muscle were detected using three separate accelerometers. The peak cross-correlations were used to quantify the cross-talk between two muscles.

Results: The magnitude of cross-talk in the MMG signals among the muscle groups ranged from, $R^2_{x,y}$ = 2.45–62.28%. Linear regression analysis showed that the magnitude of cross-talk increased linearly (r^2 = 0.857–0.90) with the levels of grip force for all the muscle groups. The amount of cross-talk showed weak positive and negative correlations (r^2 = 0.016–0.216) with the circumference and length of the forearm respectively, between the muscles at 100% MVIC. The cross-talk values significantly differed among the MMG signals due to: limb tremor (MMG_{TF}), slow firing motor unit fibers (MMG_{SF}) and fast firing motor unit fibers (MMG_{FF}) between the muscles at 100% MVIC ($p<0.05$, η^2 = 0.47–0.80).

Significance: The results of this study may be used to improve our understanding of the mechanics of the forearm muscles during different levels of the grip force.

Editor: François Hug, The University of Queensland, Australia

Funding: The authors have no support or funding to report.

Competing Interests: The authors have declared that no competing interests exist.

* E-mail: anamulsialm.phd@gmail.com

Introduction

Surface mechanomyography (MMG) is a non-invasive technique, which records low frequency skin surface vibration caused by muscle contraction and is considered to be the mechanical equivalent to surface electromyography (sEMG) [1]. The MMG signals are influenced by changes in muscle force and length, and the relationship may be further complicated by changes in force levels from sub-maximal to maximal isometric contractions [2]. Although the relationship between the force and MMG signal has been used for the assessment of the conditions of muscle function [3,4], some factors limit the applicability of the MMG technique for a comprehensive examination of muscle activity [5,6]. For example, the cross-talk that occurs between adjacent muscles is one of the more important concerns associated with both MMG [5,6] and sEMG techniques [7,8].

In the field of EMG and MMG, cross-talk refers to the contamination of the signal from the muscle of interest by the signal from another muscle or muscle group that is in close proximity [9]. Consequently, many studies have investigated the cross-talk of sEMG signals (e.g., [7,10,11]). However, very few studies [6,12] have analyzed cross-talk in MMG signals. Cramer *et al.* [12] quantified the cross-talk in MMG signals generated by the superficial quadriceps femoris muscles during maximal concentric and eccentric isokinetic muscle actions. In another study, Beck *et al.* [6] also examined cross-talk in MMG signals from the superficial quadriceps femoris muscles during sub-maximal to maximal muscle actions. These researchers [6] showed that the quadriceps femoris muscles generally provide independent activity and the exhibited cross-talk was inconsistent based on different levels of muscle action. However, these assessments may not be true for the forearm muscles because the forearm consists of many muscles in close proximity with varying degrees of common functions and because there is a relatively small area of the skin surface over these muscles for the placement of recording objects. Hence, it is expected that the forearm muscles will exhibit a higher

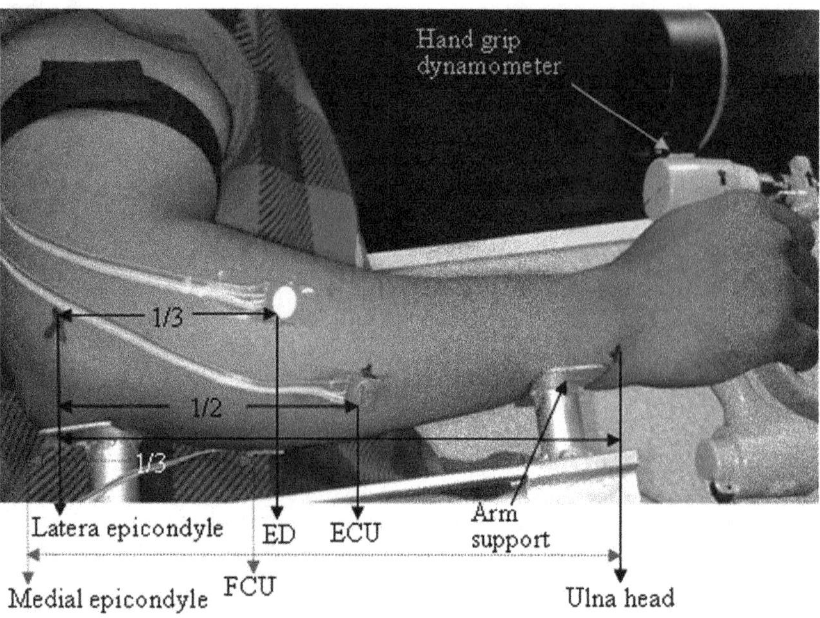

Figure 1. Schematic of an example for the placement of accelerometers used to detect the mechanomyography (MMG) signals from the bellies of extensor digitorum (ED), extensor carpi ulnaris (ECU) and flexor carpi ulnaris (FCU) muscles.

degree of cross-talk than the leg muscles. In addition, the physiological interpretation of a signal generated by the forearm muscle of interest is difficult [7,13].

To date, few studies have investigated the cross-talk in sEMG signals from the forearm muscles [7,10,11]. However, no study has carefully examined cross-talk with the MMG signal from the forearm muscles during different levels of muscle action. This is an important issue because the MMG signals are affected by muscle force, and this relationship is used in many applications [14], such as muscle function examination, prosthetic device control, and motor units control. Nonetheless, it is not clear whether the cross-talk in MMG signals changes in accordance with sub-maximal to maximal muscle actions of the grip force. Hypothetically, if cross-talk exists during muscle forces, then it should increase with the addition of muscle force because muscle activity increases with force. In addition, with an increment of force level the signal from each muscle becomes stronger.

However, the MMG signals due to the limb tremor need to be considered because the increasing force effort does not only transmit the tremor to nearby muscles but actually to the whole limb. For this reason a more precise evaluation of the MMG cross-talk need to be disclosed whether this cross-talk is the signal component due to intramuscular pressure waves produced by the motor unit fibers geometrical changes or due to the limb tremor. Under muscular contraction, mechanical vibrations occur due to three main processes [15]: (i) the inner muscular vibrations, which are the intrinsic components of the muscle contraction [16], (ii) oscillations of the human motor system, e.g. tremor and clonus [17], and (iii) artifacts. They are located in specific frequency ranges, with a certain amount of overlapping: most studies have used a filter with a 5 Hz high pass cutoff frequency to attenuate movement artifacts in MMG signals which is due to the influences of body and respiratory movements, as well as gross limb displacements [18]. The tremor frequency due to isometric contraction can go up to 12 Hz [19,20], and the mechanical inner vibrations effect falls in the range between 10 and 40 Hz due to intrinsic muscle fibers oscillations [2,16]. However, the entire frequency range of the MMG signal is widely defined between 5 and 100 Hz. It was hypothesized that the lower frequency band in the MMG signal refers to the firing rate of the slow twitching motor unit fibers whereas the higher frequency band of the signal displays the firing rate of the fast twitching motor unit fibers [21,22]. Therefore, these signals are defined as MMG_{TF}: the MMG signal due to tremor (5–12 Hz), MMG_{SF}: the MMG signal due to slow firing motor unit fibers (12–40 Hz) and MMG_{FF}: the MMG signal due to fast firing motor unit fibers (40–100 Hz) throughout the manuscript.

More importantly, the cross-talk in the MMG signals is not only dependent on just muscle effort but also on many other factors such as, the fiber composition, the distance between two muscles of interest, skin-fold thickness, and the level of activity of the two muscles [6,23]. However, no previous study has investigated the cross-talk effect on the MMG signals as a function of muscle length and circumference.

Therefore, the purpose of this study were: i) to examine the relationship between the magnitude of cross-talk in the MMG signals generated by the forearm muscles with the sub-maximal to maximal isometric muscle actions of the grip force, and with the length and circumference of the forearm, and ii) to quantify the distribution of the cross-talk in the MMG signal to determine if it appears due to the signal component of intramuscular pressure waves produced by the muscle fibers geometrical changes or due to the limb tremor. However, one marked challenge of this experimentation is the measure and quantification of cross-talk. Although the application of cross-correlation functions has been criticized in previous studies [24,25], it is currently the most powerful method for the quantification of cross-talk [6,26]. The peak correlation coefficients ($R_{x,y}$) at zero-phase shift are used as a cross-correlation function to quantify cross-talk. The cross-correlation coefficients which is the shared variance or percentage of common signal between two signals of adjacent muscle may be calculated by squaring the peak correlation to find the proportion of common signal ($R^2_{x,y}$ = % cross-talk) between two muscles [10,26].

Materials and Methods

Subjects

Twenty, healthy right-handed male volunteers (mean ± SD: age = 26.7±3.83 y; height = 174.47±6.3 cm; mass = 72.79±14.36 kg; length of the forearm = 26.95±1.47 cm; circumference of the forearm = 26.65±2.44 cm) gave written consent prior to their participation in this experiment after being fully informed of the purpose of the investigation and the experimental protocols. All of the participants were clinically healthy with no previous or ongoing records of neuromuscular or skeletomuscular disorders specific to the elbow, wrist, and/or finger joints.

Ethics

This study was approved (Ref No.: KKM/NIHSEP/P13-685) by the local Medical Research & Ethics Committee (MREC), Ministry of Health, Malaysia, and was performed in accordance with the principles of the Declaration of Helsinki.

Muscle contraction protocols

During the experiment, the subjects were seated comfortably on a chair with two adjustable arm supports attached to the chair arm. Each subject's forearm was placed on the arm supports with a neutral posture. The ulna bone positioned near the wrist and elbow (olecranon) joints was used to fix the arm supports at a height of 2 inches to ensure no contact pressure between the forearm muscles and the chair arm (Figure 1). Then the participants were requested to perform three trials of the maximum voluntary isometric contraction (MVIC) of the grip force. The participants were verbally encouraged to produce as much force as possible during each maximal trial. Each trial consisted of 6 s, and there was a resting period of 2 min between the trials. Of the three tests, the highest force was considered as the MVIC. After a resting period of 10 min, the participants were required to perform sub-maximal to maximal grip forces at approximately 20% increment of their maximum for 6 s each with a resting period of 2 min between the increments. The participants were shown visual feedback of the generated force and asked to maintain their force at the expected levels. The trials were repeated following the same resting period if any deviation of ±5% of their required forces was not achieved. All of the sub-maximal to maximal contractions was measured using a digital hand grip dynamometer (Digital Hand Dynamometer, SAEHAN Corporation, Korea). All of the muscle actions were performed at a joint angle of approximately 90° between the arm and the forearm. The distance between the medial epicondyle and distal head of ulna was considered as the length of the forearm. The circumference of the forearm was measured nearby the proximal part of the forearm, where the sensors were placed.

MMG measurements

Three accelerometers (ADXL335, Analog Devices, USA; full-scale range = ±3 g; typical frequency response = 0.5–500 Hz; sensitivity = 330 mV/g; size = 15 mm×15 mm×1.5 mm, including breakout board on which it was mounted; weight including wires and board <1.5 gram) were used to detect the MMG signals. The three accelerometers were attached on the skin surface over the muscle bellies of the ED, ECU, and FCU with double-sided adhesive tape. The anatomical position of each muscle belly was determined according to the anatomical guide for the electromyographer by Perotto 2005 [27] as follows: ED – one third of the distance from proximal end of a line from lateral epicondyle of humerus to distal head of ulna; ECU – just lateral to ulnar border on the half way of the distance between the lateral epicondyle of humerus and distal head of ulna; FCU – two fingerbreadths from the ulnar border on one third of the distance between the medial epicondyle of humerus and distal head of ulna (Figure 1).

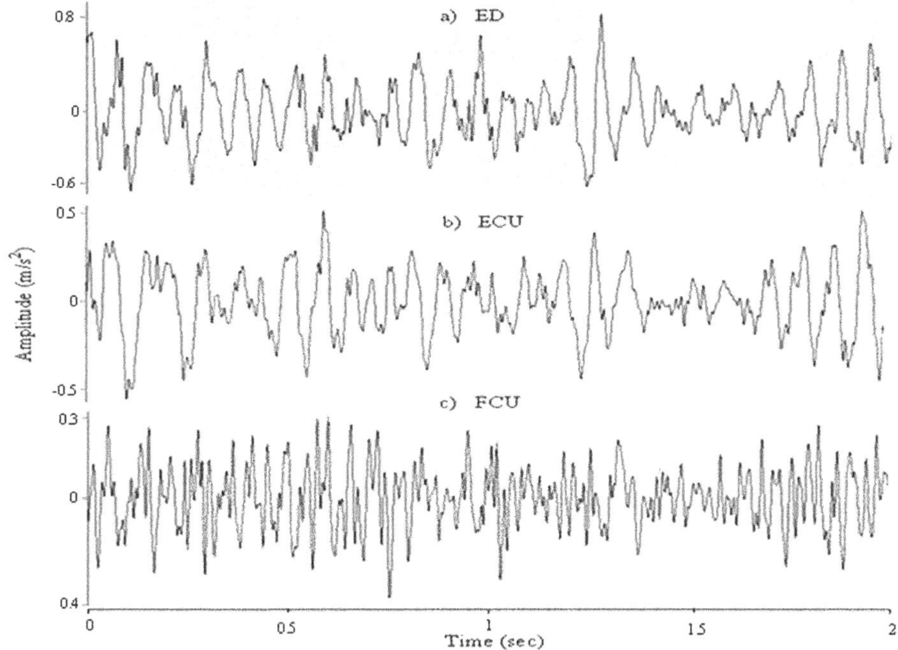

Figure 2. The mechanomyographic (MMG) signals from: a) extensor digitorum (ED), b) extensor carpi ulnaris (ECU), and c) flexor carpi ulnaris (FCU) muscles at 100% MVIC, which were used to analyze cross-talk.

Table 1. The magnitude of cross-talk in MMG signals between the ED and ECU muscle pairs for different levels of the grip force.

Subjects	% Cross-talk at different MVIC levels				
	20%	40%	60%	80%	100%
1	12.62	27.86	52.04	60.35	60.66
2	43.59	55.04	53.34	59.79	62.28
3	21.56	61.98	50.07	36.34	54.06
4	34.63	42.11	52.24	51.41	61.05
5	10.62	18.70	50.60	60.96	47.39
6	43.60	50.95	52.74	60.80	60.16
7	38.10	42.33	56.88	56.12	61.59
8	50.25	41.57	52.69	60.90	58.69
9	41.61	50.79	55.94	59.38	61.51
10	13.38	42.19	53.74	59.31	61.36
11	30.58	39.19	45.95	32.04	42.47
12	31.07	59.40	53.89	60.72	61.51
13	24.23	48.72	51.68	61.97	59.82
14	7.06	18.94	29.04	28.97	54.52
15	48.94	58.74	55.66	60.34	62.14
16	11.53	26.42	57.75	61.10	59.08
17	6.53	9.50	25.67	15.13	23.23
18	36.55	35.92	40.29	46.29	53.90
19	16.83	42.17	30.63	62.04	43.65
20	25.82	31.21	35.03	60.86	54.29

Table 2. The magnitude of cross-talk in MMG signals between the ECU and FCU muscle pairs for different levels of the grip force.

Subjects	% Cross-talk at different MVIC levels				
	20%	40%	60%	80%	100%
1	7.57	17.55	50.89	56.39	50.26
2	5.35	3.70	10.28	14.50	19.38
3	5.01	11.81	7.77	15.71	14.81
4	15.39	6.48	23.83	18.11	12.88
5	4.25	12.09	5.20	28.03	15.07
6	9.01	26.39	31.67	23.53	26.70
7	30.24	20.40	26.04	17.37	6.96
8	15.11	8.00	43.93	29.60	35.96
9	29.96	47.61	56.33	57.84	58.45
10	26.97	34.51	24.04	49.06	52.58
11	31.97	54.50	53.83	60.99	59.90
12	36.36	55.97	53.13	60.17	60.62
13	12.25	30.16	59.29	60.89	43.35
14	2.89	11.27	13.53	18.22	39.35
15	17.76	38.84	33.64	48.94	22.46
16	12.98	18.38	27.64	52.61	43.78
17	9.62	15.17	6.40	14.37	6.30
18	15.11	39.37	17.78	27.45	44.87
19	4.11	6.69	7.91	7.44	10.16
20	14.83	24.91	28.11	49.45	47.24

Table 3. The magnitude of cross-talk in MMG signals between the ED and FCU muscle pairs for different levels of the grip force.

Subjects	% Cross-talk at different MVIC levels				
	20%	40%	60%	80%	100%
1	8.73	7.19	45.53	52.52	20.33
2	6.63	5.71	10.95	11.10	17.56
3	3.32	8.78	19.59	35.08	40.40
4	15.36	4.00	23.24	40.05	36.40
5	2.45	5.48	8.72	35.69	17.58
6	8.34	20.66	28.69	24.22	20.90
7	11.01	17.33	13.01	16.86	10.91
8	13.75	7.37	24.59	56.23	58.40
9	12.87	30.68	40.72	54.23	58.31
10	27.29	20.21	11.35	35.98	44.18
11	43.58	51.98	37.33	36.77	41.31
12	19.31	38.14	49.26	45.25	53.18
13	5.70	21.08	40.64	59.00	42.62
14	3.84	5.19	6.32	6.92	21.59
15	33.83	36.46	15.58	19.77	5.45
16	10.50	12.52	14.38	26.37	38.49
17	6.79	4.22	5.19	3.56	4.09
18	14.55	19.08	11.21	13.29	14.19
19	3.92	5.90	17.18	3.09	4.78
20	12.37	37.16	31.96	21.67	35.97

Data acquisition and signal processing

The outputs of each of the three sensors were connected to the data acquisition unit (NI cDAQ 9191 wireless device and NI 9205 module with 16-bit resolution at CMMR of 100 dB, National Instruments, Austin, TX, USA), which differentially recorded the raw data at a rate of 1000 samples/s and stored the data in a computer for subsequent analyses. The raw data were bandpass-filtered (fourth-order Butterworth) at 5–100 Hz to obtain the MMG signals. Each MMG signal during the MVIC was then further passband-filtered (fourth-order Butterworth) at 5–12 Hz, 12–40 Hz and 40–100 Hz to obtain the MMG_{TF}, MMG_{SF} and MMG_{FF} signals, respectively. The MMG signals were extracted for a 2-s period corresponding to the middle 33% of each 6-s muscle action. The 2-s segments for each MMG signal were used to perform the cross-correlation. The cross-correlation values of the two signals X_t and Y_t were determined according to the following equation:

$$R_{x,y}(\tau) = \frac{1}{a \times b \times w(\tau)} \sum_{n=0}^{N-1} X_t(n)\, Y_t(n+\tau)|;\; 1-N < \tau < M \qquad (1)$$

where $a = \sqrt{\sum_{n=0}^{N-1} X_t^2(n)}$, $b = \sqrt{\sum_{n=0}^{M-1} Y_t^2(n)}$, w is the weighting factor, M and N are the lengths of X_t and Y_t, respectively, and τ represents the time lag between the signals. The peak cross-correlation coefficients were squared to obtain the magnitude of the cross-talk, $R^2_{x,\,y}$ (common signal %) between the two MMG signals generated by different muscles in the muscle group. All of

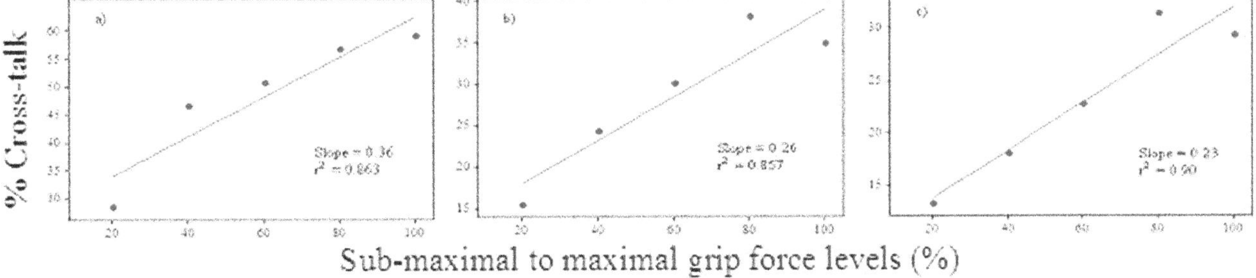

Figure 3. Correlation between the sub-maximal to maximal isometric contractions of the grip force and amount of the cross-talk (i.e., % common signal between two muscles) in the MMG signals between: a) ED and ECU, b) ECU and FCU, and c) FCU and ED muscle groups.

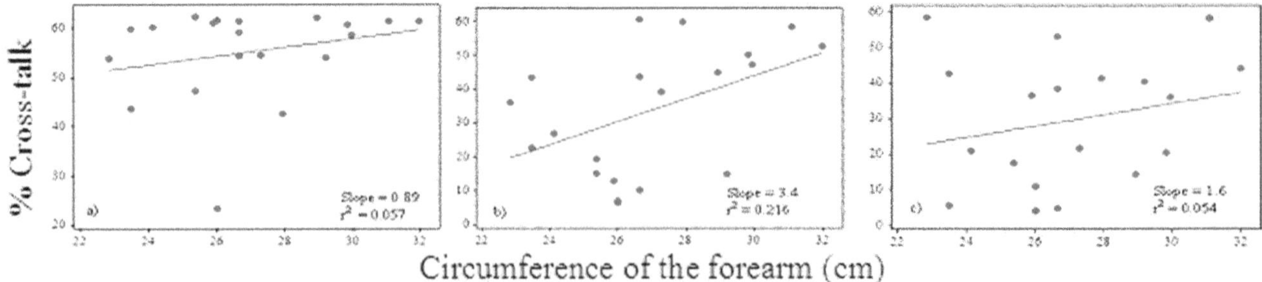

Figure 4. Correlation between circumference of the forearm and amount of the cross-talk in the MMG signals between: a) ED and ECU, b) ECU and FCU, and c) FCU and ED muscle groups at 100% MVIC.

the signal processing was performed with custom programs written in the LabVIEW programming software (version 12.0, National Instruments, Austin, TX, USA).

Data analysis

Linear regression was used to observe the relationship between different levels of the grip force and the cross-talk and between the anthropometric parameters of the forearm and the magnitude of cross-talk in the MMG signals. One-way Analysis of Variance (ANOVA) tests were used among the cross-talk values in the MMG signals between the muscle groups that were investigated. The statistical analyses were performed using Minitab (Minitab 14, Minitab Inc, PA, USA) and Microsoft Excel 2007 software tools. The critical value of F-ratio, $F_c = 3.15$ at a significance level of $\alpha = 0.05$ was affixed for statistical significant analysis. Therefore, any value of $p \leq 0.05$ was considered statistically significant.

Results

Figure 2 shows an example of the extracted MMG signals generated by the ED, ECU and FCU muscle groups at 100% MVIC for one subject. Tables 1–3 show the magnitude of cross-talk in the MMG signals between the ED and ECU, ECU and FCU, as well as FCU and ED muscle groups, which were obtained for each subject and each force level. The magnitude of the overall cross-talk in the MMG signals for all of the conditions ranged from $R^2_{x,\ y} = 2.45$–62.28%. There were strong positive correlations between the levels of the grip force and the magnitude of cross-talk in the MMG signals between the ED and ECU ($r^2 = 0.863$, m = 0.36), ECU and FCU ($r^2 = 0.857$, m = 0.26) and FCU and ED ($r^2 = 0.90$, m = 0.23) muscle groups; m representing slope in linear regression lines (Figure 3). There were weak positive correlations between the circumference of the forearm and the amount of cross-talk in the signals between the ED and ECU ($r^2 = 0.057$; m = 0.89), ECU and FCU ($r^2 = 0.216\%$; m = 3.4) as well as FCU and ED ($r^2 = 0.054$; m = 1.6) muscle groups during 100% MVIC (Figure 4). However, there were weak negative correlations between the length of the forearm and the amount of cross-talk in the signals between the ED and ECU ($r^2 = 0.067$; m = −1.7), ECU and FCU ($r^2 = 0.082\%$; m = −3.7) as well as FCU and ED ($r^2 = 0.016$; m = −1.5) muscle groups during 100% MVIC (Figure 5).

Tables 4–6 show the magnitude of the cross-talk in the MMG_{TF}, MMG_{SF} and MMG_{FF} signals generated by the muscle groups at 100% MVIC. The MMG_{TF} (range: 11.09–95.17%) and MMG_{FF} (range: 2.18–26.10%) signals showed higher and lower cross-talk values, respectively for all the muscle groups (Tables 4 and 6). The cross-talk (range: 6.12–66.24%) also occurred in the MMG_{SF} signals for all the muscle groups (Table 7). We also found that there were statistically significant differences in the cross-talk values among all the MMG signals due to tremor, slow and fast firing motor unit fibers for any of the muscle groups at 100% MVIC (Table 7) ($F = 113.44$, $p = 0.0001$, $\eta^2 = 0.80$ between the ED and ECU; $F = 30.74$, $p = 0.0001$, $\eta^2 = 0.52$ between the ECU and FCU; $F = 25.59$, $p = 0.0001$, $\eta^2 = 0.47$ between ED and FCU muscle groups).

Discussion

The present study quantified and correlated the magnitude of the cross-talk in MMG signals between the ED, ECU, and FCU muscles during the sub-maximal to maximal isometric muscle actions of the grip force. This study also examined the relationship between the amount of cross-talk in the MMG signals and the anthropometric parameters of the forearm during 100% MVIC. Furthermore, this study analyzed the cross-talk in the MMG

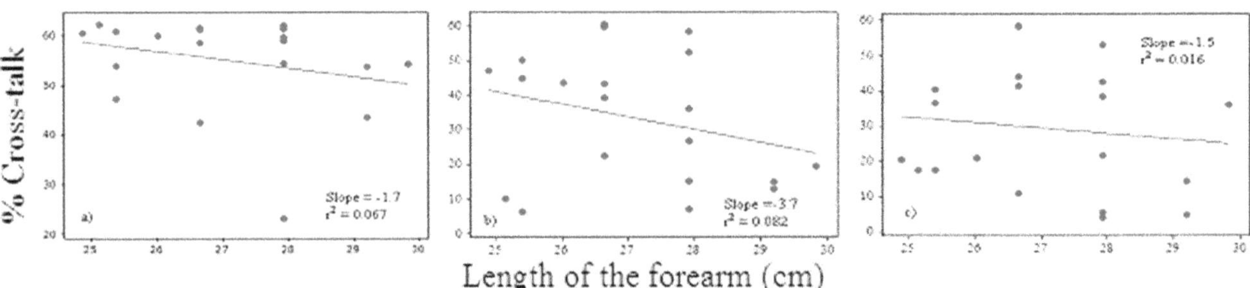

Figure 5. Correlation between length of the forearm and amount of the cross-talk in the MMG signals between: a) ED and ECU, b) ECU and FCU, and c) FCU and ED muscle groups at 100% MVIC.

Table 4. The magnitude of cross-talk in the MMG_{TF} signals between the muscle groups at 100% MVIC.

Subjects	% Cross-talk		
	ED-ECU	ECU-FCU	FCU-ED
1	80.27	56.48	21.09
2	87.59	37.33	44.68
3	84.19	62.08	33.15
4	84.60	11.09	23.08
5	80.71	46.94	48.25
6	90.59	34.69	21.93
7	76.68	25.84	18.19
8	94.30	88.63	81.58
9	22.93	86.92	26.60
10	53.13	14.70	19.26
11	85.78	92.77	69.78
12	95.17	88.74	81.69
13	67.08	90.99	56.78
14	89.19	84.33	78.30
15	86.13	59.61	68.26
16	67.40	58.68	21.04
17	76.25	62.76	29.96
18	73.31	18.44	14.25
19	91.34	80.82	76.71
20	78.09	27.81	26.22

Table 5. The magnitude of cross-talk in the MMG_{SF} signals between the muscle groups at 100% MVIC.

Subjects	% Cross-talk		
	ED-ECU	ECU-FCU	FCU-ED
1	64.56	51.26	24.54
2	64.28	6.16	6.44
3	37.50	6.30	23.63
4	66.24	20.16	41.27
5	55.70	19.07	23.03
6	57.24	24.38	9.92
7	50.27	27.16	25.75
8	53.95	54.08	21.41
9	31.09	65.50	19.96
10	16.56	8.62	32.20
11	58.28	61.87	50.23
12	63.61	49.89	42.88
13	37.25	66.13	40.72
14	65.89	63.39	53.10
15	57.17	22.98	22.67
16	31.17	52.50	14.90
17	64.57	50.34	36.63
18	14.65	8.94	6.12
19	49.19	40.19	31.00
20	35.54	18.55	9.83

signals due to the tremor, slow and fast firing motor unit fibers. In all of the measured cross-correlations, almost all of the peak coefficients appeared at a time shift of approximately 0 s (i.e., $\tau = 0$ s). Cross-talk was observed in the MMG signals generated by the forearm muscles for all of the conditions that were performed. The magnitude of cross-talk in the MMG signals ranged from, $R^2_{x,y} = 2.45\%$ to 62.28% considering all of the conditions that were performed (Tables 1–3). In addition, the cross-talk also appeared in all the MMG_{TF} (range: 11.09–95.17%), MMG_{SF} (range: 6.12–66.24%) and MMG_{FF} (range: 2.18–26.10%) signals between the muscle groups during 100% MVIC. This assessment supports the observation that the complete differentiation of muscle activities of the different forearm muscles is difficult [13]. This may be because there are more than ten individual muscles in the forearm, which act to flex and extend the phalanges and hand (e.g., extensor carpi radialis longus, extensor carpi radialis brevis, extensor carpi ulnaris, extensor pollicis brevis, flexor carpi ulnaris, and flexor pollicis longus). Together, these muscles may contribute to the MMG signals due to their close proximity and the small surface area to which the sensors were placed.

Despite the intricacy of association among studies because of diverse experimental conditions and cross-talk quantification indices, the magnitude of the cross-talk obtained in this study can be compared to the findings reported by Beck *et al.* [6] who found that the peak correlation coefficients between the superficial quadriceps femoris muscles ranged from 0.124 to 0.714 (i.e., 1.5 to 51% common signal) during sub-maximal to maximal isometric contractions. As expected, the forearm muscles experienced higher cross-talk compared with the quadriceps muscle groups because the forearm muscles are relatively smaller in size and thus closer in proximity which may be influenced to generate the greater cross-talk. Kong et al. [7] revealed that the amounts of cross-talk with sEMG generally ranged from 4 to 50% in the forearm flexors. In another study, Mogk and Keir [11] reported that the amount of cross-talk in sEMG signals were up to 64% for flexors and 58% for extensors during gripping tasks. The findings of these studies [7,11] may also be compared to the findings of the present study.

The present study also observed that there were strong positive correlations between the different levels of the grip force and the amount of cross-talk in the MMG signals between the between the ED and ECU, ECU and FCU, as well as FCU and ED muscle groups. The slopes for the cross-talk between the ED and ECU ($m = 0.36$), ECU and FCU ($m = 0.26$) as well as FCU and ED ($m = 0.23$) muscle groups indicate that an increment of 20% grip force also increased the amount of cross-talk by 7.2%, 5.2% and 4.6%, respectively. This assessment supports the findings reported by Solomonow *et al.* [28] who reported that the cross-talk with the wire EMG between the lateral gastrocnemius and tibialis anterior increased linearly during increasing force contraction from 10 to 100% of the maximal force. However, the findings of the present study is contrary to the findings reported by Beck *et al.* [6] who examined the quadriceps femoris muscles and described that "........., and the cross-correlation coefficients generally did not increase with isometric torque".

It can be pointed out that an increment of 20% force level refers to orderly recruitment of the motor unit in the MMG signals. Therefore, the results of this study have practical meaning, specifically in the application of MMG technique for the examination of motor control and muscle mechanics during various degrees of muscle action. Hence, the amount of cross-talk

Table 6. The magnitude of cross-talk in the MMG_{FF} signals between the muscle groups at 100% MVIC.

Subjects	% Cross-talk		
	ED-ECU	ECU-FCU	FCU-ED
1	16.17	8.24	10.70
2	5.30	11.96	3.05
3	3.11	4.71	2.18
4	2.97	12.19	6.61
5	10.47	3.95	3.81
6	13.17	6.47	4.30
7	26.10	5.11	5.15
8	16.24	3.75	4.85
9	17.72	8.51	5.08
10	4.86	3.72	3.59
11	3.87	3.46	2.98
12	3.69	4.47	4.67
13	6.19	3.50	3.78
14	7.57	7.36	6.12
15	12.21	3.09	5.29
16	19.81	6.71	19.88
17	4.00	3.76	3.41
18	5.73	5.73	6.23
19	25.55	6.87	6.09
20	14.85	5.12	7.15

needs to be accounted when different levels of the force measurement are of interest. Further, there were weak positive correlations between the circumference of the forearm and the amount of cross-talk in the MMG signals between the ED and ECU, ECU and FCU as well as FCU and ED muscle groups at 100% MVIC. This assessment is contrary to the finding reported by Yung and Wells [10], who stated that "Individuals with larger forearm would be expected to push the cross-correlations towards lower values while higher correlations would be seen in the smaller individuals". The results that the present study observed are possibly due to the fact that most of the forearms considered in this experiment were large due to larger musculature, which might produce larger cross-talk values instead of larger forearms due to higher levels of fat, which may attenuate the MMG signal and consequently produce smaller cross-talk values. However, there were weak negative correlations between the length of the forearm and the amount of cross-talk in the signals between the ED and ECU, ECU and FCU as well as FCU and ED muscle groups during 100% MVIC. The slopes indicate that 1 cm changes in the forearm length decreased the cross-talk values by 1.7%, 3.7% and 1.5% from the MMG signals between the ED and ECU, ECU and FCU and FCU and ED muscle groups respectively (Figure 5). This is possibly due to the fact that the muscle contraction originates from the proximal part and attenuates throughout the propagation path towards the distal end and is thus expected to lower the cross-talk values in longer forearms. It is interesting to point out that there are other factors such as muscle fibers composition, skin-fold thickness, and distance between the muscles of interest that may equally affect the MMG signal other than the size and length of the forearm [6,23].

We also found that there were statistically significant differences in the cross-talk values among the MMG_{TF}, MMG_{SF} and MMG_{FF} signals in the muscle groups at 100% MVIC. According to Cohen's interpretation of effect size for *F*-ratio statistics when $p \leq 0.05$, Eta Squared (η^2) is used to determine effect size: 0.01 = small, 0.06 = medium and 0.138 = large [29]. Thus, the present study observed a large effect size on the cross-talk values among the different bands of the MMG signals between the muscle groups at 100% MVIC (Table 7).

Post-hoc analysis was used to analyze the statistical significance of the cross-talk values between each individual groups of the three different band MMG signals (i.e., between the MMG_{TF} and MMG_{SF}; between the MMG_{SF} and MMG_{FF} and between the MMG_{TF} and MMG_{FF}). For all the cases the mean differences of the cross-talk values were much higher than the related standard error. Therefore, this study further confirmed that the amount of cross-talk significantly differed among the MMG_{TF}, MMG_{SF} and MMG_{FF} signals at 100% MVIC for all the muscle groups that were investigated.

The present study has several possible limitations. This study did not consider the skin-fold thickness of the forearm muscles, which cannot be ruled out because tissue thickness (e.g., subcutaneous fat, skin, and bone) influences the amount of cross-talk in both MMG and sEMG signals [23,28]. This study also did not consider muscle fatigue and/or stiffness due to repeatedly produced muscle force. It is expected that the rest breaks between trials performed in this study may reduce these effects. In addition,

Table 7. Statistical analysis of the mean cross-talk among the MMG_{TF}, MMG_{SF} and MMG_{FF} signals between the muscle groups at 100% MVIC.

Muscle pairs	MMG bands	Mean (SD)	Mean square	Standard error	*F*	*p*-value	Effect size, η^2
ED & ECU	MMG_{TF}	78.24 (16.61)	22732.70	4.48	113.44	0.0001	0.80
	MMG_{SF}	48.73 (16.43)					
	MMG_{FF}	10.98 (7.44)					
ECU & FCU	MMG_{TF}	56.48 (28.01)	12921.59	6.48	30.74	0.0001	0.52
	MMG_{SF}	35.87 (21.67)					
	MMG_{FF}	5.93 (2.66)					
ED & FCU	MMG_{TF}	43.04 (24.68)	6991.60	5.23	25.59	0.0001	0.47
	MMG_{SF}	26.81 (14.00)					
	MMG_{FF}	5.75 (3.83)					

the present study also used cross-correlation based index rather than amplitude based because the former is easier to use in practice, since it can quantify the amount of cross-talk between two muscles without collecting information of the contaminated signal. However, cross-correlation does not necessarily always mean cross-talk. There is evidence that the cross-correlation method being used to determine motor unit synchrony as common neural input between two muscles [30]. If two muscles receive common input and response similarly with the muscle action, then it is reasonable to expect that they would exhibit high cross-correlations instead of cross-talk. Therefore, cross-correlations can represent cross-talk, but it can also represent other mechanisms. It is also documented that both amplitude- and correlation-based indices were not statistically significant in the case of cross-talk magnitude quantification [25]. Therefore, the results of this study may be used in certain applications where precise measurements of motor unit control are essential, such as externally powered prosthetics.

Conclusions

In summary, the present study observed the following: First, the MMG signals generated by the forearm muscles exhibited cross-talk regardless of the levels of the grip force that were performed. The cross-talk also appeared in the MMG signals oscillated only by the muscle motor unit fibers regardless of the tremor signal. Thus, it can be concluded that MMG signals cannot be used to completely differentiate the activities of the forearm muscles during sub-maximal to maximal muscle contractions. Second, the magnitude of cross-talk in the MMG signals showed strong positive correlation with the different levels of the grip force for all the muscle groups that were examined. Therefore, the amount of cross-talk in the MMG signals needs to be accounted when the condition of muscle function measurements using different levels of the grip force from the forearm muscles are concerned. Third, the amount of cross-talk was also influenced by the circumference and length of the forearm for all the muscle groups. Therefore, anthropometric parameters of the forearm may influence the amount of cross-talk in the MMG signals. Further investigation is needed to determine the cross-talk effects on the MMG signals from different muscle groups using various types of static and dynamic muscle actions.

Acknowledgments

The authors would like to thank the participants for their efforts.

Author Contributions

Conceived and designed the experiments: MAI KS RBA. Performed the experiments: MAI SS MAA. Analyzed the data: MAI NUA. Wrote the paper: MAI KS.

References

1. Orizio C, Gobbo M (2006) Mechanomyography Wiley Encyclopedia of Biomedical Engineering. Brescia: John Wiley & Sons, Inc. pp. 1–23.
2. Orizio C, Perini R, Veicsteinas A (1989) Muscular sound and force relationship during isometric contraction in man. Eur J Appl Physiol Occup Physiol 58: 528–533.
3. Islam MA, Sundaraj K, Ahmad RB, Ahamed NU (2013) Mechanomyogram for Muscle Function Assessment: A Review. PLoS One 8: 11.
4. Beck TW (2010) Applications of Mechanomyography for examining muscle function. In: T. W. . Beck, editor editors. Technical aspects of surface mechanomyography. Kerala, India: Transworld Research Network.pp. 95–107.
5. Ebersole KT, Housh TJ, Johnson GO, Evetovich TK, Smith DB (2001) The mechanomyographic and electromyographic responses to passive leg extension movements. Isokinet Exerc Sci 9: 11–18.
6. Beck TW, DeFreitas JM, Stock MS (2010) An examination of cross-talk among surface mechanomyographic signals from the superficial quadriceps femoris muscles during isometric muscle actions. Hum Movement Sci 29: 165–171.
7. Kong YK, Hallbeck MS, Jung MC (2010) Crosstalk effect on surface electromyogram of the forearm flexors during a static grip task. J Electromyogr Kinesiol 20: 1223–1229.
8. Hagg GM, Milerad E (1997) Forearm extensor and flexor muscle exertion during simulated gripping work - an electromyographic study. Clin Biomech 12: 39–43.
9. Basmajian JV, De Luca CJ (1985) Muscles alive: Their functions revealed by electromyography. Baltimore: Lippincott Williams & Wilkins. 495 p.
10. Yung M, Wells RP (2013) Changes in muscle geometry during forearm pronation and supination and their relationships to EMG cross-correlation measures. J Electromyogr Kinesiol 23: 664–672.
11. Mogk JP, Keir PJ (2003) Crosstalk in surface electromyography of the proximal forearm during gripping tasks. J Electromyogr Kinesiol 13: 63–71.
12. Cramer JT, Housh TJ, Weir JP, Ebersole KT, Perry-Rana SR, et al. (2003) Cross-correlation analyses of mechanomyographic signals from the superficial quadriceps femoris muscles during concentric and eccentric isokinetic muscle actions. Electromyogr Clin Neurophysiol 43: 293–300.
13. Riek S, Carson RG, Wright A (2000) A new technique for the selective recording of extensor carpi radialis longus and brevis EMG. J Electromyogr Kinesiol 10: 249–253.
14. Islam MA, Sundaraj K, Ahmad RB, Ahamed NU, Ali MA (2013) Mechanomyography Sensor Development, Related Signal Processing, and Applications: A Systematic Review. IEEE Sens J 13: 2499–2516.
15. Tarata MT (2003) Mechanomyography versus electromyography, in monitoring the muscular fatigue. Biomed Eng Online 2: 3.
16. Barry DT (1992) Vibrations and sounds from evoked muscle twitches. Electromyogr Clin Neurophysiol 32: 35–40.
17. Iaizzo PA, Pozos RS (1992) Analysis of multiple EMG and acceleration signals of various record lengths as a means to study pathological and physiological oscillations. Electromyogr Clin Neurophysiol 32: 359–367.
18. Wee AS, Ashley RA (1989) Vibrations and sounds produced during sustained voluntary muscle contraction. Electromyogr Clin Neurophysiol 29: 333–337.
19. McAuley JH, Marsden CD (2000) Physiological and pathological tremors and rhythmic central motor control. Brain 123: 1545–1567.
20. Christakos CN, Papadimitriou NA, Erimaki S (2006) Parallel neuronal mechanisms underlying physiological force tremor in steady muscle contractions of humans. J Neurophysiol 95: 53–66.
21. Beck TW, Housh TJ, Johnson GO, Cramer JT, Weir JP, et al. (2007) Does the frequency content of the surface mechanomyographic signal reflect motor unit firing rates? A brief review. J Electromyogr Kinesiol 17: 1–13.
22. Boron WF, Boulpaep EL (2008) Medical Physiology. Elsevier Health Sciences.
23. Jaskolska A, Brzenczek W, Kisiel-Sajewicz K, Kawczynski A, Marusiak J, et al. (2004) The effect of skinfold on frequency of human muscle mechanomyogram. J Electromyogr Kinesiol 14: 217–225.
24. Lowery MM, Stoykov NS, Kuiken TA (2003) A simulation study to examine the use of cross-correlation as an estimate of surface EMG cross talk. J Appl Physiol 94: 1324–1334.
25. Farina D, Merletti R, Indino B, Nazzaro M, Pozzo M (2002) Surface EMG crosstalk between knee extensor muscles: experimental and model results. Muscle Nerve 26: 681–695.
26. Winter DA, Fuglevand AJ, Archer SE (1994) Crosstalk in surface electromyography: Theoretical and practical estimates. J Electromyogr Kinesiol 4: 15–26.
27. Perotto A, Delagi EF (2005) Anatomical Guide for the Electromyographer: The Limbs and Trunk. Charles C Thomas.
28. Solomonow M, Baratta R, Shoji H, D'Ambrosia R (1990) The EMG-force relationships of skeletal muscle; dependence on contraction rate, and motor units control strategy. Electromyogr Clin Neurophysiol 30: 141–152.
29. Cohen J (1988) Statistical Power Analysis for the Behavioral Sciences. In: J Cohen, editor editors. New Jersey: Lawrence Erlbaum Associates Inc. Hillsdale.
30. Keenan KG, Farina D, Meyer FG, Merletti R, Enoka RM (2007) Sensitivity of the cross-correlation between simulated surface EMGs for two muscles to detect motor unit synchronization. J Appl Physiol 102: 1193–1201.

Genetic Variations in the Androgen Receptor Are Associated with Steroid Concentrations and Anthropometrics but Not with Muscle Mass in Healthy Young Men

Hélène De Naeyer[1,2], Veerle Bogaert[1], Annelies De Spaey[1], Greet Roef[1], Sara Vandewalle[1], Wim Derave[2], Youri Taes[1], Jean-Marc Kaufman[1,3]*

1 Department of Endocrinology, Ghent University Hospital, Ghent, Belgium, **2** Department of Movement and Sport Sciences, Ghent University, Ghent, Belgium, **3** Unit for Osteoporosis and Metabolic bone diseases, Ghent University Hospital, Ghent, Belgium

Abstract

Objective: The relationship between serum testosterone (T) levels, muscle mass and muscle force in eugonadal men is incompletely understood. As polymorphisms in the androgen receptor (*AR*) gene cause differences in androgen sensitivity, no straightforward correlation can be observed between the interindividual variation in T levels and different phenotypes. Therefore, we aim to investigate the relationship between genetic variations in the *AR*, circulating androgens and muscle mass and function in young healthy male siblings.

Design: 677 men (25–45 years) were recruited in a cross-sectional, population-based sibling pair study.

Methods: Relations between genetic variation in the *AR* gene (CAGn, GGNn, SNPs), sex steroid levels (by LC-MS/MS), body composition (by DXA), muscle cross-sectional area (CSA) (by pQCT), muscle force (isokinetic peak torque, grip strength) and anthropometrics were studied using linear mixed-effect modelling.

Results: Muscle mass and force were highly heritable and related to age, physical activity, body composition and anthropometrics. Total T (TT) and free T (FT) levels were positively related to muscle CSA, whereas estradiol (E_2) and free E_2 (FE_2) concentrations were negatively associated with muscle force. Subjects with longer CAG repeat length had higher circulating TT, FT, and higher E_2 and FE_2 concentrations. Weak associations with TT and FT were found for the rs5965433 and rs5919392 SNP in the *AR*, whereas no association between GGN repeat polymorphism and T concentrations were found. Arm span and 2D:4D finger length ratio were inversely associated, whereas muscle mass and force were not associated with the number of CAG repeats.

Conclusions: Age, physical activity, body composition, sex steroid levels and anthropometrics are determinants of muscle mass and function in young men. Although the number of CAG repeats of the *AR* are related to sex steroid levels and anthropometrics, we have no evidence that these variations in the *AR* gene also affect muscle mass or function.

Editor: Joseph Devaney, Children's National Medical Center, Washington, United States of America

Funding: This study is supported by grants from the Research Foundation - Flanders (FWO-Vlaanderen grants #G.0332.02 and # G.0404.00) and an unrestricted grant from Roche and GSK Belgium. S.V. is holder of a PhD fellowship and Y.T. is holder of a postdoctoral fellowship from the Research Foundation Flanders (FWO) (http://www.fwo.be/). The funders had no role in study design, data collection and analysis, decision to publish, or preparation of the manuscript.

Competing Interests: The authors have declared that no competing interests exist.

* E-mail: Jean.Kaufman@ugent.be

Introduction

Skeletal muscle mass and function are highly heritable [1] and influenced by age, anthropometrics, sex steroid status and lifestyle-related factors [2–4]. The clinical relationship between androgens and muscle mass is well-described. Androgen deficiency (i.e. hypogonadism) leads to significant muscle loss and weakness [5], whereas testosterone (T) supplementation has dose-dependent anabolic effects [6,7]. Moreover, impaired steroid production or low androgen sensitivity could interfere with normal bone development and closure of the epiphyseal growth plates at the end of puberty.

However, the interrelationship between T levels, muscle mass and muscle force in eugonadal men is less clear [8]. Serum T levels are maintained at appropriate levels by the hypothalamic-pituitary-gonadal feedback loop. In healthy men, a large interindividual variation in serum T levels exists [9]. This between-subjects variability in T levels has been related to environmental conditions such as age, body mass index and smoking [10], and is considerably influenced by genetic factors [11,12]. The sensitivity to circulating T is determined in part by the transcriptional activity of the androgen receptor (*AR*). Polymorphisms in the *AR* gene have been described to alter this activity. We have previously shown that diminished androgen feedback, and consequently higher serum T concentrations, are associated with the CAG repeat length, and to a lesser extend with the GGN repeat length [9,13]. Furthermore, some single nucleotide polymorphisms (SNP) in the *AR* gene, resulting in an altered binding with cofactors, have been linked with the androgen insensitivity syndrome (AIS) [14–16] and could therefore affect androgen action and circulating androgen levels.

In order to gain more insight into the between subject variation in muscle mass in young healthy men, we investigated the relationship between androgens and muscle mass and function, as well as the influence of genetic components. We hypothesized that genetic variations in the *AR*, causing differences in androgen sensitivity, contribute to the variation in muscle mass in young healthy men.

Materials and Methods

Ethics statement

The study protocol was conducted according to the Helsinki Declaration and was approved by the ethical committee of the Ghent University Hospital. All participants gave their written informed consent and questionnaires about previous illness and medication use were completed. Physical activity was scored using the questionnaire as proposed by Baecke *et al.* [17].

Study design and population

This population-based cross-sectional study is part of a larger study, from which inclusion criteria and study design were described previously [18]. Participants were recruited from the population registries of 3 semi-rural to suburban communities around Ghent, Belgium. Men (n = 12446), 25–45 years of age were contacted by direct mailing, briefly describing the study purpose and asking if they had a brother within the same age range also willing to participate (maximal age difference between brothers was set at 12 yrs). The overall response rate was 30.2%. Finally, a sample of 768 young healthy men who fulfilled the primary inclusion criterion of having a brother within the same age range agreed to participate. After exclusions, 677 men in total were included in the study. Two hundred ninety six pairs of brothers (for a total of 592 men) were included in addition to 64 men as single participants, when their brother could not participate in the study; 19 men were included as third brother in a family and 2 as fourth brother. Exclusion criteria were defined as illnesses or medication use affecting body composition, hormone levels or bone metabolism.

Body composition and muscle strength

Body weight and anthropometrics (arm span, hand and finger length) were measured in light indoor clothing without shoes. Sternum height was measured using a wall-mounted Harpenden stadiometer (Holtain, Crymych, UK). Lean and fat mass of the whole body were measured using dual-energy x-ray absorptiometry (DXA) with a Hologic QDR-4500A device (software version 11.2.1; Hologic, Bedford, MA, USA). Isokinetic peak torque of biceps and quadriceps muscles was assessed at the dominant limbs using an isokinetic dynamometer (Biodex, New York, NY, USA). Grip strength at the dominant hand was measured using an adjustable hand-held standard grip device (JAMAR hand dynamometer; Sammons & Preston, Bolingbrook, IL, USA). Their maximum performance was assumed to best reflect the current status and the history of their musculoskeletal adaptation.

Cross-sectional muscle area

A peripheral quantitative computed tomography (pQCT) device (XCT-2000, software version 5.4; Stratec Medizintechnik, Pforzheim, Germany) was used to scan the dominant leg (tibia) and forearm (radius). Muscle cross-sectional area (CSA) was estimated using a threshold below water equivalent linear attenuation set at 0.22/cm. This threshold eliminated skin and fat mass with lower linear attenuation in the cross-sectional slice. From the remaining area, bone area was subtracted, revealing the muscle at its maximum CSA.

Biochemical determinations

Venous blood samples were obtained between 08:00 and 10:00 AM after overnight fasting. All serum samples were stored at −80°C until batch analysis. Serum total testosterone (TT) and estradiol (E_2) levels were determined by liquid chromatography tandem mass spectrometry (LC-MS/MS) (AB Sciex 5500 triple-quadrupole mass spectrometer; AB Sciex, Toronto, Canada). Serum limit of quantification was <0.5 pg/mL (1.9 pmol/L) for E_2 and 1.2 ng/dL for T. The interassay coefficients of variation (CV) were 4.0% at 21 pg/mL (77 pmol/L) for E_2, and 8.3% at 36.7 ng/dL and 3.1% at 307.8 ng/dL for T [19]. Commercial radioimmunoassays were used to determine serum levels of sex hormone binding globulin (SHBG) (Orion Diagnostica, Espoo, Finland), luteinizing hormone (LH) and follicle-stimulating hormone (FSH) (ECLIA; Roche Diagnostics, Mannheim, Germany). Free testosterone (FT) and free estradiol (FE_2) concentrations were calculated from serum TT, E_2, SHBG and albumin concentrations using a previously validated equation derived from the mass action law [20,21].

Genotyping of the androgen receptor

Genomic DNA was extracted from EDTA-treated blood using a commercial kit (Puregene kit; Gentra Systems, Minneapolis, MN, USA). The CAG and GGN repeats were determined as previously described [13].

Genotyping data for the AR gene for the Caucasian CEPH population was downloaded from the International Haplotype Mapping Project web site (http://www.hapmap.org) and the data was incorporated into the Haploview program [22]. The tagger function within Haploview was used to assign Tag SNPs. The tagging SNPs were chosen, by aggressive tagging (use 2- or 3-marker haplotypes), to capture the variations within the gene and the surrounding area with minor allele frequency (MAF) 0.01 and a minimum r^2 of 0.80 (for their location and the SNPs which they tag). For the SNP analyses, SNPlex [23] was carried out on fragmented gDNA at a final concentration of 25 ng/µl (total volume of 9 µl). Samples were run on an ABI 3730xl DNA Analyzer (Applied Biosystems, Foster City, CA, USA) and data were analysed using Gene Mapper v. 3.7 software (Applied Biosystems). Genotype analysis was performed based on the SNPlex_Rules_3730 method following the factory default rules. Missing genotypes in the SNPlex analysis were obtained using TagMan Pre-Designed SNP Genotyping Assays® (Applied Biosystems) which were run on the StepOne System (Applied Biosystems). In total, 5 SNPs of the AR gene were genotyped.

Statistics

Descriptives are expressed as mean ± standard deviation or median [1st–3rd quartile] when criteria for normality were not fulfilled (Kolmogorov-Smirnov) and variables were log-transformed in subsequent linear models. Linear mixed-effects modelling with random intercepts and a simple residual correlation structure was used to study the effect of anthropometrics, sex steroid concentrations and genetic variations in the *AR* on muscle mass and function, with adjustment for the confounding effect of age, adult height and weight or fat mass and taking into account the interdependence of measurements between brothers. Parameters of fixed effects were estimated via restricted maximum likelihood estimation and reported as estimates of effect size (β) with their respective standard error. A sample size of 677 subjects allowed us a 81% power to detect a minimum effect size of 0.01 at a two-sided significance level of 5%. Validity of the models was assessed by exploring normality of distribution of the residuals. SNPs were considered as a categorical variable, whereas CAG and GGN lengths were analysed as continuous variables for assessing association, and as categorical variable (quartiles) with groups compared by one-way analysis of variance (ANOVA). Associations were considered significant at p-values less than 0.05. Statistical analyses were performed using S-Plus 7.0 (Insightful, Seattle, WA, USA). The polygenic program in SOLAR 2.0 (Southwest Foundation for Biomedical Research, San Antonio, TX, USA) was used to estimate heritability, using a variance component model.

Results

Study population and characteristics

Six hundred seventy seven subjects with a mean age of 34.5±5.5 years are included in the study. Mean height is 1.79±0.06 m and mean weight 81.4±11.8 kg, with a body mass index of 25.3±3.5 kg/m^2. Body composition and muscle function parameters are given in Table 1.

As expected, the level of physical activity was associated with muscle mass. Biceps force was positively associated with the level of physical activity during work (β : 0.18±0.03; $p<0.0001$) but not related to physical activity during sports ($p=0.96$), whereas quadriceps force was related to sports (β : 0.11±0.04; $p=0.004$) and not to physical activity during work ($p=0.52$), independent from age, height and weight.

Age, weight and height in relation to muscle mass and force

Both fat (β : 0.2±0.05 kg/y; $p=0.0001$) and lean mass (β : 0.1±0.05 kg/y; $p=0.03$) increased with age, as well as muscle CSA at the radius (β : 21 mm^2/y±4; $p<0.0001$) and tibia (β : 32 mm^2/y±8; $p=0.0001$), which remained positive after additional adjustment for height, physical activity level and body fat (radius: $p<0.0001$ and tibia: $p=0.004$). With increasing age, lower limb muscle force indices slightly decreased after adjustment for height and weight ($p=0.02$). Biceps muscle force and maximal grip strength were unrelated to age.

Whole body lean mass was positively associated with height (β : 0.22±0.02; $p<0.0001$) and weight (β : 0.78±0.02; $p<0.0001$). Also a close relationship between muscle CSA and weight (β : 0.54±0.03; $p<0.0001$ for radius, and β : 0.56±0.03; $p<0.0001$ for tibia) was found. Moreover, maximal grip strength and muscle force indices at upper (biceps) and lower limb (quadriceps) were all positively related to height (all $p<0.0001$) and weight (all $p<0.001$).

Whole body lean mass exhibited a strong positive association with muscle CSA and muscle function (all $p<0.0001$), whereas whole body fat mass was inversely related to muscle CSA at radius ($p<0.0001$) and grip strength and muscle force of biceps ($p<0.001$).

Table 1. General characteristics and hormone concentrations of all study participants (n = 677).

	Mean ± SD
Age (yr)	34.5±5.5
Weight (kg)	81.4±11.8
Height (m)	1.79±0.06
BMI (kg/m^2)	25.3±3.5
Testosterone (ng/dL)	579 [467.0–703.8]
Free testosterone (ng/dL)	14.2 [11.9–17.0]
Estradiol (ng/dL)	2.12 [1.67–2.57]
Free estradiol (ng/dL)	0.04 [0.03–0.05]
SHBG (nmol/L)	23 [18.4–29.7]
LH (U/L)	4.3 [3.1–5.5]
FSH (U/L)	3.8 [2.7–5.4]
Whole body lean mass (kg)	62.2±6.6
Whole body fat mass (kg)	16.4±6.4
Radius 66% muscle area (cm^2)	45.2±5.9
Tibia 66% muscle area (cm^2)	82.6±11.1
Grip strength (kg)	51.7±8.0
Biceps force (Nm)	57.3±10.5
Quadriceps force (Nm)	203±42
Arm span (cm)	182.7±7.3
Hand length (cm)	20.5±1.0
Digit 2 finger length (cm)	7.4±0.5
Digit 4 finger length (cm)	7.6±0.5
Sternum height (cm)	61.5±2.7

Non-Gaussian distribution: data presented as median [1st–3rd quartile]. Free testosterone and free estradiol serum concentrations were calculated using previously validated equations [20,21].

The relationship of muscle CSA and muscle force (grip, biceps and quadriceps) with height and weight are represented in Figure 1.

Heritability of muscle mass and function

Table 2 illustrates the heritabilities of muscle mass and function parameters. All parameters are highly heritable ($p<0.0001$), with the highest h^2 observed for whole body lean mass.

Muscle mass and force in relation to anthropometric measurements

Whole body lean mass and muscle CSA at the radius were positively associated with arm span (β : 0.29±0.05; $p<0.0001$ and β : 0.31±0.07; $p<0.0001$ respectively) as well as with finger ($p=0.0001$ to 0.04) and hand length (all $p<0.0001$) adjusted for height, weight and age. Fat mass was negatively associated with arm span (β : −0.23±0.03; $p<0.0001$). Moreover, biceps flexion and hand grip force were related to arm span (β : 0.46±0.06; $p<0.0001$ for biceps and β : 0.48±0.07; $p<0.0001$ for grip), even more strongly than to hand length (β : 0.32 to 0.34±0.05; $p<0.0001$ for biceps and β : 0.33±0.05; $p<0.0001$ for grip) and finger length (β : 0.19 to 0.24±0.04 ; $p<0.0001$ for biceps and β : 0.25 to 0.30±0.04; $p<0.0001$ for grip). Muscle force and muscle CSA were unrelated to sternum height (data not shown). All

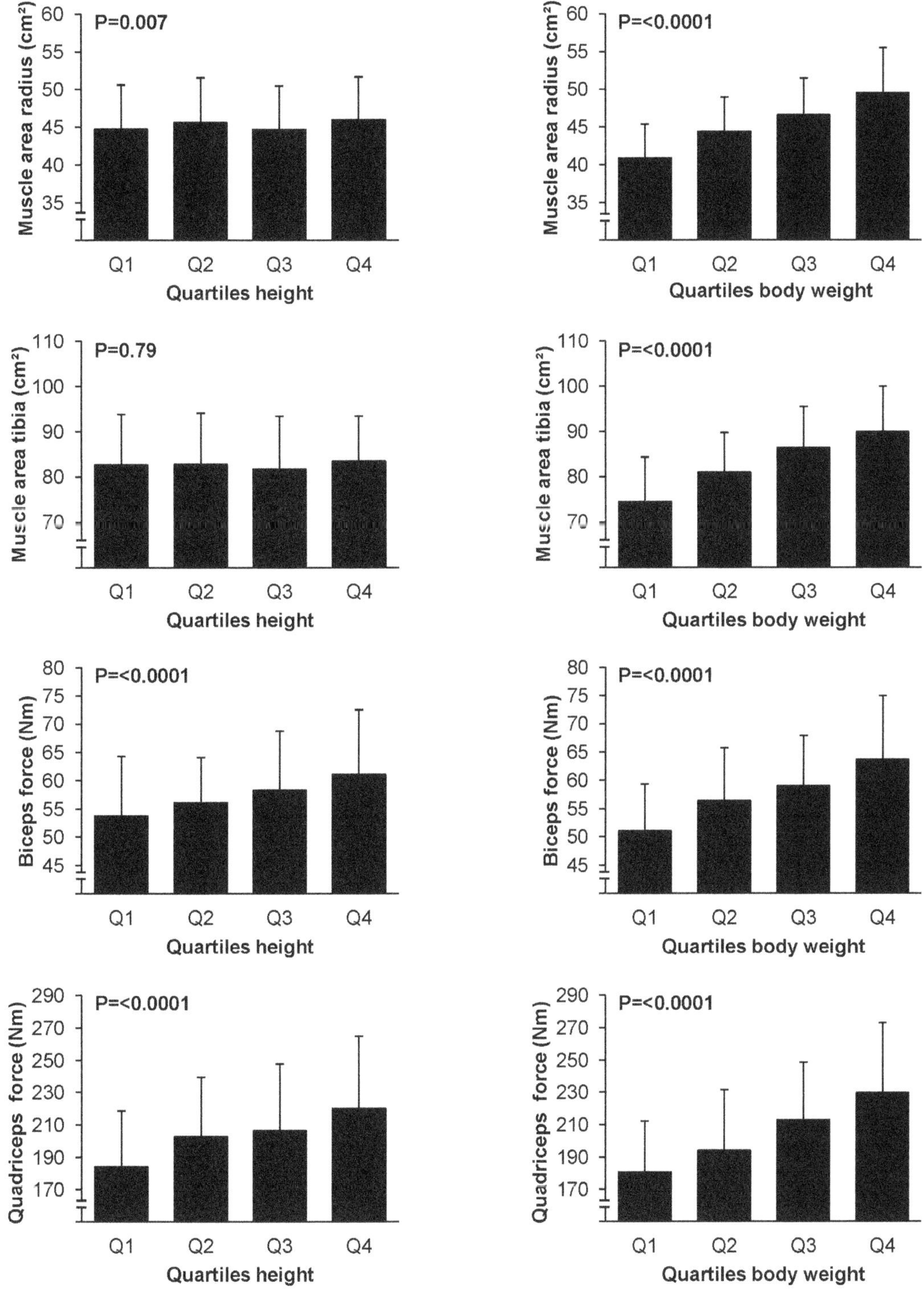

Figure 1. Muscle CSA and muscle force (grip, biceps and quadriceps) according to quartiles of height and weight. P-values result from ANOVA (overall difference between categories). Each bar represents the mean ± standard deviation (SD).

associations remained positive after additional adjustment for fat or lean mass.

Sex steroids in relation to muscle mass and function

TT and FT concentrations were positively related to whole body lean mass (β : 0.07±0.02; p = 0.0002 and β : 0.08±0.02; p<0.0001 respectively) and inversely to fat mass (β : −0.07±0.02; p = 0.0001 and β : −0.08±0.02; p<0.0001 respectively), adjusted for age, weight and height. TT concentrations were positively related to muscle CSA at the tibia (β : 0.07±0.04; p = 0.04), and FT was positively associated with muscle CSA at the radius (β : 0.07±0.04; p = 0.03). E_2 and FE_2 concentrations were negatively associated with maximal grip strength (β : −0.08±0.04; p = 0.04 and β : −0.10±0.04; p = 0.007 respectively) and quadriceps force

Table 2. Heritability estimates of selected muscle parameters.

	h^2
Whole body lean mass (kg)	0.86±0.09
Whole body fat mass (kg)	0.73±0.10
Radius 66% muscle area (mm^2)	0.67±0.10
Tibia 66% muscle area (mm^2)	0.63±0.10
Grip strength (kg)	0.56±0.10
Biceps force (Nm)	0.76±0.10
Quadriceps force (Nm)	0.67±0.10

(β : -0.08 ± 0.04; $p=0.02$ and β : -0.11 ± 0.04; $p=0.002$ respectively), even after additional adjustment for T. No influence of TT or FT on muscle force was observed (data not shown). The 2D:4D finger length ratio and arm span were unrelated to circulating steroid concentrations (data not shown).

Genetic variation in AR in relation to circulating sex steroids, anthropometrics and muscle mass and function

The influence of genetic variation in the *AR* on circulating gonadal steroids, body composition and muscle function is shown in Table 3. The CAG repeat demonstrated a positive association with circulating TT and FT concentration, as well as with E_2 and FE_2 concentrations. Weak associations were found for the rs5965433 and rs5919392 polymorphisms in the *AR*. However, only the association between CAG repeat and TT and FT remained significant after Bonferroni correction. No associations between GGN repeat polymorphism and TT or FT concentrations, as determined by LC-MS/MS, were found.

No consistent effects of the *AR* polymorphisms or CAG/GGN repeats were found on either body composition, muscle mass or muscle force (Table 3). Figure 2 illustrates the influence of the CAG repeat polymorphism on anthropometrics. Arm span was inversely associated with the number of CAG repeats (β : -0.09 ± 0.02; $p=0.0001$). Adult height (Figure 2), hand and digit 4 length (data not shown) were unrelated to CAG length, but digit 2 length at both left and right hand was inversely related to the CAG polymorphism (right β : -0.04 ± 0.01; $p=0.0002$ and left β : -0.04 ± 0.01; $p=0.002$ adjusted for age and height). From the 7 genetic variations analysed, only the CAG repeat length was found to be negatively related to the 2D:4D finger length ratio (right β : -0.05 ± 0.01; $p=0.0006$ and left β: -0.03 ± 0.01; $p=0.01$).

Discussion

In this cross-sectional study we investigated the interrelation between androgen sensitivity, heritability, circulating sex steroids, anthropometrics and muscle mass and function in a cohort of young men. We observed that the number of CAG repeats is associated with TT, FT, E_2 and FE_2 levels, and the 2D:4D finger length ratio and arm span. In contrast with the observed associations with circulating sex steroids, these genetic variations in the *AR* did not influence muscle mass or function in this cohort of young healthy men.

Our results are in agreement with twin studies reporting that muscle mass and strength are highly heritable [1]. Some of the remaining variance in muscle mass might be explained by antropometry, which is also under genetic control [2–4]. Height and weight were closely related to lean mass in our study. As taller subjects have longer bones, it is reasonable that they have longer muscles and thus higher muscle mass. Biceps force and hand grip force were also found to be related with anthropometric measurements, demonstrating that the strength of an individual is strongly determined by its body size.

Age has also an influence on skeletal muscle mass and function [3]. However, few studies have examined the relationship between age and lean mass in (young) adults [24,25]. In our study, we found a small but positive association between lean mass, muscle CSA and age. The association of age with grip and biceps force, and the small inverse relationship with quadriceps force supports the results of Janssen *et al.* [25] which state that the muscle strength of the upper body is preserved better with increasing age than the muscle strength of the lower body.

The alterations in body composition with aging are thought to be related to changes in sex steroid levels [26]. A loss of lean mass and an increase in fat mass are observed in elderly and hypogonadal men, whereas puberty in boys is associated with a remarkable gain in muscle mass [3,5]. However, the clinical relationship between androgens and muscle mass for variations within the normal range is less clear. In this cohort of eugonadal men, we demonstrated that whole body lean mass and muscle CSA are positively associated with both TT and FT. It is noteworthy that physical activity was also positively associated with serum T concentrations, indicating a higher impact of physical activity on muscle mass in men with higher serum T levels. However, and in agreement with Folland *et al.* [8], further analysis revealed that neither TT nor FT had any relation with muscle strength.

As mentioned earlier, between-subject differences in serum T levels within the physiological range are related in part to differences in androgen sensitivity and hypothalamus-pituitary feedback setpoint [9]. Genetic variations in the *AR* gene, in particulary CAG repeat polymorphisms, have been associated with disorders linked to a reduced androgen activity [27]. We have previously shown that serum T levels are positively associated with the CAG and GGN repeat length in young, middle-aged and elderly men [9,13]. This is in contrast with the present study, in which we did not find any correlation between TT or FT and the GGN repeat length. It is noteworthy that the subjects of the current study are partly overlapping (358 unrelated men i.e. a single representative of the nuclear families out of 677 men) with the cohort of young men published by Crabbe *et al.* [9] and Bogaert *et al.* [13]. However, the serum concentrations of T have been re-determined by a highly precise LC-MS/MS method, as these were previously determined using less specific commercial immunoassay kits. Reports on associations between the GGN repeat and AR function are limited and inconsistent, with one study describing a positive association in a cohort of men with prostate cancer [28], whereas another study in young men could not find an association between the GGN repeat and serum T levels [29].

Based on studies reporting mutations in the *AR* gene related to AIS [14–16] we further screened for genetic polymorphisms in the *AR* that may affect the AR activity and thus circulating androgen levels. Interestingly, two SNPs (rs5965433 and rs5919392) were found to be significantly associated with FT, with the first also borderline significantly associated with TT. However, it is noteworthy that these associations did not remained significant after Bonferroni correction. Two recent genome-wide association studies [30,31] have identified several SNPs at different loci that were associated with serum T levels in middle-aged and elderly men. However, the *AR* gene was not described in these studies. Considering our relatively limited sample size, we suggest that

Table 3. Androgen receptor polymorphisms in relation to circulating gonadal steroids and muscle parameters.

	CAG repeat	GGN repeat	rs17217069	rs5965433	rs5919392	rs6152	rs12011793
Testosterone (ng/dL)	**0.10±0.04 (p=0.004)**	0.06±0.04 (p=0.09)	0.44±0.26 (p=0.10)	−0.28±0.14 (p=0.05)	0.27±0.16 (p=0.10)	0.16±0.11 (p=0.12)	0.03±0.14 (p=0.84)
Free testosterone (ng/dL)	**0.17±0.04 (p<0.0001)**	0.06±0.04 (p=0.08)	0.41±0.28 (p=0.14)	**−0.30±0.14 (p=0.04)**	**0.35±0.17 (p=0.04)**	0.19±0.11 (p=0.08)	0.12±0.14 (p=0.40)
Estradiol (ng/dL)	**0.08±0.04 (p=0.05)**	0.07±0.04 (p=0.07)	0.32±0.30 (p=0.029)	0.07±0.15 (p=0.65)	0.16±0.18 (p=0.39)	0.11±0.12 (p=0.36)	0.25±0.15 (p=0.09)
Free estradiol (ng/dL)	**0.10±0.04 (p=0.014)**	0.07±0.04 (p=0.07)	0.29±0.29 (p=0.33)	0.06±0.15 (p=0.68)	0.17±0.18 (p=0.35)	0.10±0.12 (p=0.37)	0.26±0.15 (p=0.08)
SHBG (nmol/L)	−0.05±0.04 (p=0.21)	0.02±0.04 (p=0.52)	0.40±0.27 (p=0.14)	−0.13±0.14 (p=0.35)	0.02±0.17 (p=0.89)	0.04±0.11 (p=0.69)	−0.14±0.14 (p=0.31)
LH (U/L)	0.06±0.04 (p=0.14)	0.05±0.04 (p=0.23)	0.22±0.30 (p=0.45)	−0.12±0.15 (p=0.42)	−0.05±0.18 (p=0.80)	0.23±0.12 (p=0.05)	0.22±0.15 (p=0.14)
FSH (U/L)	−0.07±0.04 (p=0.07)	0.06±0.04 (p=0.15)	−0.34±0.29 (p=0.24)	0.29±0.15 (p=0.05)	−0.12±0.18 (p=0.49)	−0.04±0.11 (p=0.70)	0.10±0.15 (p=0.51)
Whole body lean mass (kg)	−0.004±0.017 (p=0.80)	0.02±0.02 (p=0.20)	−0.17±0.12 (p=0.17)	−0.08±0.07 (p=0.24)	0.10±0.08 (p=0.22)	0.09±0.05 (p=0.08)	0.10±0.06 (p=0.11)
Whole body fat mass (kg)	−0.005±0.018 (p=0.80)	−0.02±0.02 (p=0.30)	0.23±0.13 (p=0.08)	0.06±0.07 (p=0.40)	−0.08±0.08 (p=0.34)	−0.10±0.05 (p=0.05)	−0.12±0.07 (p=0.07)
Radius 66% muscle area (mm^2)	−0.04±0.03 (p=0.17)	0.04±0.03 (p=0.22)	−0.03±0.24 (p=0.89)	−0.07±0.12 (p=0.57)	0.33±0.15 (p=0.02)	0.15±0.09 (p=0.11)	0.17±0.12 (p=0.15)
Tibia 66% muscle area (mm^2)	0.005±0.033 (p=0.90)	0.01±0.03 (p=0.75)	−0.05±0.24 (p=0.84)	−0.11±0.12 (p=0.36)	−0.07±0.15 (p=0.66)	0.08±0.10 (p=0.39)	0.07±0.12 (p=0.59)
Grip strength (kg)	−0.02±0.04 (p=0.53)	−0.002±0.036 (p=0.97)	−0.004±0.271 (p=0.99)	−0.002±0.140 (p=0.99)	−0.02±0.17 (p=0.90)	0.09±0.11 (p=0.41)	0.14±0.14 (p=0.32)
Biceps force (Nm)	−0.05±0.04 (p=0.21)	0.03±0.03 (p=0.42)	−0.09±0.27 (p=0.73)	−0.18±0.13 (p=0.17)	0.29±0.16 (p=0.07)	0.04±0.10 (p=0.69)	0.04±0.13 (p=0.77)
Quadriceps force (Nm)	−0.02±0.04 (p=0.51)	0.03±0.04 (p=0.38)	−0.16±0.28 (p=0.56)	−0.07±0.14 (p=0.59)	0.19±0.16 (p=0.24)	−0.007±0.104 (p=0.95)	0.02±0.13 (p=0.87)

Data are presented as standardized estimate ± SD (p-value). Results from mixed effects accounted for family structure and adjusted for age, height and weight.

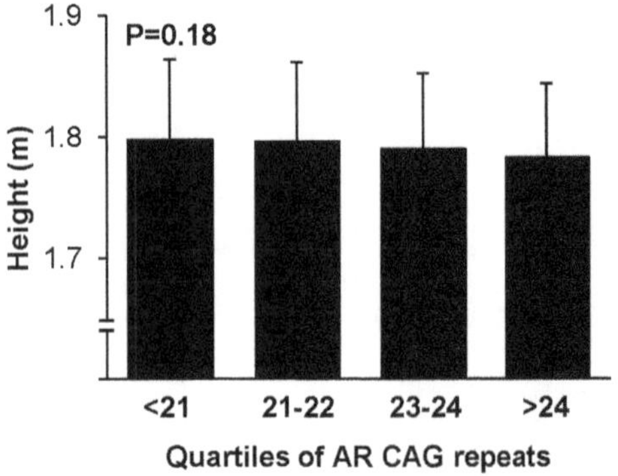

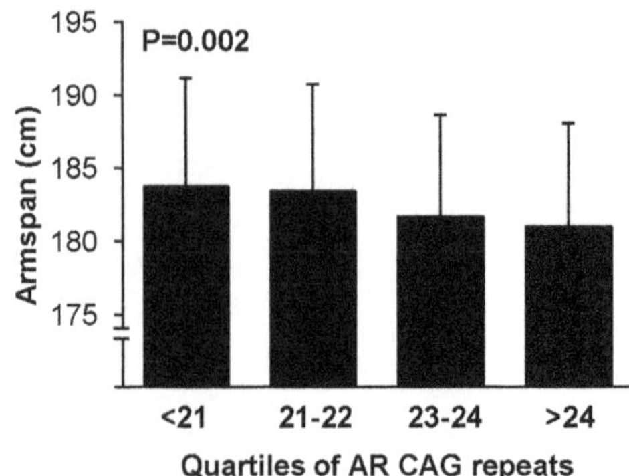

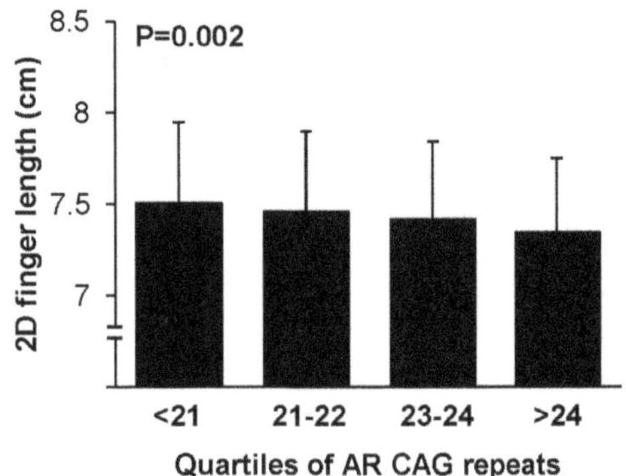

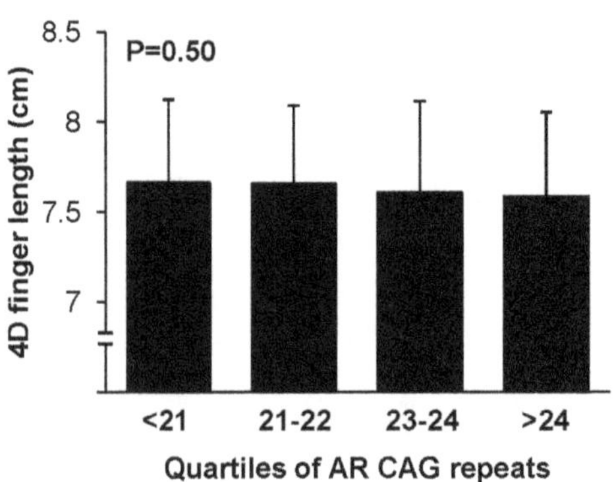

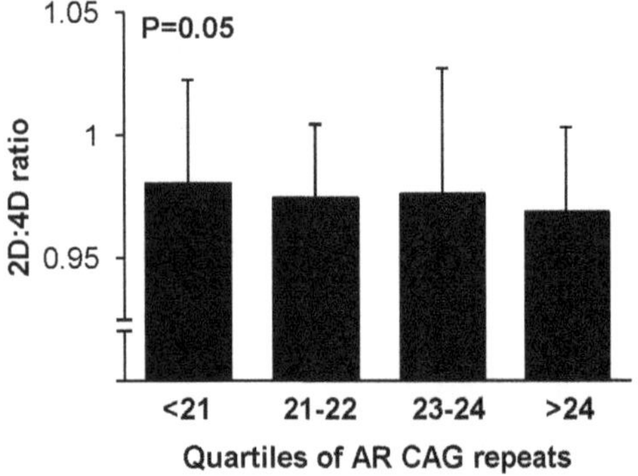

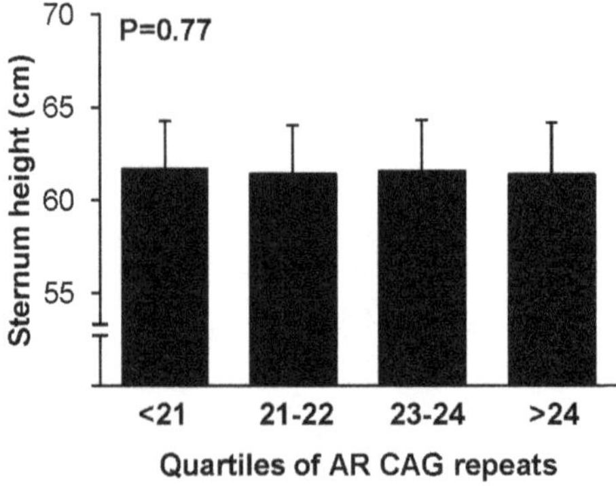

Figure 2. Anthropometrics according to quartiles of AR CAG repeat polymorphism. P-values result from ANOVA (overall difference between categories). Each bar represents the mean ± standard deviation (SD).

analysis of our SNPs in those larger study populations may be required to confirm our findings.

Genetic variation in the *AR* gene influences circulating androgen levels, but may also affect body composition, muscularity or anthropometrics. Data on the association between CAG repeat length and muscle mass is limited and has been contradictory [8,32,33]. In our study, we could not find any relationship of CAG, GGN repeat length or the analysed SNPs in the *AR* with either body composition or measurements of muscularity. This might indicate that the relation of T with the muscle CSA is not related to genetic factors influencing androgen sensitivity, most likely because lower androgen sensitivity is compensated by elevated T levels.

Interestingly, we found that arm span and the 2D:4D finger length ratio were inversely associated with the number of CAG repeats, but not with the GGN repeat lenght or the analysed SNPs. The 2D:4D finger length ratio has been proposed as a marker of prenatal androgen action and of sensitivity to T, with a lower 2D:4D being associated with high androgen exposure [34,35]. Given the hypothesis that elevated T levels in men with lower androgen sensitivity do not necessary show differences in androgen action, we can speculate that the negative effects on arm span and finger length might be mediated by the higher levels of FE_2 levels found in men with longer CAG repeat length, as suggested by Huhtamieni IT *et al.* [36]. As most E_2 produced in normal men is formed by aromatization of androgens [37], the higher T substrate availability in men with lower androgen sensitivity can explain the higher serum E_2 levels. E_2 is considered to be the main sex steroid involved in the development and maintenance of bone mass [18]. In addition, it is also important to initiate epiphyseal closure of long bones [38]. Therefore, we speculate that the presence of higher levels of E_2 in men with lower androgen sensitivity, but preserved estrogen action, resulted in earlier termination of longitudinal bone growth during puberty, an event wich is clearly observed in boys with aromatase excess syndrome or familiar hyperestrogenism [39,40].

To date, several studies have examined the possible relation of adult sex hormone concentrations [41,42] and *AR* CAG number [43–45] with 2D:4D, but results are controversial. To our knowledge, there is only one study that has examined the relationship between GGN repeat variation in the *AR* and 2D:4D ratios [46], but no reports on the relationship between SNPs in *AR* and 2D:4D ratios exist.

The higher serum E_2 levels found in men with a higher CAG repeat number might also play a direct role on muscle force since the negative association between E_2 and grip strength and biceps force, and between FE_2 and grip strength and biceps force in our study persisted after adjustment for T. Also Auyeung *et al.* [47] reported that E_2 levels, though positively related to muscle mass, were negatively related to muscle strength. However, it should be noted that the participants of the latter study were much older, with lower T levels.

Possible effects of E_2 on the regulation of muscle mass and function are still poorly understood. As skeletal muscle myoblasts and mature fibers express functional estrogen receptors (ER), a direct effect of E_2 in muscle cells may occur [48,49]. Although some studies have shown that E_2 is involved in muscle recovery [50,51] and has anabolic effects [52,53], a negative role of E_2 on the musculature has also been suggested by others. Several studies observed a decrease in muscle mass and force after E_2 administration of ovariectomized rats [54–57], and Brown M *et al.* [50] found an increase in muscle mass and function in *ER* knockout mice. However, the exact mechanism by which estrogens regulate muscle mass still has to be elucidated.

We recognize that our study has some limitations. First, our study may have been limited by the relatively small sample size, by which small but significant associations might have been missed, especially for the genetics analysis. Secondly, observations within brothers are not completely independent from each other. However, all analyses in this study were performed using linear mixed-effects modelling with random intercepts to account for this interdependence. Furthermore, the cross-sectional design of this study does not allow us to draw conclusions on causality.

A major strength of this study is that we have used a highly precise LC-MS/MS method to determine T and E_2 serum concentrations. Most other studies used direct immunoassays, which are thought to have a reduced specificity at lower concentrations, especially those for serum E_2 [58,59], which could explain some of the conflicting results reported. Also, our cohort of healthy men in a well-defined age range may have strengthened our results.

In summary, in this study we showed that age, physical activity, body composition, sex steroid levels and anthropometrics are all determinants of muscle mass and function in young men. Although the number of CAG repeats were related to sex steriod levels and anthropometrics, we have no evidence that variations in the *AR* gene also contributes to the between subject variation in muscle mass or muscle function in young healthy men.

Acknowledgments

The authors are indebted to K. Toye, K. Mertens, and I. Bocquart for their excellent technical assistance.

Author Contributions

Conceived and designed the experiments: HDN YT JMK. Performed the experiments: HDN VB ADS GR SV. Analyzed the data: HDN WD YT. Wrote the paper: HDN.

References

1. Arden NK, Spector TD (1997) Genetic influences on muscle strength, lean body mass, and bone mineral density: a twin study. J Bone Miner Res 12: 2076–2081.
2. Gallagher D, Heymsfield SB (1998) Muscle distribution: variations with body weight, gender, and age. Appl Radiat Isot 49: 733–734.
3. Baumgartner RN, Waters DL, Gallagher D, Morley JE, Garry PJ (1999) Predictors of skeletal muscle mass in elderly men and women. Mech Ageing Dev 107: 123–136.
4. Geirsdottir OG, Arnarson A, Briem K, Ramel A, Tomasson K, et al. (2012) Physical function predicts improvement in quality of life in elderly Icelanders after 12 weeks of resistance exercise. J Nutr Health Aging 16: 62–66.
5. Bhasin S, Storer TW, Berman N, Yarasheski KE, Clevenger B, et al. (1997) Testosterone replacement increases fat-free mass and muscle size in hypogonadal men. J Clin Endocrinol Metab 82: 407–413.
6. Bhasin S, Storer TW, Berman N, Callegari C, Clevenger B, et al. (1996) The effects of supraphysiologic doses of testosterone on muscle size and strength in normal men. N Engl J Med 335: 1–7.
7. Storer TW, Woodhouse L, Magliano L, Singh AB, Dzekov C, et al. (2008) Changes in muscle mass, muscle strength, and power but not physical function are related to testosterone dose in healthy older men. J Am Geriatr Soc 56: 1991–1999.
8. Folland JP, Mc Cauley TM, Phypers C, Hanson B, Mastana SS (2012) The relationship of testosterone and AR CAG repeat genotype with knee extensor muscle function of young and older men. Exp gerontol 47: 437–443.
9. Crabbe P, Bogaert V, De Bacquer D, Goemaere S, Zmierczak H, et al. (2007) Part of the interindividual variation in serum testosterone levels in healthy men reflects differences in androgen sensitivity and feedback set point: contribution of the androgen receptor polyglutamine tract polymorphism. J Clin Endrocrinol Metab 92: 3604–3610.
10. Ukkola O, Gagnon J, Rankinen T, Thompson PA, Hong Y, et al. (2001) Age, body mass index, race and other determinants of steroid hormone variability: the HERITAGE Family Study. Eur J Endocrinol 145: 1–9.
11. Meikle AW, Stringham JD, Bishop DT, West DW (1988) Quantitating genetic and nongenetic factors influencing androgen production and clearance rates in men. J Clin Endocrinol Metab 67: 104–109.
12. Ring HZ, Lessov CN, Reed T, Marcus R, Holloway L, et al. (2005) Heritability of plasma sex hormones and hormone binding globulin in adult male twins. J Clin Endocrinol Metab 90: 3653–3658.
13. Bogaert V, Vanbillemont G, Taes Y, De Bacquer D, Deschepper E, et al. (2009) Small effect of the androgen receptor gene GGN repeat polymorphism on serum testosterone levels in healthy men. Eur J Endocrinol Societies 161: 171–177.
14. Li W, Cavasotto CN, Cardozo T, Ha S, Dang T, et al. (2005) Androgen receptor mutations identified in prostate cancer and androgen insensitivity syndrome display aberrant ART-27 coactivator function. Mol Endocrinol 19: 2273–2282.
15. Black BE, Vitto MJ, Gioeli D, Spencer A, Afshar N, et al. (2004) Transient, ligand-dependent arrest of the androgen receptor in subnuclear foci alters phosphorylation and coactivator interactions. Mol Endocrinol 18: 834–850.
16. Quigley CA, Tan J, He B, Zhou Z, Mebarki F, et al. (2004) Partial androgen insensitivity with phenotypic variation caused by androgen receptor mutations that disrupt activation function 2 and the NH(2)- and carboxyl-terminal interaction. Mech Ageing Dev 125: 683–695.
17. Baecke JA, Burema J, Frijters JE (1982) A short questionnaire for the measurement of habitual physical activity in epidemiological studies. Am J Clin Nutr 36: 936–942.
18. Lapauw BM, Taes Y, Bogaert V, Vanbillemont G, Goemaere S, et al. (2009) Serum estradiol is associated with volumetric BMD and modulates the impact of physical activity on bone size at the age of peak bone mass: a study in healthy male siblings. J Bone Miner Res 24: 1075–1085.
19. Fiers T, Casetta B, Bernaert B, Vandersypt E, Debock M, et al. (2012) Development of a highly sensitive method for the quantification of estrone and estradiol in serum by liquid chromatography tandem mass spectrometry without

derivatization. J Chromatogr B Analyt Technol Biomed Life Sci 893–894: 57–62.
20. Vermeulen A, Verdonck L, Kaufman JM (1999) A critical evaluation of simple methods for the estimation of free testosterone in serum. J Clin Endocrinol Metab 84: 3666–3672.
21. Szulc P, Claustrat B, Munoz F, Marchand F, Delmas PD (2004) Assessment of the role of 17beta-oestradiol in bone metabolism in men: does the assay technique matter? The MINOS study. Clin endocrinol 61: 447–457.
22. Barret JC (2009) Haploview: Visualization and analysis of SNP genotype data. Cold Spring Harb Protoc 2009:pdb.ip71.
23. Tobler AR, Short S, Andersen MR, Paner TM, Briggs JC, et al. (2005) The SNPlex genotyping system: a flexible and scalable platform for SNP genotyping. J Biomol Tech 16: 398–406.
24. Lowndes J, Carpenter RL, Zoeller RF, Seip RL, Moyna NM, et al. (2009) Association of age with muscle size and strength before and after short-term resistance training in young adults. J Strength Cond Res 23: 1915–1920.
25. Janssen I, Heymsfield SB, Wang Z, Ross R, Janssen IAN, et al. (2000) Skeletal muscle mass and distribution in 468 men and women aged 18–88 yr. J Appl Physiol 89: 81–88.
26. Kaufman JM, Vermeulen A (2005) The decline of androgen levels in elderly men and its clinical and therapeutic implications. Endocr Rev 26: 833–876.
27. Davis-Dao CA, Tuazon ED, Sokol RZ, Cortessis VK (2007) Male infertility and variation in CAG repeat length in the androgen receptor gene: a meta-analysis. J Clin Endocrinol Metab 92: 4319–4326.
28. Giwercman YL, Abrahamsson PA, Giwercman A, Gadaleanu V, Ahlgren G (2005) The 5alpha-reductase type II A49T and V89L high-activity allelic variants are more common in men with prostate cancer compared with the general population. Eur Urol 48: 679–685.
29. Lundin KB, Giwercman YL, Rylander L, Hagmar L, Giwercman A (2006) Androgen receptor gene GGN repeat length and reproductive characteristics in young Swedish men. Eur J Endocrinol 155: 347–354.
30. Jin G, Sun J, Kim ST, Feng J, Wang Z, et al. (2012) Genome-wide association study identifies a new locus JMJD1C at 10q21 that may influence serum androgen levels in men. Hum Mol Genet 21: 5222–5228.
31. Ohlsson C, Wallaschofski H, Lunetta KL, Stolk L, Perry JR, et al. (2011) Genetic determinants of serum testosterone concentrations in men. PLoS Genet 7: e1002313.
32. Nielsen TL, Hagen C, Wraae K, Bathum L, Larsen R, et al. (2010) The impact of the CAG repeat polymorphism of the androgen receptor gene on muscle and adipose tissues in 20–29-year-old Danish men: Odense Androgen Study. Eur J Endocrinol 162: 795–804.
33. Guadalupe-Grau A, Rodríguez-González FG, Dorado C, Olmedillas H, Fuentes T, et al. (2011) Androgen receptor gene polymorphisms lean mass and performance in young men. Br J Sports Med 45: 95–100.
34. Manning J, Bundred P, Flanagan B (2002) The ratio of 2nd to 4th digit length: a proxy for transactivation activity of the androgen receptor gene? Med Hypotheses 59: 334–336.
35. McIntyre MH (2006) The use of digit ratios as markers for perinatal androgen action. Reprod Biol Endocrinol 4: 10.
36. Huhtaniemi IT, Pye SR, Limer KL, Thomson W, O'Neill TW, et al. (2009) Increased estrogen rather than decreased androgen action is associated with longer androgen receptor CAG repeats. J Clin Endocrinol Metab 94: 277–284.
37. MacDonald PC, Madden JD, Brenner PF, Wilson JD, Siiteri PK (1979) Origin of estrogen in normal men and in women with testicular feminization. J Clin Endocrinol Metab 49: 905–916.
38. Weise M, De-Levi S, Barnes KM, Gafni RI, Abad V, et al. (2001) Effects of estrogen on growth plate senescence and epiphyseal fusion. Proc Natl Acad Sci USA 98: 6871–6876.
39. Stratakis CA, Vottero A, Brodie A, Kirschner LS, DeAtkine D, et al. (1998) The aromatase excess syndrome is associated with feminization of both sexes and autosomal dominant transmission of aberrant P450 aromatase gene transcription. J Clin Endocrinol 83: 1348–1357.
40. Martin RM (2003) Familial Hyperestrogenism in Both Sexes: Clinical, Hormonal, and Molecular Studies of Two Siblings. J Clin Endocrinol 88: 3027–3034.
41. Hönekopp J, Watson S (2010) Meta-analysis of digit ratio 2D:4D shows greater sex difference in the right hand. Am J Hum Biol 22: 619–630.
42. Muller DC, Giles GG, Bassett J, Morris HA, Manning JT, et al. (2011) Second to fourth digit ratio (2D:4D) and concentrations of circulating sex hormones in adulthood. Reprod Biol Endocrinol 9: 57.
43. Butovskaya ML, Vasilyev VA, Lazebny OE, Burkova VN, Kulikov AM, et al. (2012) Aggression, digit ratio, and variation in the androgen receptor, serotonin transporter, and dopamine D4 receptor genes in African foragers: the Hadza. Behav Genet 42: 647–662.
44. Hurd PL, Vaillancourt KL, Dinsdale NL (2011) Aggression, digit ratio and variation in androgen receptor and monoamine oxidase a genes in men. Behav Genet 41: 543–556.
45. Knickmeyer RC, Woolson S, Hamer RM, Konneker T, Gilmore JH (2011) 2D:4D ratios in the first 2 years of life: Stability and relation to testosterone exposure and sensitivity. Horm Behav 60: 256–263.
46. Zhang C, Dang J, Pei L, Guo M, Zhu H, et al. (2013) Relationship of 2D:4D finger ratio with androgen receptor CAG and GGN repeat polymorphism. Am J Hum Biol 25: 101–106.
47. Auyeung TW, Lee JS, Kwok T, Leung J, Ohlsson C, et al. (2011) Testosterone but not estradiol level is positively related to muscle strength and physical performance independent of muscle mass: a cross-sectional study in 1489 older men. Eur J Endocrinol 164: 811–817.
48. Kahlert S, Grohe C, Karas RH, Lobbert K, Neyses L, et al. (1997) Effects of estrogen on skeletal myoblast growth. Biochem Biophys Res Commun 232: 373–378.
49. Barros RP, Machado UF, Warner M, Gustafsson JA (2006) Muscle GLUT4 regulation by estrogen receptors ERbeta and ERalpha. Proc Natl Acad Sci USA 103: 1605–1608.
50. Brown M, Ning J, Ferreira JA, Bogener JL, Dennis B, et al. (2009) Estrogen receptor- α and - β and aromatase knockout effects on lower limb muscle mass and contractile function in female mice. Am J Physiol Endocrinol Metab 296: E854-E861.
51. McClung JM, Davis JM, Wilson MA, Goldsmith EC, Carson JA (2006) Estrogen status and skeletal muscle recovery from disuse atrophy. J Appl Physiol 100: 2012–2023.
52. Phillips SK, Rook KM, Siddle NC, Bruce SA, Woledge RC (1993) Muscle weakness in women occurs at an earlier age than in men, but strength is preserved by hormone replacement therapy. Clin Sci (Lond) 84: 95–98.
53. Moran AL, Nelson SA, Landisch RM, Warren GL, Lowe DA (2007) Estradiol replacement reverses ovariectomy-induced muscle contractile and myosin dysfunction in mature female mice. J Appl Physiol 102: 1387–1393.
54. Ihemelandu EC (1981) Comparison of effect of oestrogen on muscle development of male and female mice. Acta Anat (Basel) 110: 311–317.
55. Kobori M, Yamamuro T (1989) Effects of gonadectomy and estrogen administration on rat skeletal muscle. Clin Orthop Relat Res 243: 306–311.
56. McCormick KM, Burns KL, Piccone CM, Gosselin LE, Brazeau GA (2004) Effects of ovariectomy and estrogen on skeletal muscle function in growing rats. J Muscle Res Cell Motil 25: 21–27.
57. Suzuki S, Yamamuro T (1985) Long-term effects of estrogen on rat skeletal muscle. Exp Neurol 87: 291–299.
58. Wang C, Catlin DH, Demers LM, Starcevic B, Swerdloff RS (2004) Measurement of total serum testosterone in adult men: comparison of current laboratory methods versus liquid chromatography-tandem mass spectrometry. J Clin Endocrinol Metab 89: 534–543.
59. Lee JS, Ettinger B, Stanczyk FZ, Vittinghoff E, Hanes V, et al. (2006) Comparison of methods to measure low serum estradiol levels in postmenopausal women. J Clin Endocrinol Metab 91: 3791–3797.

15

Spinal Loads during Cycling on an Ergometer

Antonius Rohlmann*, Thomas Zander, Friedmar Graichen, Hendrik Schmidt, Georg Bergmann

Julius Wolff Institute, Charitè – Universitätsmedizin Berlin, Berlin, Germany

Abstract

Cycling on an ergometer is an effective exercise for improving fitness. However, people with back problems or previous spinal surgery are often not aware of whether cycling could be harmful for them. To date, little information exists about spinal loads during cycling. A telemeterized vertebral body replacement allows *in vivo* measurement of implant loads during the activities of daily living. Five patients with a severe compression fracture of a lumbar vertebral body received these implants. During one measurement session, four of the participants exercised on a bicycle ergometer at various power levels. As the power level increased, the maximum resultant force and the difference between the maximum and minimum force (force range) during each pedal revolution increased. The average maximum-force increases between the two power levels 25 and 85 W were 73, 84, 225 and 75 N for the four patients. The corresponding increases in the force range during a pedal revolution were 84, 98, 166 and 101 N. There were large variations in the measured forces between the patients and also within the same patient, especially for high power levels. In two patients, the maximum forces during high-power cycling were higher than the forces during walking measured on the same day. Therefore, the authors conclude that patients with back problems should not cycle at high power levels shortly after surgery as a precaution.

Editor: Amir A. Zadpoor, Delft University of Technology (TUDelft), Netherlands

Funding: Funding for this study was obtained from the Deutsche Forschungsgemeinschaft, Bonn, Germany (Ro 581/18-1) and the Deutsche Arthrose-Hilfe, Frankfurt, Germany. The funders had no role in study design, data collection and analysis, decision to publish, or preparation of the manuscript.

Competing Interests: The authors have declared that no competing interests exist.

* E-mail: antonius.rohlmann@charite.de

Introduction

Sport is usually associated with physical activity and is thus an important factor for the prevention and palliation of various diseases. After spinal surgery, the physical performance of patients is often drastically reduced because of preoperative sparing and postoperative decline in fitness due to pain or reduced mobility. This is especially the case in elderly people. Physical exercise is also an effective way to improve the fitness of such patients. Patients often do not know which exercises can be performed without overloading an implant or bone and consequently endangering surgical success (e.g., implant subsidence). Cycling is one of the most popular sports, along with swimming, aerobic exercise and jogging [1]. Patients with low back pain and those who have undergone spinal surgery are often unsure whether exercising on a bicycle ergometer will interfere with their recovery. In contrast to jogging, cycling does not lead to impact loading of the spine; however, there have been few experimental studies of the actual spinal loads during cycling [2] and how they compare to those during walking.

Direct measurement of the complete spinal load is currently not possible. However, there are a variety of ways to indirectly measure spinal loads. Intradiscal pressure has been measured *in vivo* for many activities [3–5], but no data for cycling are available. Another way to quantify spinal loads is to measure the induced change in spinal length, termed 'spinal shrinkage'. Measurements indicate that after 1 h of cycling at a constant speed of 12 km/h, the shrinkage is only half of that after 1 h of erect standing [2]. However, this method of measurement provides only relative values and does not predict the real spinal forces acting on an implant during different activities.

A severe fracture of a vertebral body and tumors of the spine are often surgically treated by implantation of a vertebral body replacement (VBR) [6]. The vertebral body and the adjacent intervertebral discs are at least partially removed and replaced with the metallic implant. Several studies have used a telemeterized VBR to investigate the forces and moments on the implant during different activities [7–12]. However, no data were reported for cycling. Knowledge about VBR loads will be useful for the validation of computer models created to predict spinal loads.

Therefore, the aim of the current study was to document the effect of power level on the forces on a VBR during ergometer cycling.

Materials and Methods

Ethics Statement

The Ethics Committee of Charité – Universitätsmedizin Berlin approved the clinical implantation of the modified VBR in patients and subsequent measurements (registry number: 213-01/225-20). The procedure was explained to the patients prior to surgery, and they gave their written consent to the implantation of an instrumented VBR, the subsequent measurements and publication of their images. Measurements were permitted within a maximum period of 6 years.

Telemeterized VBR

To measure implant loads, the clinically used VBR Synex (Sythes Inc., Bettlach, Switzerland) was modified. Six strain gauges, a 9-channel telemetry unit and a coil for the inductive power supply were integrated within a hermetically closed cylindrical tube. Endplates of various heights that were attached using screws allowed for intraoperative adaptation of the implant height to the defect dimensions. After extensive calibration by applying 21 different load combinations, the implant was used to measure the 3 force and 3 moment components acting on it. The average errors were lower than 2% for the force and 5% for the moment components relative to the maximum applied force (3,000 N) and moment (20 Nm), respectively. The sensitivity of the implant was less than 1 N for the forces and 0.01 Nm for the moments. The telemetry was only active within a magnetic field of 4 kHz. The implant and the measurement accuracy have been described in detail elsewhere [13].

Patients

Within a period of more than 2 years, only 5 patients were found who required surgical stabilization of their spine and were qualified for a telemeterized VBR. The patients (WP1 to WP5) were suffering from an A3 type compression fracture [14] of a lumbar vertebral body. In four patients, the vertebral body L1 was fractured, and in one patient (WP5), L3 was fractured. The fractures were first stabilized from the posterior using an internal fixation device. In a second surgery, parts of the fractured vertebral body and the adjacent intervertebral discs were removed, and the instrumented VBR was inserted into the corpectomy defect. Autologous bone material was added to enhance interbody fusion. At the time of surgery, the patients were between 62 and 71 years of age. More information about the patients and the surgical procedure is provided in Table 1.

Measurements

For the load measurements, a coil was placed around the patient's trunk at the level of the implant, and an antenna was secured on the patient's back. The coil and the antenna did not restrain the patient during the exercises. During the measurements, the patient's images were synchronously recorded on a digital videocassette with the load-dependent telemetry signals [15]. This allowed for later analysis of implant loads and motions without the patient being present. The signals were also transferred to a notebook where the forces and moments were calculated and displayed online on a monitor.

The main aim of the study of the telemeterized VBRs was to measure the loads on the implant for a wide variety of activities under daily living conditions. Thus, in 97 measuring sessions within a period of 65 months, the loads were measured for approximately 1,000 activity and parameter combinations. Approximately 25 activities, such as standing, walking, bending (forward, backward, and lateral) of the upper body while sitting and standing, were evaluated several times during almost every measuring session. Other activities, such as whole body vibration, walking on a treadmill, and cycling on an ergometer, were performed only once. Keep in mind that the patients were over 60 years old at the time of surgery, were involved in several other load measurement studies, and were not paid for the measurements. Therefore, the number of repetitions and the time-demanding measurement of additional parameters were very limited.

Four of the 5 patients agreed to cycle during one session on an ergometer. Patient WP3 did not accept our invitation because she did not feel strong enough for this exercise. The ergometer session occurred between 13 and 65 months after surgery, depending on the availability of the patients. All 4 patients were male, felt fit on that day of the session and reported no pain.

Exercises

The patients sat upright on the bicycle ergometer with their hands on the handlebar and attempted to maintain a cadence of 40 rpm. The pedal resistance was initially 25 W and was automatically increased every 60 sec to the next power level up to 95 W. The power levels were 35, 50, 60, 70 or 75, and 85 W. Two patients were only able to cycle up to 85 W. The bicycle ergometer had a crank length of 17.5 cm. The height of the saddle was adjusted to the patient's leg length. No straps were used on the pedals.

Evaluation

The resultant force acting on the VBR is presented here as the geometric sum of the three measured force components. The maximum force during a single pedal revolution is the 'peak force', and the difference between the maximum and minimum force magnitude is the 'force range'. For each power level, the medians of the peak forces and the force ranges were determined from an average of 20 pedal revolutions. The values obtained during cycling at 85 W were compared with the values during level walking and relaxed standing that were measured on the same day. The cycling values were also compared to those during the lifting of a 10 kg weight from the ground. Walking is an important regular daily activity with high spinal loads. Relaxed standing is one of the best reproducible positions and was measured an average of 9 times during each measurement session. Lifting a weight from the ground is the activity that caused the highest forces on the VBR.

Only descriptive statistics could be applied because no more than 4 patients with a telemeterized VBR could be included in the study and not all of them cycled at all power levels.

During cycling, the power generated is the product of the angular velocity and the crank torque (the crank length multiplied by the average mostly vertical pedal force during a revolution).

Table 1. Data on the patients and surgical procedures.

Parameter	Patient			
	WP1	WP2	WP4	WP5
Age at the time of surgery (years)	62	71	63	66
Height (cm)	168	169	170	180
Body mass (kg)	66	74	60	63
Fractured vertebra	L1	L1	L1	L3
Level of the internal fixation device	T12-L2	T12-L2	T11-L3	L2-L4
Time between implantation and measurement session (months)	65	13	49	15

The ergometer displays the power and the cadence (cadence multiplied by 2×Pi delivers the angular velocity), while the crank length is constant and known. With these data, the average pedal force during a pedal revolution can be calculated. For the various power levels, the average pedal forces were estimated and compared with the corresponding force ranges on the VBR. It was assumed that the changes in the forces of those muscles that span the hip region correlate with the average pedal force and with the force range on the VBR.

Results

Figure 1 shows a typical example of the measured components and the resultant loads on the VBR for 5 successive randomly chosen pedal revolutions at a cadence of approximately 40 rpm and a power of 85 W. The peak values and the force ranges varied considerably.

The peak resultant force on the VBR generally increased as the cycling power was increased (Figure 2). However, the increase varied for the different patients. For patients WP1 and WP4, there was a nearly constant force increase; the increase was progressive for patient WP2; and no increase was observed below 60 W for patient WP5. The average force increases between 25 and 85 W were 73, 84, 225 and 75 N for patients WP1, WP2, WP4 and WP5, respectively. The peak force usually occurred in the first half of the downward motion of the pedal. For two patients (WP1 and WP2), the median of the peak values for cycling was lower than that for walking measured on the same day, but for the other two patients (WP4 and WP5), the value for cycling was higher (Table 2) [8]. The peak value for cycling was higher than the average value for standing for all 4 patients [9]. By comparison, the maximum force on the VBR measured when patient WP4 lifted a weight of 10 kg from the ground was 1650 N.

Similar to the peak force, the force range during a pedal revolution also generally increased with increasing cycling power (Figure 3). The average range increases between the power levels 25 and 85 W were 84, 98, 166 and 101 N for patients WP1, WP2, WP4 and WP5, respectively. There were large intra- (Figure 1) and inter-individual (Figures 2 and 3) variations in the measured peak forces and the force ranges during a revolution. The magnitudes of the calculated average pedal force for the various power levels were similar to those of the average VBR force ranges during a pedal revolution of the four patients (Figure 3).

Discussion

The loads on a VBR during cycling at various power levels were measured in four patients. The peak force and the force range during a pedal revolution increased with increasing cycling power. There were large intra- and inter-individual variations in the measured forces.

One limitation of the study is that these unique measurements were performed in a small cohort of only four patients. The forces were measured within one session, but the values for an average of 20 revolutions were evaluated for each power level. Thus, the median value should be representative. However, repeating the measurements on a different day may lead to slightly different values due to small differences in the overall muscle tone, the orientation of the upper body or the position of the hands on the handlebar. In 2 patients the power level 70 W instead of 75 W was chosen. The higher power levels were chosen depending on the patient's behavior during the exercise in order not to overstress them. Only the cadence of 40 rpm was studied to avoid overstressing the patients, who were involved in many other load measurement studies [7–12]. Measurements of telemeterized knee joints showed that higher cadences lead to smaller forces in the knee joint [16]. We expected the same trend for spinal loads.

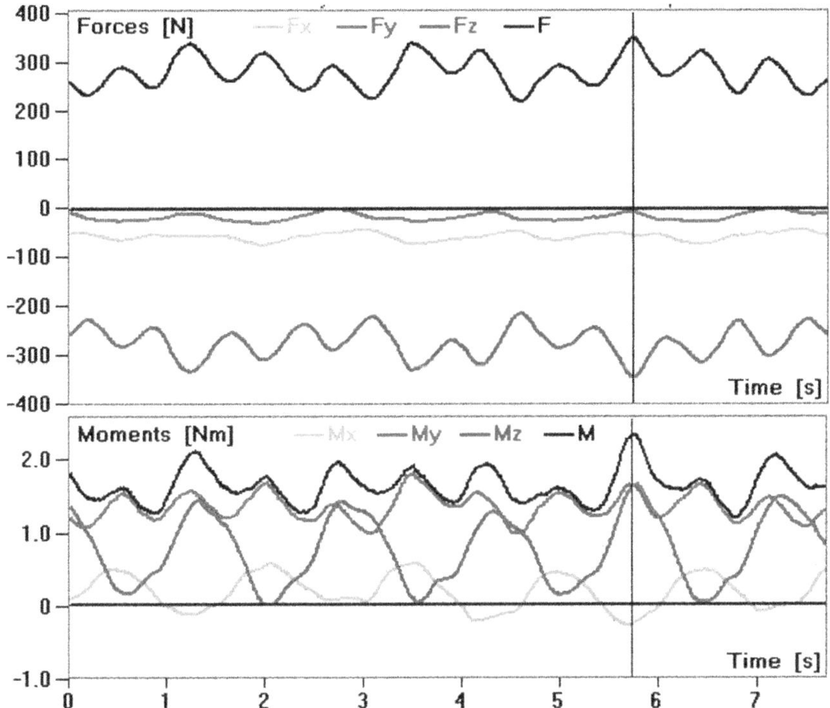

Figure 1. Measured loads. Force and moment components and the resultant values during cycling on an ergometer at approximately 40 rpm and a power level of 85 W. The loading curves for 5 pedal revolutions of patient WP1 are shown.

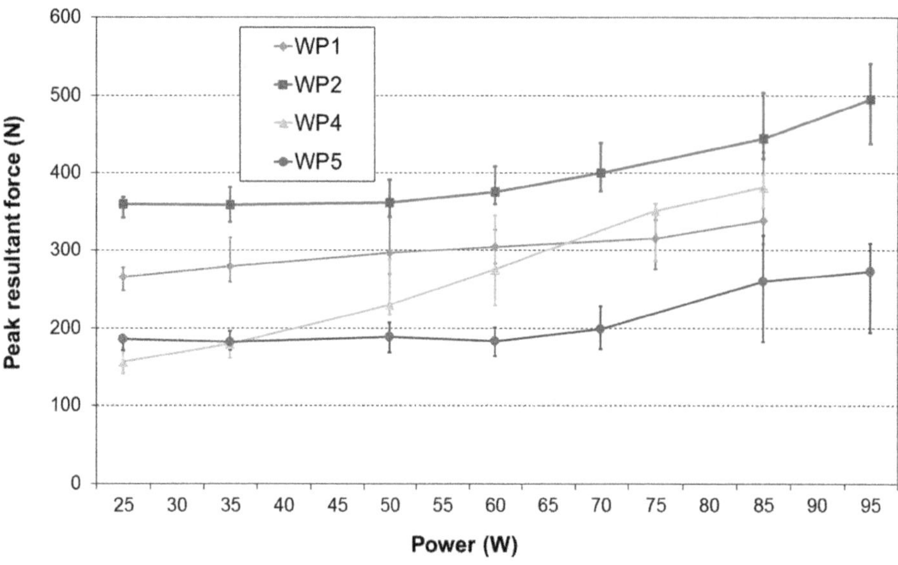

Figure 2. Peak resultant force versus power. The influence of the power level on the peak resultant force on the implant during cycling. The medians and ranges are shown for various power levels for the four patients (WP1, WP2, WP4 and WP5).

During the measurements, the patients sat upright on the ergometer with their hands on the handlebar. This may affect the magnitude of the measured force; however, this and the other limitations should not affect the general trend of the results.

Three of the VBRs were implanted at level L1 and one (in WP5) at level L3. The spinal loads at the lower level should be higher because a greater part of the upper body weight is acting there. However, the peak force on the VBR and the measured forces for other activities were mostly lower in WP5 than in the other patients. Thus, other factors such as the percentage of load taken over by the internal fixators and possible implant subsidence have a stronger influence on the VBR peak force.

Measurement of the loads during cycling was performed between 13 and 65 months after surgery. At the time of measurement, the muscle activation pattern should have normalized, and all patients felt fit. All measurements of a patient presented here were acquired in one day, except weight lifting. Thus, these measurements do not provide information about the influence of the postoperative time on the results.

The maximum spinal load during an activity varies strongly [8,11,17,18]. Even for the reproducible position 'relaxed standing', the force on the VBR varied on average by approximately ±50 N when measured 10 times within 1 h [9]. Similar variations were found in intradiscal pressure measurements [4] and in a previous study on internal spinal fixation devices [19]. The spinal loads obviously depend on several factors such as small variations in the posture, muscle co-contractions and psychic stress, which are all difficult to control.

The pedal forces during cycling are much lower than the reaction on the foot during walking although the forces on the VBR were similar. This demonstrates that for the spinal load, muscle forces are more relevant than external forces. With increasing cycling power, the forces in the muscles that span the hip region increase. Higher trunk muscle forces lead to higher spinal forces. The trunk muscle forces also depend strongly on the location of the center of mass (CoM) of the upper body [12,20]. An anterior shift of the CoM requires higher back muscle force to keep a stable position, which in turn leads to higher spinal forces. The position of the CoM of the upper body in relation to the spine has the strongest effect on the spinal loads.

The peak forces during cycling on an ergometer at a power of 85 W were higher than the maximum values for walking measured on the same day in 2 patients. The exact load which places a considerable risk on the spine is unknown. Walking is considered to be the most important regularly performed activity in daily life. If patients are allowed to walk then all activities with lower maximum forces than during walking should be allowed. But, to be safe, people with back problems or previous spinal surgery should not exercise on a bicycle ergometer at high power levels. However, in general, our results suggest that cycling is a suitable

Table 2. Comparison of the average peak force values (in N) for cycling at a power of 85 W, level walking [8] and relaxed standing [9] measured on the same day and for lifting of a 10 kg weight from the ground.

Patient	Cycling	Walking	Standing	Lifting 10 kg
WP1	339 (308–426)	422 (352–464)	318 (294–347)	944 (578–1230)
WP2	444 (419–503)	578 (520–674)	320 (288–351)	1225 (1050–1452)
WP4	381 (356–397)	365 (325–430)	210 (196–227)	1380 (1131–1649)
WP5	260 (183–320)	166 (139–232)	92 (80–114)	1129 (732–1361)

The values in parenthesis represent the ranges.

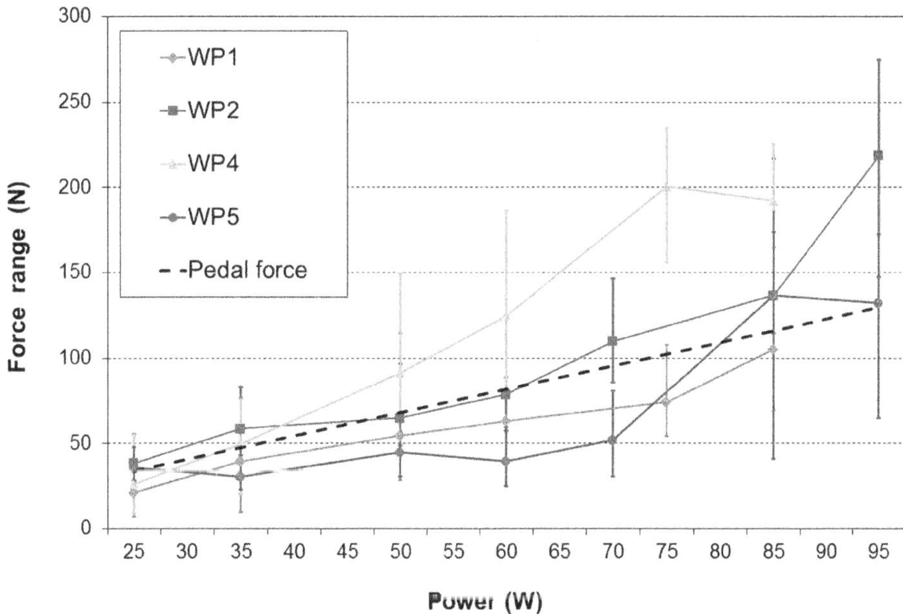

Figure 3. Force range versus power. The influence of the power level during cycling on the force ranges during a pedal revolution. The medians and ranges are shown for various power levels for the four patients (WP1, WP2, WP4 and WP5). The calculated average pedal force is represented by the dashed line.

activity for people with back problems. For the first time, loads acting on a spinal implant were directly measured *in vivo* during cycling. These data may also be used for the validation of computer models for estimating spinal loads.

Acknowledgments

The authors greatly appreciate the cooperation of their patients. We thank Dr. A. Bender, J. Dymke, and H. Razi for technical support.

Author Contributions

Conceived and designed the experiments: AR FG GB. Performed the experiments: AR TZ FG. Analyzed the data: AR TZ HS. Contributed reagents/materials/analysis tools: FG GB. Wrote the paper: AR TZ HS FG GB.

References

1. Weber J, Schonfeld C, Spring A (2009) [Sports after surgical treatment of a herniated lumbar disc: a prospective observational study]. Z Orthop Unfall 147: 588–592.
2. van Deursen LL, van Deursen DL, Snijders CJ, Wilke HJ (2005) Relationship between everyday activities and spinal shrinkage. Clin Biomech 20: 547–550.
3. Nachemson AL (1981) Disc pressure measurements. Spine 6: 93–97.
4. Sato K, Kikuchi S, Yonezawa T (1999) In vivo intradiscal pressure measurement in healthy individuals and in patients with ongoing back problems. Spine 24: 2468–2474.
5. Wilke H-J, Neef P, Hinz B, Seidel H, Claes L (2001) Intradiscal pressure together with anthropometric data - a data set for the validation of models. Clin Biomech 16: S111–126.
6. Lange U, Knop C, Bastian L, Blauth M (2003) Prospective multicenter study with a new implant for thoracolumbar vertebral body replacement. Arch Orthop Trauma Surg 123: 203–208.
7. Dreischarf M, Bergmann G, Wilke HJ, Rohlmann A (2010) Different arm positions and the shape of the thoracic spine can explain contradictory results in the literature about spinal loads for sitting and standing. Spine 35: 2015–2021.
8. Rohlmann A, Dreischarf M, Zander T, Graichen F, Bergmann G (2014) Loads on a vertebral body replacement during locomotion measured in vivo. Gait Posture 39: 750–755.
9. Rohlmann A, Dreischarf M, Zander T, Graichen F, Strube P, et al. (2013) Monitoring the load on a telemeterised vertebral body replacement for a period of up to 65 months. Eur Spine J 22: 2575–2581.
10. Rohlmann A, Hinz B, Bluthner R, Graichen F, Bergmann G (2010) Loads on a spinal implant measured in vivo during whole-body vibration. Eur Spine J 19: 1129–1135.
11. Rohlmann A, Zander T, Graichen F, Bergmann G (2013) Lifting up and laying down a weight causes high spinal loads. J Biomech 46: 511–514.
12. Rohlmann A, Zander T, Graichen F, Dreischarf M, Bergmann G (2011) Measured loads on a vertebral body replacement during sitting. Spine J 11: 870–875.
13. Rohlmann A, Gabel U, Graichen F, Bender A, Bergmann G (2007) An instrumented implant for vertebral body replacement that measures loads in the anterior spinal column. Med Eng Phys 29: 580–585.
14. Magerl F, Aebi M, Gertzbein SD, Harms J, Nazarian S (1994) A comprehensive classification of thoracic and lumbar injuries. Eur Spine J 3: 184–201.
15. Graichen F, Arnold R, Rohlmann A, Bergmann G (2007) Implantable 9-channel telemetry system for in vivo load measurements with orthopedic implants. IEEE Trans Biomed Eng 54: 253–261.
16. Kutzner I, Heinlein B, Graichen F, Rohlmann A, Halder AM, et al. (2012) Loading of the knee joint during ergometer cycling: telemetric in vivo data. J Orthop Sports Phys Ther 42: 1032–1038.
17. Rohlmann A, Schmidt H, Gast U, Kutzner I, Damm P, et al. (2013) In vivo measurements of the effect of whole body vibration on spinal loads. Eur Spine J. 23: 666–672.
18. Rohlmann A, Zander T, Graichen F, Bergmann G (2013) Effect of an orthosis on the loads acting on a vertebral body replacement. Clin Biomech 28: 490–494.
19. Rohlmann A, Graichen F, Weber U, Bergmann G (2000) 2000 Volvo Award winner in biomechanical studies: Monitoring in vivo implant loads with a telemeterized internal spinal fixation device. Spine 25: 2981–2986.
20. Rohlmann A, Zander T, Graichen F, Schmidt H, Bergmann G (2014) How does the way a weight is carried affect spinal loads? Ergonomics 57: 262–270.

16

Model Sensitivity and Use of the Comparative Finite Element Method in Mammalian Jaw Mechanics: Mandible Performance in the Gray Wolf

Zhijie Jack Tseng[1,2*], Jill L. Mcnitt-Gray[1,3], Henryk Flashner[1,4], Xiaoming Wang[1,2], Reyes Enciso[1,5]

1 Integrative and Evolutionary Biology Program, Department of Biological Sciences, University of Southern California, Los Angeles, California, United States of America, **2** Department of Vertebrate Paleontology, Natural History Museum of Los Angeles County, Los Angeles, California, United States of America, **3** Departments of Kinesiology, Biological Sciences, and Biomedical Engineering, University of Southern California, Los Angeles, California, United States of America, **4** Department of Aerospace and Mechanical Engineering, University of Southern California, Los Angeles, California, United States of America, **5** Ostrow School of Dentistry, University of Southern California, Los Angeles, California, United States of America

Abstract

Finite Element Analysis (FEA) is a powerful tool gaining use in studies of biological form and function. This method is particularly conducive to studies of extinct and fossilized organisms, as models can be assigned properties that approximate living tissues. In disciplines where model validation is difficult or impossible, the choice of model parameters and their effects on the results become increasingly important, especially in comparing outputs to infer function. To evaluate the extent to which performance measures are affected by initial model input, we tested the sensitivity of bite force, strain energy, and stress to changes in seven parameters that are required in testing craniodental function with FEA. Simulations were performed on FE models of a Gray Wolf (*Canis lupus*) mandible. Results showed that unilateral bite force outputs are least affected by the relative ratios of the balancing and working muscles, but only ratios above 0.5 provided balancing-working side joint reaction force relationships that are consistent with experimental data. The constraints modeled at the bite point had the greatest effect on bite force output, but the most appropriate constraint may depend on the study question. Strain energy is least affected by variation in bite point constraint, but larger variations in strain energy values are observed in models with different number of tetrahedral elements, masticatory muscle ratios and muscle subgroups present, and number of material properties. These findings indicate that performance measures are differentially affected by variation in initial model parameters. In the absence of validated input values, FE models can nevertheless provide robust comparisons if these parameters are standardized within a given study to minimize variation that arise during the model-building process. Sensitivity tests incorporated into the study design not only aid in the interpretation of simulation results, but can also provide additional insights on form and function.

Editor: Kenneth Carpenter, Utah State University-College of Eastern Utah, United States of America

Funding: The work was supported by a University of Southern California Zumberge Grant (to JM, HF, XW, and RE), NSF Graduate Research Fellowship and Doctoral Dissertation Improvement Grant (DEB-0909807) and American Society of Mammalogists Grant-in-Aid of Research to ZJT. The funders had no role in study design, data collection and analysis, decision to publish, or preparation of the manuscript.

Competing Interests: The authors have declared that no competing interests exist.

* E-mail: jtseng@nhm.org

Introduction

Finite element analysis (FEA), the discretization of structures and approximation of their mechanical behavior (the response of structure to load), has traditionally been an analytical technique in the engineering disciplines as an important component of the development process to improve design. More recently, however, its use in functional studies of biological structures has become more common [1–4]. FEA has been applied in vertebrate biomechanics research across diverse taxonomic groups, including crocodiles [5], non-avian dinosaurs [6–11], birds [12], lizards [13,14], fishes [15], and a variety of mammals [16–26]. FEA complements *in vivo* experimental studies by allowing simulations using user-defined input assumptions regarding the study system, which could otherwise be impossible to implement. Currently, most studies of this type address the mechanical behavior of the craniodental system.

Given the diverse functional questions that could be examined using the FE approach, the current available data from FE publications are largely incomparable across studies precisely because of the comparative nature of current applications. Even within narrow clades of closely related genera and species, lack of absolute values from FE results means published stress and strain values cannot be used to evaluate relative performance of models across different studies (e.g. models of felid species in McHenry et al., 2007 versus those in Slater and Van Valkenburgh, 2009) [18,22]. In many studies, different approaches in how muscles and constraints are modeled also make comparisons difficult. Furthermore, the diversity of taxonomic groups that can potentially be studied using this technique, accompanied by the different software programs and protocols used by researchers in FE model construction, further complicates any attempts at the synthesis of current FE knowledge across vertebrate groups. The current diversity of input assumptions in FE models used in comparative biology suggests a need to quantify the sensitivity of performance measures to those parameters, in order to build a general context for comparing results within and across different studies.

Several previous studies have addressed the choice of model parameters and their implications for comparing FE analytical results to those obtained from *in vivo* experiments for masticatory muscle forces [27], bite forces [28], and elastic bone properties [29]. However, few have addressed the comparison of relative values in the growing literature on vertebrate FE models, which is becoming more numerous given the flexibility of this approach in allowing tests of form and function [30]. In one attempt, Sellers and Crompton [31] conducted a sensitivity study of human bite force prediction with FEA using a large number of combinations of model parameters and found that masticatory muscle insertion points, as well as the modeled mobility of the temporomandibular joints (TMJ), had a large effect on resulting jaw forces. Even if current FEA applications in vertebrate functional morphology cannot provide accurate mechanical values for comparing to experimental results, and in most cases FE models do not have corresponding *in vivo* data for validation tests, standardized comparisons can nevertheless be highly informative [30]. Furthermore, a comparative approach has the advantage of being able to include extinct forms for which material properties and other parameters cannot be directly obtained.

In order to provide this context with which to evaluate the effect of different modeling parameters on the resulting stresses and strains in comparative mammalian mandible FE models, we conducted sensitivity analyses on a model of the carnivoran *Canis lupus* by testing a range of values for seven required parameters that vary among comparative FE studies (Table 1, Fig. 1). The effects of variation in those parameters on performance measures were evaluated by examining bite force output, strain energy, temporomandibular joint reaction forces, and stress distribution [30]. Bite force output (or other related measures, such as mechanical advantage) is a key performance variable in evaluating and comparing masticatory function of the craniodental system, as larger bite forces permit a species to consume harder and tougher foods, as well as predating on large prey. Both of these adaptations mediate the ecological interactions within the predator guild and across trophic levels. Strain energy has been used as a measure of the work-efficiency of the craniodental system under simulated loads [30]. Selection should favor such work efficiency given the functional demands and trade-offs of achieving maximum stiffness with a given structural quantity and weight (i.e. bone). Joint reaction forces have been shown to exhibit consistent patterns during the mastication cycle, and represent indicators of whether the joint region is being properly modeled [32]. Distributions of von Mises stress is used to show likely areas of failure when the bone undergoes ductile fracture [19,33]. This study aims to test how input assumptions in FE models affect these performance measures, which are in turn used to test functional hypotheses and in comparisons of functional capability across species.

Materials and Methods

We used the Gray Wolf *Canis lupus* mandible model from Tseng and Binder [26] for sensitivity tests. The structure of interest included both dentaries of the specimen. The specimen was CT-scanned with a Siemens Definition 64 scanner (Siemens Medical Solutions, Forcheim, Germany) with 0.6 mm slice thickness, 0.37 mm pixel resolution, and a size of 512×512 pixels. 499 images were obtained. We chose the mandible for modeling and sensitivity analysis because of the simplicity of the lower jaw, which is composed of two dentary bones with three joints and no sutures [34]. Compared to the cranium, the function of the mandible is not complicated by the multitude of roles, such as the protection of several sensory organs, played by the former structure. In addition, cranial sutures render the cranium a composite structure, and may mediate the location and magnitude of strain during muscle contraction and mastication [35]. Fewer anatomical features need to be accounted for when modeling the mandible, therefore allowing us to focus on the choices in model resolution, material properties, and boundary conditions and their effects on analysis results.

Models were constructed following the protocol used in Dumont et al. [19,30] and Tseng and Binder [26]. The starting point for the tests was a base model with 383,319 4-noded tetrahedral elements, 0.6 balancing-working side ratio, 55%-26(9)%-10% temporalis-masseter(zygomaticomandibularis)-pterygoid muscle ratio, single-node bite point and TMJ constraints, and a single material property (E = 20 GPa, Poisson ratio = 0.3). All models simulated the biological phenomenon of a unilateral bite with the left lower first molar (the carnassial tooth). We isolated seven main parameters in FE model-building for our sensitivity tests: number of finite elements used to represent the mandibular morphology, balancing- versus working-side muscle activation ratios, relative muscle forces among the masticatory muscle groups, the number of sub-groups within each masticatory muscle group, the size of the bite point constraint, the constraint used at the temporomandibular joints, and number of material properties assigned (Table S1). All models had linear elasticity, and static equilibrium equations were solved in analyses. The variations tested within each category are described in more detail below.

1. Number of finite elements

Craniodental FE models in the current literature are mainly built from four-noded tetrahedral elements; these constant stress

Table 1. Sensitivity tests performed in this study.

Parameter	# Models	Tests
Number of elements	8	Increasing element quantity from 101,674 to 1,404,279
Balancing-Working Ratio	11	+0.1 increment of ratio from 0 to 1.0
Muscle ratio	8	PCSA, mass, dry skull estimates plus individual muscle groups
Muscle number	7	Temporalis only to 6 subgroups of the temporalis and masseter
Bite point constraint	6	Single node constraint to area with 66 nodes
TMJ constraint	4	single node, single link, row of nodes, row of links
Material properties	6	Homogeneous model to 10-property heterogeneous model

A total of 44 models of the same mandible were used in the analyses; some models were used in multiple test categories.

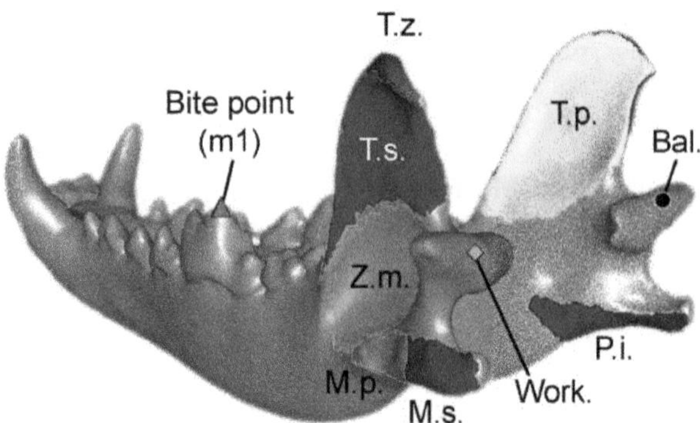

Figure 1. Mandible model used in the study. Bal., balancing-side joint; **Work.**, working-side joint; **m1**, lower first molar (carnassial); **M.p.**, deep masseter; **M.s.**, superficial masseter; **P.i.**, internal pterygoid; **T.p.**, deep temporalis; **T.s.**, superficial temporalis; **T.z.**, zygomatic part of temporalis; **Z.m.**, zygomaticomandibularis. Temporalis and masseter muscle subgroups were used incrementally in the sensitivity test on number of muscles. All other models used a four-muscle input: temporalis-masseter-zygomaticomandibularis-pterygoid.

elements have three degrees of translation freedom per node. Likewise, all models analyzed in this study used four-noded tetrahedrals only. In contrast, ten-noded tetrahedral elements provide more detailed information regarding the distribution of stress and strain within each element, but craniodental FE models built at ~250,000 elements showed variation in results with 10% between four- versus ten-noded elements [19]. This observation has been cited to justify using four-noded tetrahedral models built with large numbers of elements (>1,000,000) as being sufficient for the general functional questions being asked. Given the current widespread use of four-noded elements in craniodental and in fact most other FE models, we ran eight tests with the more commonly used four-noded tetrahedral elements. Number of triangular elements in each model were adjusted in Geomagic Studio 10 (Geomagic, Inc.) before they were meshed into 4-noded tetrahedral elements in Strand7 2.4.1 (G+D Computer Pty Ltd, Sydney, Australia). The number of tetrahedral elements ranged from ~100,000 to ~1,400,000, typical of the resolution seen in most published FE studies (Table S2).

2. Muscle activation schemes

Many of the currently published craniodental FE models use symmetrical bilateral muscle forces, even in unilateral biting simulations. Electromyography studies have shown, however, that at least in *Canis*, mastication of bone and meat is achieved without maximum bilateral recruitment of the jaw muscles [36]. Feedback from periodental nerves also plays a role in mediating the use of muscle forces to produce large bite forces, at the same time maintaining joint stability [36]. Therefore, unilateral bite simulations with maximum bilateral muscle recruitment may represent theoretical maxima and not realistic voluntary maxima [37]. Among mammals, a range of muscle recruitment ratios is present both within individuals and across clades; the adaptation of the mandible to particular modes of muscle loading may be informative in themselves in reflecting typical loading scenarios in a given species [36,38]. We tested unilateral bites at the carnassial tooth (lower molar 1) with 11 models ranging from no balancing side muscle contribution to fully bilateral muscle activation. Working- and balancing-side muscle differences were tested in 10% increments (Table S3). This range encompasses the ratios observed in several mammalian groups [36,38].

3. Muscle proportions

The relative contributions of the three main jaw-closing muscles (temporalis, masseter, and pterygoid) have been estimated in craniodental FE models using either physiological cross-sectional area (PCSA), an estimated of muscle cross-sectional area using dry skulls [39], or by mass of dissected muscles. PCSA has been shown to be a good predictor of muscle force and bite force in bats [28], but in most cases this information is not available for living vertebrates, let along fossil species. We tested a wide range of muscle proportions which encompasses several estimates that have been made for *Canis* [40,41]. Eight models were made, including muscle activation of each of the three major jaw-closing muscle groups in isolation (represented by numbers in the order of temporalis-masseter-pterygoid; Table S4). Even though the masticatory muscle groups do not activate in isolation in reality, their contribution to, and effects on, the resulting biomechanical performance measures can nevertheless reflect potential adaptations [42]. The lateral pterygoid muscle is proportionally smaller than the other jaw muscles mentioned, accounting for about 3% of total PCSA or <0.6% by wet weight in *Canis lupus* [40]; thus, this relatively minor muscle was not included in our analysis.

4. Number of muscles

The main jaw-closing muscles temporalis, masseter, and pterygoid can be subdivided into subgroups based on their gross anatomy, and mammalian craniodental models have been made with a range of muscle groups from temporalis and masseter muscles only [19] to all three muscles and their subgroups [22]. We tested for the effect of number of muscle groups on model outcomes by building seven models ranging from a single jaw closing muscle to seven muscle groups, including subgroups of the temporalis and masseter muscles (Fig. 1, Table S5). The total input force remained the same, and the relative contributions of muscle groups are calculated from the initial 55%-26(9)%-10% temporalis-masseter(zygomaticomandibularis)-pterygoid muscle ratio used in other test categories. Forces among additional subgroups within each major muscle group (when present) are distributed by their respective surface areas.

5. Bite point constraint

The evaluation of bite force in craniodental FE models is often done by sampling reaction forces of nodal constraints at the bite points; however, the range of variation in bite force magnitude estimated by a single node constraint versus constraint distributed over an area is unknown. In carnivorans with self-sharpening carnassial teeth, the cusps remain pointed through time, and thus the first point of contact during mastication is situated near the tip of the crown. Therefore, we varied the number of nodes representing the bite point, starting with a single constraint at the tip of the carnassial protoconid. We tested a range of nodal constraint quantity from a single node to ~65 nodes (covering the entire cusp) using six models (Table S6).

6. The temporomandibular joint (TMJ)

The TMJ has been modeled as rotating around single nodes [19], a row of nodes along the condyloid fossa/mandibular condyle [25], or around a beam through the axis of rotation connected to the joints by rigid links [22]. The use of single nodes creates artificially elevated stress values immediately around the constraint, but the overall distribution of stress in the structure is not affected further away from those constraints. We tested four ways of constraining the TMJ in order to examine their differences: (1) single node constraint at each TMJ; (2) a row of nodal constraints along the mandibular condyle; (3) a single rigid link between the mandibular condyle and a beam in the axis of the TMJ with no translation or rotation other than rotation in the dorsoventral plane; (4) rows of rigid links connecting the mandibular fossa to the axial beam with dorsoventral rotational freedom (Table S7). More recently, Dumont et al. [43] used another method to constrain the TMJ, namely allowing translation in the axis connecting the left and right TMJ, in addition to rotational freedom in the sagittal plane. This alternative was not tested in the current study.

7. Number of material properties

Two main methods of material property assignments in the current literature on craniodental FEA are (1) assigning properties of a single material to the entire model, or (2) assigning multiple categories of materials based on Hounsfield Units (HU), the gray values representing densities in CT image data. We tested six models ranging from homogeneous single-property to heterogeneous 10-property models (Table S8). Bone properties were assigned based on HU intervals obtained during examination of the CT data using published HU-density and density modulus equations [44,45], and tooth enamel and dentine were assigned properties based on published values [46–48]. No calibration standard was available from the CT data; the density and modulus equations were applied assuming similar relationships existed for the data (for example, cortical bone properties calculated using unadjusted HU from the CT data provided a density of 1.77 g/cm^3 and Young's modulus of 19.39 GPa, well within measured range of typical mammalian cortical bone). All materials were treated as isotropic, and all analyses were linear static (Tables S8, S9).

Three-dimensional reconstructions were built from CT image data in Mimics 13.1 (Materialise N.V., Leuven, Belgium), reconstructions were cleaned in Geomagic Studio 10 (Geomagic, Inc., Research Triangle Park, North Carolina, USA), and then remeshed in Mimics. The solid mesh FE models were built in Strand7 2.4.1. The cranium of the specimen was used as reference to identify the direction of muscle forces on the mandible; the relative positions of the cranium and mandible were modified from zero load state (full occlusion, 0° gape) by a 10° rotation of the mandible about the TMJ. This modification created a 10° gape angle that simulated mastication of a small food item between the carnassial teeth. Segmentation of the reconstruction from image data was done using both automated functions in Mimics, as well as manual delineation of bone boundaries. Meshes represented the overall macrostructure of the mandible, without differentiation of microstructural architecture in bone or teeth. Masticatory muscle forces were modeled using the Boneload program written by Grosse et al. [49]. 1000 N of total muscle force was used for all models tested. The model results used for comparison of sensitivity tests were the reaction forces (in Newtons) at the carnassial bite position and the working- and balancing-side joint constraints. Total strain energy (equivalent to the work done in deforming the mandible) values were also compared [30]. In addition, the von Mises stress distributions were visualized on the models. A total of 44 models of the *Canis lupus* mandible were constructed, each given a unique identification number (Table 1, S1; models deposited at Dryad: doi:10.5061/dryad.8961).

Results

1. Number of finite elements

Reaction forces at the bite point and balancing-side joint were lower in the low resolution model (101,674 elements), and working-side joint forces higher, than all of the other models. Higher-resolution models showed no clear trend in increasing or decreasing reaction forces, although some variation is present (Fig. 2). Strain energy values showed small increase with tetrahedral element quantity, but the slope was on the order of 10^{-9} and does not represent a significant trend. Model solution time increased exponentially between ~100,000 and ~1,200,000 tetrahedral elements. The low-resolution model showed lower von Mises stress distributions across the ascending ramus than all other models, which do not show visible differences in stress distribution (Fig. 2D)

2. Muscle activation schemes

Balancing-side reaction forces increased, and working-side decreased, with increasing ratio of balancing-working side muscle activation (Fig. 3). Bite force remained largely invariant. Joint reaction forces are lower than the bite force on both working- and balancing-sides between the ratios 0.4 to 0.6. Balancing-side joint reaction forces are higher than working-side reaction forces, a pattern consistent with experimental values, at ratios larger than 0.5 [32]. Strain energy values are lowest between ratios of 0.3 to 0.5, and are elevated in both higher and lower ratios. Higher balancing-side muscle activation is correlated with decreased von Mises stress on the working-side ascending ramus, but increased stress in the mandibular corpus below the premolars (Fig. 3C).

3. Muscle proportions

Using the internal pterygoideus or the masseter muscle in isolation created elevated working-side TMJ reaction forces (Fig. 4). Strain energy values increased when the pterygoideus and temporalis muscles were used in isolation. All other muscle ratios exhibited comparable levels of reaction forces and strain energy values, with the lowest bite force in the 55-30-15 (temporalis-masseter-pterygoideus) model. The ventral side of the mandibular corpus is more stressed in masseter- and pterygoideus-only models, and the ascending ramus is more stressed in temporalis-only models. All other models showed little difference in von Mises stress distribution (Fig. 4C).

4. Number of muscles

Reaction forces and strain energy values decreased with increasing number of muscle subgroups modeled. Reaction forces decreased by 20% from the one-muscle model to the 2–4 muscle models, and the latter showed little difference among themselves. A further decrease of ~15% was observed from the 2–4 muscle models to the 5–7 muscle models; again, the latter group showed little difference among themselves. A larger drop in strain energy (40%) was observed from one-muscle to 2–4 muscle models, and a ~25% drop from 2–4 muscle models to 5–7 muscle models. Models with more muscle subgroups showed lower stresses in the ascending ramus and the corpus ventral of the premolars (Fig. 5).

5. Bite point constraint

Bite force increased by 60% from a single-node bite point to a 66-node bite point, whereas joint reaction forces stayed constant. Strain energy decreased by <10% from a single-node to a 6-node constraint, but stayed constant for higher numbered constraints. Components of the bite force vector show no significant increases with node number, indicating that the directions of the vector were instead becoming more aligned in the dorsoventral direction, increasing the magnitude of the resultant (Fig. 6B). No differences in stress patterns are observed across the models in areas other than immediately around the bite point, which showed more widespread stress with higher numbered node constraints (Fig. 6).

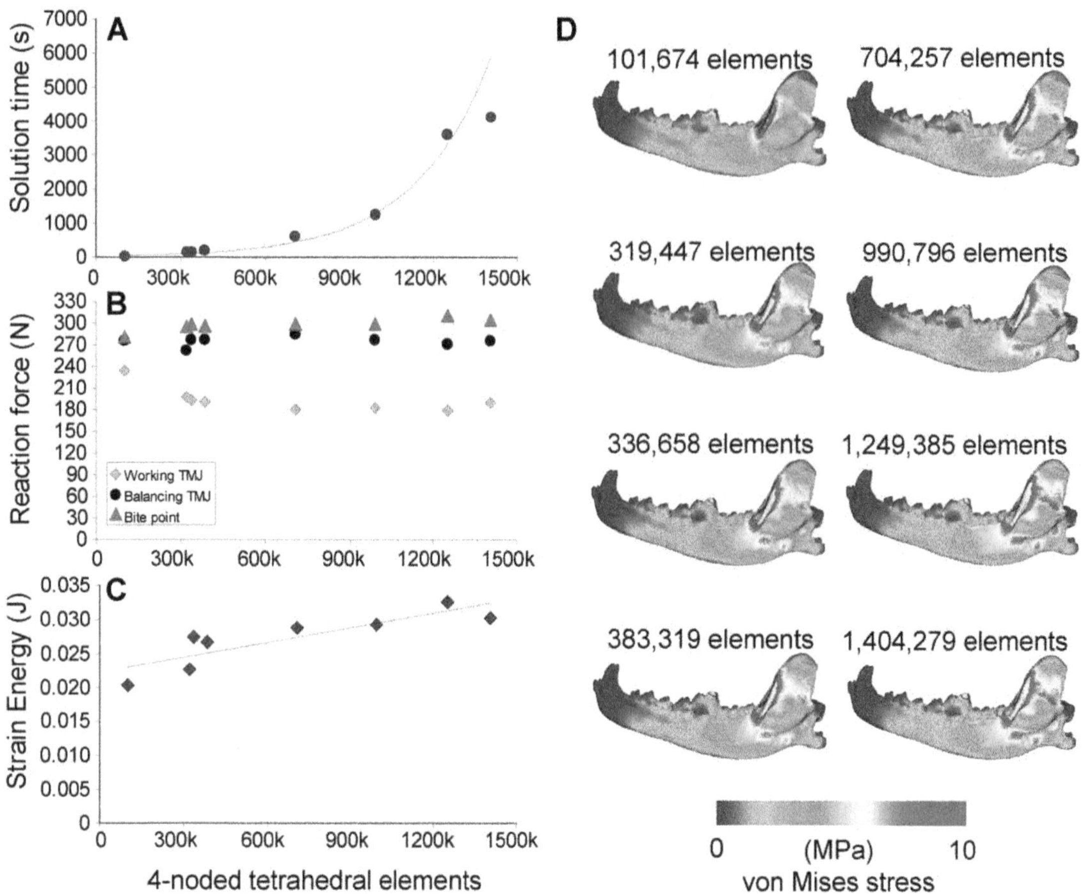

Figure 2. Sensitivity test on tetrahedral element quantity. A. Element quantity plotted against solution time (in seconds), with exponential curve in background. **B.** Element quantity plotted against reaction force (in Newtons). **C.** Element quantity plotted against strain energy (in Joules), with linear regression line. **D.** von Mises stress distribution in the working-side dentary in test models; lateral view (in Megapascals).

6. The temporomandibular joint (TMJ)

The 10-node model had similar bite force to the 1-node model, but the former had elevated joint reaction forces that exceeded the bite force, and higher working-side TMJ forces than balancing side forces. Bite force decreased <10% in the link models, which had no joint reaction forces at the nodes. Strain energy values decreased by ~50% from single-node/single-link models to 10-node/10-link models, respectively. Von Mises strain is higher in the link models than in the node models. The single-node/single-link models showed higher von Mises stress in the caudal half of the mandible compared to the other models (Fig. 7).

7. Number of material properties

Bite force increased by 30%, and joint reaction forces decreased by 20%, from 1–3 property models to 6–8 property models. Strain energy values increased more than 20 fold between those models. The modeling of enamel and dentin had a significant effect on the stress distribution of the models, with most of the stress being contained at the biting tooth in the 6–10 property models (Fig. 8C).

Discussion

We conducted sensitivity tests on performance measures by altering seven input parameters that are required in FE modeling building, but which vary among comparative studies in the literature. Results showed that varying the values of initial parameters had a wide range of effects on bite force (1% to 60% maximum difference) and strain energy (14.7% to >100% maximum difference). The balancing-working muscle activation ratio had the smallest effect on bite force output over the range tested (0.0–1.0), and for estimates of unilateral bite force one might be tempted to discount its influence on the results. However, plots of changes in joint reaction forces showed that only above a ratio of 0.5 were working-side reaction forces smaller than balancing side reaction forces, as predicted by experimental data (Fig. 3A) [32]. Furthermore, the joint reaction forces were lowest relative to the bite force, and therefore the simulated bite was least stressful to the TMJ, in the 0.4–0.6 ratio range. This range overlaps with the 0.6 ratio obtained experimentally by Dessem [36], who suggested that balancing-side muscle is not fully activated during maximum bite force production, partly because of the need to stabilize the jaw joints. The lowered joint reaction forces observed in the FE models are consistent with this hypothesis. In addition, strain energy values are also lowest in the 0.4–0.5 range, suggesting that this configuration provides optimal mandible performance on the basis of work-efficiency [30]. Even though von Mises stress distributions on the mandible showed no significant differences across the range of ratios tested, using an activation ratio of 0.4 to 0.6 between the balancing- and working-side jaw musculature returned lower joint reaction forces and higher work-efficiency (Fig. 3A) [25,50].

Bite force output showed most significant changes in models that differed in number of bite point constraints (Fig. 6).

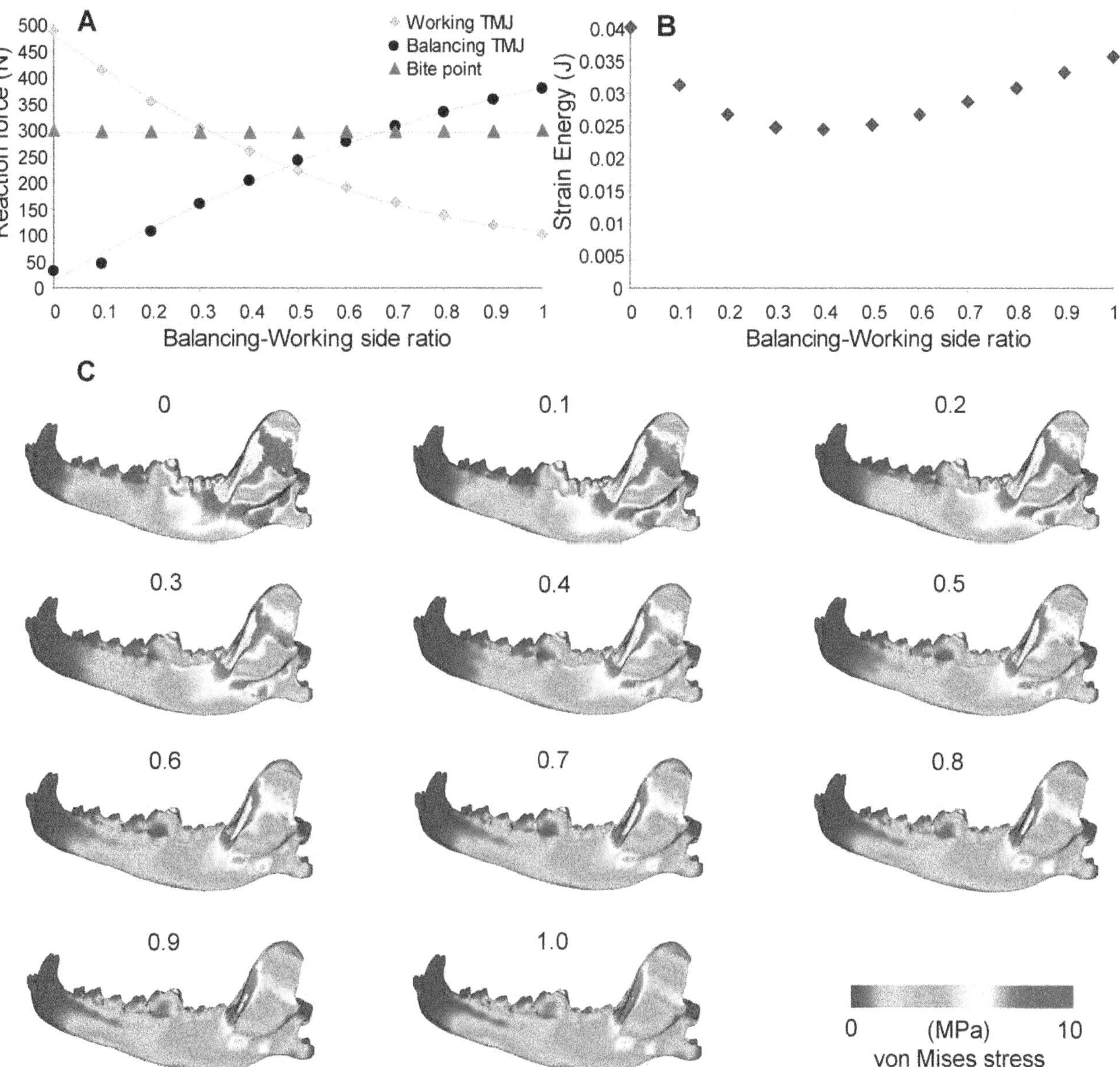

Figure 3. Sensitivity test on balancing-working side ratio. A. Ratio plotted against reaction force, with second-order polynomial curves fitted onto the working and balancing reaction forces. **B.** Ratio plotted against strain energy. **C.** von Mises stress distribution in the working-side dentary in test models.

Constraints that cover a larger area of contact produced higher bite forces than single-node constraints, and this difference approached 60%. In estimating bite forces, comparative FEA studies have used both a distributed area of bite point constraints [22] and single nodes [28]. Results from our analyses showed that, everything being equal, sum of forces from a multi-node constraint would be larger than in the single-node estimate. In most cases comparative FEA are consistent in their model constraints within each study, but care must be taken when one attempts to evaluate bite forces estimated from different studies with different approaches. This is especially true for extinct taxa; where possible, taxon-specific validation should be coupled with modeling different bite constraints to test the range of reasonable bite force estimates that can be made by FE models [28]. It remains difficult to use FEA for bite force estimates of extinct organisms before generalizations are made on how best to model bite points. Furthermore, the increasing number of constraints placed at the biting tooth could have over-constrained the models beyond realistic scenarios, and this would partially explain the large differences in bite force observed.

Strain energy values were least affected by the type of bite point constraint (Fig. 6C), but were significantly more variable in models that differed in number of material properties (Fig. 8B). This is to be expected because increased number of material properties also created more elements that have lower density and modulus values in the model. Interestingly, very high strain energy (i.e. low work efficiency) was observed in models that had more than six material properties, and von Mises stress in those models are concentrated in the biting tooth (Fig. 8C). The stress distribution indicates that most of the deformation in models with more material properties was concentrated on and within the biting tooth, which was modeled with a plate covering of enamel, and a single-element

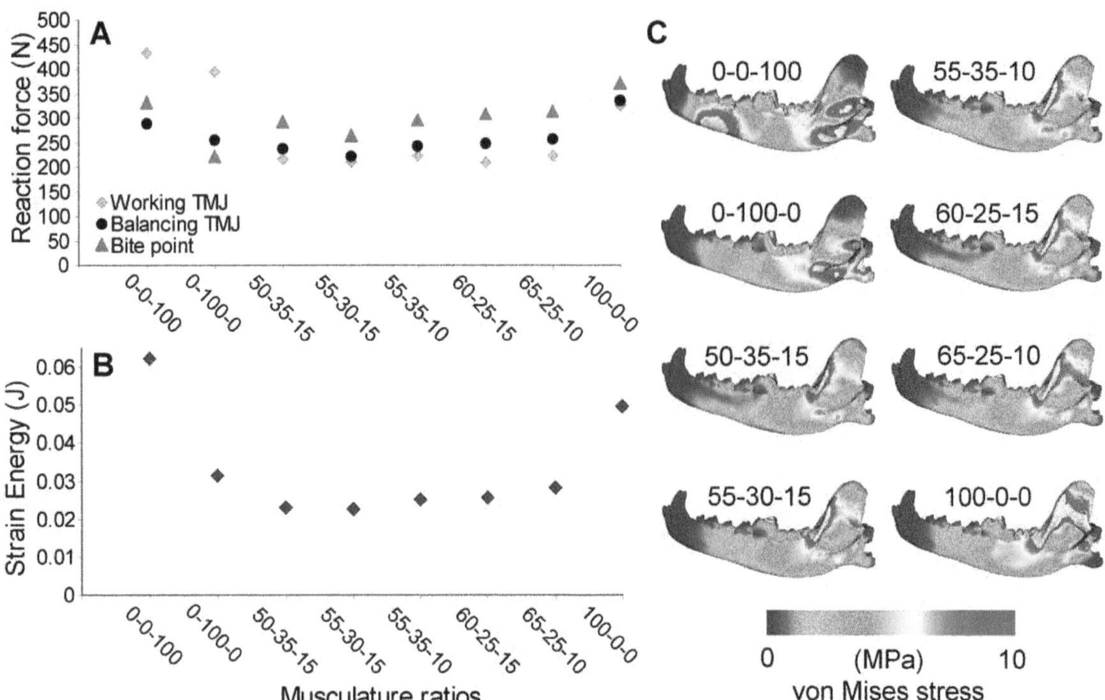

Figure 4. Sensitivity test on musculature ratio. A. Ratio plotted against reaction force. **B**. Ratio plotted against strain energy. **C**. von Mises stress distribution in the working-side dentary in test models. Ratios are given by temporalis-masseter-pterygoid sequences, with zygomaticomandibularis considered part of the masseter group.

thick layer of dentine. The large difference that exists in material properties between the tooth and the surrounding bone may explain stress concentration in the former. Evolutionary specializations of enamel microstructure in durophagous carnivorans are consistent with increased selection for stronger teeth, which are required to withstand large stresses incurred from contact against hard food [51,52]. However, increased stress concentration in the biting tooth was not observed until at least four material properties were present (Fig. 8C), indicating that sufficient differentiation in tooth-bone material properties are required to model this effect. For applications in extinct taxa, fossilized bone often does not provide enough resolution or faithful reproduction of relative bone

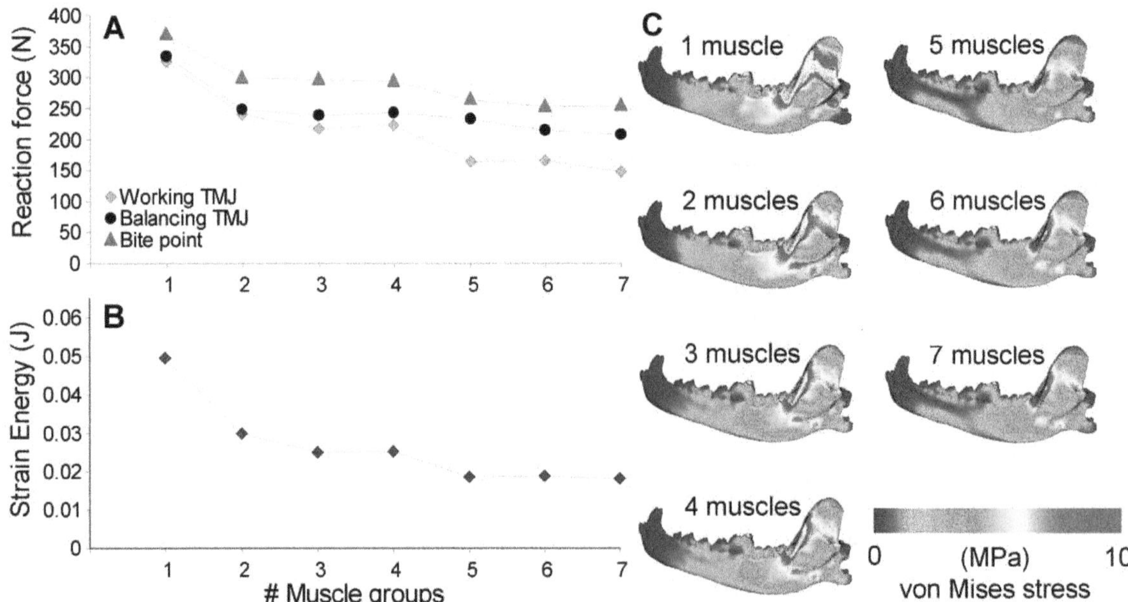

Figure 5. Sensitivity test on number of muscle groups. A. Number of groups plotted against reaction force, connected by lines to show trend. **B**. Number of groups plotted against strain energy. **C**. von Mises stress distribution in the working-side dentary in test models.

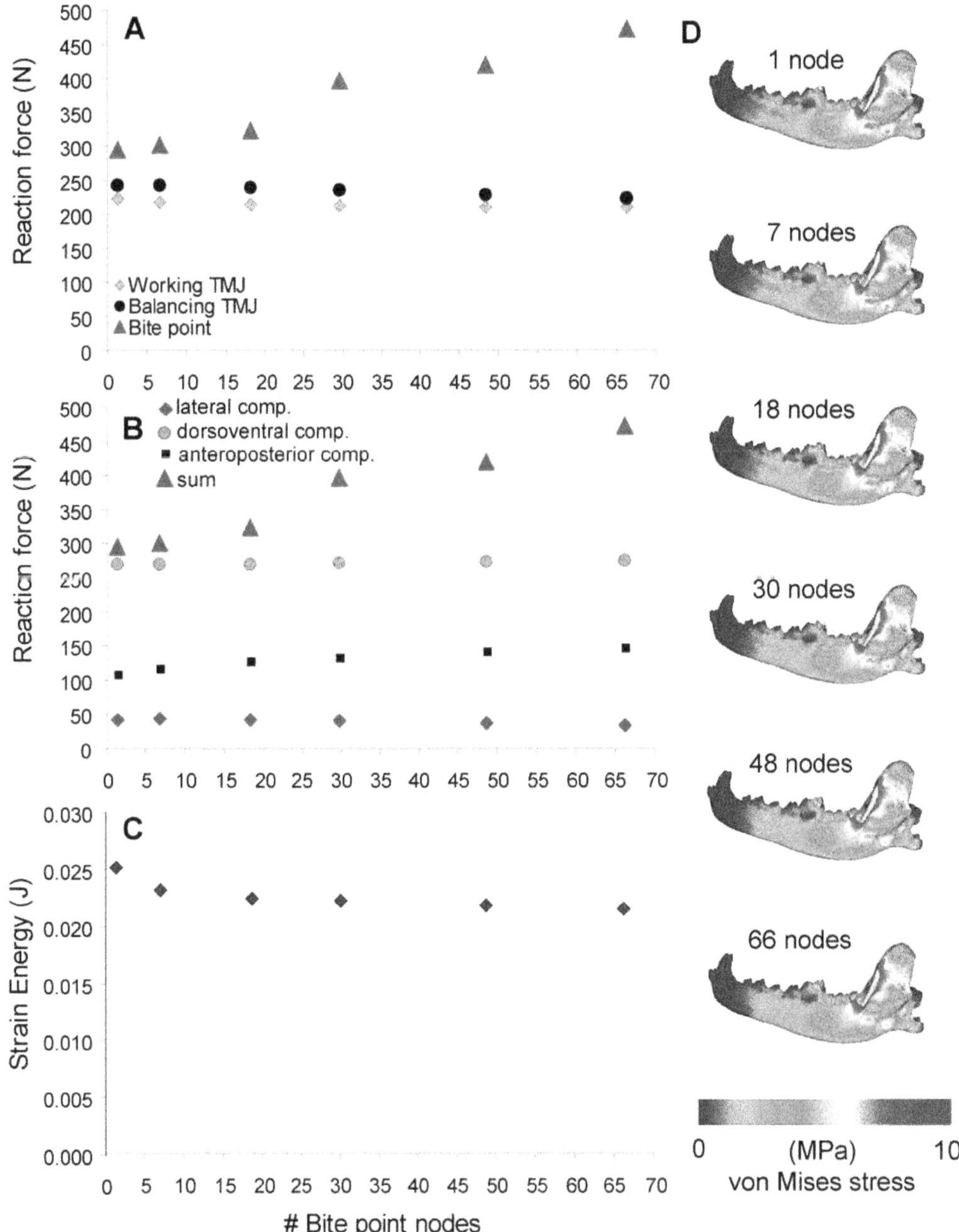

Figure 6. Sensitivity test on nodes at the bite point constraint. A. Nodal constraints plotted against reaction force. **B.** Nodal constraints plotted against reaction force, showing components of the bite force vector. **C.** Nodal constraints plotted against strain energy. **D.** von Mises stress distribution in the working-side dentary in test models.

densities to enable such tests [53]. In cases where such differentiation is possible, however, multiple-property models would tend to increase bite force and also strain energy, and would need to be standardized before comparisons are made across homogeneous and heterogeneous models. The current study did not explicitly consider variation in the ranges of material properties represented in multi-property models. Models with increasing number of material properties also had increasing ranges of densities and modulus values represented by those properties; it remains to be seen how wider or narrower ranges of material properties for a given multi-property model can affect results. An additional factor that has been validated in FE models recently is the localized effect of periodontal ligament on strain in the alveolus; the effect of excluding this tissue from FE models on overall results appear to be small, however [54].

A summary of maximum changes in bite force and strain energy is shown in Table 2. In all but one case, variation in model parameters had larger effects on strain energy than on bite force. In addition, increasing the complexity and magnitude of the values within each parameter can either increase or decrease the performance variables. Theoretically, using a mosaic combination of values in comparisons of any two species models can produce differences where there is none (false positive), or a result of no difference when a difference actually exists (false negative). Functional factors behind a two-model comparison can, therefore, be confounded with variation in input parameters. Whereas

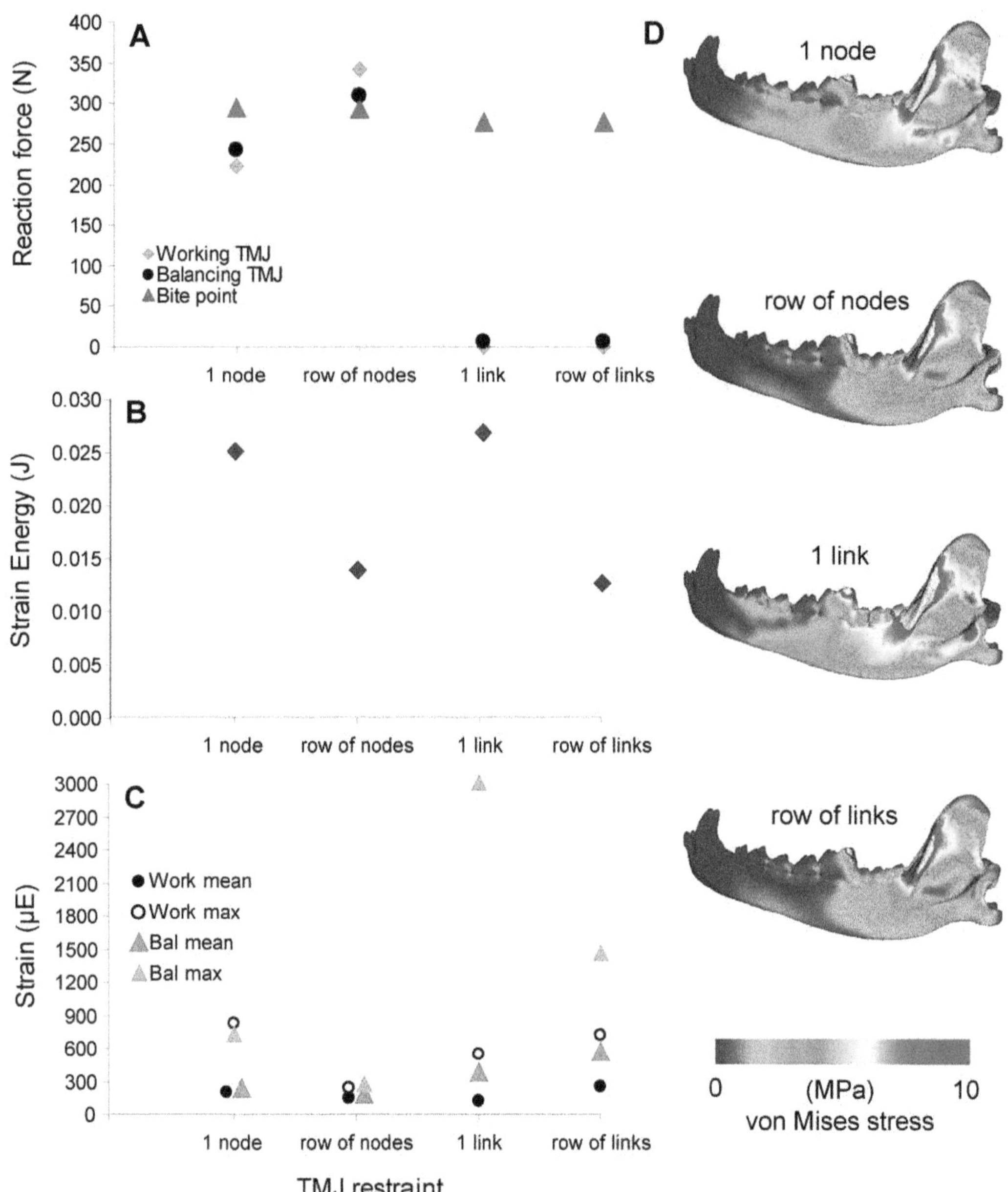

Figure 7. Sensitivity test on temporomandibular joint constraint. A. Constraint type plotted against reaction force. **B.** Constraint type plotted against strain energy. **C.** Constraint type plotted against von Mises strain, showing mean and maximum strain for the working- and balancing-side joints, respectively. **D.** von Mises stress distribution in the working-side dentary in test models.

balancing-working muscle ratios, bite point and joint constraints, and number of material properties are often standardized across species models, and therefore should not constitute as large a source of error, the number of elements and musculature ratios are rarely identical among currently published models. On average, the doubling of tetrahedral elements in the mandible model led to a ~12% increase in strain energy. One reason that differences in element numbers change the magnitude of performance measures is the different internal densities of elements as dictated by automated meshing functions in the FE software program. In the program used for this study (Strand7), coarse models are calculated by minimizing steps required to transition to the maximum element size (which is determined by the initial surface mesh), whereas fine models are built without much constraint on numbers of elements with maximum size. As a result, finer models contain larger quantity of small elements. Compounded with the fact that the number of small elements tend to be higher within each model in regions of high curvature or shape change, stress increases can be observed without changing inputs other than element quantity. The number of elements required to consistently represent a model of complex morphology can only be acquired through convergence analyses of each unique model, and a recent study by Bright and Rayfield [55] provides a specific example of convergence analysis in mammalian cranium models.

Findings also show that musculature ratios that span the available estimates for *Canis* can produce a ~20% difference in bite force and 25% difference in strain energy in otherwise identical models. PCSA has been shown to be a good predictor of

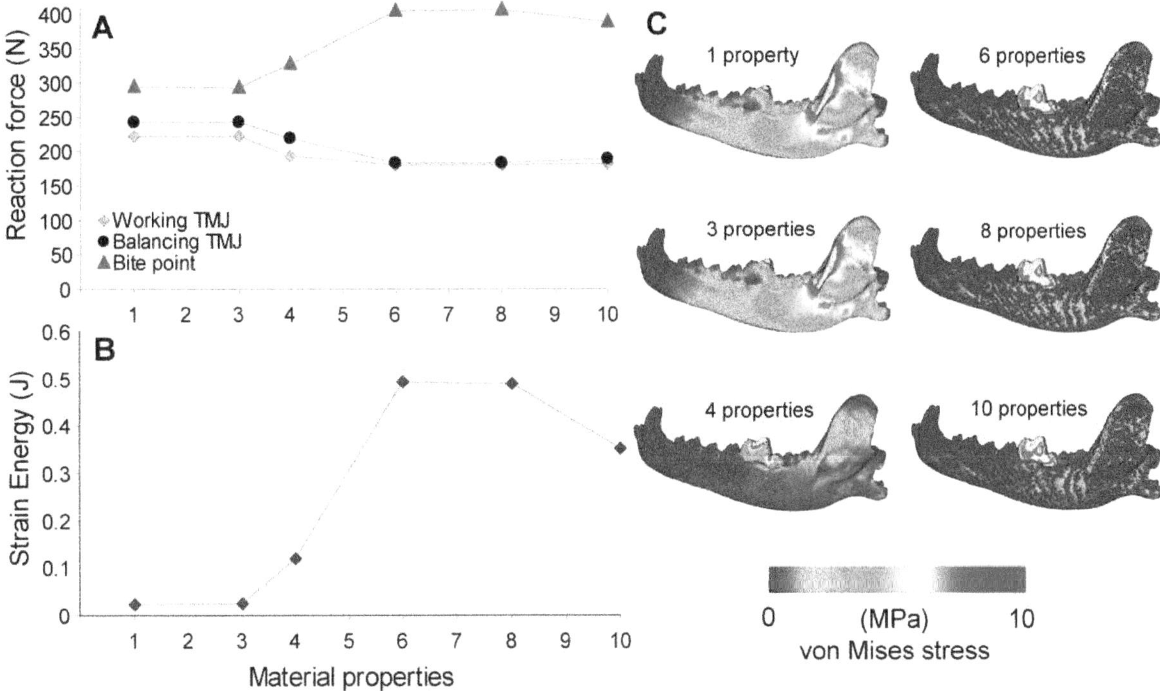

Figure 8. Sensitivity test on number of material properties. A. Number of properties plotted against reaction force, connected by lines to show trend. **B**. Number of properties plotted against strain energy. **C**. von Mises stress distribution in the working-side dentary in test models.

bite force in bats [28], but in comparisons where PCSA is not available, the results indicate that higher estimates of temporalis would tend to return higher bite force and strain energy values. The pattern of performance changes with changing musculature ratios is inherently interesting, and may reveal functional traits not apparent with comparisons of single models [42]. In these cases building multiple models from the same individual with different musculature ratios would be more informative than choosing among the available means of estimates of masticatory muscle force to build a single model.

In summary, the variations that arise in FEA results from changing initial parameters can be confounded with functional differences in model comparisons. More confidence can be placed in model comparisons where these factors are examined by sensitivity and convergence analyses, and in some cases standardized. In standardizing models, it is more important to keep bite point constraints and the number and range of material properties constant in evaluating bite force outputs, and keeping material properties, musculature ratios, and muscle subgroups constant for strain energy comparisons. The relationship between TMJ joint reaction forces on the balancing- versus working side jaw should be examined along with bite forces to ensure the forces acting on the models are reasonably comparable to experimental results. Visual stress distributions are affected more by number of material properties than by any other factor examined. Comparisons between different modeling protocols, if they are to be made, should consider these influences.

Table 2. Maximum % changes in bite force and strain energy in the sensitivity tests.

Parameter	ΔValue	maxΔ Bite force	maxΔ Strain Energy
Number of elements	102 k–1404 k	+10.2%	+60.0%
Balancing-Working Ratio	0.0–1.0	−1.1%	−39.2%
Muscle ratio	Ptery.-Temp.	+12.0%	−63.7%
Muscle number	1–7	−31.6%	−63.3%
Bite point constraint	1–66	+60.0%	−14.7%
TMJ constraint	nodes-links	−6.3%	−49.6%
Material properties	1–10	+38.2%	+>100%

Value ranges given are for the full range of tests conducted. Changes in bite force and strain energy are maximum differences within the range of each test. **Ptery.**, pterygoid muscles; **temp.**, temporalis muscles.

Other parameters

The cross-sectional shape of mandibles is an important predictor of feeding performance and bending strength in carnivorans [56]. However, in studies of fossil species the internal structures of the skull may not be preserved, and in some cases filled models can provide reasonable estimates of mechanical behavior in the original morphology [26]. In cases where internal morphology simply cannot be reconstructed with any confidence, the filled models may be sufficient for broad comparison purposes. However, researchers may wish to reconstruct the internal cavity by approximating its boundary if the evolution of corpus cortical thickness is of interest.

The mandibular symphysis, which exhibits variation in composition and gross anatomy across mammal species, is a key location that affects the distribution of stresses across the dentaries [34]. Tseng and Stynder [57] tested a range of material properties to approximate the mechanical behavior of the mandibular symphysis in their carnivoran models, and found that in most cases the stress is conducted through the symphysis, but modeling the joint as cortical bone can increase regional stress. Their results are superficially similar to those presented by McHenry et al. [22] and Wroe et al. [21], and suggest that at least for the symphysis, those models show elevated stress compared to ones constructed with material properties closer to ligament or fibrocartilage.

Homogeneous models, which are built using a single set of material properties, usually representing average cortical bone, are common in comparative studies [21,23,25]. A sensitivity test of typical elastic modulus and Poisson ratio values used in construction of homogeneous models was conduced by Tseng et al. [53], who showed that the middle range of elastic modulus (15–30 GPa) and Poisson ratio (0.1–0.4) used by many studies gave comparable results in stress and strain. Thus, stress distributions of homogeneous models built with values within those ranges are not expected to be significantly influenced by modeling artifacts when used in comparisons.

The sensitivity tests performed in this study are by no means exhaustive, and the range of input assumptions represented by the current set of models can be expanded upon to include more extensive or specific tests that pertain to specific research questions. The models discussed in this study are available in the Dryad Digital Repository (doi:10.5061/dryad.8961).

Conclusions

We conducted a series of sensitivity tests to evaluate the range of variation among the modeling parameters required in studies of functional morphology using FEA. Findings indicate that not all parameters are equally variable, and consideration needs to be given to particular sets of parameters, based on the research question being asked. In a purely comparative context, a Gray Wolf mandible model required only ~300,000 elements to produce reaction forces and strain energy values close to those obtained from higher-resolution models (>1,400,000 elements). Whereas PCSA, mass, or other estimates of muscle ratios did not greatly affect the results, the adjustment of the balancing-working side ratio in unilateral biting simulation does have an effect on joint reaction forces. For comparative purposes, the number of muscle subgroups, the area of bite point constraints, the TMJ constraint, and the number and range of material properties should be kept consistent across models within a single study. Across different studies, the compound effects of variation among those factors may be large, and differences up to 50% can be observed by extreme values in a single parameter. Validation of FE models of living species is needed to determine the set of input parameters that would give the most realistic results in a given study, but comparative studies can nevertheless be highly informative especially if sources of variation can be identified within the particular set of values used to construct the models. Lastly, the pattern of variation obtained through tests of a given parameter within each model may be instructive in itself, thus researchers may wish to consider sensitivity tests as part of a study design of comparative form and function using FEA.

Supporting Information

Table S1 Models used in the sensitivity tests. Models and their descriptions are available at Dryad Digital Repository:

Table S2 Data for sensitivity test 1: Number of tetrahedral elements. Tet4, number of 4-noded tetrahedral elements; **SE**, strain energy.

Table S3 Data for sensitivity test 2: balancing-working muscle ratios.

Table S4 Data for sensitivity test 3: musculature ratios.

Table S5 Data for sensitivity test 4: number of muscle subgroups.

Table S6 Data for sensitivity test 5: bite point constraint. m1.ap, anteroposterior component, **m1.dv**, dorsoventral component, **m1.lat**, lateral component.

Table S7 Data for sensitivity test 6: temporomandibular joint constraints.

Table S8 Data for sensitivity test 7: number of material properties.

Table S9 Material properties used in sensitivity test 7. HU, Hounsfield Units; **E**, elastic (Young's) modulus; **v**, Poisson ratio. Material properties of bone were derived from the regression equation of Schneider et al. (1996): Density (g/cm^3) = 0.0007*HU+0.3489, $R^2=0.9994$, and modulus values were calculated from the regression equation of Rho et al. (1995) as E (GPa) = $5.05*\rho^{1.269}$ for $\rho<1$ g/cm3 and E (GPa) = $9.11*\rho^{1.326}$ for $\rho>1$ g/cm^3. The lowest density material was arbitrarily assigned $\rho=0.01$ g/cm^3 as a low-end value.

Acknowledgments

We thank J. Dines (LACM) for providing the specimen used in the study. M. McNitt-Gray (UCLA) CT-scanned the specimen. J. Liu provided valuable comments on the content of the manuscript. The editor and anonymous reviewers provided constructive criticism that improved the content of the paper.

Author Contributions

Conceived and designed the experiments: ZJT JM HF. Performed the experiments: ZJT. Analyzed the data: ZJT JM HF XW RE. Contributed reagents/materials/analysis tools: JM HF XW RE. Wrote the paper: ZJT JM.

References

1. Rayfield EJ (2007) Finite element analysis and understanding the biomechanics and evolution of living and fossil organisms. Annual Review of Earth and Planetary Science 35: 541–576.
2. Ross CF (2005) Finite element analysis in vertebrate biomechanics. The Anatomical Record 283A: 253–258.
3. Kupczik K (2008) Virtual biomechanics: basic concepts and technical aspects of finite element analysis in vertebrate morphology. Journal of Anthropological Sciences 86: 193–198.
4. Fastnacht M, Hess N, Frey E, Weiser H-P (2002) Finite element analysis in vertebrate palaeontology. Senckenbergiana lethaea 82: 195–206.
5. McHenry C, Clausen PD, Daniel WJT, Meers MB, Pendharkar A (2006) Biomechanics of the rostrum in crocodilians, a comparative analysis using finite element modeling. The Anatomical Record 288A: 827–849.
6. Bell PE, Snively E, Shychoski L (2009) A comparison of the jaw mechanics in hadrosaurid and ceratopsid dinosaurs using finite element analysis. The Anatomical Record 292: 1338–1351.

7. Xing L, Ye Y, Shu C, Peng G, You H (2009) Structure, orientation and finite element analysis of the tail club of *Mamenchisaurus hochuanensis*. Acta Geologica Sinica 83: 1031–1040.
8. Arbour VM, Snively E (2009) Finite element analyses of ankylosaurid dinosaur tail club impacts. The Anatomical Record 292: 1412–1426.
9. Rayfield EJ, Norman DB, Jorner CC, Horner JR, Smith PM, et al. (2001) Cranial design and function in a large theropod dinosaur. Nature 409: 1033–1037.
10. Rayfield EJ (2004) Cranial mechanics and feeding in *Tyrannosaurus rex*. Proceedings of the Royal Society of London, Series B 271: 1451–1459.
11. Rayfield EJ (2005) Aspects of comparative cranial mechanics in the theropod dinosaurs *Coelophysis*, *Allosaurus*, and *Tyrannosaurus*. Zoological Journal of the Linnean Society 144: 309–316.
12. Soons J, Herrel A, Genbrugge A, Aerts P, Podos J, et al. (2010) Mechanical stress, fracture risk and beak evolution in Darwin's ground finches (*Geospiza*). Philosophical Transactions of the Royal Society of London B Biological Sciences 365: 1093–1098.
13. Moazen M, Curtis N, Evans SE, O'Higgins P, Fagan MJ (2008) Combined finite element and multibody dynamics analysis of biting in a *Uromastyx hardwickii* lizard skull. Journal of Anatomy 213: 499–508.
14. Moreno K, Wroe S, Clausen PD, McHenry C, D'Amore DC, et al. (2008) Cranial performance in the Komodo dragon (*Varanus komodoensis*) as revealed by high-resolution 3-D finite element analysis. Journal of Anatomy 212: 736–746.
15. Hulsey CD, Roberts RJ, Lin ASP, Guldberg R, Streelman JT (2008) Convergence in a mechanically complex phenotype: Detecting structural adaptations for crushing in cichlid fish. Evolution 62: 1587–1599.
16. Tanner JB, Dumont ER, Sakai ST, Lundrigan BL, Holekamp KE (2008) Of arcs and vaults: the biomechanics of bone-cracking in spotted hyenas (*Crocuta crocuta*). Biological Journal of the Linnean Society 95: 246–255.
17. Strait DS, Weber GW, Neubauer S, Chalk J, Richmond BG, et al. (2009) The feeding biomechanics and dietary ecology of *Australopithecus africanus*. Proceedings of the National Academy of Sciences 106: 2124–2129.
18. Slater GJ, Van Valkenburgh B (2009) Allometry and performance: the evolution of skull form and function in felids. Journal of Evolutionary Biology 22: 2278–2287.
19. Dumont ER, Piccirillo J, Grosse IR (2005) Finite-element analysis of biting behavior and bone stress in the facial skeletons of bats. The Anatomical Record 283A: 319–330.
20. Wroe S (2008) Cranial mechanics compared in extinct marsupial and extant African lions using a finite-element approach. Journal of Zoology 274: 332–339.
21. Wroe S, Clausen PD, McHenry C, Moreno K, Cunningham E (2007) Computer simulation of feeding behaviour in the thylacine and dingo as a novel test for convergence and niche overlap. Proceedings of the Royal Society B: Biological Sciences 274: 2819–2828.
22. McHenry C, Wroe S, Clausen PD, Moreno K, Cunningham E (2007) Supermodeled sabercat, predatory behavior in *Smilodon fatalis* revealed by high-resolution 3D computer simulation. Proceedings of the National Academy of Sciences 104: 16010–16015.
23. Slater GJ, Dumont ER, Van Valkenburgh B (2009) Implications of predatory specialization for cranial form and function in canids. Journal of Zoology 278: 181–188.
24. Farke AA (2008) Frontal sinuses and head-butting in goats: a finite element analysis. The Journal of Experimental Biology 211: 3085–3094.
25. Tseng ZJ (2009) Cranial function in a late Miocene *Dinocrocuta gigantea* (Mammalia: Carnivora) revealed by comparative finite element analysis. Biological Journal of the Linnean Society 96: 51–67.
26. Tseng ZJ, Binder WJ (2010) Mandibular biomechanics of *Crocuta crocuta*, *Canis lupus*, and the late Miocene *Dinocrocuta gigantea* (Carnivora, Mammalia). Zoological Journal of Linnean Society 158: 683–696.
27. Ross CF, Patel BA, Slice DE, Strait DS, Dechow PC, et al. (2005) Modeling masticatory muscle force in finite element analysis: sensitivity analysis using principal coordinates analysis. The Anatomical Record 283A: 288–299.
28. Davis JL, Santana SE, Dumont ER, Grosse I (2010) Predicting bite force in mammals: two-dimensional *versus* three-dimensional lever models. Journal of Experimental Biology 213: 1844–1851.
29. Strait DS, Wang Q, Dechow PC, Ross CF, Richmond BG, et al. (2005) Modeling elastic properties in finite-element analysis: how much precision is needed to produce an accurate model? The Anatomical Record 283A: 275–287.
30. Dumont ER, Grosse I, Slater GJ (2009) Requirements for comparing the performance of finite element models of biological structures. Journal of Theoretical Biology 256: 96–103.
31. Sellers WI, Crompton RH (2004) Using sensitivity analysis to validate the predictions of a biomechanical model of bite forces. Annals of Anatomy 186: 89–95.
32. Hylander WL (1979) An experimental analysis of temporomandibular joint reaction force in macaques. American Journal of Physical Anthropology 51: 433–456.
33. Nalla RK, Kinney JH, Ritchie RO (2003) Mechanistic failure criteria for the failure of human cortical bone. Nature Materials 2: 164–168.
34. Scapino RP (1965) The third joint of the canine jaw. Journal of Morphology 116: 23–50.
35. Herring SW, Teng S (2000) Strain in the braincase and its suture during function. American Journal of Physical Anthropology 112: 575–593.
36. Dessem D (1989) Interactions between jaw-muscle recruitment and jaw-joint forces in *Canis familiaris*. Journal of Anatomy 164: 101–121.
37. Ellis JL, Thomason JJ, Kebreab E, France J (2008) Calibration of estimated biting forces in domestic canids: comparison of post-mortem and *in vivo* measurements. Journal of Anatomy 212: 769–780.
38. Hylander WL, Ravosa MJ, Ross CF, Wall CE, Johnson KR (2000) Symphyseal fusion and jaw-adductor muscle force: An EMG study. American Journal of Physical Anthropology 112: 469–492.
39. Thomason JJ (1991) Cranial strength in relation to estimate biting forces in some mammals. Canadian Journal of Zoology 69: 2326–2333.
40. Schumacher GH (1961) Funktionelle Morphologie der Kaumuskulatur. Jena, Germany: VEB Gustav Fischer Verlag. 262 p.
41. Turnbull WD (1970) Mammalian masticatory apparatus. Fieldiana: Geology 18: 149–356.
42. Tseng ZJ, Wang X (2010) Cranial functional morphology of fossil dogs and adaptation for durophagy in *Borophagus* and *Epicyon* (Carnivora, Mammalia). Journal of Morphology 271: 1386–1398.
43. Dumont ER, Davis JL, Grosse I, Burrows AM (2011) Finite element analysis of performance in the skulls of marmosets and tamarins. Journal of Anatomy 218: 151–162.
44. Rho JY, Hobatho MC, Ashman RB (1995) Relations of mechanical properties to density and CT numbers in human bone. Medical Engineering and Physics 17: 347–355.
45. Schneider U, Pedroni E, Lomax A (1996) The calibration of CT Hounsfield units for radiotherapy treatment planning. Physics in Medicine and Biology 41: 111–124.
46. Qin Q-H, Swain MV (2004) A micro-mechanics model of dentin mechanical properties. Biomaterials 25: 5081–5090.
47. Habelitz S, Marshall SJ, Marshall Jr. GW, Balooch M (2001) Mechanical properties of human dental enamel on the nanometre scale. Archives of Oral Biology 46: 173–183.
48. Haines DJ (1968) Physical properties of human tooth enamel and enamel sheath material under load. Journal of Biomechanics 1: 117–125.
49. Grosse I, Dumont ER, Coletta C, Tolleson A (2007) Techniques for modeling muscle-induced forces in finite element models of skeletal structures. The Anatomical Record 290: 1069–1088.
50. Slater GJ, Figueirido B, Louis L, Yang P, Van Valkenburgh B (2010) Biomechanical consequences of rapid evolution in the polar bear lineage. PLoS ONE 5: e13870. doi:13810.11371/journal.pone.0013870.
51. Stefen C (1997) Chapter 7. Differentiations in Hunter-Schreger bands of carnivores. In: Koenigswald Wv, Sander PM, eds. Tooth enamel microstructure. Rotterdam: A.A. Balkema. pp 123–136.
52. Rensberger JM (1995) Determination of stresses in mammalian dental enamel and their relevance to the interpretation of feeding behaviors in extinct taxa. In: Thomason JJ, ed. Functional morphology in vertebrate paleontology. New York: Cambridge University Press. pp 151–172.
53. Tseng ZJ, Antón M, Salesa MJ (2011) The evolution of the bone-cracking model in carnivorans: Cranial functional morphology of the Plio-Pleistocene cursorial hyaenid *Chasmaporthetes lunensis* (Mammalia: Carnivora). Paleobiology 37: 140–156.
54. Panagiotopoulou O, Kupczik K, Cobb SN (2011) The mechanical function of the periodontal ligament in the macaque mandible: a validation and sensitivity study using finite element analysis. Journal of Anatomy 218: 75–86.
55. Bright JA, Rayfield EJ (2011) The response of cranial biomechanical finite element models to variations in mesh density. The Anatomical Record 294: 610–620.
56. Biknevicius AR, Ruff CB (1992) The structure of the mandibular corpus and its relationship to feeding behaviors in extant carnivorans. Journal of Zoology 228: 479–507.
57. Tseng ZJ, Stynder D (2011) Mosaic functionality in a transitional ecomorphology: skull biomechanics in stem Hyaeninae compared to modern South African carnivorans. Biological Journal of the Linnean Society 102: 540–559.

17

A National Survey of Musculoskeletal Impairment in Rwanda: Prevalence, Causes and Service Implications

Oluwarantimi Atijosan[1], Dorothea Rischewski[1], Victoria Simms[1], Hannah Kuper[1], Bonaventure Linganwa[2], Assuman Nuhi[2], Allen Foster[1], Chris Lavy[1,3]*

1 Department of Infectious and Tropical Diseases, London School of Hygiene & Tropical Medicine, London, United Kingdom, **2** CBMI, Kigali, Rwanda, **3** Nuffield Department of Orthopaedic Surgery, University of Oxford, Oxford, United Kingdom

Abstract

Background: Accurate information on the prevalence and causes of musculoskeletal impairment (MSI) is lacking in low income countries. We present a new survey methodology that is based on sound epidemiological principles and is linked to the World Health Organisation's International Classification of Functioning.

Methods: Clusters were selected with probability proportionate to size. Households were selected within clusters through compact segment sampling. 105 clusters of 80 people (all ages) were included. All participants were screened for MSI by a physiotherapist and medical assistant. Possible cases plus a random sample of 10% of non-MSI cases were examined further to ascertain diagnosis, aetiology, quality of life, and treatment needs.

Findings: 6757 of 8368 enumerated individuals (80.8%) were screened. There were 352 cases, giving an overall prevalence for MSI of 5.2%. (95% CI 4.5–5.9) The prevalence of MSI increased with age and was similar in men and women. Extrapolating these estimates, there are approximately 488,000 MSI diagnoses in Rwanda. Only 8.2% of MSI cases were severe, while the majority were moderate (43.7%) or mild (46.3%). Diagnostic categories comprised 11.5% congenital, 31.3% trauma, 3.8% infection, 9.0% neurological, and 44.4% non-traumatic non infective acquired. The most common individual diagnoses were joint disease (13.3%), angular limb deformity (9.7%) and fracture mal- and non-union (7.2%). 96% of all cases required further treatment.

Interpretation: This survey demonstrates a large burden of MSI in Rwanda, which is mostly untreated. The survey methodology will be useful in other low income countries, to assist with planning services and monitoring trends.

Editor: William Taylor, University of Otago, New Zealand

Funding: CBMI was the main funder of this study, but was not involved in the work or writing of the paper.

Competing Interests: The authors have declared that no competing interests exist.

* E-mail: christopher.lavy@ndos.ox.ac.uk

Introduction

There is a global lack of accurate information on the prevalence and causes of physical disability in low income countries [1,2]. There are two main reasons for this deficiency. Firstly, there have not been many surveys and secondly there is no universally accepted definition of physical disability. The surveys that have been undertaken have used a variety of definitions of physical disability, and a range of methodologies for measuring disability so that comparisons cannot be made between countries [3,4] . For example one survey which asked detailed questions about difficulties in different aspects of life, showed that Norway had a prevalence of physical disability of 35% while the national census in India, which merely asked whether there was a "physically handicapped" person in the household estimated that the prevalence was 0.2% [5]. With such different ways of measuring and defining disability there is little benefit in making comparisons between countries, or over time within a country. Where there has been a tighter definition of a specific impairment or symptom such as has been used in the COPCORD programme (Community-Oriented Program for the Control of Rheumatic Diseases) [6] then it has been possible to standardise a data collection methodology, with scope for international comparison. The COPCORD programme is of great value in comparing rheumatic and joint conditions in different countries, however it does not include trauma or non painful congenital or acquired musculoskeletal deformities.

The difficulty in defining physical disability stems from its many anatomical, physiological and pathological presentations and causes, and its intimate relation to society and the environment. Terminology has also been confusing, and different groups in society have different reasons for the varied used of the word disability. This debate is of more than just academic interest as in order to plan effective services it is important to estimate the prevalence and causes of physical disability, which requires a definition of the disability being measured and a survey methodology. There have been many attempts to reach a common understanding of disability, and the World Health Organisation's (WHO) publication of the International Classification on Functioning (ICF) is a major step forward [7]. The ICF classifies impairment of body structure and function, and also includes domains that measure activity and participation in society.

Rwanda as a country is in the process of rebuilding its rehabilitation services and facilities for people with musculoskeletal impairment (MSI) after its genocide and war of 1994 with all the demographic and structural destruction that took place. In order to plan effective services it is important to estimate the prevalence and causes of MSI that exist in the country. The WHO estimates that the prevalence of all types of disability on a global level is around 10% [8], but this estimate is of limited use for planning services in specific situations. Realising this difficulty, Helander developed a 'Rapid Calculation of Disability Prevalence' for less developed regions of the world and estimated that 4.8% of a population will need some rehabilitation service [9]. Several physical disability surveys have been conducted in Rwanda since the 1994 war, but all have their limitations. Handicap International carried out a nationwide survey in 1995 into 'physical disability' [10], and found a very low prevalence of 0.58%. Its own researchers noted that this was low and questioned whether many sections of the population might have been inaccessible so soon after the war. A Community Based Rehabilitation project in Kigali carried out a similar survey in 1997 and estimated that the prevalence was 1.8% (personal communication), but the sampling methodology was inadequate, and the researchers believed that many households withheld information about family members with physical disabilities.

In view of the lack of accurate data on the prevalence and causes of MSI, we worked with the Ministry of Health of Rwanda to develop a survey of MSI of all ages that involved a reliable sampling methodology and a case definition and diagnostic criteria that could clearly map onto the classification system used in the ICF. Our aim was to develop a reliable survey tool that could be used to plan and monitor MSI services in Rwanda and other developing countries.

Methods

Sample selection – (see also diagram in Appendix S1)

The survey was designed to be nationally representative, including people of all ages. The expected prevalence of MSI in this group was estimated at approximately 3% [9,11]. Allowing for a required confidence of 95%, a precision of 20%, a population size of 8,441,000 in 2005 [11], a design effect of 2.3, and 15% non-response, the required sample size was estimated to be 8399 subjects (Epi Info 6.04). In total, 105 clusters of 80 people were needed for this survey. A cluster size of 80 people was chosen for logistical reasons, as it was considered to be the number a team could complete in one day.

A nationally representative sample of the population was selected through cluster sampling with probability proportionate to size. A list was produced of all the enumeration areas and their respective populations, and a column was created with the cumulative population across the settlements. The total population (i.e. 8,441,000) was divided by the number of clusters required (i.e. 105) to derive the sampling interval (i.e. 80,390). The first cluster was selected by multiplying the sampling interval with a random number between 0 and 1. The resulting number was traced in the cumulative population column and the first cluster was taken from the corresponding enumeration area. The following clusters were identified by adding the sampling interval to the previous number.

Households within clusters were selected through compact segment sampling [12]. Maps of each selected cluster (i.e. enumeration area) were obtained from the census bureau. These maps included the locations of the head of ten-household communities, thus showing approximate population distribution. The enumeration area was visited two to three days before the survey and the village leaders were asked to update the map. The enumeration area was then divided into segments, so that each segment included approximately 80 people. For instance, if an enumeration area comprised 400 people then it would be divided into five segments. One of the segments was chosen at random by drawing lots and all households in the segment were included in the sample sequentially until 80 people were identified. People were eligible for inclusion if they lived in the household at least three months of the year. All the individuals in the final household were screened, and the number of people needed to complete the cluster was randomly selected for inclusion (e.g. if the final household included 5 people but only 3 were required to complete the cluster then 3 out of the 5 were randomly selected for inclusion). If the segment did not include 80 people then another segment was chosen at random and sampling continued. If an eligible person was absent the survey team returned to the household to examine him/her before leaving the area. If after repeated visits the person could not be examined, information about his/her presumed MSI status was collected from relatives or neighbours.

Musculoskeletal impairment assessment

The fieldwork was carried out between October and December, 2005. The survey team visited households door-to-door and conducted the MSI screening in the household. The survey team consisted of a physiotherapist and an assistant, and they were assisted in the clusters by a village guide, appointed by the village leaders. The purpose of the study and the examination procedure were explained to the subjects and verbal consent was obtained before examination.

A standardised protocol was used for the screening and assessment of MSI [13]. A survey record was filled for each eligible person that included:

- Demographic information (all participants);
- A screening examination for MSI (all participants);
- A standardised interview and examination protocol for MSI (cases and 10% random sample of non-cases)
- History of MSI (if not examined)

Screening for musculoskeletal impairment

The team physiotherapist screened all participants for MSI by asking them seven questions about difficulties using their musculoskeletal system, whether they used a mobility aid, whether they felt they had any physical deformity, and how long they had had these symptoms. Participants over 5 years of age were questioned directly, while participants under 5 years were asked through proxy, by the child's main carer. Participants who answered "yes" to any of the questions were classified as cases, provided that the condition had lasted for more than one month or was considered permanent. This screening tool was developed by orthopaedic surgeons together with physiotherapists and has been shown to have 99% sensitivity and 97% specificity with interobserver Kappa scores of 0.90 for the diagnostic group [13].

Standardised interview and examination protocol

All cases were examined in more detail by the physiotherapist using a standardised interview and examination protocol. A random 10% sample of non-cases was also examined further, to confirm their non-case status. The standardised examination protocol assessed the aetiology, duration, severity, anatomical location, diagnosis, and treatment, both received and required.

The standardised interview and examination protocol included the following sections:

a) Physical examination

The physiotherapist observed the participant as they carried out physical tasks that required use of the musculoskeletal system (i.e. walking, crouching and upper limb motor skills)

b) Diagnosis

The physiotherapist categorized the diagnosis as: congenital, traumatic, infective, neurological, or acquired non traumatic non infective. Within these categories an algorithm was used to give a specific diagnosis. Up to two diagnoses were permissible per identified case of MSI [13].

c) Area affected and nature of problem

The physiotherapist recorded information on the area of the body affected (e.g. arm) and the nature of the problem (e.g. amputation).

d) Aetiology

Where this was known it was recorded. It was determined by questioning the case about when the impairment developed and how it came about. The physiotherapists were trained as to what questions to ask for each aetiology available, which included road traffic accidents, war, infection, and familial.

e) Severity

Severity was determined using ICF parameters for the amount of function which has been lost through the presence of the MSI. This was classified as "mild", "moderate" or "severe" [6].

f) EQ-5D

Generic quality of life was measured using the EQ-5D scale, which is a public domain health-related quality of life questionnaire [14]. This was translated and back translated from English into Kinyarwandan by two medical translators, independently of each other. However, because of time restrictions, this was carried out independently from the Euroqol group, and the translated version of EQ-5D used in this study has therefore *not* been approved by the Euroqol group

g) Treatment given

Current treatment received by the participant (if any) was recorded.

h) Barriers to treatment

Cases were asked an open-ended question about why they had not accessed treatment for their MSI. Up to four responses were recorded per case on pre-coded forms.

i) Treatment needed

Treatment needed was assessed by the physiotherapist according to standard protocols, appropriate for Rwanda.

Training and quality control

There were three teams, each consisted of a physiotherapist a medical assistant, a village guide and a driver. The teams received three weeks of training. Inter-observer agreement for case definition, diagnosis, severity classification and treatment required was assessed between the teams to ensure that it was of an acceptable standard (i.e. kappa≥0.60). A pilot survey was undertaken of 480 people in 9 clusters (6 rural and 3 urban) to assess examination process and procedures. During the main survey, teams were accompanied by a field supervisor at least one day per week, to ensure that a high quality was maintained. Each day the supervisors checked items of all completed forms in the field.

Statistical analysis

A database was constructed for data entry using EpiData 3.1. The data were double-entered and validated, and inconsistencies were checked. Stata 9.0 was used for analysis. The prevalence and causes of MSI was estimated, taking into account the design effect (DEFF) when estimating the confidence intervals. (see appendix S1 for details of estimation of DEFF)

Ethical approval

Ethical approval for this survey was granted by the Independent Ethics Committee in Rwanda and the London School of Hygiene & Tropical Medicine. Permission to proceed was granted by the government, and consent was granted for each cluster visited from the community leader at the province, district, sector and cell level. Informed verbal consent was obtained from the subjects after explanation of the nature and possible consequences of the study. Written consent was obtained for any photographs that were taken. All people with treatable MSI were referred to a central community rehabilitation centre where clinical members of the study team reviewed and referred the participants for further treatment, as appropriate. The research followed the tenets of the Declaration of Helsinki.

Role of funding source.

The funding for this study was provided by CBM international. One of the authors (OR) was supported by Cure International. The funding organisations played no part in, and had no influence on the design of the study, or the data, collection, analysis or interpretation.

Results

Sampled population (table 1)

A total of 8368 individuals were enumerated and 6757 were screened (Response rate = 80.8%), 1596 (19.1%) were absent, 10 (0.1%) refused and 5(0.1%) were unable to communicate. The response rate was higher in women (84.8%) than in men (76.3%). Among the participants that were enumerated but not examined, 88 were believed to have MSI (5.5%). The age- and gender-distribution of the sampled population was very similar to that of the national population (Table 1).

Prevalence of MSI

Of the 6757 individuals screened there were 352 cases of MSI giving an overall prevalence of MSI of 5.2% (CI 4.5–5.9) (Table 2). The prevalence of MSI fell after early childhood and then increased rapidly with age so that it was almost nine-fold higher in people aged over 60 years compared to those aged 0–5 years (OR = 8.9, 6.0–13.4). The prevalence of MSI was similar in men (5.1%) and women (5.3%). People in rural areas were more likely to have an MSI (5.4%) than urban dwellers (4.1%), while those without formal education were more likely to have an MSI (5.6%) than those with formal education (4.5%), although these associations disappeared after adjustment for age and gender.

Prevalence of MSI by Severity and Gender

The majority of cases of MSI were mild (47.1%) or moderate (44.5%), and few were severe (8.4%) (Table 3). This pattern was very similar in men and women.

MSI Diagnoses

There were a total of 390 diagnoses for 352 people with MSI (Table 4). The most common causes of MSI were joint problems (13.3% of MSI diagnoses), other acquired (12.3%), fracture non or malunion (7.2%) and other chronic joint injury (6.2%). Overall 44% of MSI were due to acquired non-traumatic non-infective causes, 31% due to trauma, 9% neurological were in origin, 4% due to infection and 12% congenital. Extrapolating these estimates to the total population of Rwanda there were 488,000 MSI diagnoses.

With increasing age, the prevalence of MSI increased rapidly (Figure 1). The greatest proportional increase was in MSI diagnoses

Table 1. Age and gender composition of national* and screened sample population.

Age Groups	Male			Female			Total		
	49.7%	47%	44.3%	50.3%	52%	55.7%			
	National (%)	Enumerated Sample	Screened Sample (%)	National (%)	Enumerated Sample	S Screened ample (%)	National (%)	Enumerated Sample	Screened Sample (%)
0–10	1 302 000 (31.1)	1394 (35.4)	1222 (40.7)	1 287 000 (30.3)	1420 (32.1)	1295 (34.5)	2 589 000 (30.7)	2816 (33.7)	**2519 (37.3)**
11–20	964 000 (23.0)	1029 (26.2)	723 (24.1)	964 000 (22.7)	1081 (24.4)	832 (22.2)	1 929 000 (22.9)	2116 (25.3)	**1559 (23.1)**
21–30	807 000 (19.2)	601 (15.3)	386 (12.9)	808 000 (19.0)	724 (16.4)	567 (15.1)	1 616 000(19.1)	1325 (15.8)	**953 (14.1)**
31–40	482 000 (11.5)	335 (8.5)	234 (7.8)	467 000 (11.0)	422 (9.5)	358 (9.5)	949 000 (11.2)	757 (9.1)	**592 (8.8)**
41–50	326 000(7.7)	275 (7.0)	195 (6.5)	327 000 (7.7)	330 (7.5)	292 (7.8)	654 000 (7.7)	605 (7.2)	**487 (7.2)**
51–60	182 000(4.3)	160 (4.1)	126 (4.2)	205 000 (4.8)	231 (5.2)	203 (5.4)	387 000 (4.6)	392 (4.69)	**329 (4.9)**
>60	129 000 (3.1)	140 (3.6)	114 (3.8)	190 000 (4.5)	216 (4.9)	204 (5.4)	289 000 (3.4)	356 (4.3)	**318 (4.7)**
Total	**4 193 000 (100.0)**	**3934 (100.0)**	**3000 (100.0)**	**4 248 000 (100.0)**	**4424 (100.0)**	**3751 (100.0)**	**8 441 000 (100.0)**	**8367 (100.0)**	**6757$ (100.0)**

*based on us census bureau data for Rwanda population 2005 as this has age group divisions
$missing gender data for 6 individuals

Table 2. Prevalence of MSI by age, gender, location and educational level of head of household.

Categories*		total no screened.	No of MSI cases in that group	Prevalence of MSI (95% CI)	Age and sex adjusted Odds Ratios (95%CI)
	Total	**6757**	**352**	**5.2% (4.5–5.9%)**	
Age groups	0–5 years	1520	52	3.4% (2.3–4.5%)	1
	6–16 years	2006	39	1.9% (1.2–2.7%)	0.6 (0.4–0.9)
	17–60 years	2913	185	6.4% (5.3–7.4%)	1.9 (1.4–2.7)
	>60 years	318	76	23.9% (18.5–29.3%)	8.9 (6.0–13.4)
Gender	Male	3000	153	5.1% (4.3–6.0%)	1
	Female	3751	199	5.3% (4.5–6.2%)	0.9 (0.8–1.2)
Location	Rural	5806	312	5.4% (4.6–6.1%)	1
	Urban	938	39	4.1% (2.7–5.6%)	0.9 (0.6–1.4)
Educational Level of Head of household	No formal education	4346	244	5.6% (4.8–6.5%)	1
	Formal education	2399	108	4.5% (3.5–5.5%)	0.9 (0.7–1.2)

*There were some missing values

Table 3. Distribution of MSI according to severity and gender, and its association with quality of life.

	Male		Female		Total		
MSI status	Number	Proportion of MSI cases	Number	Proportion of MSI cases	Number	Proportion of MSI cases	EQ-5D VAS Score (95% CI)
Mild MSI	69	46.0%	94	48.0%	163	47.1%	44.4 (40.5–47.8)
Moderate MSI	65	43.3%	89	45.4%	154	44.5%	37.7.(35.4–40.0)
Severe MSI	16	10.7%	13	6.6%	29	8.4%	16.9 (11.7–22.0)
No MSI	2847		3552		6399		63.1 (61.4–64.7)

related to trauma and acquired non-traumatic non-infective. Congenital diagnoses were relatively more common in the youngest age group than in older people and the proportion of neurological diagnoses remained relatively constant with increasing age.

Aetiology of MSI

The aetiology of almost one third (32.1%) of the cases was unknown. A further 28.1% were due to trauma, 15.1% due to infection, 11.4% due to family history. Other aetiologies, including

Table 4. Cause of MSI in survey, and extrapolated to population of Rwanda.

	Diagnosis	Number	Total in category (%)	Extrapolated number of that diagnostic category in Rwanda to nearest 1000 (95%CI)
A	**Congenital deformity**		45 (12%)	59,000 (95% CI 39,000–74,000)
	Polydactyly	16		
	Syndactyly	2		
	Other upper limb deformity	4		
	Club foot	4		
	Other lower limb deformity	12		
	Spine deformity	1		
	Cleft lip or cleft palate	2		
	Multiple abnormalities	2		
	Other congenital deformity	2		
B	**Trauma**		122 (31%)	156,000 (95% CI 125,000–187,000)
	Fracture non or malunion	28		
	Burn contracture	4		
	Spine injury	3		
	Head injury	3		
	Joint chronic dislocation	6		
	Other chronic joint injury	24		
	Tendon, muscle or nerve injury	12		
	Amputation	20		
	Other traumatic MSI	22		
C	**Infective**		15 (4%)	20,000 (95% CI 9,000–29,000)
	Joint infection	4		
	Bone infection limb	8		
	Bone infection spine	1		
	Skin/soft tissue infection/wound	2		
D	**Neurological**		35 (9%)	44,000 (95% CI 27,000–60,000)
	Polio	8		
	Para/quadri/tetraplegia	11		
	Cerebral palsy or developmental delay	5		
	Peripheral nerve palsy	4		
	Other neurological MSI	7		
E	**Other acquired non-traumatic non-infective**		173 (44%)	216,000 (95% CI 182,000–245,000)
	Joint problem	52		
	Angular limb deformity	38		
	Skin/soft tissue tumour/swelling	12		
	Spine deformity	2		
	Spine pain	11		
	Limb pain	5		
	Limb swelling	5		
	Other acquired	48		
	TOTAL	390		488,000

congenital without family history (5.4%), iatrogenic (1.7%), and perinatal hypoxia (0.3%) were relatively rare.

Quality of life

The mean quality of life score was significantly higher in people without MSI (63.1, 95%CI 61.4–64.7) than among the cases (37.7, 35.4–40.0, p value<0.001. Severe cases had significantly poorer quality of life (16.9, 11.7–22.0) than moderate (34.9, 31.8–38.0), and mild cases (44.0, 40.5–47.8) (p-value 0.003).

Treatment needed

In total, 641 treatments were needed for the 390 diagnoses (table 5). The most common treatments needed were physical therapy (44.5%), surgery (22.9%) or medication (16.1%). Extrap-

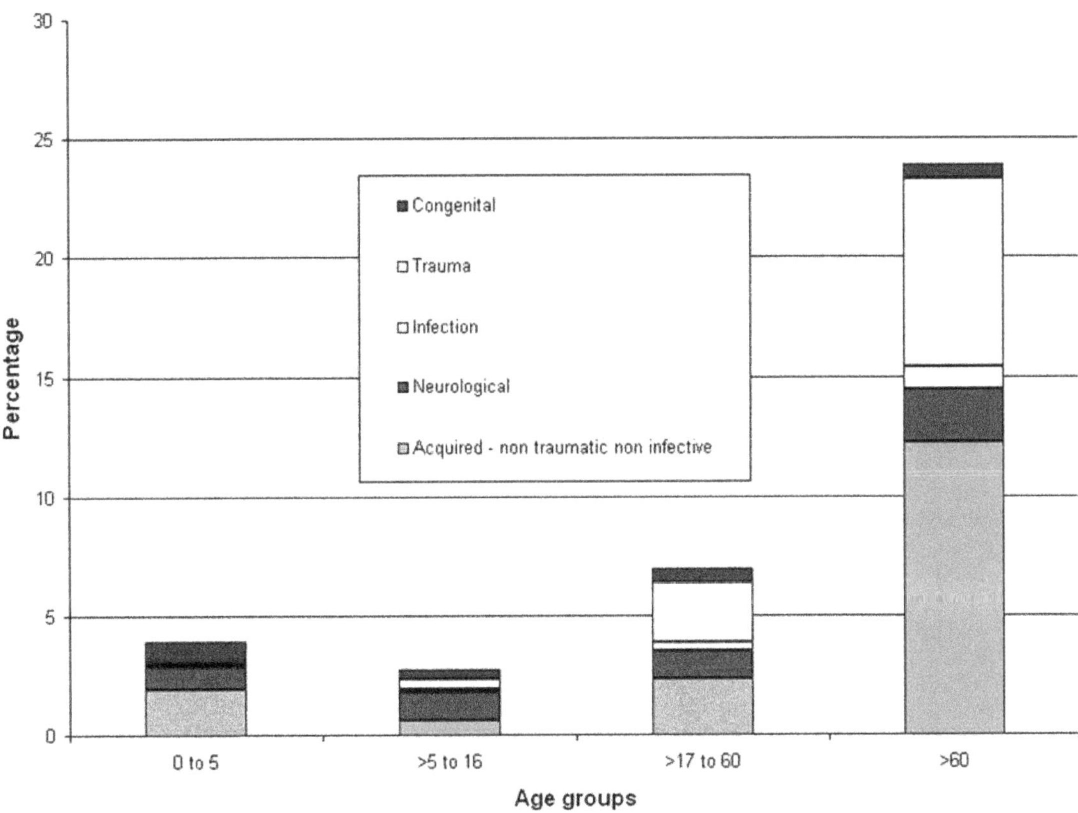

Figure 1. Prevalence and diagnostic categories of MSI, by age group.

olating these estimates to the entire Rwandese population, approximately 814,000 treatments are required, including 356,000 courses of physical therapy, 184,000 operations and 129,000 courses of medicine.

Table 5. Treatment needed among cases with MSI in survey, and extrapolated to population of Rwanda.

Treatment modality	Number of cases in survey needing that treatment modality	Extrapolated number in country needing that treatment modality (based on 2005 population estimates) (95% CI)
Medication	103	132,000 (104,000–159,000)
POP / Splintage	53	68,000 (44,000–91,000)
Physical therapy	285	362,000 (340,000–383,000)
Mobility aid	12	15,000 (6,000–25,000)
Appliance	6	8,000 (2,000–14,000)
Orthosis	16	21,000 (10,000–30,000)
Prosthesis	5	6,000 (1,000–12,000)
Wheelchair	8	10,000 (3,000–17,000)
Surgery	147	187,000 (162,000–212,000)
Permanent care	6	5,000 (0–10,000)
TOTAL	641	814,000

Discussion

This study estimates that the prevalence of MSI in Rwanda is 5.2% (95% CI 4.5–5.9). The prevalence of MSI is similar in men and women, but is much higher in older people as a result of an increase in cases caused by trauma, and degenerative changes (classified under the category ' acquired non traumatic non infective causes'), that are more prevalent in this age group. The overall prevalence for the population is higher than might be expected when compared to previous studies in Rwanda, but is in line with expectations of WHO and other prevalence estimations for other countries in the region [8,9]. In addition to comparisons with other historical surveys and estimations, the accuracy of this survey can be measured against studies of common congenital abnormalities such as club foot. In this case the measured prevalence of 0.07% for club foot is consistent with an incidence of around 1 in 1000 live births as has been measured in other international studies [15].

53% of cases of MSI were moderate or severe according to the ICF classification, thus they significantly affect the life of the individuals concerned and their communities, and will have implications for the development of rehabilitation and other services in Rwanda.

The survey has produced results that will be of use in planning rehabilitation and other services in Rwanda. For example good estimations can be drawn as to the need for appliances, orthoses, prostheses and wheelchairs. This knowledge of need can be used as a target for production and supply of these items. Similarly accurate estimations of the need for medical services such as physiotherapy and surgery can be used to measure the capacity of existing services, and for advocacy and planning of future service provision. The estimations can be used to plan both building of medical facilities, and training of personnel such as physical therapists, orthotists, prosthetists, clinicians and surgeons, to treat the burden of musculoskeletal impairment.

Some MSIs are potentially preventable, in particular those involving trauma, and to a lesser extent infection. This survey was not intended to show how such prevention might be carried out, but it helps in planning as it gives an indication of the reduction in overall burden of disability in the community if particular MSIs can be prevented or at least reduced.

The study had many strengths, which lend confidence to the estimates obtained. A major strength is that a nationally representative sample of people of all ages was enumerated and examined. There is unlikely to have been serious selection bias, as the response rate was high and the sample was representative of the national population in terms of age- and sex- distribution. Furthermore, the reported prevalence of MSI among the sample and non-responders was very similar at 5.2% and 5.5% respectively. Information bias was also unlikely as outcome definition was undertaken by experienced physiotherapists, using a sensitive screening tool [13], and a robust questionnaire and examination protocol. There was good inter-observer agreement between the examiners and sensitivity and specificity of diagnosis was high. Furthermore, the specific diagnoses of MSI could be mapped on to ICF impairment categories for comparison with other ICF linked studies. The survey methodology was practical for use in a low-income country after a relatively short in-country training programme.

There were also limitations to the study. Since the examinations were carried out door-to-door, the diagnostic tools were limited to history and a clinical examination. It is also intentionally limited to MSI and does not give an estimate of other areas of impairment such as blindness, deafness or mental impairment. The in-country study costs were in the region of $100,000 and this may limit its use in other low income countries. This sum may seem high, but it reflects the real costs in mobilising a local survey team and giving logistic support over two months.

In conclusion, this survey demonstrates a large burden of MSI in Rwanda, which is mostly untreated. The demonstrated need will be useful in planning services. The survey methodology will also be useful in other low income countries.

Author Contributions

Conceived and designed the experiments: OA HK AF CL. Performed the experiments: OA Dr VS BL AN. Analyzed the data: OA VS HK CL. Contributed reagents/materials/analysis tools: OA VS HK. Wrote the paper: OA HK CL.

References

1. Biritwum RB, Devres JP, Ofosu-Amaah S, Marfo C, Essah ER (2001) Prevalence of children with disabilities in central region, Ghana. West Afr J Med 20: 249–255.
2. Tamrat G, Kebede Y, Alemu S, Moore J (2001) The prevalence and characteristics of physical and sensory disabilities in Northern Ethiopia. Disabil Rehabil 23: 799–804.
3. Disler PB, Jacks E, Sayed AR, Rip MR, Hurford S, et al. (1986) The prevalence of locomotor disability and handicap in the Cape Peninsula. Part I. The coloured population of Bishop Lavis. S Afr Med J 69: 349–52.
4. McLaren PA, Gear JS, Irwig LM, Smit AE (1987) Prevalence of motor impairment and disability in a rural community in KwaZulu. Int Rehabil Med 8: 98–104.
5. United Nations (2008) Human Functioning and Disability. Available: http://unstats.un.org/unsd/demographic/sconcerns/disability/ Accessed 2007 Dec 12.
6. Chopra A (2004) COPCORD—an unrecognised fountainhead of community rheumatology in developing countries. J Rheumatol 31: 2320–2321.
7. World Health Organisation (2001) International Classification of Functioning disability and Health. Geneva: World Health Organisation.
8. World Health Organisation (2002) Disability and Rehabilitation: Future Trends and Challenges in Rehabilitation. Geneva: World Health Organisation.
9. Helander E (1999) Prejudice and Dignity: an introduction to Community Based Rehabilitation. New York: UNDP.
10. Handicap International, Ministère de la Réhabilitation et l'Intégration Sociale, Ministère du Travail et des Affaires Sociales (1995) Enquête Nationale sur l'Ampleur du Handicap au Rwanda : Résultats et recommandations pour l'élaboration d'un plan. Kigali: Handicap International.
11. Government of Rwanda (2003) Third General Census of Population and Housing of Rwanda. Final results: Statistical Tables. Kigali, Government of Rwanda.
12. Turner AG, Magnani RJ, Shuaib M (1996) "A not quite as quick but much cleaner alternative to the Expanded Programme on Immunization (EPI) Cluster Survey design." Int J Epidemiol 25: 198–203.
13. Atijosan O, Kuper H, Rischewski D, Simms V, Lavy C (2007) Musculoskeletal impairment survey in Rwanda: Design of survey tool, survey methodology, and results of pilot study (a cross sectional survey) BMC Musculoskeletal Disorders 8: 30.
14. Rabin R, de Charro F (2001) EQ-5D: a measure of health status from the EuroQol Group. Ann Med 33: 337–43.
15. Mkandawire NC, Kaunda E (2004) Incidence and patterns of congenital talipes equinovarus (clubfoot) deformity at Queen Elizabeth Central Hospital, Malawi. East Cent Afr J Surg 2: 2–31.

18

Are Subject-Specific Musculoskeletal Models Robust to the Uncertainties in Parameter Identification?

Giordano Valente[1]*, Lorenzo Pitto[1], Debora Testi[2], Ajay Seth[3], Scott L. Delp[3,4], Rita Stagni[5], Marco Viceconti[6], Fulvia Taddei[1]

1 Medical Technology Laboratory, Rizzoli Orthopaedic Institute, Bologna, Italy, 2 BioComputing Competence Centre, SCS s.r.l., Bologna, Italy, 3 Department of Bioengineering, Stanford University, Stanford, California, United States of America, 4 Department of Mechanical Engineering, Stanford University, Stanford, California, United States of America, 5 Department of Electrical, Electronic and Information Engineering, University of Bologna, Bologna, Italy, 6 Department of Mechanical Engineering and INSIGNEO Institute for *In Silico* Medicine, University of Sheffield, Sheffield, United Kingdom

Abstract

Subject-specific musculoskeletal modeling can be applied to study musculoskeletal disorders, allowing inclusion of personalized anatomy and properties. Independent of the tools used for model creation, there are unavoidable uncertainties associated with parameter identification, whose effect on model predictions is still not fully understood. The aim of the present study was to analyze the sensitivity of subject-specific model predictions (i.e., joint angles, joint moments, muscle and joint contact forces) during walking to the uncertainties in the identification of body landmark positions, maximum muscle tension and musculotendon geometry. To this aim, we created an MRI-based musculoskeletal model of the lower limbs, defined as a 7-segment, 10-degree-of-freedom articulated linkage, actuated by 84 musculotendon units. We then performed a Monte-Carlo probabilistic analysis perturbing model parameters according to their uncertainty, and solving a typical inverse dynamics and static optimization problem using 500 models that included the different sets of perturbed variable values. Model creation and gait simulations were performed by using freely available software that we developed to standardize the process of model creation, integrate with OpenSim and create probabilistic simulations of movement. The uncertainties in input variables had a moderate effect on model predictions, as muscle and joint contact forces showed maximum standard deviation of 0.3 times body-weight and maximum range of 2.1 times body-weight. In addition, the output variables significantly correlated with few input variables (up to 7 out of 312) across the gait cycle, including the geometry definition of larger muscles and the maximum muscle tension in limited gait portions. Although we found subject-specific models not markedly sensitive to parameter identification, researchers should be aware of the model precision in relation to the intended application. In fact, force predictions could be affected by an uncertainty in the same order of magnitude of its value, although this condition has low probability to occur.

Editor: Monica Soncini, Politecnico di Milano, Italy

Funding: This study was supported by the EU-funded NMS Physiome project (FP7-ICT-248189), and supported in part by the EU-funded VPHOP project (FP7-ICT-223865). The funders had no role in study design, data collection and analysis, decision to publish, or preparation of the manuscript. Co-author Debora Testi is employed by BioComputing Competence Centre, SCS s.r.l. BioComputing Competence Centre, SCS s.r.l. provided support in the form of salary for author DT, but did not have any additional role in the study design, data collection and analysis, decision to publish, or preparation of the manuscript. The specific roles of these authors are articulated in the 'author contributions' section.

Competing Interests: Debora Testi is affiliated to the BioComputing Competence Centre, SCS s.r.l. commercial company.

* Email: valente@tecno.ior.it

Introduction

Advances in computing power and numerical methods for modeling and simulation of movement are expanding the use of computational models of the musculoskeletal system in research and clinical applications [1,2]. Calculation of muscle and joint forces represent a challenging modeling application [3,4]. Because musculoskeletal geometry and tissue properties can vary markedly among individuals, the accuracy of generic models has been questioned [5,6], particularly when studying musculoskeletal disorders [7,8]. Conversely, subject-specific models allow inclusion of individual musculoskeletal anatomy and properties, providing an alternative approach to calculating muscle moment arms [9,10], muscle and joint forces [11,12], bone and cartilage stresses [13,14].

In general, analyses of musculoskeletal dynamics require the use of musculoskeletal models and the application of rigid body dynamics and optimization methods to calculate muscle forces [2,15]. Until now, the creation of subject-specific musculoskeletal models and simulations of movement has represented a time-consuming process, and there has been limited modeling software available to standardize the process and make musculoskeletal modeling more efficient. Consequently, few attempts have been made to create subject-specific models and study musculoskeletal pathological conditions (e.g., [16–18]). In fact, model creation requires data collections from different technology (e.g., MRI, gait analysis), and processing the data to create a model of musculoskeletal dynamics. The process involves the definition and calculation of subject-specific modeling parameters from imaging data, including the identification of: tissue volumes and densities to calculate body inertial properties; body landmark positions to define joint reference frames and constraints; muscle attachment points to define the geometry of muscles; and muscle architecture parameters to calculate muscle force-generating capacities.

Independent of the software used, there are unavoidable uncertainties in parameter identification during the process of model creation. These uncertainties have different sources: they can be operator-dependent (e.g., when a user identifies body landmark positions and point positions of musculotendon actuators), or related to the unavailability of measurements *in vivo*, such as maximum muscle tension and musculotendon architecture parameters (e.g., muscle physiological cross-sectional area, fiber length and tendon slack length). Sensitivity analyses to different parameters have been performed to assess variations in model predictions and determine which parameters have the most influence (e.g., [19–21]). However, these analyses have not assessed how the uncertainties associated with the creation of subject-specific musculoskeletal models, and their combined effect, may affect model predictions.

Therefore, the aim of the present study is to analyze the sensitivity of subject-specific model predictions (i.e., joint angles, joint moments, muscle and joint contact forces) during walking to the uncertainties in the values for model parameters. To achieve this aim, we first created a musculoskeletal model of the lower limbs from MRI of a healthy subject. We then performed a Monte-Carlo probabilistic analysis accounting for the uncertainties associated with the creation of the model, including body landmark positions, maximum muscle tension and musculotendon geometry. The analysis was performed by using freely available musculoskeletal modeling software that we developed in an effort to standardize subject-specific model creation and generate accurate models using an efficient workflow. The modeling software integrates with OpenSim [22], a widely used multi-body-dynamics solver adopted in musculoskeletal applications (e.g., [19,23,24]).

Materials and Methods

Ethics statement

This study was approved by the Bioethical Committee of the University of Bologna, Italy (July 7, 2012). Written informed consent was obtained from the participant.

Experimental data

One healthy subject (male; age: 31 years; height: 183 cm; weight: 70.5 kg) volunteered to participate in this study. The experimental data collection included lower-body MRI scans and gait analysis data, freely available at the dedicated SimTK.org project page (https://simtk.org) and described as follows.

Pelvis and lower limbs were imaged using a 1.5 T MR scanner (Intera, Koninklijke Philips N.V., The Netherlands). Four series of images were obtained at different resolutions: a full lower-body scan (T1-weighted Magnetization Transfer, 5 mm slice thickness, 5.5 mm slice spacing, resolution of 512×512 pixels), and three higher resolution acquisitions at the hip (T1-weighted High Resolution Turbo Spin Echo, 5 mm slice thickness, 5.5 mm slice spacing, resolution of 864×864 pixels), at the knee (T1-weighted Turbo Spin Echo, 3 mm slice thickness, 3.3 mm slice spacing, resolution of 560×560 pixels) and at the ankle (T1-weighted Turbo Spin Echo, 3 mm slice thickness, 3.3 mm slice spacing, resolution of 1024×1024 pixels) joint regions.

The subject was assessed by means of gait analysis. The experiment was carried out using a stereophotogrammetric system (SMART-D BTS, Milano, Italy) and two force platforms (Bertec Corporation, USA). Twenty-nine retro-reflective markers were attached to the pelvis, thighs, shanks and feet of the analyzed subject. A trial of level walking at self-selected speed was carried out. Joint neutral position was collected from a standing posture, as well as joint flexion position from a seated posture. All data were collected at 200 samples per second. Relevant anatomical landmarks [25] were calibrated in standing and flexed posture using the pointer technique illustrated in Cappozzo et al. [26]. Segmental kinematics of the pelvis and lower limbs was reconstructed via a C.A.S.T. approach [26] with double calibration [27] to minimize soft tissue artifact propagation.

Workflow of subject-specific musculoskeletal modeling

We investigated the robustness of model predictions to the uncertainties in the identification of the parameters needed to create an image-based musculoskeletal model of the lower limbs, using MRI and gait data (Figure 1). To the purpose, freely available software that we developed, i.e., NMSBuilder and the Probabilistic Musculoskeletal Modeling module (PMM), was used to create the baseline subject-specific model and perform probabilistic simulations of gait, leveraging OpenSim. Additional details on the software system can be found in the Appendix S1. All of the software is available at the dedicated SimTK.org project page (https://simtk.org).

Baseline subject-specific model

The model used in this study was defined as a 7-segment, 10-degree-of-freedom (DOF) articulated system, actuated by 84 musculotendon units, and referred to as the baseline model. The seven rigid bodies included pelvis, thighs, shanks and feet. Each body volume was derived from the MR images, and the inertial properties (mass, center of mass and moments of inertia) were calculated assuming each body composed of two parts, the bone and soft tissue, having uniform densities of 1.42 g/cm^3 and 1.03 g/cm^3 [28], respectively. Each hip was modeled as a 3 DOF ball-and-socket joint, each knee and ankle as a 1 DOF hinge joint. Body and joint coordinate systems were identified according to the ISB standards [29]. The hip joint was defined at the center of the femoral head, the knee axis of rotation was defined as the trans-epcondylar line [30], and the ankle axis of rotation was defined as the trans-malleolar line [31]. The number and paths of the musculotendon actuators were defined according to the generic model proposed by Delp and co-workers [32]. The model includes one or more lines of action per muscle, acting between origin points on the proximal body and insertion points on the distal body. Intermediate via-points are included to model the paths of muscles wrapping over underlying structures. The maximum isometric force (F_{max}) of each musculotendon unit (i) was estimated, assuming muscle fiber length proportional to musculotendon length [33], as:

$$F_{\max i} = (PCSA)_i \cdot \sigma = \left(\frac{Vol}{l_0}\right)_i \cdot \sigma = \left(\frac{Vol}{l_0^{(gen)} \cdot \frac{l_{MT}}{l_{MT}^{(gen)}}}\right)_i \cdot \sigma \qquad (1)$$

where $PCSA$ is the muscle physiological cross-sectional area, Vol is the muscle volume calculated from MRI, l_0 and l_{MT} are the optimal fiber length (unknown) and the musculotendon length (calculated from MRI) for the subject-specific model, respectively, $l_0^{(gen)}$ and $l_{MT}^{(gen)}$ are the corresponding quantities for the generic model [32], and σ is the maximum muscle tension set to 61 N/cm^2 [34].

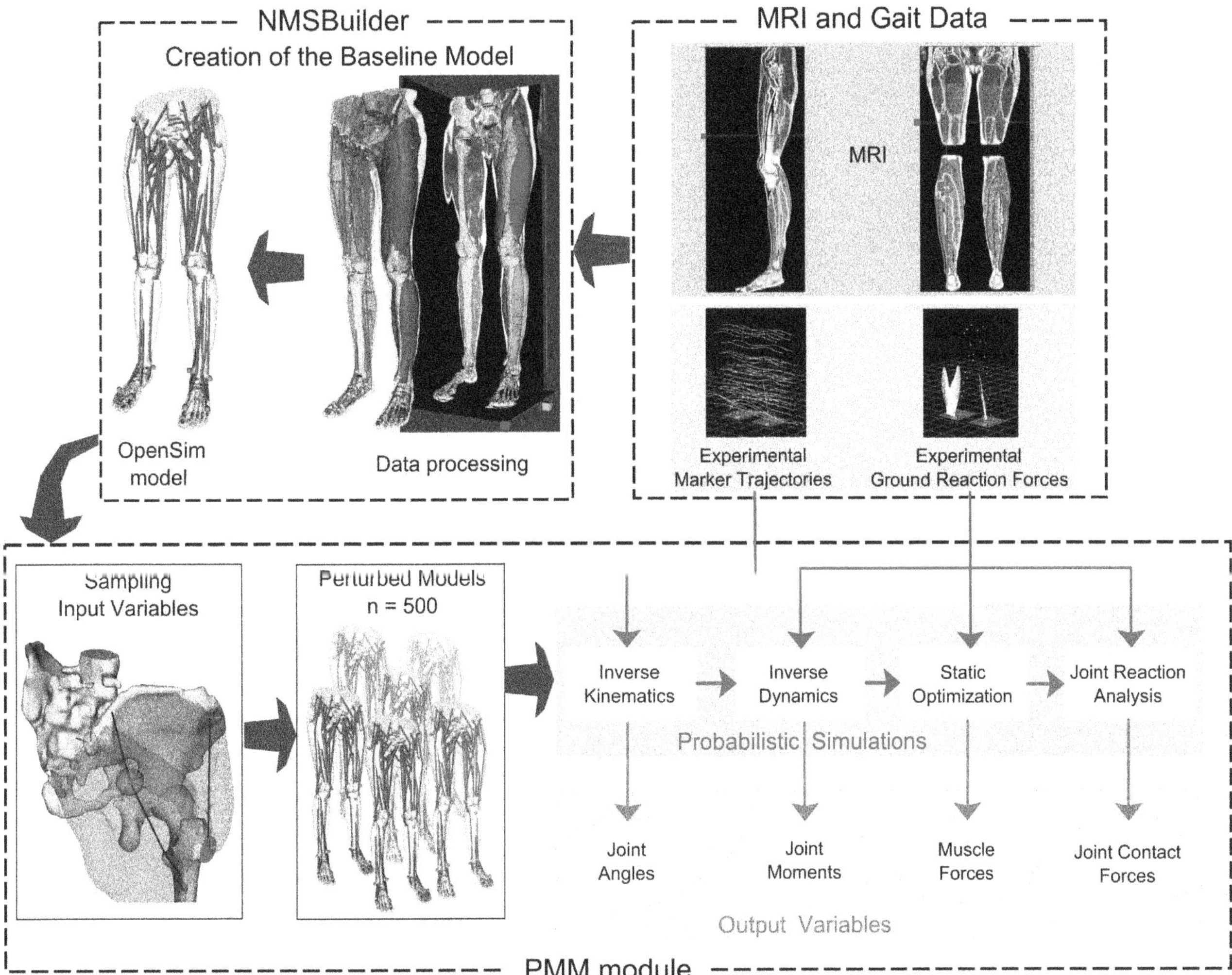

Figure 1. Workflow of subject-specific musculoskeletal modeling. The modeling software systems were applied to study the sensitivity of model predictions to the uncertainties in parameter identification. Lower-body MRI and gait analysis data were acquired for a healthy subject. NMSBuilder was used to create the baseline subject-specific model leveraging OpenSim. The Probabilistic Musculoskeletal Modeling module (PMM) was used to create probabilistic simulations of gait through a Monte-Carlo analysis, by interfacing Matlab and OpenSim. The input variables were perturbed according to their uncertainties, and the corresponding OpenSim models were created that included the different sets of perturbed variables. Using each model and the recorded gait analysis data, simulations of gait were run to calculate the stochastic output variables.

To create the baseline model, bone and soft tissue meshes (pelvis, thighs, shanks and feet) were segmented semi-automatically using Amira (Visage Imaging, Berlin, Germany). NMSBuilder was then used to create the subject-specific musculoskeletal model. The segmented surfaces were imported in NMSBuilder as STL files, and were divided into seven body districts, each made of bone and soft tissue parts [35]. The data were organized into a hierarchical structure. Different density values were then assigned to each part as metadata attributes, to calculate the inertial properties of each body. The necessary anatomical landmarks were virtually palpated [36] on the body surfaces with the help of the superimposed MR images. Subsequently, the landmark positions were used to define the reference frames of each body and the joint positions and orientations (in the parent and child bodies). The positions of musculotendon origin, via and insertion points were assigned as close as possible to those in the generic model [32]. This was done by applying an affine registration based on the body landmarks to initialize the musculotendon point positions, and then adjusting the points according to a centroid approach [37] and visually comparing their positions in the MR images. Next, the values of maximum isometric muscle force were assigned to each musculotendon unit as metadata attributes. Finally, the C++ commands of the OpenSim application programming interface (API) were generated and compiled to create the baseline OpenSim model.

Probabilistic simulations of gait

A probabilistic study was performed to analyze the sensitivity of model predictions to the uncertainties associated with the creation of the baseline model, given the specific articulated linkage actuated by musculotendon units represented by line segments. Therefore, three categories of variable parameters were defined (Figure 2), resulting in a total of 312 stochastic input variables:

1. Body landmark positions. The x-, y- and z-coordinates of the 21 landmarks in each corresponding body reference frame were assumed as normally distributed variables. The standard deviations of each variable (Table 1) were calculated via an experimental study. In this experiment, five expert modelers used NMSBuilder to virtually palpate the landmarks on the bone

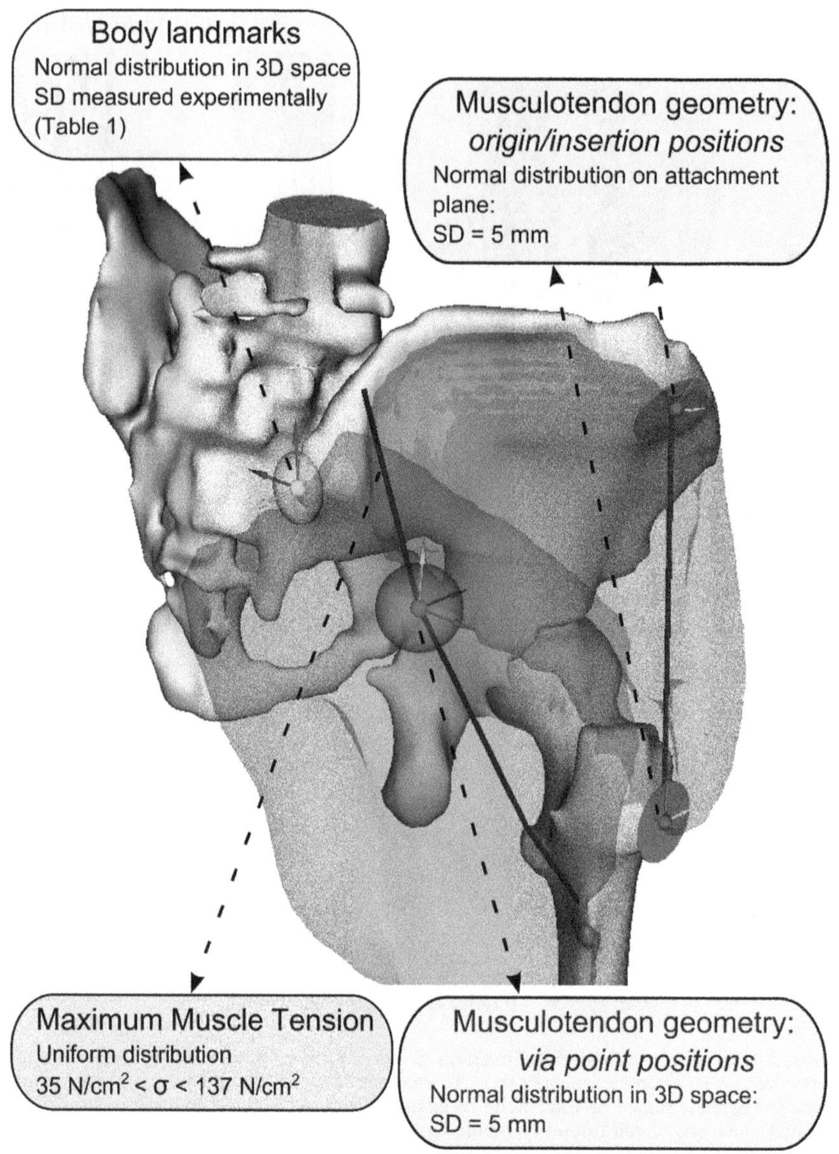

Figure 2. Schematic of statistical perturbation of the input variables. To analyze the sensitivity of model predictions to the uncertainties in parameter values, three categories of stochastic input variables were identified (for a total of 312 input variables): body landmark positions (affecting position and orientation of body reference frames and joints, inertial tensors and joint kinematics), musculotendon geometry (position of origin/insertion and via points defining musculotendon paths and affecting muscle moment arms) and maximum muscle tension (affecting maximum force-generating capacity of the muscles). Each variable was assumed as normally or uniformly distributed, and a Latin Hypercube Sampling strategy was applied to efficiently sample the variables from their distribution.

surfaces three times within a time interval of two weeks. Landmark positions affect calculation of body reference frames, inertial tensors, joint positions and orientations, and joint kinematics.

2. Musculotendon geometry. The positions of the 89 points of the musculotendon paths affecting moment arm lengths were assumed as normally distributed variables. The points included origins, pseudo-origins (most distal via point on the proximal body), pseudo-insertions (most proximal via point on the distal body), and insertions, according to the definition of the different musculotendon paths. A plane approximating each musculotendon attachment area was calculated, so that each origin and insertion point position could be perturbed along two directions on the plane. Points belonging to attachment areas with large length/width ratio were approximated by a line and perturbed along one direction only. Conversely, each position of pseudo-origin and pseudo-insertion points was perturbed along the three directions of the body reference frame. Therefore, a total of 209 normally distributed variables were defined. Mean values were assumed those of the baseline model and standard deviations were set to 5 mm, as derived from the error in locating muscle attachment points from the measurement of surface landmarks [38].

3. Maximum muscle tension. The maximum muscle tension (σ) was assumed as a uniformly distributed variable, ranging from 35 N/cm^2 to 137 N/cm^2 [39]. Consequently, the maximum isometric force of each musculotendon unit was calculated, using equation (1), as:

Table 1. Standard deviations of the body landmark positions measured experimentally.

		Standard Deviation (mm)		
		X	Y	Z
Body landmarks	SACRUM	0.7	0.6	1.8
	RASIS	1.6	0.4	2.6
	RPSIS	0.8	0.3	2.1
	LASIS	1.2	0.6	2.3
	LPSIS	0.9	0.4	2.8
	RGT	1.0	1.4	1.1
	RME	0.4	0.7	1.3
	RLE	0.6	1.6	1.3
	RHC	0.6	0.8	1.5
	RHF	2.2	0.8	0.3
	RTT	3.5	1.3	4.2
	RLC	0.7	3.5	1.2
	RMC	0.5	1.5	0.6
	RMM	1.6	0.9	0.5
	RLM	0.7	0.5	0.3
	RCA	1.1	1.0	0.3
	RFM	0.8	1.6	0.1
	RSM	0.8	0.7	1.0
	RVM	0.7	0.7	0.4
	RPAI	0.6	1.4	0.1
	RPAII	0.6	0.5	0.0

Values were measured through virtual palpation using NMSBuilder by 5 operators in 3 trials each. X, Y and Z indicate antero-posterior, cranio-caudal and medio-lateral directions of the body reference frames, respectively. Body landmark acronyms indicate: sacrum (SACRUM), right anterior superior iliac spine (RASIS), right posterior superior iliac spine (RPSIS), left anterior superior iliac spine (LASIS), left posterior superior iliac spine (LPSIS), right great trochanter (RGT), right medial epicondyle (RME), right lateral epicondyle (RLE), right hip center (RHC), right head of fibula (RHF), right tibial tuberosity (RTT), right lateral tibial condyle (RLC), right medial tibial condyle (RMC), right medial malleolus (RMM), right lateral malleolus (RLM), right calcaneus (RCA), right first metatarsus (RFM), right second metatarsus (RSM), right fifth metatarsus (RVM), right superior plantar aspect of calcaneus (RPAI), right inferior plantar aspect of calcaneus (RPAII).

$$F_{\max i,j} = \left(\frac{Vol}{l_0^{(gen)} \cdot \frac{l_{MT}}{l_{MT}^{(gen)}}} \right)_i \cdot \sigma_j \tag{2}$$

where i is the musculotendon unit and j the sample of muscle specific tension within the specified range.

Uncertainties introduced by volume segmentation were not included, being segmentation a time-consuming process and hence performed by a single operator. The stance phase of one gait cycle was selected to be included in the analysis, as it is the most interesting phase from the musculoskeletal loading standpoint. PMM allowed us to perform a Monte-Carlo analysis that included kinematic and dynamic simulations of the stance phase of gait (Figure 1), leveraging the OpenSim API. The baseline model was opened in PMM, and a Latin Hypercube Sampling (LHS) strategy [40,19] was applied to generate an efficient sampling of the input variables from their distribution. This made possible the generation of OpenSim models that included the different sets of perturbed variable values. Using each model, Inverse Kinematics, Inverse Dynamics, Static Optimization (minimizing the sum of muscle activations squared and neglecting the force-length-velocity relationships of muscle [41]) and Joint Reaction analysis were run to calculate the following stochastic output variables: joint angles, joint moments, muscle forces and joint contact forces. A convergence criterion was defined as a stopping rule for the Monte-Carlo simulations. Five-hundred simulations ensured that the output variables reached convergence. Specifically, over the last 10% of the simulations, the means and standard deviations of each output variable were within the 2% of each final mean and standard deviation [11,19,20]. A perturbed simulation was considered unsuccessful if joint dynamic equilibrium could not be achieved. Specifically, unsuccessful simulations occurred if the use of reserve actuators on any joint DOF exceeded 5% of the peak joint moment [24] in at least one frame of the stance phase. Preliminary analysis of the results showed that the 0.8% of the simulations run was unsuccessful, suggesting that muscle forces were generally able to generate the required joint moments. The unsuccessful simulations were excluded from the subsequent data analysis.

Data analysis

The analysis was focused on joint angles, joint moments, major muscle forces, i.e. gluteus medius anterior (*GMedA*), middle (*GMedM*) and posterior (*GMedP*), gluteus maximus anterior (*GMaxA*), tensor fascia latae (*TFL*), *psoas*, *iliacus*, semimbranosus (*Semimem*), rectus femoris (*Rec Fem*), vastus medialis (*Vas Med*), lateralis (*Vas Lat*) and intermedius (*Vas Int*), medial (*Med Gas*) and

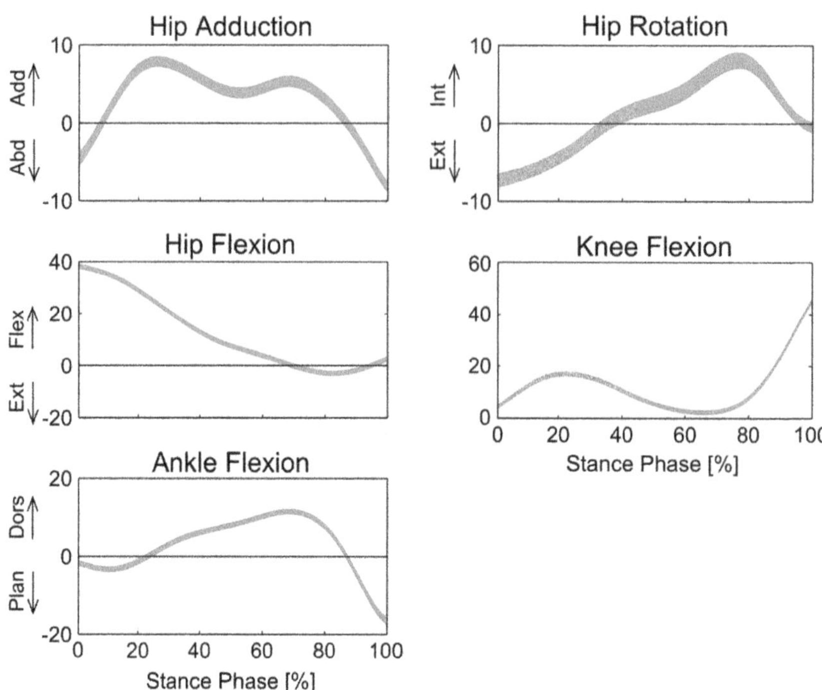

Figure 3. Variability in joint angles due to the perturbation of model variables. Bands represent mean values ±1 standard deviation (in degrees) during the stance phase of gait.

lateral (*Lat Gas*) gastrocnemius, *soleus*, tibialis anterior (*Tib Ant*), and joint contact forces, i.e. hip, knee and ankle force magnitude. First, all quantities were expressed in percentage of the stance phase, and the force values were normalized to the subject body-weight and thus expressed in multiples of body-weight (BW). The data were then post-processed to evaluate the statistical variability in the output variables and the correlations between output and input variables. The variability was analyzed as maximum and mean standard deviation (among the output samples at each time step), and range (difference between maximum and minimum values at each time step) during the stance phase of gait. A correlation analysis was performed that evaluated the statistically significant ($p<0.001$) coefficients of determination (R^2) between all output and input variables.

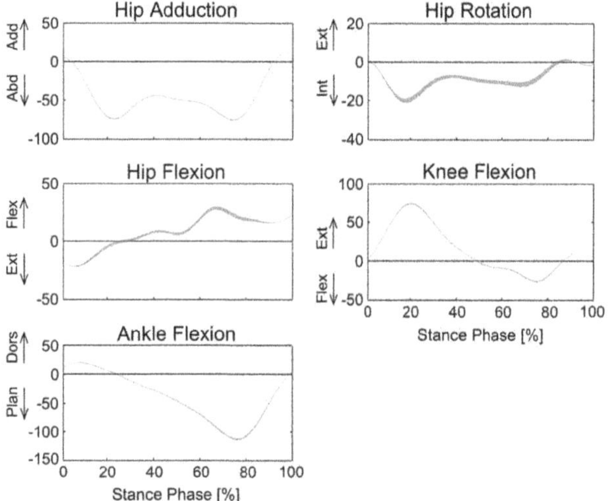

Figure 4. Variability in net joint moments due to the perturbation of model variables. Bands represent mean values ±1 standard deviation (in Nm) during the stance phase of gait.

Results

The joint angles and joint moments were relatively insensitive to the expected variation in musculoskeletal parameters. We found that the maximum standard deviation among joint angles during the stance phase of gait was only 1°, and the maximum range was 7° (Figure 3). Similarly, the maximum standard deviation among joint moments from perturbation of model parameters was only 1.4 Nm, and the maximum range was 9.1 Nm (Figure 4). Joint contact forces and muscle forces presented a more marked variability compared to joint angles and joint moments. Joint contact forces showed a maximum standard deviation of 0.26 BW and a maximum range of 2.14 BW at the knee (Figure 5, Table 2). Although the standard deviations of joint contact forces were 10 times smaller than the corresponding force values, the maximum ranges presented the same order of magnitude. Muscle forces showed larger variability in *Soleus*, *Med Gas*, *Rec Fem* and *Psoas* (Figure 6, Table 2), resulting in a maximum standard deviation of 0.23 BW and a maximum range of 1.54 BW in *Soleus*.

Given the relatively small variability in joint kinematics and kinetics, we analyzed only the correlations between joint contact forces and input variables during the stance phase of gait. Among these correlations, only 6.3% showed significant R^2 ($p<0.001$). In

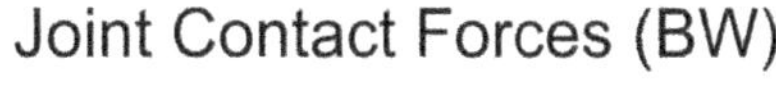

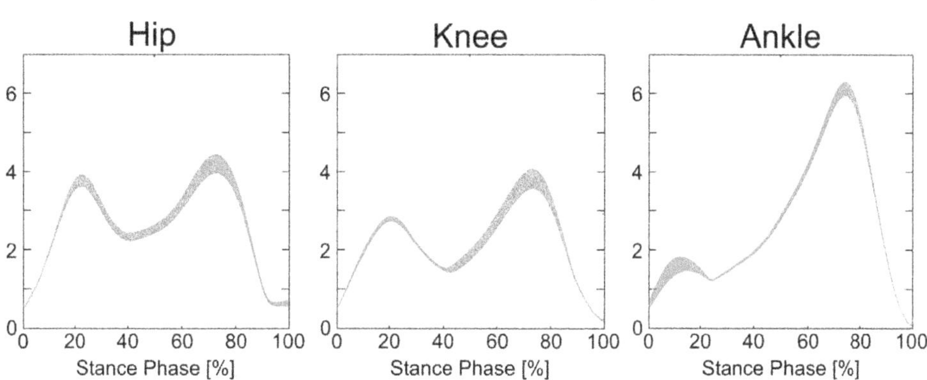

Figure 5. Variability in joint contact forces due to the perturbation of model variables. Bands represent mean values ±1 standard deviation (in BW) during the stance phase of gait.

addition, 1.3% showed significant R^2 greater than 0.2 and never exceeding 0.7, where only seven input variables out of 312 were involved (Figure 7). The hip contact force mostly correlated with the point positions defining the geometry of *GMedA*, *Iliacus* and *Psoas*, and with the maximum muscle tension in the early stance phase. The knee contact force mostly correlated with the geometric definition of *Vas Lat*, *Iliacus* and *GMedA*, and with that of *Med Gas*, *Rec Fem* and *Soleus* for a less extended portion of stance phase. The ankle contact force mostly correlated with the geometric definition of *Soleus* and with the maximum muscle tension for a less extended portion of stance phase. The significant R^2 between joint contact forces and body landmark positions were all less than 0.1 during the stance phase. These results (Figure 7) showed a weak correlation between output and input variables,

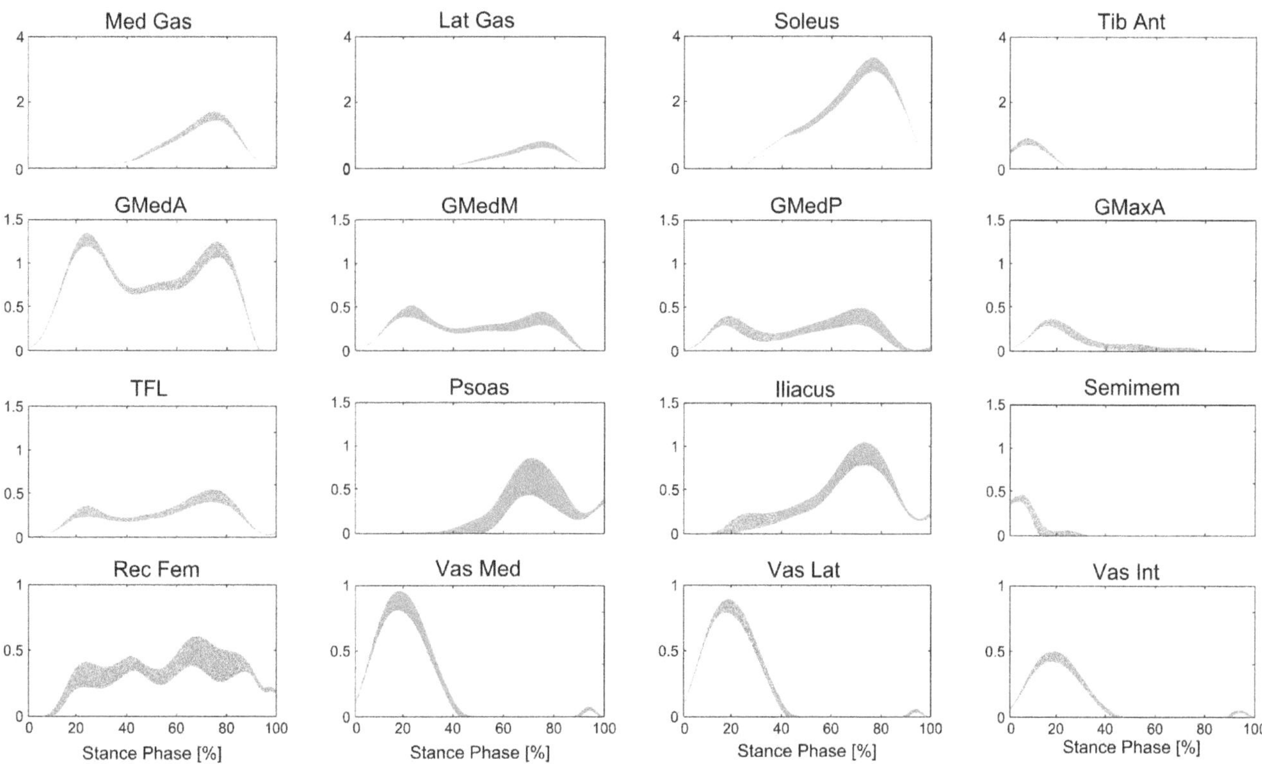

Figure 6. Variability in the major muscle forces due to the perturbation of model variables. Bands represent mean values ±1 standard deviation (in BW) during the stance phase of gait. Muscles shown are: medial (*Med Gas*) and lateral (*Lat Gas*) gastrocnemius, soleus, tibialis anterior (*Tib Ant*), gluteus medius anterior (*GMedA*), middle (*GMedM*) and posterior (*GMedP*), gluteus maximus anterior (*GMaxA*), tensor fascia latae (*TFL*), psoas, iliacus, semimembranosus (*Semimem*), rectus femoris (*Rec Fem*), vastus medialis (*Vas Med*), lateralis (Vas Lat) and intermedius (*Vas Int*).

Table 2. Variability in joint contact and muscle forces.

		Standard Deviation (BW)		Range (BW)	
		Mean	**Max**	**Mean**	**Max**
Joint Contact Forces	Hip	0.13	0.25	0.75	1.51
	Knee	0.11	0.26	0.84	2.14
	Ankle	0.10	0.23	0.62	1.58
Muscle Forces	Med Gas	0.05	0.14	0.33	0.95
	Lat Gas	0.03	0.10	0.21	0.67
	Soleus	0.08	0.23	0.54	1.54
	Tib Ant	0.02	0.10	0.11	0.68
	GMedA	0.05	0.09	0.32	0.66
	GMedM	0.04	0.08	0.25	0.51
	GmedP	0.05	0.10	0.31	0.59
	GMaxA	0.03	0.06	0.17	0.40
	TFL	0.01	0.03	0.08	0.17
	Psoas	0.05	0.15	0.33	0.89
	Iliacus	0.07	0.13	0.42	0.79
	Semimem	0.01	0.03	0.04	0.19
	Rec Fem	0.07	0.14	0.44	0.88
	Vas Med	0.01	0.04	0.07	0.24
	Vas Lat	0.02	0.07	0.11	0.35
	Vas Int	0.01	0.02	0.04	0.13

Standard deviations and ranges of the magnitudes of joint contact forces and the major muscle forces are reported as mean and maximum values across the stance phase of gait.

without a marked influence of specific input variables. The sampled input variables and the complete set of post-processed output variables are available at the dedicated SimTK.org project page (https://simtk.org).

Discussion

In this study, we analyzed the sensitivity of the predictions of an MRI-based musculoskeletal model (i.e., joint angles, joint moments, muscle and joint contact forces) during walking to the unavoidable uncertainties in parameter identification, i.e., body landmark positions, maximum muscle tension and musculotendon geometry (Figure 1).

Overall, the unavoidable uncertainties in parameter identification during the process of model creation have a moderate effect on model predictions during gait. In fact, we found that the main outcomes of model predictions, i.e., joint contact forces and muscle forces, had a maximum standard deviation of 0.26 BW across the stance phase of gait (Figure 5 and 6, Table 2). In addition, there were no critical parameters that markedly affected model predictions. We performed a correlation analysis between joint contact forces and input variables (Figure 7), and found few significant R^2, whose values never exceeded 0.7. The input variables involved were the point positions defining the geometry of few musculotendon actuators that presented larger force-generating capacities and the maximum muscle tension in limited portions of the stance phase.

Although we found that subject-specific models are not markedly sensitive to the uncertainties in parameter identification, there is no conclusive answer to the robustness of subject-specific models. In fact, the precision of model predictions should be evaluated with regards to specific applications. For example, we found ranges (differences between maximum and minimum of the predicted value) that reached 2.1 BW in joint contact forces at the knee during the gait cycle (Table 2). In this case, the result could be affected by an uncertainty in the same order of magnitude of its value, although this condition has low probability to occur. Therefore, one should be aware of the uncertainty in musculoskeletal force predictions according to their intended application (e.g., investigation of risk of bone fracture and bone stress distribution).

To our knowledge, this is the first study investigating how the combined effect of the uncertainties in model parameters affects the predictions of a subject-specific musculoskeletal model, using a probabilistic approach. Therefore, this represents the most extended sensitivity analysis of musculoskeletal modeling predictions, providing an overall scenario of robustness of subject-specific musculoskeletal models to the uncertainties in parameter identification. Consequently, only partial or indirect comparisons with the literature were possible. We found an effect of anatomical landmark positions on predicted joint moments weaker than that showed in a previous probabilistic study limited to inverse dynamics results [21]. The uncertainties that we assigned to the landmark positions (Table 1) were lower than those in the prior study (i.e., standard deviations of 2 mm for all landmarks in each direction). We evaluated experimentally the standard deviations of the distribution by using an accurate method for landmark virtual palpation [36] implemented in NMSBuilder, which allowed us to

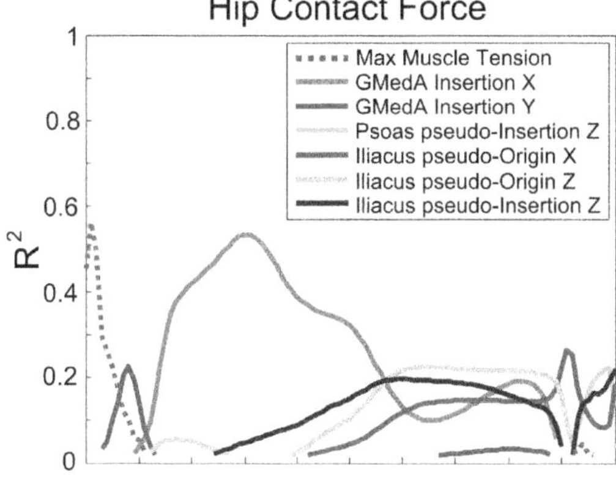

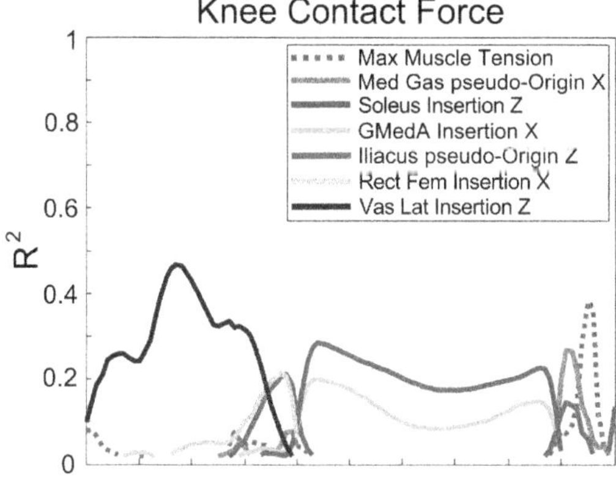

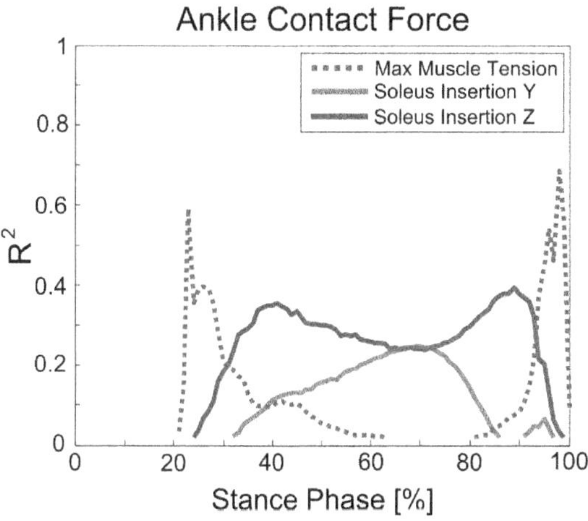

Figure 7. Significant R^2 between joint contact forces and input variables during the stance phase of gait. Correlations between hip, knee and ankle joint contact forces and input variables: only statistically significant ($p<0.001$) R^2 exceeding 0.2 at least in one frame during the stance phase of gait are plotted.

improve the uncertainty in the identification of landmark positions. Similarly, we found a weaker effect of musculotendon geometry on predicted muscle forces compared to a previous study [42] that used a fixed-size perturbation (±10 mm) applied to each musculotendon point position along each direction of the local reference frames. Differently from that study, we assigned an uncertainty (standard deviation of 5 mm) derived from the range of landmark location errors [38], we adopted a probabilistic approach to analyze all possible configurations of musculotendon point positions, and we constrained the muscle attachment points to vary on the bone surfaces. In addition, our results generally confirm the weak influence of maximum muscle tension on the calculated muscle forces, when minimizing a cost function in static optimization problems [20,43,44]. We additionally found that the maximum muscle tension played a more relevant role on joint contact forces during transient phases of the gait cycle (Figure 7). Differently from previous studies, our approach explored the range of maximum muscle tension found in the literature [39] using a uniform distribution, rather than an arbitrary-size perturbation of a baseline value. However, the portions of stance phase showing larger correlations were not biomechanically relevant, as most muscles were inactive or exerted low forces.

The results of our study are affected by some limitations. We limited the study to a healthy subject and we investigated only the task of level walking as the most common daily activity. Model robustness might be different in pathological conditions and for other motor tasks such as sit-to-stand, stair ascent or descent. Although further investigations might extend our findings, the healthy subject included in this study can be considered representative of physiological conditions, and adding greater complexity was beyond the aim of the study. We did not include musculotendon parameters describing force-length-velocity relationships (i.e., optimal fiber length, tendon slack length and pennation angle). Changes in these parameters, and particularly in tendon slack length of some muscles, can markedly affect model dynamics predictions [20,44]. However, measurements and corresponding uncertainties of these parameters are difficult to obtain *in vivo* and even by dissection studies [2]; in addition, the lack of implementation of musculotendon force-length-velocity relationships has a small influence on force predictions during walking [41]. Further, we did not consider the uncertainty introduced by representing the musculotendon units by deformable line segments in the model. However, our aim was to analyze the effect of the uncertainties in the parameters identifying a specific state-of-the art model, and including more accurate muscle path representation (e.g., [45]) would have introduced large computational costs and additional uncertainty not compatible with our analysis.

This study has relevant potentials within the computational biomechanics community. We assessed robustness of musculoskeletal models to the uncertainties in parameter identification using a probabilistic approach. Although in presence of the limitation regarding the impossibility to validate muscle forces, our results confirm that musculoskeletal models represent a promising tool that is heading towards clinical applicability, particularly to improve treatment of orthopaedic and neurological diseases [1,15]. The analysis has been facilitated by the use of an efficient workflow (Figure 1), whose software tools allowed us to reduce time and effort. The freely available modeling software may provide a marked contribution to create subject-specific models and simulations of movement more efficiently, saving time and effort, and without necessarily requiring high skilled expertise.

In summary, our study revealed that the uncertainties in parameter identification of subject-specific musculoskeletal models have a moderate effect on model predictions, and there are not specific parameters considered crucial for the degree of model robustness. However, the precision of model predictions should be considered carefully with regards to the intended application. In fact, model predictions such as joint contact forces may present maximum ranges of variability that are in the same order of magnitude of their values.

Author Contributions

Conceived and designed the experiments: GV LP FT. Performed the experiments: GV LP. Analyzed the data: GV LP FT. Wrote the paper: GV. Contributed software design and development: GV LP DT AS SLD MV FT. Produced gait analysis data: RS. Edited the manuscript: GV LP DT AS SLD RS MV FT.

References

1. Fregly BJ, Besier TF, Lloyd DG, Delp SL, Banks SA, et al. (2012) Grand Challenge Competition to Predict In Vivo Knee Loads. Journal of Orthopaedic Research 30: 503–513.
2. Pandy MG, Andriacchi TP (2010) Muscle and joint function in human locomotion. Annu Rev Biomed Eng 12: 401–433.
3. Fregly BJ (2009) Design of Optimal Treatments for Neuromusculoskeletal Disorders using Patient-Specific Multibody Dynamic Models. Int J Comput Vis Biomech 2: 145–155.
4. Fernandez JW, Pandy MG (2006) Integrating modelling and experiments to assess dynamic musculoskeletal function in humans. Experimental physiology 91: 371–382.
5. Wagner DW, Stepanyan V, Shippen JM, DeMers MS, Gibbons RS, et al. (2013) Consistency Among Musculoskeletal Models: Caveat Utilitor. Annals of Biomedical Engineering 41: 1787–1799.
6. Scheys L, Spaepen A, Suetens P, Jonkers I (2008) Calculated moment-arm and muscle-tendon lengths during gait differ substantially using MR based versus rescaled generic lower-limb musculoskeletal models. Gait & posture 28: 640–648.
7. Correa TA, Schache AG, Graham HK, Baker R, Thomason P, et al. (2012) Potential of lower-limb muscles to accelerate the body during cerebral palsy gait. Gait & posture 36: 194–200.
8. Lenaerts G, Bartels W, Gelaude F, Mulier M, Spaepen A, et al. (2009) Subject-specific hip geometry and hip joint centre location affects calculated contact forces at the hip during gait. Journal of Biomechanics 42: 1246–1251.
9. Scheys L, Desloovere K, Suetens P, Jonkers I (2011) Level of subject-specific detail in musculoskeletal models affects hip moment arm length calculation during gait in pediatric subjects with increased femoral anteversion. Journal of Biomechanics 44: 1346–1353.
10. Valente G, Martelli S, Taddei F, Farinella G, Viceconti M (2012) Muscle discretization affects the loading transferred to bones in lower-limb musculoskeletal models. Proceedings of the Institution of Mechanical Engineers, Part H: Journal of Engineering in Medicine 226: 161–169.
11. Martelli S, Valente G, Viceconti M, Taddei F (2014). Sensitivity of a subject-specific musculoskeletal model to the uncertainties on the joint axes location. Comput Methods Biomech Biomed Engin Jun 25:1–9 [Epub ahead of print].
12. Lenaerts G, Mulier M, Spaepen A, Van der Perre G, Jonkers I (2009) Aberrant pelvis and hip kinematics impair hip loading before and after total hip replacement. Gait & posture 30: 296–302.
13. Besier TF, Gold GE, Beaupre GS, Delp SL (2005) A Modeling Framework to Estimate Patellofemoral Joint Cartilage Stress In Vivo. Medicine & Science in Sports & Exercise 37: 1924–1930.
14. Jonkers I, Sauwen N, Lenaerts G, Mulier M, Van der Perre G, et al. (2008) Relation between subject-specific hip joint loading, stress distribution in the proximal femur and bone mineral density changes after total hip replacement. Journal of Biomechanics 41: 3405–3413.
15. Erdemir A, McLean S, Herzog W, van den Bogert AJ (2007) Model-based estimation of muscle forces exerted during movements. Clinical Biomechanics (Bristol, Avon) 22: 131–154.
16. Taddei F, Martelli S, Valente G, Leardini A, Benedetti MG, et al. (2012) Femoral loads during gait in a patient with massive skeletal reconstruction. Clinical Biomechanics (Bristol, Avon) 27: 273–280.
17. Correa TA, Baker R, Graham HK, Pandy MG (2011) Accuracy of generic musculoskeletal models in predicting the functional roles of muscles in human gait. Journal of Biomechanics 44: 2096–2105.
18. Gerus P, Sartori M, Besier TF, Fregly BJ, Delp SL, et al. (2013) Subject-specific knee joint geometry improves predictions of medial tibiofemoral contact forces. Journal of Biomechanics 46: 2778–2786.
19. Valente G, Taddei F, Jonkers I (2013) Influence of weak hip abductor muscles on joint contact forces during normal walking: probabilistic modeling analysis. Journal of Biomechanics 46: 2186–2193.
20. Ackland DC, Lin Y-C, Pandy MG (2012) Sensitivity of model predictions of muscle function to changes in moment arms and muscle–tendon properties: A Monte-Carlo analysis. Journal of Biomechanics 45: 1463–1471.
21. Langenderfer JE, Laz PJ, Petrella AJ, Rullkoetter PJ (2008) An efficient probabilistic methodology for incorporating uncertainty in body segment parameters and anatomical landmarks in joint loadings estimated from inverse dynamics. Journal of Biomechanical Engineering 130: 014502.
22. Delp SL, Anderson FC, Arnold AS, Loan P, Habib A, et al. (2007) OpenSim: open-source software to create and analyze dynamic simulations of movement. IEEE Transactions on Biomedical Engineering 54: 1940–1950.
23. Crossley KM, Dorn TW, Ozturk H, van den Noort J, Schache a G, et al. (2012) Altered hip muscle forces during gait in people with patellofemoral osteoarthritis. Osteoarthritis and cartilage 20: 1243–1249.
24. van der Krogt MM, Delp SL, Schwartz MH (2012) How robust is human gait to muscle weakness? Gait & posture 36: 113–119.
25. Benedetti MG, Catani F, Leardini A, Pignotti S, Giannini S (1998) Data management in gait analysis for clinical applications. Clinical Biomechanics (Bristol, Avon) 13: 204–215.
26. Cappozzo A, Catani F, Della Croce U, Leardini A (1995) Position and orientation in space of bones during movement: anatomical frame definition and determination. Clinical Biomechanics (Bristol, Avon) 10: 171–178.
27. Cappello A, Stagni R, Fantozzi S, Leardini A (2005) Soft Tissue Artifact Compensation in Knee Kinematics by Double Anatomical Landmark Calibration: Performance of a Novel Method During Selected Motor Tasks. IEEE Transaction on Biomedical Engineering 52: 992–998.
28. Dumas R, Aissaoui R, Mitton D, Skalli W, Guise JAD (2005) Personalized Body Segment Parameters From Biplanar Low-Dose Radiography. IEEE Transactions on Biomedical Engineering 52: 1756–1763.
29. Wu G, Siegler S, Allard P, Kirtley C, Leardini A, et al. (2002) ISB recommendation on definitions of joint coordinate system of various joints for the reporting of human joint motion—part I: ankle, hip, and spine. Journal of Biomechanics 35: 543–548.
30. Churchill DL, Incavo SJ, Johnson CC, Beynnon BD (1998) The transepicondylar axis approximates the optimal flexion axis of the knee. Clinical Orthopaedics and Related Research 356: 111–118.
31. Lundberg A, Svenson OK, Nemeth G, Selvik G (1989) The axis of rotation of the ankle joint. Journal of Bone and Joint Surgery 71: 94–99.
32. Delp SL, Loan JP, Hoy MG, Zajac FE, Topp EL, et al. (1990) An interactive graphics-based model of the lower extremity to study orthopaedic surgical procedures. IEEE Transactions on Biomedical engineering 37: 757–767.
33. Correa TA, Pandy MG (2011) A mass-length scaling law for modeling muscle strength in the lower limb. Journal of Biomechanics 44: 2782–2789.
34. Arnold EM, Ward SR, Lieber RL, Delp SL (2010) A model of the lower limb for analysis of human movement. Annals of biomedical engineering 38: 269–279.
35. Clauser CE, McConville JT, Young JW (1969) Weight, volume, and center of mass of segments of the human body. AMRL-TR-69-70 Wright Patterson Air Force Base, Ohio.
36. Taddei F, Ansaloni M, Testi D, Viceconti M (2007) Virtual palpation of skeletal landmarks with multimodal display interfaces. Medical informatics and the Internet in medicine 32: 191–198.
37. Scheys L, Jonkers I, Loeckx D, Maes F, Spaepen A, et al. (2006) Image based musculoskeletal modeling allows personalized biomechanical analysis of gait. Lecture notes in computer science 4072: 58–66.
38. Pal S, Langenderfer JE, Stowe JQ, Laz PJ, Petrella AJ, et al. (2007) Probabilistic modeling of knee muscle moment arms: effects of methods, origin-insertion, and kinematic variability. Annals of biomedical engineering 35: 1632–1642.
39. Buchanan TS, Lloyd DG, Manal K, Besier TF (2004) Neuromusculoskeletal modeling: estimation of muscle forces and joint moments and movements from measurements of neural command. Journal of applied biomechanics 20: 367–395.
40. McKay MD, Beckman RJ, Conover WJ (1979) Comparison of Three Methods for Selecting Values of Input Variables in the Analysis of Output from a Computer Code. Technometrics 21: 239–245.
41. Anderson FC, Pandy MG (2001) Static and dynamic optimization solutions for gait are practically equivalent. Journal of Biomechanics 34: 153–161.
42. Carbone V, van der Krogt MM, Koopman HFJM, Verdonschot N (2012) Sensitivity of subject-specific models to errors in musculo-skeletal geometry. Journal of Biomechanics 45: 2476–2480.
43. Xiao M, Higginson J (2010) Sensitivity of estimated muscle force in forward simulation of normal walking. J Appl Biomech 26, 142–149.
44. De Groote F, Van Campen A, Jonkers I, De Schutter J (2010) Sensitivity of dynamic simulations of gait and dynamometer experiments to Hill muscle model parameters of knee flexors and extensors. Journal of Biomechanics 43: 1876–1883.
45. Blemker SS, Delp SL (2005) Three-dimensional representation of complex muscle architectures and geometries. Annals of biomedical engineering 33: 1433–1437.

Permissions

All chapters in this book were first published in PLOS ONE, by The Public Library of Science; hereby published with permission under the Creative Commons Attribution License or equivalent. Every chapter published in this book has been scrutinized by our experts. Their significance has been extensively debated. The topics covered herein carry significant findings which will fuel the growth of the discipline. They may even be implemented as practical applications or may be referred to as a beginning point for another development.

The contributors of this book come from diverse backgrounds, making this book a truly international effort. This book will bring forth new frontiers with its revolutionizing research information and detailed analysis of the nascent developments around the world.

We would like to thank all the contributing authors for lending their expertise to make the book truly unique. They have played a crucial role in the development of this book. Without their invaluable contributions this book wouldn't have been possible. They have made vital efforts to compile up to date information on the varied aspects of this subject to make this book a valuable addition to the collection of many professionals and students.

This book was conceptualized with the vision of imparting up-to-date information and advanced data in this field. To ensure the same, a matchless editorial board was set up. Every individual on the board went through rigorous rounds of assessment to prove their worth. After which they invested a large part of their time researching and compiling the most relevant data for our readers.

The editorial board has been involved in producing this book since its inception. They have spent rigorous hours researching and exploring the diverse topics which have resulted in the successful publishing of this book. They have passed on their knowledge of decades through this book. To expedite this challenging task, the publisher supported the team at every step. A small team of assistant editors was also appointed to further simplify the editing procedure and attain best results for the readers.

Apart from the editorial board, the designing team has also invested a significant amount of their time in understanding the subject and creating the most relevant covers. They scrutinized every image to scout for the most suitable representation of the subject and create an appropriate cover for the book.

The publishing team has been an ardent support to the editorial, designing and production team. Their endless efforts to recruit the best for this project, has resulted in the accomplishment of this book. They are a veteran in the field of academics and their pool of knowledge is as vast as their experience in printing. Their expertise and guidance has proved useful at every step. Their uncompromising quality standards have made this book an exceptional effort. Their encouragement from time to time has been an inspiration for everyone.

The publisher and the editorial board hope that this book will prove to be a valuable piece of knowledge for researchers, students, practitioners and scholars across the globe.

List of Contributors

Viola F. Gnocchi, Juergen Scharner, Zhe Huang, Jaclyn S. Lee, Robert B. White, Yin-Biao Sun, Juliet A. Ellis and Peter S. Zammit
The Randall Division of Cell and Molecular Biophysics, King's College London, New Hunt's House, Guy's Campus, London, United Kingdom

Ken Brady
Centre for Ultrastructural Imaging, King's College London, New Hunt's House, Guy's Campus, London, United Kingdom

Jennifer E. Morgan
The Dubowitz Neuromuscular Centre, Institute of Child Health, University College, London, United Kingdom

Eduardo Gallatti Yasumura, Roberta Sessa Stilhano, Vı´vian Yochiko Samoto, Priscila Keiko Matsumoto, Leonardo Pinto de Carvalho, Valderez Bastos Valero Lapchik, Sang Won Han
Research Center for Gene Therapy, Department of Biophysics, Universidade Federal de São Paulo, São Paulo, São Paulo, Brazil

Bernadett Kalmar, James Dick and Linda Greensmith
Sobell Department of Motor Neuroscience and Movement Disorders, MRC Centre for Neuromuscular Disorders, UCL Institute of Neurology, University College London, London, United Kingdom

Axel Petzold
Department of Neuroinflammation, UCL Institute of Neurology, University College London, London, United Kingdom
VU Medical Centre, Dept. of Neurology, Amsterdam, The Netherlands

Ching-Hua Lu
Sobell Department of Motor Neuroscience and Movement Disorders, MRC Centre for Neuromuscular Disorders, UCL Institute of Neurology, University College London, London, United Kingdom
Trauma and Neuroscience Centre, Blizard Institute, Barts and The School of Medicine and Dentistry, Queen Mary University of London, London, United Kingdom

Andrea Malaspina
Trauma and Neuroscience Centre, Blizard Institute, Barts and The School of Medicine and Dentistry, Queen Mary University of London, London, United Kingdom
North-East London and Essex MND Care and Research Centre, London, United Kingdom

Dejia Li, Jin-Hong Shin and Dongsheng Duan
Department of Molecular Microbiology and Immunology, University of Missouri, Columbia, Missouri, United States of America

Hannes Höppner
Institute of Robotics and Mechatronics, German Aerospace Center, Wessling, Germany

Joseph McIntyre
Centre d'Etudes de la Sensorimotricité , Centre National de la Recherche Scientifique and Université Paris Descartes, Paris, France

Patrick van der Smagt
Faculty for Informatics, Technische Universität München, Munich, Germany

Stéphanie Bissonnette and Myléne Vaillancourt
Axe Neurosciences, Centre de recherche du CHU de Québec, CHUL, Québec, Canada

Sébastien S. Hébert, Guy Drolet and Pershia Samadi
Axe Neurosciences, Centre de recherche du CHU de Québec, CHUL, Québec, Canada
Département de psychiatrie et de neurosciences, Université Laval, Québec, Canada

Yi-Ching Chen
School of Physical Therapy, Chung Shan Medical University, Taichung City, Taiwan
Physical Therapy Room, Chung Shan Medical University Hospital, Taichung City,Taiwan

Yen-Ting Lin
Physical Education Office, Asian University, Taichung City, Taiwan

Chien-Ting Huang and Zong-Ru Yang
Institute of Allied Health Sciences, College of Medicine, National Cheng Kung University, Tainan City, Taiwan

Ing-Shiou Hwang
Institute of Allied Health Sciences, College of Medicine, National Cheng Kung University, Tainan City, Taiwan
Department of Physical Therapy, College of Medicine, National Cheng Kung University, Tainan City, Taiwan

Chia-Li Shih
Department of Physical Therapy, College of Medicine, National Cheng Kung University, Tainan City, Taiwan

Juan Del Coso, Cristina González-Millán, Juan José Salinero, Javier Abián-Vicén, Lidón Soriano, Sergio Garde, Benito Pérez-González
Exercise Physiology Laboratory, Camilo José Cela University, Madrid, Spain

Abdallah I. Hassaballah, Azizi N. Mardi and Mohd Hamdi
Department of Mechanical Engineering, Faculty of Engineering, University of Malaya, Kuala Lumpur, Malaysia
Center of Advanced Manufacturing & Material processing, Faculty of Engineering, University of Malaya, Kuala Lumpur, Malaysia

Mohsen A. Hassan
Department of Mechanical Engineering, Faculty of Engineering, University of Malaya, Kuala Lumpur, Malaysia
Center of Advanced Manufacturing & Material processing, Faculty of Engineering, University of Malaya, Kuala Lumpur, Malaysia
Department of Mechanical Engineering, Faculty of Engineering, Assiut University, Assiut, Egypt

Tibor Istvan Toth and Silvia Daun-Gruhn
Emmy Noether Research Group of Computational Biology, Department of Animal Physiology, University of Cologne, Cologne, Germany

Joachim Schmidt and Ansgar Büschges
Department of Animal Physiology, University of Cologne, Cologne, Germany

Pierre Joanne and Onnik Agbulut
Université Paris Diderot, Sorbonne Paris Cité , CNRS EAC4413, Unit of Functional and Adaptive Biology, Laboratory of Stress and Pathologies of the Cytoskeleton, Paris, France

Christophe Hourdé, Yvain Caudéran, Fadia Medja, Alban Vignaud, Etienne Mouisel, Wahiba Hadj-Said, Ludovic Arandel, Luis Garcia, Aurélie Goyenvalle and Gillian Butler-Browne
Université Pierre et Marie Curie-Paris, Sorbonne Universités, UMR S794, INSERM U974, CNRS UMR7215, Institut de Myologie, Paris, France

Arnaud Ferry
Université Pierre et Marie Curie-Paris, Sorbonne Universités, UMR S794, INSERM U974, CNRS UMR7215, Institut de Myologie, Paris, France
Université Paris Descartes, Sorbonne Paris Cité, Paris, France

Julien Ochala
Department of Neuroscience, Uppsala University, Uppsala, Sweden

Rémi Mounier
Université Paris Descartes, Sorbonne Paris Cité , INSERM U1016, CNRS UMR8104, Institut Cochin, Paris, France

Daria Zibroba and Kei Sakamato
MRC Protein Phosphorylation Unit, College of Life Sciences, University of Dundee, Dundee, United Kingdom

Lei Ren
School of Mechanical, Aerospace and Civil Engineering, University of Manchester, Manchester, United Kingdom

Dan Hu
School of Mechanical, Aerospace and Civil Engineering, University of Manchester, Manchester, United Kingdom
State Key Laboratory of Automotive Simulation and Control, Jilin University, Changchun, P.R. China

David Howard
School of Computing, Science and Engineering, University of Salford, Manchester, United Kingdom

Md. Anamul Islam, Kenneth Sundaraj, R. Badlishah Ahmad, Nizam Uddin Ahamed and Md. Asraf Ali
AI-Rehab Research Group, Universiti Malaysia Perlis (UniMAP), Arau, Perlis, Malaysia

Sebastian Sundaraj
Medical Officer, Malaysian Ministry of Health, Klang, Selangor, Malaysia

Veerle Bogaert, Annelies De Spaey, Greet Roef, Sara Vandewalle and Youri Taes
Department of Endocrinology, Ghent University Hospital, Ghent, Belgium

Hélène De Naeyer
Department of Endocrinology, Ghent University Hospital, Ghent, Belgium
Department of Movement and Sport Sciences, Ghent University, Ghent, Belgium

Wim Derave
Department of Movement and Sport Sciences, Ghent University, Ghent, Belgium

Jean-Marc Kaufman
Unit for Osteoporosis and Metabolic bone diseases, Ghent University Hospital, Ghent, Belgium

Antonius Rohlmann, Thomas Zander, Friedmar Graichen, Hendrik Schmidt and Georg Bergmann
Julius Wolff Institute, Charitè - Universitätsmedizin Berlin, Berlin, Germany

Zhijie Jack Tseng and Xiaoming Wang
Integrative and Evolutionary Biology Program, Department of Biological Sciences, University of Southern California, Los Angeles, California, United States of America
Department of Vertebrate Paleontology, Natural History Museum of Los Angeles County, Los Angeles, California, United States of America

Jill L. Mcnitt-Gray
Integrative and Evolutionary Biology Program, Department of Biological Sciences, University of Southern California, Los Angeles, California, United States of America
Departments of Kinesiology, Biological Sciences, and Biomedical Engineering, University of Southern California, Los Angeles, California, United States of America

Henryk Flashner
Integrative and Evolutionary Biology Program, Department of Biological Sciences, University of Southern California, Los Angeles, California, United States of America
Department of Aerospace and Mechanical Engineering, University of Southern California, Los Angeles, California, United States of America

Reyes Enciso
Integrative and Evolutionary Biology Program, Department of Biological Sciences, University of Southern California, Los Angeles, California, United States of America
Ostrow School of Dentistry, University of Southern California, Los Angeles, California, United States of America

Hwasil Moon, Changki Kim, Minhyuk Kwon, Yen Ting Chen, Tanya Onushko and Neha Lodha
Department of Applied Physiology and Kinesiology, University of Florida, Gainesville, FL, United States of America

Evangelos A. Christou
Department of Applied Physiology and Kinesiology, University of Florida, Gainesville, FL, United States of America
Department of Physical Therapy, University of Florida, Gainesville, FL, United States of America

Giordano Valente, Lorenzo Pitto and Fulvia Taddei
Medical Technology Laboratory, Rizzoli Orthopaedic Institute, Bologna, Italy

Debora Test
BioComputing Competence Centre, SCS s.r.l., Bologna, Italy

Ajay Seth
Department of Bioengineering, Stanford University, Stanford, California, United States of America

Scott L. Delp
Department of Bioengineering, Stanford University, Stanford, California, United States of America
Department of Mechanical Engineering, Stanford University, Stanford, California, United States of America

Rita Stagni
Department of Electrical, Electronic and Information Engineering, University of Bologna, Bologna, Italy

Marco Viceconti
Department of Mechanical Engineering and INSIGNEO Institute for In Silico Medicine, University of Sheffield, Sheffield, United Kingdom

Index

CPSIA information can be obtained
at www.ICGtesting.com
Printed in the USA
BVHW02*0448020218
506942BV00003B/28/P